www.harcourt-international.com

Bringing you products from all Harcourt Health Sciences companies including Baillière Tindall, Churchill Livingstone, Mosby and W.B. Saunders

- ▶ **Browse** for latest information on new books, journals and electronic products

- ▶ **Search** for information on over 20 000 published titles with full product information including tables of contents and sample chapters

- ▶ **Keep up to date** with our extensive publishing programme in your field by registering with eAlert or requesting postal updates

- ▶ **Secure online ordering** with prompt delivery, as well as full contact details to order by phone, fax or post

- ▶ **News** of special features and promotions

If you are based in the following countries, please visit the country-specific site to receive full details of product availability and local ordering information

USA: www.harcourthealth.com

Canada: www.harcourtcanada.com

Australia: www.harcourt.com.au

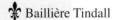 Baillière Tindall 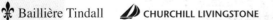 CHURCHILL LIVINGSTONE Mosby 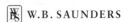 W.B. SAUNDERS

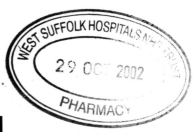

Medical
Pharmacology
and Therapeutics

Dedication
To our families

For W. B. Saunders:

Commissioning Editor: Timothy Horne
Project Development Manager: Ruth Swan
Project Manager: Nancy Arnott
Designer: Sarah Russell

Medical Pharmacology and Therapeutics

Derek G. Waller BSc (Hons), DM, MBBS (Hons), FRCP
Consultant Physician and Senior Lecturer in Medicine and Clinical Pharmacology
Southampton University Hospitals Trust

Andrew G. Renwick OBE, BSc, PhD, DSc
Professor of Biochemical Pharmacology
School of Medicine
University of Southampton

Keith Hillier BSc, PhD, DSc
Senior Lecturer in Pharmacology
School of Medicine
University of Southampton

Illustrations by Hardlines, Oxford

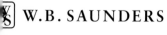

W.B. SAUNDERS

Edinburgh • London • New York • Philadelphia • St Louis • Sydney • Toronto 2001

W. B. SAUNDERS
An imprint of Harcourt Publishers Limited

 logo is a registered trademark of Harcourt Publishers Limited

First published 2001

ISBN 0 7020 2272 1

British Library Cataloguing in Publication Data
A catalogue record for this book is available from the British Library

Library of Congress Cataloging in Publication Data
A catalog record for this book is available from the Library of Congress

The
publisher's
policy is to use
**paper manufactured
from sustainable forests**

Printed in Spain

Contents

Preface

Effective and safe prescribing of medicines and monitoring patient responses to prescribed and non-prescribed drugs underpins the day-to-day activities of doctors and other health professionals. Effective prescribing stems from a sound understanding of the nature and mechanisms of drug actions and effects. Influences such as age, disease and the increasing potential for drug interactions when drugs are being given together, need to be taken into account.

The initial chapters of this book give information about basic principles of drug development and drug action, and the ways in which drugs are absorbed, distributed and excreted by the body. A chapter is devoted to the autonomic nervous system and to the range of receptors that are important targets for drug action, both now and in the future.

Other chapters are laid out to include:

- a basic introduction to the mechanisms of disease or condition, to help the reader understand how medicines achieve their effects
- a comprehensive review of the major classes of drugs used with selected examples to illustrate important principles, including sites and mechanisms of drug actions, pharmacokinetics and unwanted effects.

The chapter content is then put into a clinical context by discussing the broad therapeutic approaches to major diseases.

Many chapters conclude with self-assessment exercises, case studies, references and a drug compendium.

The authors would be pleased to receive comments about this book.

Derek Waller
Andrew Renwick
Keith Hillier   Southampton 2001

Acknowledgements

We are indebted to Frances Lowman for her patience and skilled secretarial assistance in preparing this manuscript.

Drug dosage and nomenclature

Drug nomenclature

Directive 92/27/EEC requires use of the Recommended International Non-proprietary Name (rINN) for medicinal substances. In most cases the British Approved Name (BAN) and rINN are identical but where they differ the rINN has been used with the old BAN in parentheses.

The names 'adrenaline' and 'noradrenaline' are used when referring to the natural hormones, but 'epinephrine' and 'norepinephrine' are applied to these hormones when used as drugs. Similarly, 'oestrogen' is used to refer to the naturally occurring hormone, whereas synthetic hormone, as in the contraceptive pill, is referred to as 'estrogen'.

Drug dosages

Medical knowledge is constantly changing. As new information becomes available, changes in treatment, procedures, equipment and the use of drugs become necessary. The editors and the publishers have taken care to ensure that the information given in the text is accurate and up to date. However, readers are strongly advised to confirm that the information, especially with regard to drug usage, complies with the latest legislation and standards of practice.

GENERAL PRINCIPLES

1

Sites and mechanisms of drug action

Modern clinical and biological sciences have provided a detailed understanding of the interaction of many therapeutic drugs with biological systems at a molecular level. Many medical students find it difficult to evaluate the depth of information necessary for them to achieve in order to use drugs effectively. Understanding may range from the general (e.g. it paralyses the patient) to the highly specific (e.g. it alters the tertiary structure of the receptor protein by interfering with the hydrogen bonding between certain specific amino acids). The former is totally inadequate because it allows no possibility of predicting any problems, while the latter is excessive (but may be fascinating, e.g. such detailed information could explain why some patients show abnormal responses). The depth of understanding necessary is that which provides:

- a suitable framework to allow comparison of the relative benefits and risks of alternative drugs (drug selection)
- an ability to predict possible problems in a particular patient owing to other disease processes, other medicines, etc.

Sites of drug action

The actions of drugs can be divided into those occurring at specific sites and those that are non-specific.

Non-specific effects. The response is mediated via a generalised effect in many organs, such as an osmotic effect, and the response observed depends on the distribution of the drug, with a response in the organ(s) with the highest concentrations.

Specific sites. The effect is produced by interaction of the drug with a specific site(s) either on the cell membrane or inside the cell; for example, the drug may act only at acetylcholine receptors. In some cases, the site of action may involve one (or more) member of a group, or a family, of receptors. Under such circumstances, the drug may act preferentially on one member of the group and it is said to be *selective*; for example, a drug that has a higher affinity for β-adrenoceptors (β-adrenergic receptors) than for α-adrenoceptors would be selective for β-adrenoceptors. Alternatively, the drug may show a similar affinity for all adrenoceptors and would be described as *non-selective*. The context for the use of the term *selective* must be defined because a drug may be selective for β-adrenoceptors compared with α-adrenoceptors, but it could also exhibit a level of selectivity among β-adrenoceptors being selective for β_1-adrenoceptors compared with β_2-adrenoceptors.

Specific sites of action

The activities of most cellular processes are controlled in order to produce the optimum homeostatic conditions for the cell in relation to the prevailing physiological and metabolic requirements. For example, the heart rate and force of contraction increase during exercise, and this is accompanied by modification of energy sources. Such reflex actions require the appropriate response of different cells in the body to a signal (or signals) produced as a result of the altered physiological states. The signals typically take the form of specific chemicals (such as noradrenaline), which are either released into the circulation or released locally and which are recognised by the cell. Therefore, homeostasis is dependent on

1. the generation of a signal
2. the recognition of specific signals
3. the production of appropriate cellular changes.

Each of these three steps provides important targets for drug action.

Receptor-mediated mechanisms

The critical recognition step involves the chemical signal binding to a specific and specialised macromolecule of the cell, and it is this binding that triggers the cellular response. The chemical forming the signal is termed a *ligand*, because it ligates to (ties itself to) the specialised cellular macromolecule. The cellular macromolecule is termed a *receptor*, because it receives the ligand.

Receptors may be either in the cell membrane, in order to react with extracellular ligands that cannot cross the cell membrane (such as peptides) or cross only slowly, or in the cytoplasm, for lipid-soluble ligands that can cross the cell membrane. The binding of the ligand to the receptor results in a ligand–receptor complex, which triggers the intracellular changes. These changes may be brought about directly, for example by inhibiting a process, indirectly, by interacting with DNA to alter the synthesis of the enzymes *etc.* involved in the process, or by changing a normal intracellular chemical signal (a 'second messenger') that controls the process.

A drug that binds to a specific type of receptor may:

- mimic the normal endogenous ligand and produce the same cellular response: such drugs have a 'positive' effect and are called *agonists*

- block the binding and actions of the normal receptor ligand: such drugs are called *antagonists*.

Properties of receptors

Receptor binding

The binding of the ligand to the receptor is normally reversible; consequently, the intensity and duration of the intracellular changes are dependent on the continuing presence of the ligand. The interaction between the ligand and its receptor does not involve permanent covalent bonds but weaker, reversible forces such as:

- ionic bonding between ionisable groups in the ligand (e.g. $-NH_3^+$) and in the receptor (e.g. $-COO^-$)
- hydrogen bonding between amino-, hydroxyl-, keto- functions, etc.
- hydrophobic interactions between lipid-soluble sites in the ligand and receptor.
- van der Waals forces, which are very weak interatomic attractions.

Receptor specificity

There are numerous possible extracellular and intracellular chemical signals produced in the body, which can affect different processes. Therefore, a fundamental property of a receptor is its *specificity*, i.e. the extent to which it can recognise and respond to only one signal. Some receptors show high specificity and bind a single endogenous ligand (e.g. acetycholine is the only endogenous ligand that binds to N_1 nicotinic receptors; see Ch. 4), whereas other receptors are less specific and will bind a number of related endogenous ligands (e.g. the β_1-adrenoceptors on the heart will bind noradrenaline, adrenaline and to some extent dopamine, which are all catecholamines). The ability of receptors to recognise and bind the correct ligand depends on an interaction between the receptor molecule and certain specific characteristics of the chemical structure of the ligand. The formulae of representative chemical signals and, therefore, receptor ligands are shown in Figure 1.1, and it is clear that the differences between them may be subtle. Receptor specificity occurs because the different sites for reversible binding interactions (such as anion and cation sites, lipid centres and hydrogen bonding sites; see above) are present in a specific three-dimensional organisation, which corresponds to the three-dimensional structure of the endogenous ligand. Receptors are proteins that are folded into a tertiary structure such that the necessary specific arrangement of bonding types is brought together within a small volume – the receptor site (Fig. 1.2).

Three-dimensional aspects

Receptors have a three-dimensional organisation in space and, therefore, the ligand has to be presented to the receptor in the correct configuration (rather like

(a)

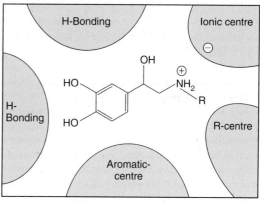

Dopamine

Noradrenaline

5-Hydroxytryptamine (5HT)

Histamine

(b)

Glycine

Glutamate

Aspartate

γ-Aminobutyrate (GABA)

(c)

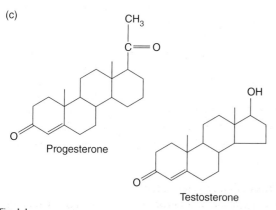

Progesterone

Testosterone

Fig. 1.1

Groups of chemicals using different receptors in spite of similar structure. (a) Biogenic amines; (b) amino acids; (c) steroids.

ADRENOCEPTOR

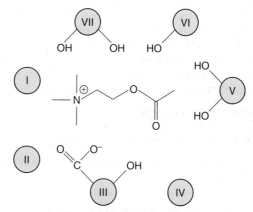

MUSCARINIC RECEPTOR

Fig. 1.2

Receptor ligand-binding sites. The coloured areas are schematic cross-sections of the transmembrane segments of the receptor protein. Different segments provide different properties (hydrogen bonding, anionic site, etc.) to make up the active site.

fitting a hand into the correct glove). Because some drugs are a mixture of stereoisomers (the same chemical structures but with different three-dimensional configurations), the different isomers may show very different binding characteristics and biological properties. For example, the different stereoisomers of the drug labetalol bind to different types of receptor. A drug that is an equal mixture of *levo-* and *dextro*-isomers (or *S*- and *R*- forms; a racemate) could be a mixture of 50% active compound plus 50% inactive, or in some cases, a mixture of 50% therapeutic drug and 50% inactive but toxic compound. In consequence, there has been a trend in recent years for the development of single isomers for therapeutic uses; one of the earliest examples was the use of levodopa (the *levo*-isomer of dopa) in Parkinson's disease (Ch. 24).

Receptor types and subtypes

Different types of receptor recognise different ligands, for example noradrenaline receptors bind catecholamines, such as noradrenaline, but do not bind acetylcholine (see receptor specificity above). There may be a number of subtypes of a receptor each of which specifically recognises or binds the same particular ligand. For example α_1, α_2, β_1, β_2 and β_3 are all subtypes of noradrenaline receptors but produce different intracellular changes (see below). The different subtypes of receptor often show a different tissue or organ distribution within the body and produce different effects (see below); these characteristics allow selective drugs to show selective actions, with fewer unwanted effects. Acetylcholine acts via different receptors on ganglia (nicotinic N_1), the neuromuscular junction of skeletal muscle (nicotinic N_2) and at smooth muscle (muscarinic). This aspect is discussed in detail in Chapter 4. Until recently, receptor subtypes were 'discovered' when a pharmaceutical company developed a new agonist or antagonist that was found to alter some, but not all, of the activities of a currently known receptor class. Recent developments in molecular biology have enhanced our abilities to detect receptor subtypes; for example, it is now recognised that there are multiple types of muscarinic receptors. The recognition and cloning of subtypes of receptors is important in that it should facilitate the development of drugs showing greater selectivity and hopefully fewer unwanted effects.

Receptor numbers

The number of receptors present in a cell is not static, and there is a high turnover of receptors as they are being formed and removed continuously. The numbers of receptors within the cell membrane may be altered during repeated drug treatment, with either an increase (*upregulation*) or a decrease (*downregulation*) in receptor numbers. The changes in receptor numbers that may occur following treatment with some drugs can be an important part of the therapeutic response. A well-recognised example is the therapeutic benefit of tricyclic antidepressants, which develops slowly during regular therapy despite their rapid inhibition of the reuptake of 5-hydroxytryptamine (5HT) and noradrenaline; the delayed response is probably related to adaptive downregulation of receptor numbers rather than the recognised acute effects of these drugs. Tolerance to the effects of some drugs (e.g. opiates) may arise from downregulation of opioid receptor numbers; as a result, there is the need for increased doses to produce the same activity.

Transmembrane ion channels

The intracellular concentrations of ions such as Na^+, K^+, Ca^{2+} and Cl^- are controlled by a combination of ion pumps that move specific ions from one side of the membrane to the other and ion channels, which open to allow the selective transfer of ions down their concentration gradients. Both Na^+ and Ca^{2+} will diffuse into the cell, making the cytosol more positive and causing depolarisation of excitable tissues; K^+ will diffuse out of a cell making the cytosol more negative and inhibiting depolarisation; Cl^- diffuses into the cell making the cytosol more negative and inhibiting depolarisation.

Some ion channels show voltage-dependent opening (e.g. the Na^+ channel, which opens in response to a nerve impulse), while others open in response to the presence of a ligand (e.g. the Na^+ channel linked to acetycholine and Cl^- channels linked to GABA; see Ch. 4). Voltage-dependent and ligand-operated channels can be intimately linked in facilitating the transfer of ions and in maintaining cellular homeostasis.

Voltage-gated ion channels consist of a number of subunits (Fig. 1.3) each of which is a transmembrane protein that crosses the membrane in a number of loops. The central unit contains the pore through which the ions pass and is largely responsible for the specificity of the channel for a particular ion. Ion specificity is determined by the amino acid composition of a short segment of the pore, which is different for each type of ion channel. Both Na^+ and K^+ channels show fast inactivation after opening; this is produced by an intracellular loop of the channel, which blocks the open channel from the intracellular end (Fig. 1.3). The activity of voltage-gated channels may be modulated by drugs, either indirectly via intracellular events or directly, for example local anaesthetics bind to and block activated Na^+ channels.

There are a number of different subtypes for each of the main types of cation channels (Na^+, K^+ and Ca^{2+}). These subtypes have different characteristics, and this allows the possibility of selective drug actions. There are at least five different voltage-gated Ca^{2+} channels (L, N, P/Q, R and T) only one of which, the L-type, binds drugs. The differences arise from the nature of the α_1-subunits and that for L-type channels has three high-affinity, stereoselective binding sites for dihydropyridines, verapamil and diltiazem-type Ca^{2+} channel antagonists. The different types of Ca^{2+} and K^+ channels are described in Chapter 5 in relation to the clinical use of selective drugs. Sodium channels are of vital importance in excitable tissues, and different types of channel are present in the membrane of the axon of nerves (Ch. 18), and at the neuromuscular junction (Ch. 27). Chloride channels are described in Chapter 20.

Ligand-gated channels are often complex in nature and may consist of a number of transmembrane subunits, which cluster around a central channel. Each peptide subunit is orientated so that hydrophilic chains face towards the channel and hydrophobic chains towards the membrane lipid bilayer. The ligand binding is usually present on one of the subunits or is produced by the juxtaposition of subunits. The nicotinic acetylcholine receptor is a good example of this type of structure since it comprises five transmembrane subunits and requires the binding of two molecules of acetylcholine for channel opening. Channel opening is a very

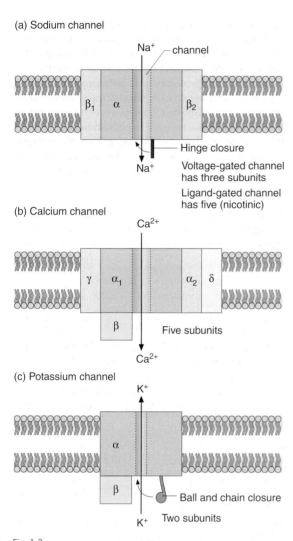

(a) Sodium channel

Na⁺ channel

β₁   α   β₂

Hinge closure

Na⁺   Voltage-gated channel has three subunits

Ligand-gated channel has five (nicotinic)

(b) Calcium channel

Ca²⁺

γ   α₁   α₂   δ

β   Five subunits

Ca²⁺

(c) Potassium channel

K⁺

α

β   Ball and chain closure

K⁺   Two subunits

Fig. 1.3
Typical transmembrane ion channels. (The different subunits (α, β, γ) in different channels are not the same peptide sequences.) Ions diffuse down their concentration gradients when the channel is open. Two types of inactivation of open channels have been described (hinged and ball and chain), which involve an intracellular loop of the channel. The ligand-gated γ-aminobutyric acid (GABA)-linked Cl⁻ channel is shown in Figure 20.1, p. 236.

rapid process lasting only milliseconds and is usually short lived because the ligand is rapidly inactivated (Ch. 4). Prolonged occupancy of the ligand-binding site by an agonist, such as succinylcholine, leads to a loss of channel opening owing to a further conformational change in the receptor protein, which is associated with both receptor occupancy and a closed channel (see muscle relaxants; Ch. 27). Other ligand-gated ion channels that mediate fast synaptic transmission are linked to γ-aminobutyric acid type A (GABA_A) receptors, glycine receptors and 5HT₃ receptors.

Ion channels may be influenced by transmembrane receptors linked to guanosine-binding proteins (G-proteins) (see below) in two ways:

- indirectly via the second messenger system affecting the status of the channel
- directly via the G-protein subunits (α or βγ, see below) interacting with the channel.

G-protein-linked transmembrane receptors and second messenger systems

The structure of a hypothetical G-protein-linked transmembrane receptor is shown in Figure 1.4. Most transmembrane receptors have the N-terminals on the extracellular side and cross the membrane seven times with helical segments (heptahelical) so that the C-terminal is on the inside of the cell. The outer loops produce the active site for ligand binding and the inner loops are involved in coupling to the second messenger system, usually via a guanosine-binding protein (G-protein). The binding of an appropriate agonist (natural ligand or agonist drug) to the ligand-binding site, on the extracellular side of the membrane, alters the three-dimensional conformation of the receptor protein. The consequences of the change in conformation depend on the nature of the receptor, and the intracellular enzymes and other systems to which it is linked. The intracellular enzyme systems produce an intracellular signal, the second messenger, which alters the functioning of the cell.

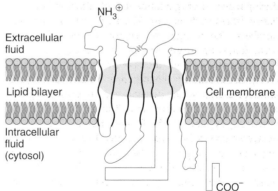

NH₃⊕

Extracellular fluid

Lipid bilayer   Cell membrane

Intracellular fluid (cytosol)

COO⁻

Fig. 1.4
Hypothetical transmembrane receptor based on the β-adrenoceptor. The receptor is a glycoprotein in which sites of glycosylation are indicated by a straight line. The orientation of the receptor within the membrane is achieved by folding of the polypeptide chain plus the presence of hydrophilic centres (such as the extracellular polysaccharide chain) and the transmembrane segments (shown as thick regions), which orientate the peptide within the cell membrane. The receptor is stabilised across the membrane by the presence of polar amino groups where the chains leave the lipid bilayer that can interact with the phospholipid end of the bilayer. The ligand-binding site (Fig. 1.2) represents a small volume in space (coloured pink in this diagram) in which the parts of the polypeptide are orientated in such a way as to bind specific ligands only. Other possible ligands may be too large for the site or may show much weaker binding characteristics.

Second messenger systems

There are two complementary second messenger systems (Fig. 1.5).

Cyclic nucleotide system. One system is based on cyclic nucleotides such as cyclic adenosine monophosphate (cAMP), which is synthesised from ATP via the enzyme adenylate cyclase, and cyclic guanosine monophosphate (cGMP), which is synthesised from GTP via guanylate cyclase. There are many isoforms of adenylate cyclase; these show different tissue distributions and could be important sites of drug action in the future. The cyclic nucleotide second messenger is inactivated by hydrolysis by a phosphodiesterase enzyme to give AMP or GMP.

The phosphatidylinositol system. The other system is based on inositol 1,4,5-trisphosphate (IP_3) and diacylglycerol (DAG), which are synthesised from the membrane phospholipid phosphatidylinositol 4,5-bisphosphate (PIP_2), by the enzyme phospholipase C_β. There are a number of isoenzymes of phospholipase C, and these may be activated by the α-subunits of G-proteins (phospholipase $C_{\beta1}$) or the βγ-subunits of G-proteins (phospholipase $C_{\beta2}$) (see below). The second messengers produced by phospholipase C (IP_3 and DAG) are inactivated and then converted back to PIP_2.

The G-protein system

The G-protein system (Fig. 1.6) consists of three different subunits (i.e. it is a heterotrimer).

- **The α-subunit.** There are 23 different types that have been identified. These belong to four families (α_s, α_i, α_q and α_{12}). The α-subunit is important because it binds GDP/GTP; it also has GTPase

activity, which is involved in terminating the activity. When an agonist binds to the receptor, GDP (which is normally present) is replaced by GTP and the α-subunit dissociates from the βγ-subunits. The α-subunit/GTP complex is active while GTP is bound to it, but it is inactivated when the GTP is hydrolysed to GDP.

- **The β-subunit.** There are five different closely related forms that have been identified. The β-subunit remains associated with the γ-subunit when the receptor is occupied and the combined βγ-subunit may activate cellular enzymes, e.g. phospholipase C.

- **The γ-subunit.** Ten different forms are known. The γ-subunit remains associated with the β-subunit when the receptor is occupied.

The sequence from receptor binding to activation of second messenger systems is illustrated in Figure 1.6. Binding of an agonist to the receptor stimulates the replacement of GDP by GTP, and the α- and βγ-subunits of the G-protein are activated. GDP binds more strongly than GTP to the non-activated receptor, but the reverse is true once the ligand binds to the receptor. The subunits disassociate from the receptor protein and exert their intracellular effects via activation of second messenger systems. The α-subunit has GTPase activity, which converts the active α-subunit/GTP complex to an inactive α-subunit/GDP complex. The GDP-α- and βγ-subunits recombine with the receptor protein to give the inactive form of the receptor G-protein complex.

There are three main types of G-proteins, the properties of which are largely determined by the nature of the α-subunit:

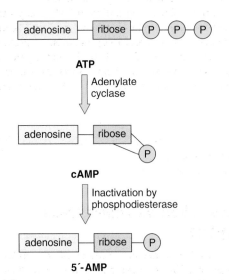

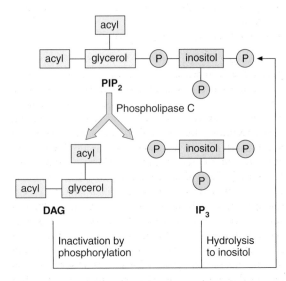

Fig. 1.5
Second messenger systems. The transmembrane receptor (see Fig. 1.4) produces intracellular changes normally by either activating or inhibiting the formation of intracellular second messengers such as cAMP (produced from ATP via the enzyme adenylate cyclase), cGMP (produced from GTP via the enzyme guanylate cyclase) or diacylglycerol (DAG) and inositol trisphosphate (IP_3) (produced from membrane phospholipid by phospholipase C). The receptor acts on the enzymes in the cell membrane via G-proteins (see Fig. 1.6).

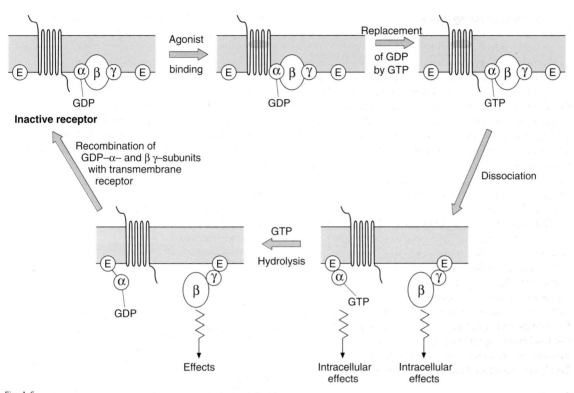

Fig. 1.6
The functioning of G-protein subunits. Ligand binding results in replacement of GDP on the α-subunit by GTP and this is followed by dissociation of the α- and βγ-subunits, which affect a range of intracellular systems (shown as E on the figure) such as second messenger systems (e.g. adenylate cyclase and phospholipase C), other enzymes and ion channels (see Fig. 1.5). Hydrolysis of GTP inactivates the α-subunit, which then reforms the inactive transmembrane receptor.

- G_s: stimulates membrane-bound adenylate cyclase to increase cAMP
- G_i (and G_o): inhibits adenylate cyclase to decrease cAMP
- G_q (and G_{12}): activates phospholipase C.

Activation of the receptor/G-protein complex can produce a number of intracellular events (Fig. 1.7), which affect many cellular processes such as enzyme activity (via the enzyme protein per se or via gene transcription), contractile proteins, ion channels (affecting depolarisation of the cell) and cytokine production. The intracellular effects are mediated by the GTP-α-subunit or the βγ-subunit (of which many different forms exist; see above). Depending on the type of G-protein, the GTP-α-subunit may close K^+ channels, activate phospholipase C or activate adenylate cyclase, while the βγ-subunit may open K^+ channels, close Ca^{2+} channels, activate phospholipase A or C, activate or inhibit adenylate cyclase, activate receptor kinases or activate the transmembrane Ca^{2+} pump. The effects on ion channels may be direct, for example the βγ-subunit of the acetylcholine muscarinic receptor directly opens K^+ channels in the sinoatrial node to hyperpolarise the cell. In other cases, the opening of a K^+ channel may be produced

indirectly via phosphorylation of channels through cAMP-mediated activation of protein kinase A.

The intracellular concentration of Ca^{2+} is important for many processes and this is affected by G_i and G_o proteins, which inhibit N and P/Q channels, G_s proteins, which stimulate L and P/Q channels, and G_q and G_{12} proteins, which release Ca^{2+} from intracellular stores via the action of IP_3 on its receptors on the endoplasmic reticulum.

Examples of G-protein-coupled receptors are given in Table 1.1.

Kinase-linked transmembrane receptors

Kinase-linked transmembrane receptors are similar to the G-protein linked receptors in that they have a ligand-binding domain on the surface of the cell membrane, traverse the membrane and have an intracellular 'effector' region (Fig. 1.8). However, they differ in a number of important respects.

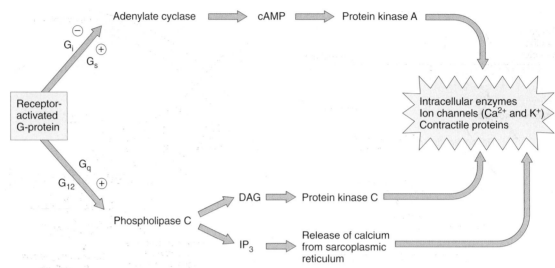

Fig. 1.7
The intracellular consequences of receptor activation and G-protein dissociation. The G-proteins affect the second messenger systems (Fig. 1.5) and the changes in cAMP, cGMP, diacylglycerol (DAG) and inositol trisphosphate (IP_3) produce a number of intracellular changes directly, indirectly via actions on protein kinases (which change the activities of other proteins by phosphorylation) or by actions on ion channels, which alter the internal environment.

Table 1.1
Examples of receptors linked to G-proteins

Ligand	Receptor	Type of G-protein
Noradrenaline	α_1	G_q
	α_2	G_i
	$\beta_1, \beta_2, \beta_3$	G_s
Acetylcholine (muscarinic)	M_1, M_3, M_5	G_q
	M_2, M_4	G_i
5-Hydroxytryptamine (5HT)	$5HT_1$ ($5HT_{1A}, 5HT_{1B}, 5HT_{1D}$)	G_i ($+G_q$?)
	$5HT_2$ ($5HT_2, 5HT_{1C}$)	G_q
	$5HT_3$	(ligand-gated ion channel)
	$5HT_4$	G_s
Dopamine	D_1	G_s
	D_2	G_i
Adenosine	A_1	G_i
	A_{2a}	G_s

G_s increases cAMP; G_i decreases cAMP and G_q activates phospholipase.

- the extracellular region associated with the ligand-binding domain is very large; this is related to the size of the endogenous ligands, which are peptides such as insulin and cytokines
- there is a single transmembrane helical region
- the intracellular region possesses tyrosine kinase activity; different receptors have different intracellular effector regions.

Ligand binding is accompanied by dimerisation of two kinase-linked receptors, and these phosphorylate each other. This activated 'pair of receptors' then phosphorylates specific intracellular protein(s), which bind to the specific activated kinase-linked receptors. The phosphorylated intracellular proteins are active enzymes, such as kinases or phospholipases, that can then bring about the relevant intracellular changes appropriate to the biological activities of the extracellular ligand. These intracellular enzymes can either act directly on metabolising enzymes or alter the gene transcription of enzymes.

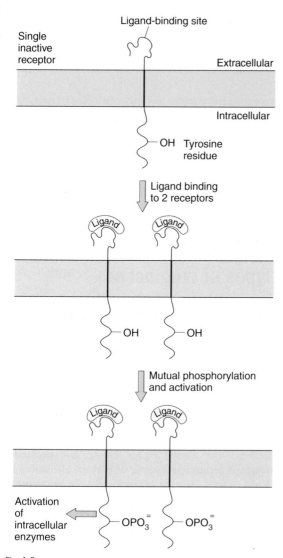

Fig. 1.8
Kinase-linked transmembrane receptor. The receptor has a large extracellular domain, a single transmembrane segment and an intracellular tyrosine kinase domain, which is responsible for intracellular effects (see text for details).

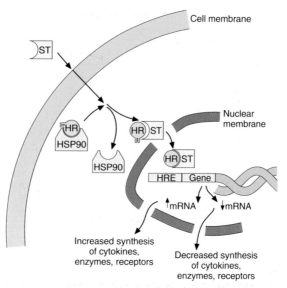

Fig. 1.9
The activation of intracellular hormone receptors. Steroid hormones (ST) are lipid soluble compounds which readily cross membranes and bind to intracellular receptors (HR). This binding displaces a protein called heat-shock protein (HSP90) and the hormone/receptor complex enters the nucleus where it alters gene expression by binding to hormone response elements (HRE) on DNA.

genome to modify the expression of downstream genes. Binding of the hormone/receptor to the hormone response element usually activates genes, but binding sometimes silences gene expression and result in a decrease in mRNA synthesis (Fig. 1.9). Steroid hormones (and some other hormones) are recognised by specific members of the steroid/thyroid receptor superfamily (Box 1.1).

Steroids, and synthetic steroid analogues, show specificity for different receptors, which then determines the spectrum of DNA gene expression that is affected. Frequently, the hormone response element needs two hormone/receptor complexes to form a

Intracellular hormone receptors

Many hormones produce long-term changes in cellular activity by altering the genetic expression of enzymes, cytokines or receptor proteins. Such actions on DNA expression are mediated by interactions with intracellular receptors. The sequence of hormone binding and actions are shown in Figure 1.9. The cytosolic hormone receptor is usually in an inactive form linked to a protein called heat shock protein (HSP). Binding of the hormone causes dissociation of the HSP and the hormone binds to its receptor. The hormone/receptor complex passes through pores in the nuclear membrane and interacts with *hormone response elements* on the

Box 1.1	
The steroid/thyroid superfamily of receptors	
Oestrogen receptor	ER
Progesterone receptor	PR
Androgen receptor	AR
Glucocorticoid receptor	GR
Mineralocorticoid receptor	MR
Thyroid hormone receptor	TR
Vitamin D receptor	VDR
Retinoic acid receptor	RAR
9-*cis*-Retinoic acid receptor	RXR

Table 1.2
The structure of steroid hormone receptors

Region	Action	Role
N-terminus		
A/B	Transactivation	Activates target genes and gives the specificity of the receptor response
C	DNA binding and dimerisation	Binds receptor to DNA by two zinc finger regions
D	Nuclear localisation	Hinge region to allow correct conformation
E	Ligand binding	Ligand specificity of receptor; a large complex region; region also binds heat shock protein
F	Unknown	Deletion of this region does not alter functioning
C-terminus		

dimer in order to alter gene expression. Some steroid hormone/receptor complexes (e.g. involving ER, PR, AR, GR and MR) tend to bind to the same hormone/receptor complex to form homodimers (e.g. ER–ER) while the others (TR, VDR, RAR and RXR) can also form heterodimers (e.g. RAR–RXR).

The steroid receptor is made up of five regions with different functions (Table 1.2). The different regions are involved in hormone recognition, DNA binding and DNA modulation.

Hormone drugs act primarily by mimicking the endogenous hormone (i.e. as an agonist) but often the drug has more appropriate pharmacokinetic characteristics than the endogenous ligand. Some drugs act as antagonists by blocking the binding of the normal ligand.

Other sites of drug action

In addition to the sites and mechanisms of actions discussed above, drugs may also bind to and either activate or inhibit other specific sites.

- **Specific cell membrane ion pumps**. For example, Na^+/K^+-ATPase in the brain is activated by the anticonvulsant phenytoin whereas that in cardiac tissue is inhibited by digoxin; K^+/H^+-ATPase in gastric parietal cells is inhibited by omeprazole.
- **Specific enzymes**. For example, a number of anticancer drugs inhibit enzymes involved in purine, pyrimidine or DNA synthesis. Some drugs act on the enzymes that synthesise or degrade the endogenous ligands for extracellular or intracellular receptors.
- **Specific organelles**. For example, some antibiotics interfere with the functioning of the bacterial ribosome.
- **Specific transport proteins**. For example, diuretics affect Na^+ transport in the renal tubules, and probenecid inhibits renal tubular secretion of anions.

Types of drug action

Drug actions can show a number of important properties:

- specificity
- selectivity
- potency
- efficacy.

Specificity

Most drugs are specific in that they act only on one type of receptor, for example noradrenergic rather than cholinergic (see above). Drugs that are not specific to one type of receptor frequently display a wide variety of adverse effects (see for example tricyclic antidepressants, Ch. 22).

Selectivity

Many drugs act preferentially on particular receptor types or subtypes and may bind to different receptor subtypes, for example β_1- and β_2-adrenoceptors, to different extents (see above). For such drugs it would be possible to determine dose–response relationships for each receptor subtype. The selectivity of the drug is the measure of the separation of the dose responses for different receptor subtypes. For example, the β-adrenoceptor antagonist propranolol is a non-selective antagonist acting equally on β_1- and β_2-adrenoceptors, whereas atenolol shows selectivity towards β_1-adrenoceptors and has less effect on β_2-adrenoceptors. The expression of selectivity is dependent on the dose and on the concentration at the receptors, because high concentrations will give a maximal blockade at both receptor subtypes (Fig. 1.10).

Potency

The potency of a drug in vitro is determined by the strength of its binding to the receptor, that is the receptor affinity. The more potent a drug, the lower will be the concentration needed to bind to the receptor and to

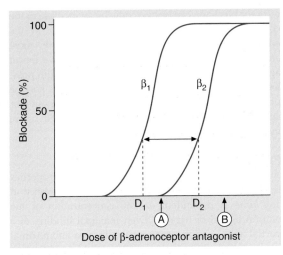

Fig. 1.10
**Effect of dose on selectivity of a β-adrenoceptor antagonist
(β-blocker).** The drug shows β_1 selectivity, because it produces
β_1-effects at doses that produce little effect on β_2-adrenoceptors (i.e. at
doses of A or less). However, this selectivity is lost when the dose is
increased above A and no selectivity is seen at dose B (which produces
a maximum response for both β_1- and β_2-adrenoceptors). The extent of
selectivity is given by the comparative potencies at each receptor type
(i.e. it is the degree of separation of the two curves). The relative
potency at each receptor subtype is given by doses giving similar
responses, e.g. D_1 and D_2 in the diagram. β_1, dose response on
β_1-adrenoceptor-mediated effects; β_2, dose response on
β_2-adrenoceptor-mediated effects.

give a response for an agonist, or to block a response for
an antagonist. Potencies of different drugs are compared using the ratio of the doses required to produce
(or block) the same response. Because dose–response
curves are usually parallel (for drugs that share a
common mechanism of action), the ratio is the same at
different response values, e.g. 10, 20 or 50% response.
(Figure 1.10 can be used to compare the potency of the
drug on β_1- and β_2-adrenoceptors). Potencies cannot be
determined by comparing the responses to similar doses
because the difference between drugs will vary with the
dose. Drugs that show the highest receptor affinities are
the most potent in vitro; however, the dose-response
relationship in vivo depends also on the delivery of the
drug to its site of action, and this can be affected by
absorption, distribution and elimination (pharmacokinetics – Chapter 2). Therefore the in vivo potencies of
a series of related drugs may not reflect their in vitro
receptor binding properties.

Efficacy

The efficacy of a drug is its ability to produce the
maximal response possible. For example, agonists can
be divided into *full agonists*, which give an increase in
response with increase in concentration until the
maximum possible response is obtained, and *partial
agonists*, which also give an increase in response with
increase in concentration but cannot produce the
maximum possible response (see later).

Classification of drug action

Specific types of drug action will be introduced
throughout this book. They can be classified as:

- agonists
- antagonists
- partial agonists
- inverse agonists
- allosteric modulators
- enzyme inhibitors/activators
- non-specific.

Agonists

An agonist binds to the receptor or site of action and
produces a conformational change in the receptor that
mimics the action of the normal ligand. The action of the
compound will be additive with the natural ligand at
low concentrations. Drugs may differ in both the affinity
(or strength) of binding and the rate of association/
dissociation.

**The affinity or strength of binding of the drug to
the receptor.** This determines the concentration necessary to produce a response and, therefore, is directly
related to the potency of the drug. In the examples in
Figure 1.11, drug A_1 is more potent than drug A_2, but
both are capable of giving a maximal response. For
some compounds a maximal response may require all of
the receptors to be occupied, but for most drugs the
maximal response is produced while some receptors
remain unoccupied, that is, there may be *spare* receptors.
The presence of spare receptors becomes important
when considering changes in receptor numbers owing
to adaptive responses during chronic treatment (tolerance) or caused by irreversible binding of an antagonist
(see below).

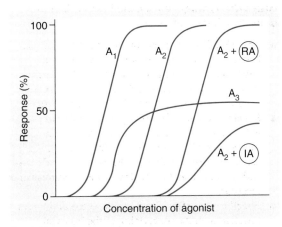

Fig. 1.11
**Dose–response curves for agonists in the absence or presence
of an antagonist.** A_1, A_2, two different agonists (A_1 more potent than
A_2); A_3, partial agonist; RA, reversible antagonist;
IA, irreversible antagonist.

The rate of binding/dissociation. This is usually of negligible importance in determining the rates of onset or termination of effect in vivo, because these depend mainly on the rates of delivery to and removal from the target organ, that is on the overall absorption or elimination rate of the drug from the body (see Ch. 2).

Changes in the number of receptors. The effect of changes in the numbers of receptors on the dose–response curve for agonists depends on their potency, receptor occupancy and efficacy. This can be illustrated by a consideration of the theoretical situation illustrated in Table 1.3, for a membrane that contains 100 receptors. Drug A is the most potent and there are spare receptors at maximal response. Drug B gives 100% response when 100% of receptors are occupied and drug C is a partial agonist (see below). With downregulation of receptors, the response obtained depends upon the extent of downregulation and also to the extent of occupancy necessary to produce a maximal response (Table 1.3). (In practice, drug effects are usually produced at concentrations that do not produce 100% receptor occupancy. Under such circumstances the extent of any effect of downregulation will depend also on the slope of the dose–response curve, but the concept illustrated in the table will still apply.)

Antagonists

An antagonist binds to the receptor but does not cause the necessary conformational change. The compound will block access to the receptor-binding site by the normal ligand. The drug effect may only be detectable when the natural agonist is present (e.g. β-adrenoceptor antagonists lower heart rate, particularly when heart rate is increased by stimulation of the sympathetic nervous system). The binding of most clinically useful antagonists is reversible and competitive; in consequence, the receptor blockade can be overcome by an increase in the concentration of the natural receptor ligand or by the administration of an agonist drug. Therefore, most antagonist drugs move the dose–response curve for an agonist to the right but do not alter the maximum possible response (Fig. 1.11). Irreversible antagonists, such as phenoxybenzamine, bind covalently to their site of action, and a full response cannot be achieved by an increase in agonist concentration.

Partial agonists

A drug showing both agonist and antagonist properties is known as a partial agonist: the activity expressed at any time is dependent on the concentration of the natural ligand or agonist. Even maximal binding of a partial agonist to the receptor produces a submaximal response, possibly because of incomplete amplification of the receptor signal via the G-proteins. A partial agonist will show agonist activity at low concentrations of the natural ligand, but the dose–response will not reach the maximal activity even when all receptors are occupied (see Fig. 1.11, drug A_3). At high concentrations of the natural ligand, a partial agonist will behave as an antagonist because it will prevent access of the natural ligand to the receptor and thereby result in a submaximal response.

Inverse agonists

The concept of an inverse agonist arose because some compounds were found to show 'negative efficacy' – in other words they acted on receptors to produce a change opposite to that caused by an agonist. This discovery gave rise to the concept that receptors exist in an equilibrium between inactive and active forms in the absence of an agonist ligand. The presence of an agonist will increase the proportion of active receptors. The

Table 1.3
Responses of a tissue containing 100 receptors

	Status of tissue receptors	Drug[a]		
		A	B	C
Percentage of maximal response when 100 receptors are occupied by the drug	Normal	100	100	50
Concentration giving 100% receptor occupancy (nmol l^{-1})	Normal	1	2	2
Numbers of receptors occupied to give greatest effect seen (100% maximal for A and B, 50% maximal for C)	Normal	40	100	100
Percentage response at concentrations giving 100% receptor occupancy in normal tissue	DR[b] 50%	100	50	25
Percentage response at concentrations given 100% receptor occupancy in normal tissue	DR[b] 20%	50	20	10

[a]A, B and C are three agonist drugs with different receptor-binding characteristics.
[b]DR, downregulated tissue so that preparation contains either 50% or 20% of the normal numbers of receptors.

presence of an inverse agonist will shift the balance towards more inactive receptors, thereby reducing the level of basal activity and actions. Antagonists (see above) bind to the receptor and will block the activity of both agonists and inverse agonists. The concept of a degree of receptor activation in the absence of an agonist ligand is supported by observations that cell lines which express increased numbers of β_2-adrenoceptors show increased basal adenylate cyclase activity (in the absence of an agonist signal). The mechanism of action of inverse agonists is not well characterised, but they may destabilise the receptor/G-protein coupling, or they may preferentially bind to the inactivated form of the receptor, thereby shifting the equilibrium away from the active form. A final complication, which awaits resolution, is that some drugs, for example β-adrenoceptor antagonists, that are normal antagonists at some tissue receptors may be inverse agonists when the receptor is expressed on a different tissue. The role of inverse agonism in the therapeutic effects of drugs remains to be fully elucidated.

Allosteric modulators

An allosteric modulator does not act directly on the ligand/receptor site but may bind elsewhere on the receptor to enhance or decrease the binding of the natural ligand to its receptor. An example is the benzodiazepine drugs, which alter the affinity of Cl⁻ channels for the neurotransmitter GABA (Ch. 20).

Enzyme inhibitors/activators

Some drugs have a site of action that is an enzyme; the drug acts either on the catalytic site or at an allosteric site.

Non-specific action

Some compounds have a generalised effect that causes the desired therapeutic outcome. Examples are the modulation of neuronal cell membrane fluidity by general anaesthetics and the action of osmotic diuretics on the kidney.

Tolerance to drug effects

Tolerance to drug effects results in a decrease in response with repeated doses. Tolerance may occur through a decrease in the concentrations of drug at the receptor or through a decrease in response of the receptor to the same concentration of drug. The relationship between drug dosage and the concentrations delivered to the receptor is discussed in Chapter 2; some drugs stimulate their own metabolism and, as a result, they are eliminated more rapidly on repeated dosage and less drug is available to produce a response. However, most clinically important examples of tolerance arise from changes in receptor numbers and concentration–response relationships.

Desensitisation is used to describe both long-term and short-term changes in dose–response relationships arising from a decrease in response of the receptor. Desensitisation can occur by a number of mechanisms:

- decreased receptor numbers (downregulation): a slow process taking hours or days
- decreased receptor binding affinity
- decreased G-protein coupling
- modulation downstream of the initial signal.

Extracellular receptors coupled to G-proteins show rapid desensitisation (within minutes) during continued activation that occurs through two mechanisms:

- *homologous desensitisation*: the enzymes activated following ligand binding to a receptor–G-protein complex include *G-protein-coupled receptor kinases* (GRKs); these interact with the $\beta\gamma$-subunit of the G-protein and inactivate the occupied receptor protein by phosphorylation (a related peptide (β-arrestin) enhances the GRK-mediated desensitisation)
- *heterologous desensitisation*: the receptor (whether occupied or not) is inactivated through phosphorylation by a cAMP-dependent kinase (protein kinase A or protein kinase C), which can be switched on by a variety of signals that increase cAMP.

Muscarinic and α_1-adrenoceptors, which are linked to phospholipase C (Table 1.1), may also undergo desensitisation via receptor phosphorylation, which uncouples the G-protein from the receptor. The phosphorylated receptor protein may then be internalised and undergo intracellular dephosphorylation prior to re-entering the cytoplasmic membrane.

Downstream modulation of the signal may also occur through feedback mechanisms or simply through depletion of some essential cofactor. A good example of the latter is the chronic administration of organic nitrates, which may deplete the SH groups necessary for the generation of nitric oxide (see angina, Ch. 5); high doses of indirectly acting sympathomimetic amines may cause depletion of neuronal noradrenaline, which is necessary for their activity (see Ch. 4).

Conclusions

The specificity and selectivity of drugs arise from their ability to interact with and affect certain target sites within a cell. In principle, high selectivity should result in safer drugs with fewer adverse effects. Our increasing knowledge of the complexity of receptor pharmacology

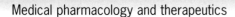
offers the promise of safer drugs in the future. However, it should be remembered that:

- not all effects seen following drug administration are caused by the drug (the placebo effect can be very powerful!)

- nearly all drugs show multiple effects no matter how receptor selective they are
- not all effects produced by a drug will be therapeutically beneficial.

FURTHER READING

Ackerman MJ, Clapham DE (1997) Ion-channels – basic science and clinical disease. *N Engl J Med* 336, 1575–1586

Catterall WA (1995) Structure and function of voltage-gated ion channels. *Annu Rev Biochem* 64, 493–531

Chuang TT, Iacovelli L, Sallese M, de Blasi A (1996) G protein-coupled receptors: heterologous regulation of homologous desensitization and its implications. *Trends Pharmacol Sci* 17, 416–421

Dohlman HG, Thomer J, Caron MG. Lefkowitz RJ (1991) Model systems for the study of seven-transmembrane-segment receptors. *Annu Rev Biochem* 60, 653–688

Gudermann T, Kalkbrenner F, Schultz G (1996) Diversity and selectivity of receptor–G-protein interaction. *Annu Rev Pharmacol Toxicol* 36, 429–459

Koenig JA, Edwardson JM (1997) Endocytosis and recycling of G protein-coupled receptors. *Trends Pharmacol Sci* 18, 276–287

Milligan G, Bond RA, Lee M (1995) Inverse agonism: pharmacological curiosity or potential therapeutic strategy. *Trends Pharmacol Sci* 16, 10–13

Polson JB (1996) Cyclic nucleotide phosphodiesterases and vascular smooth muscle. *Annu Rev Pharmacol Toxicol* 36, 403–427

Simon MI, Strathmann MP, Gautam N (1991) Diversity of G proteins in signal transduction. *Science* 252, 802–808

Strader CD, Fong TM, Tota MR, Underwood D, Dixon RAF (1994) Structure and function of G-protein-coupled receptors. *Annu Rev Biochem* 63, 101–132

Sunahara RK, Dessauer CW, Gilman AG (1996) Complexity and diversity of mammalian adenylyl cyclases. *Annu Rev Pharmacol Toxicol* 36, 461–480

Tsai M-J, O'Malley BW (1994) Molecular mechanisms of action of steroid/thyroid receptor superfamily members. *Annu Rev Biochem* 63, 451–486

Wess J (1993) Molecular basis of muscarinic acetylcholine receptor function. *Trends Pharmacol Sci* 14, 308–313

Pharmacokinetics

The nature of the response of a patient to a particular drug, for example a decrease in blood pressure, depends on the inherent pharmacological properties of the drug at its site of action. The time delay prior to a response and the duration of response are usually related to physiological and biochemical processes that determine the delivery to, and removal from, the site of action: that is the movement of drug around the body. Consequently, the overall response of the patient represents a combination of the actions of the drug on the body (*pharmacodynamics*) and the effects of the body on the drug (*pharmacokinetics*) (Fig. 2.1). Both pharmacodynamic and pharmacokinetic aspects are subject to a number of variables (Fig. 2.1), which affect the dose–response relationship. Pharmacodynamic aspects are determined by processes such as drug–receptor interaction and are specific to the class of the drug, e.g.

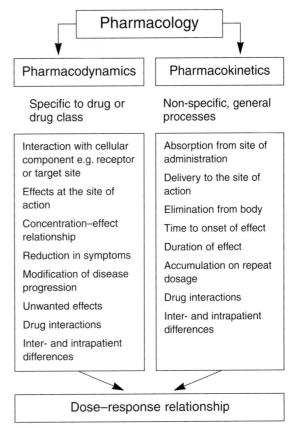

Fig. 2.1
Factors determining the response of a patient to a drug.

β-adrenoceptor blockers. Pharmacokinetic aspects are determined by general processes, such as transfer across membranes, xenobiotic (foreign compound) metabolism and renal elimination, which apply irrespective of the pharmacodynamic properties.

Pharmacokinetics may be divided into three basic processes:

absorption: the transfer of the drug from the site of administration to the general circulation
distribution: the transfer of the drug from the general circulation into the different organs of the body
elimination: the removal of the drug from the body, which may involve either excretion or metabolism.

Each of these processes can be described in terms of their chemical, biochemical and physiological basis and also in mathematical terms. The mathematical description of pharmacokinetic processes determines many of the quantitative aspects of drug prescribing:

- why oral and intravenous doses may be different
- the interval between doses during chronic therapy
- the dosage adjustment that may be necessary in hepatic and renal disease
- the calculation of dosages for the very young and the elderly.

The biological basis of pharmacokinetics

Drug structures bear little resemblance to normal dietary constituents such as carbohydrates, fats and proteins, and they are handled in the body by different processes. Although drugs may bind to the receptor for a specific endogenous neurotransmitter, they only rarely share the same carrier processes or metabolising enzymes with the natural ligand. Consequently, the movement of drugs around the body is usually by simple passive diffusion rather than specific transporters, while metabolism is usually by 'drug-metabolising enzymes', which have a low substrate specificity and can handle a wide variety of drug substrates.

General considerations

Passage across membranes

With the exception of direct intravenous or intra-arterial injections, a drug must cross at least one membrane in its movement from the site of administration into the general circulation. Drugs acting at intracellular sites must also cross the cell membrane to exert an effect. The main mechanisms by which drugs can cross membranes (Fig. 2.2) are:

- passive diffusion
- carrier-mediated processes: facilitated diffusion and active transport
- through pores or ion channels
- by pinocytosis.

Passive diffusion. Passive movement down a concentration gradient occurs for all drugs. The drug must pass into the phospholipid bilayer (Fig. 2.2) and therefore has to have a degree of lipid solubility. Eventually a state of equilibrium will be reached in which equal concentrations of the diffusible form of the drug are present in solution on each side of the membrane.

Carrier-mediated processes. In *facilitated diffusion*, energy is not consumed and the drug cannot be transported against a concentration gradient; by comparison *active transport* is an energy-dependent mechanism resulting in accumulation of the drug on one side of the membrane. In each case the drug in question resembles

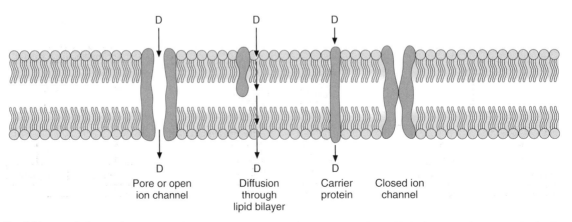

Fig. 2.2
The passage of drugs (D) across membrane bilayers.

the natural ligand for the carrier process sufficiently to bind to the carrier macromolecule, but the strength of binding is such that it is also readily released. Examples include levodopa (Ch. 24), which crosses the blood–brain barrier by facilitated diffusion, and base analogues such as 5-fluorouracil (Ch. 52), which undergoes active uptake. Drugs that bind to carrier proteins but are released only slowly act as inhibitors of the carrier; for example, probenecid inhibits the secretion of anions, such as penicillins, by the renal tubule.

Passage through membrane pores or ion channels. Movement occurs down a concentration gradient and can only occur for extremely small water-soluble molecules (<100 Da). This is applicable to therapeutic ions such as lithium and radioactive iodide.

Pinocytosis. This can be regarded as a form of carrier-mediated entry into the cell cytoplasm. Pinocytosis is normally concerned with the uptake of macromolecules, but attempts are currently underway to utilise it for targeted drug uptake by incorporating the drug into a lipid vesicle or liposome.

A number of reversible and irreversible processes can influence the total concentration of drug present on each side of the membrane (Fig. 2.3). Ionisation is a fundamental property of most drugs and will occur whenever the drug is in solution. The majority of drugs are either weak acids, such as aspirin, or weak bases, such as propranolol. The presence of an ionisable group(s) is essential for the mechanism of action of most drugs, because ionic forces represent a key part of ligand–receptor interactions. Drug receptors are formed by the three-dimensional arrangement of a specific section of a protein (Ch. 1), and drug binding requires both lipid- and water-soluble sites within the drug molecule; the latter are usually produced by an ionisable functional group.

The overall polarity of the drug and its extent of ionisation determine a number of key aspects of its fate in the body, such as distribution, entry into the brain, accumulation in adipose tissue and mechanism and route of elimination from the body. Ionisation is a fundamental

property and occurs when drugs containing acidic or basic groups dissolve in an aqueous body fluid.

$$[\text{Acidic drug}] \rightleftharpoons [\text{Acidic drug}]^- + H^+$$

$$[\text{Basic drug}] + H^+ \rightleftharpoons [\text{Basic drug} - H]^+$$

In general terms, the ionised form of the molecule can be regarded as the water-soluble form and the unionised form as the lipid-soluble form. Drugs with ionisable groups exist as an equilibrium between charged and uncharged forms. The extent of ionisation can affect both the pharmacodynamics (for example the affinity for the receptor) and the pharmacokinetics (for example the extent of uptake by adipose tissue and the route of elimination). The ease with which a drug can enter and cross a lipid bilayer is determined by the lipid solubility of its unionised form. Drugs that are fixed in their ionised form at all pH values, such as the quaternary amine d-tubocurarine, cross membranes extremely slowly or not at all; they have limited effects on the brain (because of lack of entry) and are given by injection (because of lack of absorption from the intestine).

The extent of ionisation of a drug depends on the strength of the ionisable group and the pH of the solution. The extent of ionisation is given by the acid dissociation constant K_a.

$$\text{Conjugate acid} \rightleftharpoons \text{Conjugate base} + H^+$$

$$K_a = \frac{[\text{conjugate base}]\,[H^+]}{[\text{conjugate acid}]} \tag{2.1}$$

The term conjugate acid refers to a form of the drug able to release a proton such as an unionised acid drug (Drug–COOH) or an ionised basic drug (Drug–NH_3^+). The conjugate base is the corresponding equilibrium form of the drug that has lost the proton, such as an ionised acidic drug (Drug–COO^-) or an unionised basic drug (Drug–NH_2).

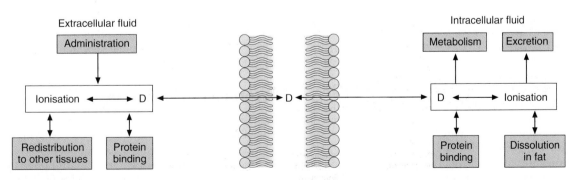

Fig. 2.3
Passive diffusion and factors that affect the concentration of drug freely available in solution (as an equilibrium between unionised and ionised forms).

The value of K_a is normally low (e.g. 10^{-5}) and therefore it is easier to compare compounds using the negative logarithm of the K_a, which is called the pK_a (e.g. 5).

For acidic functional groups, a strong acid will have a high tendency to dissociate to give H^+; this results in a high value for K_a and a low pK_a. Thus strongly acidic groups (such as Drug–SO_3H) have a pK_a of 1–2 while weakly acid groups (such as a phenolic–OH) have a pK_a of 9–10. In contrast, for basic functional groups, the stronger the base the greater will be its ability to retain the H^+ as a conjugate acid – resulting in a low K_a and a high pK_a. Thus strongly basic groups (such as R–NH_2 where R is an alkyl group) have a pK_a of 10–11 while weakly basic groups (such as R_3N) have a pK_a of 2–3.

The pH of body fluids is controlled by the buffering capacity of the ionic groups present in endogenous molecules, such as phosphate ions and proteins. When the fluids on each side of a membrane (see Fig. 2.3) have the same pH values there will be equal concentrations of both the diffusible, unionised form and the polar ionised form of the drug on each side of the membrane at equilibrium. When the fluids on each side of a membrane are at different pH values, the concentration of ionised drug in equilibrium with the unionised will be determined by the pH of the solution and the pK_a of the drug. This results in pH-dependent differences in drug concentration on each side of a membrane (pH partitioning). The pH differences between plasma (pH 7.4) and stomach contents (pH 1–2) and urine (pH 5–7) can influence drug absorption and drug elimination.

Drugs are 50% ionised when the pH of the solution equals the pK_a of the drug. Acidic drugs are most ionised when the pH of the solution exceeds the pK_a, whereas basic drugs are most ionised when the pH is lower than the pK_a (Fig. 2.4). The practical importance is that the total concentration of drug will be higher on the side of the membrane where it is most ionised (Fig. 2.5), which has implications for drug absorption from the stomach and the renal elimination of some drugs. In drug overdose, increasing the pH of the urine can enhance the renal elimination of acidic drugs, such as aspirin, by retaining the ionised drug in the urine (see below), whereas a decrease in urine pH can be useful for basic drugs, such as amphetamine. It is important to realise that if you change urine pH in the wrong direction for the type of drug taken in overdose, you will make matters worse and could kill the patient!

The low pH of the stomach contents (usually pH 1–2) means that most acidic drugs are present largely in their unionised (proton-associated) form and pH partitioning allows the drug to pass into plasma (pH 7.4) where it is more ionised. In contrast, basic drugs are highly ionised in the stomach and absorption is negligible until the stomach empties and the drug can be absorbed from the lumen of the duodenum (pH about 8).

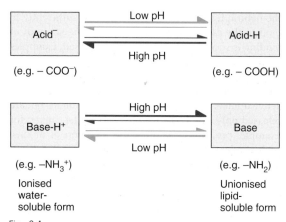

(e.g. – COO^-)   (e.g. – COOH)

(e.g. –NH_3^+)   (e.g. –NH_2)
Ionised   Unionised
water-   lipid-
soluble form   soluble form

Fig. 2.4
The effect of pH on drug ionisation.

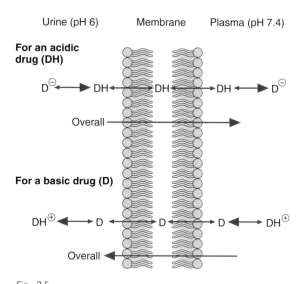

Fig. 2.5
Partitioning of acidic and basic drugs across a pH gradient.

Absorption

Absorption is the process of transfer of the drug from the site of administration into the general or systemic circulation.

Absorption from the gut

The easiest and most convenient route of administration of medicines is orally by tablets, capsules or syrups; however, this route is the most complex and presents the greatest number of barriers for the drug prior to reaching the systemic circulation. A number of factors can affect the rate and extent to which a drug can pass from the gut lumen into the general circulation.

Drug structure

Drug structure is a major determinant of absorption, distribution and elimination. Drugs need to be lipid soluble to be absorbed from the gut. Therefore, highly polar acids and bases tend to be absorbed only slowly and incompletely, with much of the dose not absorbed but voided in the faeces. High polarity may be useful for delivery of the drug to the lower bowel. The structure of some drugs can make them unstable either at the low pH of the stomach, for example penicillin G, or in the presence of digestive enzymes, for example insulin. Such compounds have to be given by injection.

Drugs that are weak acids or bases may undergo pH partitioning between the gut lumen and mucosal cells. Acidic drugs will be least ionised in the stomach lumen, and most absorption would be expected at this site. However, the potential for absorption in the stomach is decreased by its low surface area and the presence of a zone at neutral pH on the immediate surface of the gastric mucosal cells. In consequence, even weak acids, such as aspirin, tend to be absorbed mainly from the small intestine. Basic drugs are highly ionised in the stomach; as a result, absorption does not occur until the drug has passed from the stomach to the small intestine.

Formulation

Drugs cannot be absorbed until the administered tablet/capsule disintegrates and the drug is dissolved in the gastrointestinal contents to form a molecular solution. Most tablets disintegrate and dissolve rapidly and completely and all of the dose is rapidly available for absorption. However, some formulations are produced that disintegrate slowly so that the rate at which the drug is absorbed is limited by the rate of release of drug from the formulation, rather than by the transfer of the dissolved drug across the gut wall. This is the basis for *modified-release formulations* (e.g. slow-release) in which the drug either is incorporated into a complex matrix from which it diffuses or is administered in a crystallised form that dissolves only slowly. Dissolution of a tablet in the stomach can be prevented by coating it in an acid-insoluble layer, producing an *enteric-coated formulation*, for example omeprazole and aspirin.

Gastric emptying

The rate of gastric emptying determines the rate at which a drug is delivered to the small intestine, which is the major site of absorption. A delay between dose administration and the detection of the drug in the circulation is seen frequently after oral dosing and is usually caused by delayed gastric emptying. The co-administration of drugs that slow gastric emptying, for example anticholinergics, can alter the rate of drug absorption.

Food has a complex effect on drug absorption since it reduces the rate of gastric emptying and delays absorption, but it can also alter the total amount of drug absorbed.

First-pass metabolism

Metabolism of drugs (see below) can occur prior to and during absorption, and this can limit the amount of parent compound reaching the general circulation. Drugs taken orally have to pass four major metabolic barriers before they reach the general circulation.

Intestinal lumen. This contains digestive enzymes secreted by the mucosal cells and pancreas that are able to split amide, ester and glycosidic bonds. In addition, the lower bowel contains large numbers of aerobic and anaerobic bacteria, which are capable of performing a range of metabolic reactions, especially hydrolysis and reduction.

Intestinal wall. The cells of the wall are rich in enzymes such as monoamine oxidase (MAO), L-aromatic amino acid decarboxylase, CYP3A (see below) and the enzymes responsible for the phase 2 conjugation reactions (see below).

Liver. Blood from the intestine is delivered directly to the liver, which is the major site of drug metabolism in the body (see metabolism, below).

Lung. Cells of the lung have high affinity for many basic drugs and are the main site of metabolism for many local hormones via MAO or peptidase activity.

Because of metabolism at these sites, only a fraction of the administered oral dose may reach the general circulation. This process is known as *first-pass metabolism* because it occurs at the first passage through these organs. The liver is generally the most important site of first-pass metabolism. Hepatic metabolism can be avoided by administration of the drug to a region of the gut from which the blood does not drain into the hepatic portal vein, for example the buccal cavity and rectum. A good example of avoiding hepatic first-pass metabolism is the buccal administration of glyceryl trinitrate (nitroglycerin; Ch. 5).

Absorption from other routes

Percutaneous administration

The human epidermis (especially the stratum corneum) represents an effective permeability barrier to water loss and to the transfer of water-soluble compounds. Although lipid-soluble drugs are able to cross this barrier, the rate and extent of entry are very limited. In consequence, this route is only really effective for use with potent non-irritant drugs, such as glyceryl trinitrate, or to produce a local effect. The slow and continued absorption from dermal administration (e.g. patches) can be used to produce low, but relatively constant, blood concentrations.

Intradermal and subcutaneous injection

Intradermal or subcutaneous injection avoids the barrier presented by the stratum corneum, and entry into the general circulation is limited largely by the blood flow to the site of injection. However, these sites only allow the administration of small volumes of drug and tend to be used for local effects such as local anaesthesia or to limit the rate of drug absorption, for example insulin.

Intramuscular injection
The rate of absorption from an intramuscular injection depends on two variables: the local blood flow and the water solubility of the drug, both of which enhance the rate of removal from the injection site. Absorption of drugs from the injection site can be prolonged intentionally either by incorporation of the drug into a lipid vehicle or by formation of a sparingly soluble salt, such as procaine benzylpenicillin (procaine penicillin), thereby creating a depot formulation.

Inhalation
Although the lungs possess the characteristics of a good site for drug absorption (a large surface area and extensive blood flow), inhalation is rarely used to produce systemic effects. The principal reason for this is the difficulty of delivering non-volatile drugs to the alveoli. Therefore, inhalation drug administration is largely restricted to:

- Volatile compounds such as general anaesthetics
- Locally acting drugs such as bronchodilators used in asthma
- Potent agents such as ergotamine for migraine, since this route avoids the gastric stasis that is a common feature of a migraine attack.

The last two groups present technical problems for administration because the drugs are not volatile and have to be given either as aerosols containing the drug or as fine particles of the solid drug. Particles greater than 10 µm in diameter settle out in the upper airways, which are poor sites for absorption, and the drug then passes back up the airways, via ciliary motion and is eventually swallowed. The optimum particle size for airways deposition is 2–5 µm. It has been estimated that only 5–10% of the dose may be absorbed from the airways, even when the administration technique generates mostly small particles (i.e. 5 µm or less). Particles less than 1 µm in diameter are not deposited in the airways and are exhaled.

Minor routes
Although drugs may be applied to all body surfaces and orifices, this is usually to produce a local and not a systemic effect. However, absorption from the site of administration may be important in producing unwanted systemic actions.

Distribution

Distribution is the process by which the drug is transferred from the general circulation into the tissues. For most drugs this occurs by simple diffusion of the unionised form across cell membranes until equilibrium is reached (Fig. 2.3). At equilibrium, any process that removes the drug from one side of the membrane results in movement of drug across the membrane to re-establish the equilibrium (Fig. 2.3).

Administration
The concentration of drug in extracellular fluid is high immediately after drug administration and there is a net transfer of drug into tissues.

Drug ionisation
Ionisation, a simple pH-dependent equilibrium, alters the availability of drug molecules for other processes (see above).

Redistribution to other tissues
After an intravenous injection, there is a high initial plasma concentration, and the drug may rapidly enter and equilibrate with well-perfused tissues, such as the brain, liver and lung, giving relatively high concentrations in these tissues (Table 2.1). However, the drug will continue to enter poorly perfused tissues, and this will lower the plasma concentration. The high concentrations in the rapidly perfused tissues then decrease in parallel with the decreasing plasma concentrations, which results in a transfer of drug back from those tissues into the plasma (Fig. 2.6). In most cases, the uptake into well-perfused tissues is so rapid that these tissues may be assumed to equilibrate instantaneously with plasma and represent part of the 'central' compartment (see below). Redistribution from well-perfused to

Table 2.1
Relative organ perfusion rates in humans[a]

Organ	Cardiac output (%)	Blood flow (ml min^{-1} 100 g^{-1} tissue)
Well perfused organs		
Lung	100	1000
Adrenals	1	550
Kidneys	23	450
Thyroid	2	400
Liver	25	75
Heart	5	70
Intestines	20	60
Brain	15	55
Placenta (full term)	–	10–15
Poorly perfused organs		
Skin	9	5
Skeletal muscle	16	3
Connective tissue	–	1
Fat	2	1

[a] Except for the placenta, the data are for an adult male under resting conditions.

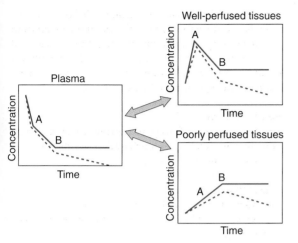

Fig. 2.6
A simplified scheme for the redistribution of drugs between tissues. The initial decrease in plasma concentrations results from uptake into well-perfused tissues, which essentially reaches equilibrium at point A. Between points A and B, the drug continues to enter poorly perfused tissues, which results in a decrease in the concentrations in both plasma and well-perfused tissues. At point B, all tissues are in equilibrium. NB The scheme has been simplified by representing the phases as discreet linear steps and also by the omission of any removal process. The presence of a removal process would produce a parallel decrease in all tissues from point B (shown as ----).

poorly perfused tissues is of clinical importance for terminating the action of some drugs that are given as a rapid intravenous injection or bolus. For example, thiopental produces rapid anaesthesia after intravenous dosage, but this is short-lived because continued uptake into muscle lowers the concentrations in the blood and in the brain (section A to B in Fig. 2.6).

Elimination processes

The processes of elimination (such as metabolism and excretion) are of major importance and are discussed in detail below. Elimination processes lower the concentration of the drug within the cells of the organ that eliminates the drug; this results in a transfer from plasma into the cells in order to maintain the equilibrium. The resultant fall in the concentration of drug in plasma results in drug transfer from other tissues into plasma in order to maintain their equilibria. Thus there is a net transfer from other tissues to the organ of elimination. Figure 2.6 illustrates how elimination (shown as a dashed line) produces a parallel decrease in drug concentrations in both plasma and tissues.

Reversible protein binding

Many drugs show an affinity for specific sites on proteins, which results in a reversible association or binding:

Drug + protein $\rightleftharpoons$ Drug–protein complex

Binding sites occur on circulating proteins such as albumin and α_1-acid glycoprotein and on intracellular

proteins (Fig. 2.3). The drug–protein binding interaction resembles the drug–receptor interaction since it is an extremely rapid, reversible and saturable process and different ligands can compete for the same site. However, it differs in two extremely important respects:

● drug–protein binding is of low specificity and does not result in any pharmacological effect but serves simply to lower the concentration of free drug in solution; such protein binding lowers the concentration of drug available to act at the receptor
● large amounts of drug may be present in the body bound to proteins such as albumin; in contrast, the amount of drug actually bound to receptors at the site of pharmacological activity is only a minute fraction of the total body load.

The rapidly reversible nature of protein binding is important because protein-bound drug can act as a depot. If the intracellular concentration of unbound drug decreases, for example through metabolism, then this will affect all the equilibria shown in Figure 2.3. Drug will dissociate from intracellular protein-binding sites, and some will transfer across the membrane from plasma until the intracellular equilibria are re-established. As a result, the extracellular (plasma) concentration of unbound drug will decrease, and drug will dissociate from plasma protein-binding sites. The ratio of the total amount of drug in the extracellular and intracellular compartments is determined by the relative affinity of the intra- and extracellular binding proteins.

Competition for protein binding can occur between different drugs (drug interaction; see Ch. 56), and also between drugs and natural, endogenous ligands. Administration of a highly protein-bound drug (such as aspirin) to a patient who is already receiving maintenance therapy with a drug that binds reversibly to plasma proteins (such as warfarin) will result in displacement of the initial drug from its binding sites; this increases the unbound concentration and therefore the biological activity (Table 2.2). In practice, such protein-binding interactions are frequently of limited duration because the extra free drug is removed by metabolism or excretion.

An important interaction involving the displacement of an endogenous compound bound to albumin occurs in jaundiced neonates. If these infants are given drugs, such as sulfonamides, that compete for the same binding sites on albumin as endogenous bilirubin, a potentially dangerous increase in the level of free bilirubin can follow.

Irreversible protein binding

Certain drugs, because of their chemical reactivity, undergo covalent binding to plasma or tissue components, such as proteins or nucleic acids. When the binding is irreversible, as for example the interaction of some cytotoxic agents with DNA, then this should be considered as an elimination process (because the parent drug

Table 2.2
Examples of drugs that undergo extensive plasma protein binding and may show therapeutically important interactions

Bound to albumin	Bound to α_1-acid glycoprotein
Clofibrate	Chlorpromazine
Digitoxin	Propranolol
Furosemide (frusemide)	Quinidine
Ibuprofen	Tricyclics
Indometacin (indomethacin)	Lidocaine
Phenytoin	
Salicylates	
Sulfonamides	
Thiazides	
Tolbutamide	
Warfarin	

cannot re-enter the circulation, as occurs after simple distribution to tissues). In contrast, the covalent binding of thiol-containing drugs (such as captopril) to proteins, via the formation of a disulfide bridge, may be slowly reversible. In such cases, the covalently bound drug will not dissociate in response to a rapid decrease in the concentration of unbound drug and such binding represents a slowly equilibrating reservoir of drug.

Distribution to specific organs

Although the distribution of drugs to all organs is covered by the general considerations discussed above,

two systems require more detailed consideration: the brain, because of the difficulty of drug entry, and the fetus, because of the potential for toxicity.

Brain

Lipid-soluble drugs, such as the anaesthetic thiopental, readily pass from the blood into the brain, and for such drugs the brain represents a typical well-perfused tissue (see Fig. 2.6, Table 2.1 and Ch. 17). In contrast, the entry of water-soluble drugs into the brain is much slower than into other well-perfused tissues, and this has given rise to the concept of a blood–brain barrier. The functional basis of the barrier (Fig. 2.7) is reduced capillary permeability owing to:

- tight junctions between adjacent endothelial cells
- a decrease in the size and number of pores in the cell membranes
- the presence of a surrounding layer of astrocytes.

Therefore, only lipid-soluble compounds can readily enter the brain. Water-soluble endogenous compounds needed for normal brain functioning, such as carbohydrates and amino acids, enter the brain via specific transport processes. Some drugs, for example levodopa, may enter the brain via these transport processes, and in such cases the rate of transport of the drug will be influenced by the concentrations of competitive endogenous substrates.

There is limited drug-metabolising ability in the brain and drugs leave by diffusion back into plasma, by active transport processes in the choroid plexus, or by elimination in the cerebrospinal fluid.

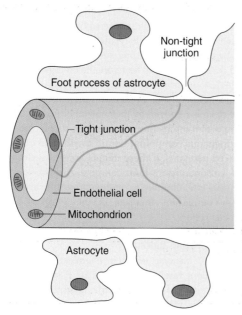

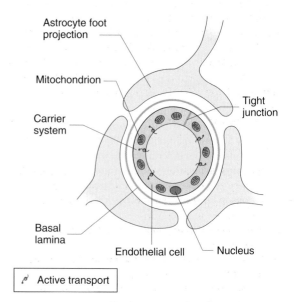

Fig. 2.7
The blood–brain barrier.

Fetus

Lipid-soluble drugs can readily cross the placenta and enter the fetus. The placental blood flow is slow compared with that in the liver, lung and spleen (Table 2.1); consequently, the fetus equilibrates slowly with the maternal circulation. Highly polar and large molecules (such as heparin) do not readily cross the placenta. The fetal liver has only low levels of drug-metabolising enzymes. The fetus relies on maternal elimination processes to lower drug concentration in the maternal circulation, which causes the drug to diffuse back across the placenta from fetal to maternal circulation.

After delivery, the baby may show effects from drugs given to the mother prior to delivery: such effects may be prolonged because the infant now has to rely on its own immature elimination processes.

Elimination

Elimination is the removal of drug from the body and may involve *metabolism*, in which the drug molecule is transformed into a different molecule, and/or *excretion*, in which the drug molecule is expelled in the body's liquid, solid or gaseous 'waste'.

Metabolism

Lipid solubility is an essential property of most drugs, since it allows the compound to cross lipid barriers and hence to be given via the oral route. Metabolism is essential for the elimination of lipid-soluble chemicals from the body, because it converts a lipid-soluble molecule (which would be reabsorbed from urine in the kidney tubule) into a water-soluble species (which is capable of rapid elimination in the urine). The drug itself is eliminated as soon as metabolism converts it into a different chemical structure. However, the elimination of the unwanted carbon skeleton of the drug may involve a complex series of biotransformation reactions (see below).

Metabolism of the parent drug produces a new chemical entity, which may show different pharmacological properties:

- loss of biological activity, which is the usual result of drug metabolism; this can increase polarity (especially phase 2 metabolism – see below) and prevent receptor binding
- decrease in activity, when the metabolite retains some activity
- increase in activity, when the metabolite is more potent than the parent drug
- change in activity, when the metabolite shows different pharmacological properties
- activation of a prodrug; in some cases, the drug molecule administered does not show biological

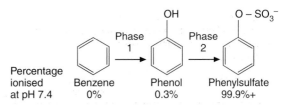

| Percentage ionised at pH 7.4 | Benzene 0% | | Phenol 0.3% | | Phenylsulfate 99.9%+ |

Fig. 2.8
The two phases of drug metabolism.

activity but is metabolised into the pharmacologically active form
- production of toxic metabolites; in some cases, drug metabolism produces a reactive or toxic product.

The various steps of drug metabolism can be divided into two phases (Fig. 2.8). Although many compounds undergo both phases of metabolism, it is possible for a chemical to undergo only a phase 1 or a phase 2 reaction. Phase 1 metabolism (oxidation, reduction and hydrolysis) is usually described as *preconjugation* because it produces a molecule that is a suitable substrate for a phase 2 or *conjugation* reaction. The enzymes involved in these reactions have low substrate specificities and can metabolise a vast range of drug substrates. In this section, drug metabolism is discussed in terms of the functional groups that may be found in different drugs, rather than individual specific compounds. (In the following tables R refers to an aliphatic or aromatic group and Ar refers specifically to an aromatic group).

Phase 1

Oxidation is by far the most important of the phase 1 reactions and can occur at carbon, nitrogen or sulfur atoms (Table 2.3). In most cases, an oxygen atom is

Table 2.3
Oxidation reactions

Oxidation at carbon atoms

Aromatic	$ArH \rightarrow ArOH$
Alkyl	$RCH_3 \rightarrow RCH_2OH \rightarrow RCHO \rightarrow RCOOH$
Dealkylation	$ROCH_3 \rightarrow ROH + HCHO$
	$RNHCH_3 \rightarrow RNH_2 + HCHO$
Deamination	$RCH_2NH_2 \rightarrow RCHO + NH_3$
	$RCH(CH_3)NH_2 \rightarrow RCO(CH_3) + NH_3$

Oxidation at nitrogen atoms

Secondary amines	$R-\overset{\overset{H}{\mid}}{N}-R \rightarrow R-\overset{\overset{OH}{\mid}}{N}-R$
Tertiary amines	$R_3N \rightarrow R_3N \rightarrow O$

Oxidation at sulphur atoms

Thioethers	$R-S-R \rightarrow R-\overset{\overset{O}{\uparrow}}{S}-R$

R, aliphatic or aromatic group; Ar, aromatic group.

retained in the metabolite, although some reactions, such as dealkylation, result in loss of the oxygen atom in a small fragment of the original molecule.

Oxidation reactions are catalysed by a diverse group of enzymes of which the cytochrome P450 system is the most important. Cytochrome P450 is a superfamily of membrane-bound enzymes (Table 2.4) that are present in the smooth endoplasmic reticulum of cells (Fig. 2.9). The liver is the major site of drug oxidation. The amounts of cytochrome P450 in extrahepatic tissues are low compared with those in liver.

Cytochrome P450 is a haemoprotein that can bind both the drug and molecular oxygen (Fig. 2.10). It cata-

lyses the transfer of one oxygen atom to the substrate while the other oxygen atom is reduced to water:

$$RH + O_2 + NADPH + H^+ \rightarrow ROH + H_2O + NADP^+$$

The reaction involves initial binding of the drug substrate to the ferric (Fe^{3+}) form of cytochrome P450 (Fig. 2.10), followed by reduction (via a specific cytochrome P450 reductase) and then binding of molecular oxygen. Further reduction is followed by molecular re-arrangement, with release of the reaction products and regeneration of ferric cytochrome P450.

Oxidations at nitrogen and sulfur atoms are frequently performed by a second enzyme of the

Table 2.4
The cytochrome P450 superfamily

Isoenzyme	Typical substrate	Comments
CYP1A	Theophylline	Induced by smoking
CYP2A	Testosterone	Induced by polycyclic hydrocarbons (e.g. smoking)
CYP2B	Numerous	Induced by phenobarbital
CYP2C	Numerous	Constitutive; 2C19 shows genetic polymorphism
CYP2D	Debrisoquine/sparteine	Constitutive; 2D6 shows genetic polymorphism
CYP2E	Nitrosamines	Induced by alcohol
CYP3A	Nifedipine/ciclosporin	Main constitutive enzyme induced by carbamazepine
CYP4	Fatty acids	Induced by clofibrate

Human liver contains at least 20 isoenzymes of cytochrome P450.
Families 1–4 are related to drugs and their metabolism; families 17, 19, 21 and 22 are related to steroid biosynthesis.

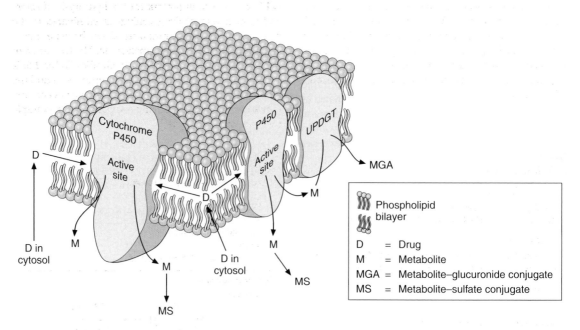

Fig. 2.9
Drug metabolism in the smooth endoplasmic reticulum. The lipid-soluble drug (D) partitions into the lipid bilayer of the endoplasmic reticulum. The cytochrome P450 oxidises the drug to a metabolite (M) that is more water soluble and diffuses out of the lipid layer. The metabolite may undergo a phase 2 (conjugation reaction) with UDP-glucuronyl transferase (UDPGT) in the endoplasmic reticulum or sulfate in the cytosol to give a glucuronide conjugate (MGA) or a sulfate conjugate (MS), respectively.

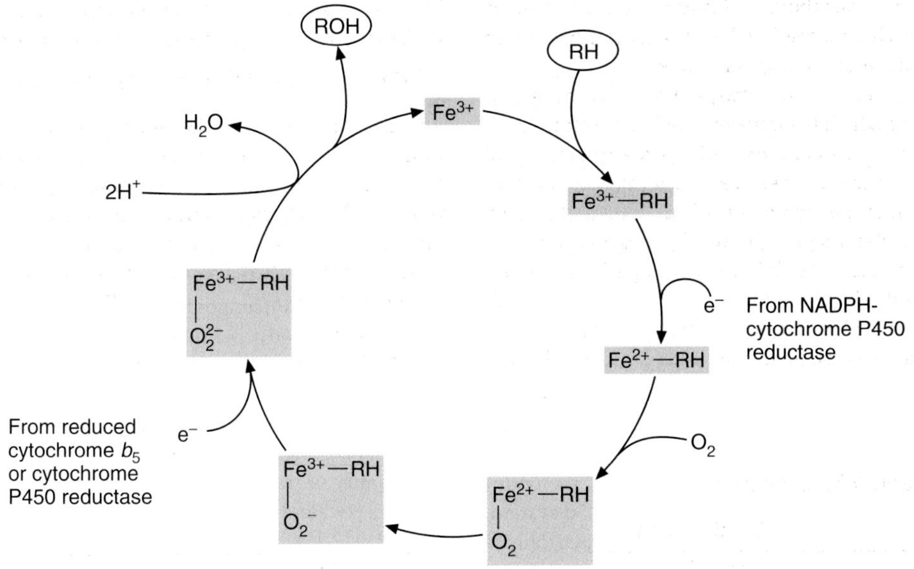

Fig. 2.10
The oxidation of substrate (RH) by cytochrome P450. Fe^{3+}, the active site of cytochrome P450 in its ferric state; RH, drug substrate; ROH, oxidised metabolite. Cytochrome b_5 is present in the endoplasmic reticulum and can transfer an electron to cytochrome P450 as part of its redox reactions.

endoplasmic reticulum, the flavin-containing mono-oxygenase, which also requires molecular oxygen and NADPH. A number of other enzymes, such as alcohol dehydrogenase, aldehyde oxidase and MAO may be involved in the oxidation of specific functional groups.

Reduction can occur at unsaturated carbon atoms and at nitrogen and sulfur centres (Table 2.5); such reactions are less common than oxidation. Reduction reactions can be performed both by the body tissues and also by the intestinal microflora. The tissue enzymes include cytochrome P450 and cytochrome P450 reductase.

Hydrolysis and *hydration* reactions (Table 2.6) involve addition of water to the drug molecule. In hydrolysis, the drug molecule is split by the addition of water. A number of enzymes present in many tissues are able to hydrolyse ester and amide bonds in drugs. The intestinal flora are also important for the hydrolysis of esters and amides and of drug conjugates eliminated in the bile (see below). In hydration reactions, the water molecule is retained in the drug metabolite. The hydration of the epoxide ring to produce a dihydrodiol (Table 2.6) is performed by a microsomal enzyme, epoxide hydrolase. This is an important reaction in the metabolism and toxicity of a number of aromatic compounds, for example the drug carbamazepine.

Table 2.5
Reduction reactions

Reduction at carbon atoms

Aldehydes	$RCHO \rightarrow RCH_2OH$
Ketones	$RCOR \rightarrow RCHOHR$

Reduction at nitrogen atoms

Nitro groups	$ArNO_2 \rightarrow ArNO \rightarrow ArNHOH \rightarrow ArNH_2$
Azo group	$ArN{=}NAr' \rightarrow ArNH_2 + H_2NAr'$

Reduction at sulphur atoms

Sulfoxides	$R{-}\overset{\overset{O}{\uparrow}}{S}{-}R \rightarrow R{-}S{-}R$
Disulphides	$R{-}S{-}S{-}R' \rightarrow RSH + HSR'$

R, aliphatic or aromatic group; Ar, aromatic group.

Table 2.6
Hydrolysis and hydration reactions

Hydrolysis reactions

Esters
$RCO.OR' \rightarrow RCOOH + HOR'$
Amides
$RCO.NHR' \rightarrow RCOOH + H_2NR'$

Hydration reactions

Epoxides

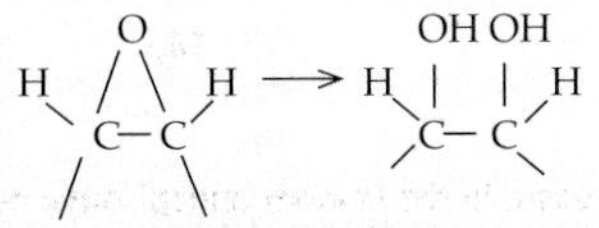

R, R', different aliphatic/aromatic groups.

Phase 2

Phase 2 or conjugation reactions involve the synthesis of a covalent bond between the drug and a normal body constituent (endogenous substrate). Energy to synthesise the bond is supplied by activation of either the drug or the endogenous substrate. The types of phase 2 reactions are listed in Table 2.7, which shows the functional group necessary in the drug molecule and the activated species for the reaction. In most cases, the reaction involves an activated endogenous substrate. The products of conjugation reactions are usually of greater water solubility and lower biological activity than the substrate.

The activated endogenous substrate for *glucuronide* synthesis is uridine-diphosphate glucuronic acid (UDPGA), which is synthesised from UDP-glucose. The enzymes that transfer the glucuronic acid moiety to the drug (UDP-glucuronyl transferases) occur in the endoplasmic reticulum close to the cytochrome P450 system, the products of which frequently undergo glucuronidation (Fig. 2.9). Glucuronide synthesis occurs in many tissues, especially the gut wall and liver, where it may contribute significantly to the first-pass metabolism of substrates such as simple phenols.

In contrast, *sulfate* conjugation is performed by a cytosolic enzyme, which utilises high energy sulfate (3'-phosphoadenosine-5'-phosphosulfate or PAPS) as the endogenous substrate. The capacity for sulfate conjugation is limited by the availability of PAPS, rather than the transferase enzyme. Sulfate conjugation is highly dose dependent, and saturation of sulfate conjugation contributes to the metabolic events involved in the liver toxicity seen in paracetamol (acetaminophen in USA) overdose (see Chapter 53).

The reactions of *acetylation* and *methylation* frequently decrease polarity because they block an ionisable functional group. These reactions mask potentially active functional groups such as amino and catechol moieties, and the enzymes are primarily involved in the inactivation of neurotransmitters such as noradrenaline or local hormones such as histamine.

The conjugation of drug carboxylic acid groups with *amino acids* is of interest because the drug is converted to a high-energy form (a CoA derivative) prior to the formation of the conjugate bond. The enzymes involved in formation of the drug CoA derivative are the mitochondrial acyl CoA synthetases, which normally deal with intermediate chain length fatty acids. Conjugation of the drug CoA derivative with the amino acid is catalysed by transferase enzymes.

An important conjugation reaction, related to drug toxicity, is that with the tripeptide *glutathione* (L-α-glutamyl-L-cysteinylglycine). This reaction is catalysed by a family of transferase enzymes and the drug metabolite is covalently bound to the thiol group in the cysteine (Fig. 2.11). This can also occur non-enzymatically. The substrates are often reactive drugs or activated metabolites, which are inherently unstable (see Ch. 53). Therefore, glutathione conjugation may be regarded as a true detoxication reaction in which glutathione acts as a scavenging agent to protect the cell from toxic damage. The initial glutathione conjugate undergoes a series of reactions, which illustrates the complexity of drug metabolism (Fig. 2.11).

A good example of a drug that undergoes a complex array of biotransformation reactions is sulfinpyrazone (Fig. 2.12). These involve oxidation by the tissues at various sites in the molecule including the sulfoxide group, reduction by the gut microflora at the sulfoxide group and conjugation with glucuronic acid of phenolic metabolites as well as at the carbon in position 4 of the heterocyclic ring (which is a very rare reaction, only found in humans). This drug also illustrates how metab-

Table 2.7
Major conjugation reactions

Reaction	Functional group	Activated species	Product
Glucuronidation	−OH −COOH −NH$_2$	UDPGA (uridine diphosphate glucuronic acid)	
Sulfation	−OH −NH$_2$	PAPS (3'-phosphoadenosine 5'-phosphosulfate)	−O−SO$_3$H −NH−SO$_3$H
Acetylation	−NH$_2$ −NHNH$_2$	Acetyl-CoA	−NH−COCH$_3$ −NHNH−COCH$_3$
Methylation	−OH −NH$_2$ −SH	S-Adenosyl methionine	−OCH$_3$ −NHCH$_3$ −SCH$_3$
Amino acid	−COOH	Drug–CoA	CO−NHCHRCOOH
Glutathione	Various	—	Glutathione conjugate

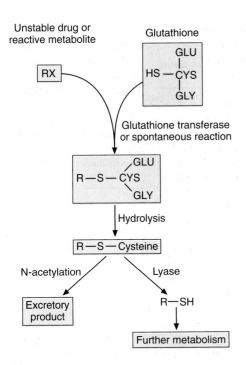

Fig. 2.11
The formation and further metabolism of glutathione conjugates.

olism can alter pharmacological properties since sulfinpyrazone is a potent uricosuric, while its sulfide metabolite has potent anti-aggregatory activity against platelets and the sulfone is inactive.

Factors affecting drug metabolism

The ability of patients to metabolise drugs is determined by their genetic constitution, their environment and their physiological status.

Genetic constitution

Wide interindividual differences in drug-metabolising ability arise from genetically determined differences in the basal level of expression of the metabolising enzyme. In most cases, there is a normal (Gaussian) distribution of enzyme activity in the population, and enzyme activities typically vary by about threefold between individuals. However, for some enzymes there is polymorphic expression of the enzyme activity and it is possible to divide the population into two groups: 'fast' metabolisers and 'slow' metabolisers. Slow metabolisers have low enzyme activity and will show higher plasma concentrations of the parent drug but lower concentrations of the metabolite(s). In some cases,

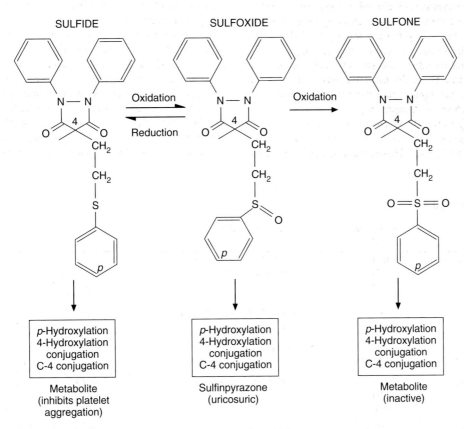

Fig. 2.12
The pathways of metabolism of sulfinpyrazone in humans and animals. This figure illustrates that a single drug may generate a large number of metabolites, which may possess different pharmacological properties.

Table 2.8
Pharmacogenetic differences in drug-metabolising enzymes

Enzyme	Incidence of deficiency[a] or slow metabolisers	Typical substrates
Plasma pseudocholinesterase[b]	1 in 3000	Suxamethonium (succinylcholine)
Alcohol dehydrogenase	5–10% (approx. 90% in Asians)	Ethanol
CYP2C19	5% (approx. 20% in Asians)	S-Mephenytoin, omeprazole
CYP2D6	5–10%	Debrisoquine, sparteine, metoprolol, dextromethorphan
CYP2C?	Very rare	Phenytoin
N-Acetyltransferase	Approx. 60% (approx. 5% in Japanese)	Isoniazid, hydralazine, procainamide
Methyltransferase	0.5%	6-Mercaptopurine

[a]For Caucasians.
[b]A number of variants are known.

the polymorphism arises from altered transcription of the normal enzyme protein, but frequently the gene in slow metabolisers codes for a modified enzyme protein that has an altered binding site and a decreased substrate affinity. Drug-metabolising enzymes showing polymorphism or enzyme deficiencies are given in Table 2.8.

Ethnic origins can affect the proportion of the population showing a genetic deficiency or polymorphism (see Table 2.8). In addition, the extent of metabolism in the general population may be different, for example subjects from the Indian subcontinent show a two- to threefold lower systemic clearance of nifedipine (a CYP3A substrate) compared with Caucasians.

Environmental influences
The activity of drug-metabolising enzymes, especially the cytochrome P450 system, can be increased or inhibited by foreign compounds such as environmental contaminants and therapeutic drugs. Induction of cytochrome P450 results in increased synthesis of the haemoprotein following exposure to the inducing agent. Environmental contaminants, such as organochlorine pesticides (such as DDT) and polycyclic aromatic hydrocarbons (such as benzo[a]pyrene in cigarette smoke), induce the CYP1A and CYP2A isoenzymes (Table 2.4). Therapeutic drugs such as phenobarbital, induce members of the CYP2, CYP3 and CYP4 families (Table 2.9). Chronic consumption of alcohol induces CYP2E. Induction of cytochrome P450 isoenzymes occurs over a period of a few days during which the additional enzyme is synthesised; the higher levels last for a few days after the removal of the inducing agent, while the extra enzyme is removed. In contrast, inhibition of drug-metabolising enzymes is by direct competition for the enzyme site and the time course follows closely the absorption and elimination of the inhibitor substance. A number of drugs (Table 2.9) can produce clinically significant drug interactions because of their induction or inhibition of cytochrome

Table 2.9
Common inducers and inhibitors of cytochrome P450

Inducers	Inhibitors
Barbiturates (esp. phenobarbital)	Cimetidine
Phenytoin	Allopurinol
Carbamazepine	Isoniazid
Griseofulvin	Chloramphenicol
Rifampicin (rifampin)	Disulfiram
Glutethimide	Quinine
	Erythromycin

P450 enzymes. Such changes in hepatic metabolism can affect both the bioavailability and clearance of drugs undergoing hepatic elimination (see below).

Physiological status
The functional capacity of the drug-metabolising enzymes is dependent on both the intrinsic enzyme activity and the delivery of drug to the site of metabolism via the circulation. Drug metabolism, and hence clearance and half-life for most drugs, is affected significantly by age (the very young and the elderly) and by liver disease. This is discussed in detail in Chapter 56.

Excretion

Drugs and their metabolites may be eliminated from the circulation by various routes:

- **in fluids (urine, bile, sweat, tears, milk, etc.):** these routes are most important for low-molecular-weight polar compounds, and the urine is the major route; milk is important because of the potential for exposure of the suckling infant
- **in solids (faeces, hair, etc.):** drugs enter the gastrointestinal tract by various mechanisms (see below) and this route is most important for high-molecular-weight compounds; the sequestration of

foreign compounds into hair is not of quantitative importance, because of the slow growth of hair, but distribution of a drug along the hair can be used to indicate the history of drug intake during the preceding weeks

- **in gases (expired air):** this route is only of importance for volatile compounds.

Excretion via the urine

There are three processes involved in the handling of drugs and their metabolites in the kidney: glomerular filtration, reabsorption and tubular secretion. The total urinary excretion of drug depends on the balance of these three processes: total excretion equals glomerular filtration plus tubular secretion less reabsorption.

Glomerular filtration. All molecules less than about 20 kDa undergo filtration through the pores of 7–8 nm in the glomerular membrane under positive hydrostatic pressure. Approximately 20% of the non-protein-bound drug enters the filtrate, together with a similar amount of plasma water. Plasma proteins and protein-bound drug are not filtered; therefore, the efficiency of glomerular filtration for a drug is influenced by the extent of plasma protein binding.

Reabsorption. The glomerular filtrate contains a number of constituents that the body cannot afford to lose. There are specific tubular uptake processes for carbohydrates, amino acids, vitamins, etc. and most of the water is also reabsorbed. Drugs may pass back from the tubule into the plasma if they are substrates for the uptake processes (very rare) or if they are lipid soluble. The urine is concentrated on its passage down the renal tubule and the tubule-to-plasma concentration gradient increases so that only the most polar and least diffusible molecules will remain in the urine. The pH of urine is usually less than that of plasma; consequently, pH partitioning, between urine (pH 5–6) and plasma (pH 7.4), may either increase or decrease the tendency of the compound to be reabsorbed (see above).

Tubular secretion. The renal tubule has secretory mechanisms for both acidic and basic compounds. Drugs and their metabolites (especially the glucuronic acid and sulfate conjugates) may undergo an active carrier-mediated elimination. Because secretion lowers the plasma concentration of unbound drug by an active process, there will be a rapid dissociation of any drug–protein complex; as a result, even highly protein-bound drugs may be cleared almost completely from the blood in a single passage through the kidney.

Excretion via the faeces

Uptake into hepatocytes and subsequent elimination in bile is the principal route of elimination of larger molecules (those with a molecular weight greater than about 500 Da). Conjugation with glucuronic acid increases the molecular weight of the substrate by almost 200 Da, and therefore bile can be an important route for the elimin-

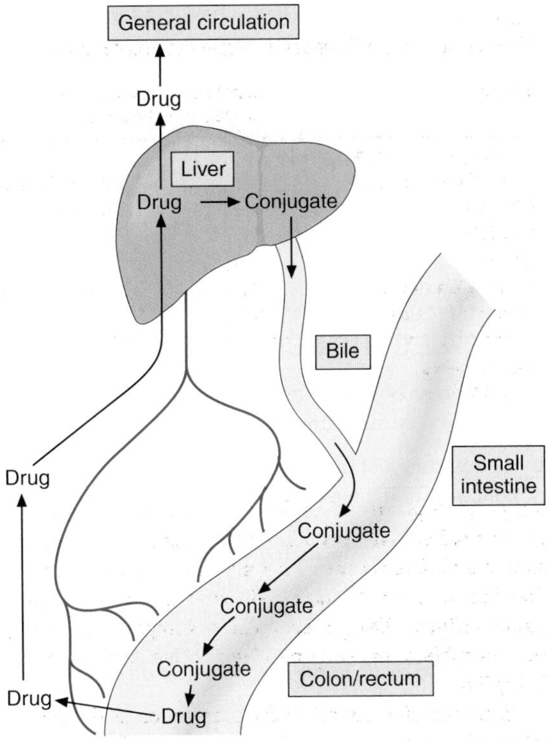

Fig. 2.13
Enterohepatic circulation of drugs.

ation of glucuronide conjugates. Once the drug, or its conjugate, has entered the intestinal lumen via the bile, it passes down the gut and eventually may be eliminated in the faeces. However, some drugs may be reabsorbed from the lumen of the gut and re-enter the hepatic portal vein. As a result, the drug is recycled between the liver, bile, gut lumen and hepatic portal vein. This is described as an enterohepatic circulation (Fig. 2.13); it can maintain the drug concentrations in the general circulation, because some of the reabsorbed drug will escape hepatic extraction. Highly polar glucuronide conjugates excreted into the bile undergo little reabsorption in the upper intestine, but the bacterial flora of the lower intestine may hydrolyse the drug conjugate back to the original drug and glucuronic acid. The original drug will have a greater lipid solubility and therefore be absorbed from the gut lumen and enter the hepatic portal vein (Fig. 2.13).

The mathematical basis of pharmacokinetics

The use of mathematics to describe the fate of a drug in the body can be complex and rather daunting for undergraduates. Nevertheless, a basic understanding is essential for an appreciation of many aspects of drug handling and for the rational prescribing of drugs. The following account gives the mathematics for the absorption, distribution and elimination of a single dose of a drug before brief consideration of chronic administration and the factors that can affect pharmacokinetic processes.

General considerations

Two different but complimentary approaches are used to describe pharmacokinetics.

- **Compartmental model analysis.** Plasma concentration–time curves are described by an equation containing one or more exponential functions. This approach gives a precise mathematical description of the concentration–time curve and can be used to predict the concentration of drug at any time after a dose. However, it is difficult to relate to the physiological disposition of the compound.
- **Model-independent analysis.** This approach may be related more closely to the physiological processes governing the disposition of the chemical. It is more useful in predicting and assessing the influence of variables such as disease, age and the administration of other compounds. However, this approach is not used to predict the concentration at any particular time after dosing.

Some undergraduate texts provide details of compartmental analysis, but the model-independent methods are of greater potential value to medical undergraduates and are the basis of the following account.

The three basic processes that need to be described mathematically are absorption, distribution and elimination. For each process it is important to know the *rate* or speed with which the drug is processed and the *extent* of the process, i.e. the amount or proportion of drug that undergoes that process.

For most physiological processes, the rate of reaction is proportional to the amount of substrate (drug) available: this is described as a *first-order reaction*. Diffusion down a concentration gradient and glomerular filtration are examples of first-order reactions. Protein-mediated reactions, such as metabolism and active transport, are also first-order at low concentrations. However, as the substrate concentration increases the enzyme or transporter can become saturated with substrate and the rate of reaction cannot increase in response to a further increase in concentration. The process then occurs at a fixed maximum rate that is independent of substrate concentration, and the reaction is described as a *zero-order reaction*, examples are the metabolism of ethanol

(Ch. 54) and phenytoin (Ch. 23). When the substrate concentration has decreased sufficiently for protein sites to become available again, then the change in concentration will proceed at a rate proportional to the concentration available, and the reaction will revert to first-order.

Zero-order reactions

If a drug is being processed (absorbed, distributed or eliminated) according to zero-order kinetics, then the change in concentration with time (dC/dt) is a fixed amount per time – independent of concentration:

$$\frac{dC}{dt} = -k \tag{2.2}$$

The units of k (the reaction rate constant) will be an amount per unit time (e.g. $\mu g\ min^{-1}$). A graph of concentration against time will produce a straight line with a slope of $-k$ (Fig. 2.14a).

First-order reactions

In first-order reactions, the change in concentration at any time (dC/dt) is proportional to the concentration present at that time:

$$\frac{dC}{dt} = -kC \tag{2.3}$$

The units of the rate constant, k, are time^{-1} (e.g. min^{-1}), and k may be regarded as the proportional change per unit of time. The rate of change will be high at high concentrations, but low at low concentrations (Fig. 2.14b) and a graph of concentration against time will produce an exponential decrease. Such a curve can be described by an exponential equation:

$$C = C_0 e^{-kt} \tag{2.4}$$

where C is the concentration at time t and C_0 is the initial concentration (when time = 0). This equation may be written more simply by taking natural logarithms:

$$\ln C = \ln C_0 - kt \tag{2.5}$$

and a graph of $\ln C$ against time will produce a straight line with a slope of $-k$ and an intercept of $\ln C_0$ (Fig. 2.14c).

The units of k (e.g. h^{-1}) are difficult to use practically, and therefore the rate of a first-order reaction is usually described in terms of its half-life (which has units of time). The half-life is the time taken for a concentration to decrease to one-half. The half-life is independent of concentration (Fig. 2.15) and is a characteristic for that particular first-order process and that particular drug. The decrease in plasma concentration after an intravenous bolus dose is shown in Figure 2.15, which has been plotted such that the concentration is halved every hour.

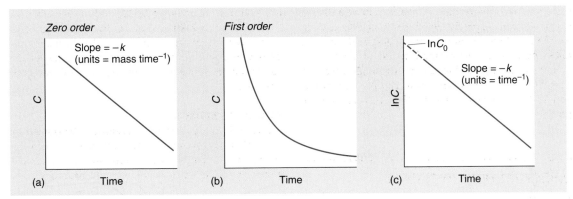

Fig. 2.14
Zero- and first-order kinetics. C, concentration; k, rate constant.

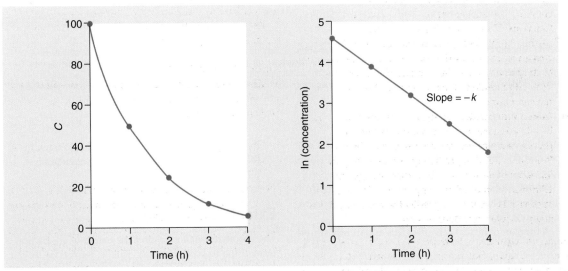

Fig. 2.15
The elimination half-life of a drug in plasma. Here the concentration (C) decreases by 50% every hour, i.e. the half-life is 1 h.

The relationship between the half-life and the rate constant is derived by substituting $C_0 = 2$ and $C = 1$ into the above equation, when the time interval t will be one half-life ($t_{1/2}$)

$$\ln 1 = \ln 2 - k t_{1/2} \tag{2.6}$$

$$0 = 0.693 - k t_{1/2}$$

$$t_{1/2} = \frac{0.693}{k}$$

A half-life can be calculated for any first-order process (e.g. for absorption, distribution or elimination); in practice, the 'half-life' reported for a drug is the half-life for the elimination rate (i.e. the slowest, terminal phase of the plasma concentration–time curve; see below).

Absorption

The mathematics of absorption apply to all 'non-intravenous' routes, for example oral, inhalation, percutaneous, etc. and are illustrated by absorption from the gut lumen.

Rate of absorption

The rate of absorption after oral administration is determined by the rate at which the drug is able to pass from the gut lumen into the systemic circulation. For lipid-soluble drugs, the rate of absorption is greater than the rate of elimination; as a result, the plasma concentration–time curve after an oral dose (Fig. 2.16) may be divided into two phases, as shown in Fig. 2.16a; the

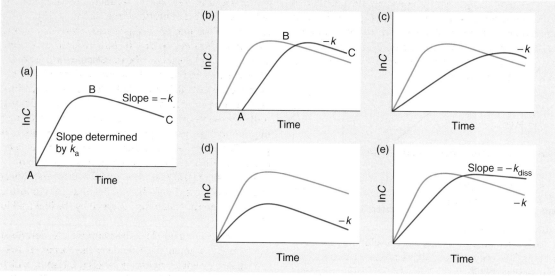

Fig. 2.16
Plasma concentration–time curves following oral administration. (a) General profile (A, start of absorption; B, end of absorption; B–C, elimination (rate = k) (this 'normal' profile is given as a green line in parts b–e). (b) Influence of gastric emptying; there is a delay between $t = 0$ and A. (c) Influence of food; slower absorption results in a reduction in the absorption rate constant (k_a) derived from A–B. (d) Decrease in bioavailability (owing to incomplete dissolution of formulation, decomposition, increased first-pass metabolism). (e) Slow-release formulation; the rate at which the drug can be eliminated is limited by the rate at which the formulation disintegrates (k_{diss}).

initial steep increase, from which the absorption rate constant (k_a) can be calculated, and the terminal slope, which gives the elimination rate constant (k). In Figure 2.16a, the absorption is essentially complete by point B since the subsequent data are fitted by a single exponential rate constant (the elimination rate).

A number of factors can affect this apparently simple pattern.

- **Gastric emptying.** Basic drugs undergo negligible absorption from the stomach (see above). In consequence, there can be a delay of up to an hour between drug administration and the detection of drug in the general circulation (Fig. 2.16b).
- **Food.** The pattern of absorption can be affected by changes in gastric emptying and food can alter the value of k_a (Fig. 2.16c).
- **Decomposition or metabolism prior to or during absorption.** This will reduce the amount of drug that reaches the general circulation but will not affect the rate of absorption (which is usually determined by lipid solubility). Therefore, the curve is parallel but at lower concentrations (Fig. 2.16d).
- **Modified-release formulation.** If a drug is eliminated rapidly, the plasma concentrations will show rapid fluctuations during regular oral dosing, and patients may have to take the drug at very frequent intervals. This can be avoided by giving a tablet that releases drug at a slow and predictable rate over many hours: a modified-release formulation. The terminal slope of the concentration–time curve is then determined by

the dissolution rate of the oral formulation, not by the elimination of the drug from the circulation (Fig. 2.16e).

Extent of absorption

The parameter that measures the extent of absorption is termed the *bioavailability* (F). This is defined as *the fraction of the administered dose that reaches the systemic circulation as the parent drug* (not as metabolites). For oral administration, incomplete bioavailability ($F < 1$) may result from:

- incomplete absorption and loss in the faeces, either because the molecule is too polar to be absorbed or the tablet did not release all of its contents
- first-pass metabolism, in the gut lumen, during passage across the gut wall or by the liver prior to the drug reaching the systemic circulation.

The bioavailability of a drug has important therapeutic implications, because it is the major factor determining the dosage requirements for different routes of administration. For example, if a drug has an oral bioavailability of 0.1, the oral dose will need to be 10 times higher than the corresponding intravenous dose.

The bioavailability of a drug is determined by comparison of data obtained after oral administration (when the fraction F enters the general circulation as the parent drug) with data following intravenous administration (when by definition 100% enters the general circulation as the parent drug). The amount in the circulation cannot be compared at only one time point, because intravenous and oral dosing show different concentration–time profiles. This is avoided by using the total area under the plasma concentration–time curve (AUC) from $t = 0$ to $t =$ infinity:

$$F = \frac{AUC_{oral}}{AUC_{iv}} \qquad (2.7)$$

if the oral and intravenous (iv) doses are equal or

$$F = \frac{AUC_{oral} \times Dose_{iv}}{AUC_{iv} \times Dose_{oral}} \qquad (2.8)$$

if different doses are used.

This calculation assumes that the elimination (clearance) is first order. The AUC is a reflection of overall body exposure and is discussed below under clearance.

An alternative method to calculate F is to measure the total urinary excretion *of the parent drug* (Aex) following oral and intravenous doses (even in situations where the urine is a minor route of elimination). Here

$$F = \frac{Aex_{oral}}{Aex_{iv}} \qquad (2.9)$$

for two equal doses.

Distribution

Distribution of a drug is the reversible movement of the parent drug from the blood into the tissues during administration and its re-entry from tissue into blood *as the parent drug* during elimination.

Rate of distribution

The rate of distribution is only occasionally of clinical relevance. The time delay between an intravenous bolus dose and the response may be caused by the time taken for distribution to the site of action. Redistribution of intravenous drugs, such as thiopental (Ch. 17), may limit the duration of action (see above). Usually the rate of distribution can only be measured following an intravenous bolus dose. Some drugs reach equilibrium between blood/plasma and tissues very rapidly and a distinct distribution phase is not apparent, only the terminal elimination phase is seen (Fig. 2.17a). Most drugs take some time to distribute into, and equilibrate with, the tissues. This is shown as a rapid distribution phase (Slope A–B in Fig. 2.17b, which has a high rate constant) prior to the terminal elimination phase (slope B–C in Fig. 2.17b; which has a lower rate constant). In Figure

2.17b, the processes of distribution are complete by point B. The concentration–time curve in Fig. 2.17b cannot be described by a single exponential term, and two first-order rates occur. The faster (distribution) rate is termed α and the slower (elimination) rate β. The distribution rate constant (α) cannot be derived directly from the slope A–B, because both distribution and elimination start as soon as the drug enters the body and A–B represents both processes. Back extrapolation of the terminal (β) phase gives an initial concentration at point D, which is the value that would have been obtained if distribution had been instantaneous. In practice the distribution rate (α) is calculated for the difference between the line D–B for each time point and the actual concentration measured (given by the line A–B in Fig. 2.17b).

Instantaneous and slow distributions are described by different mathematical models; the former is described as a *one-compartment model* (Fig. 2.17a) in which all tissues are in equilibrium instantaneously. The latter is described as a *two-compartment model* (Fig. 2.17b) in which the drug initially enters and reaches instantaneous equilibrium with one compartment (blood and possibly well-perfused tissues) prior to equilibrating more slowly with a second compartment (possibly poorly perfused tissues; refer back to Fig. 2.6). This is shown schematically in Figure 2.18.

The rate of distribution is dependent on two main variables:

- for *water-soluble drugs*, the rate of distribution depends on the rate of passage across membranes, that is the diffusion characteristics of the drug
- for *lipid-soluble drugs*, the rate of distribution depends on the rate of delivery (the blood flow) to those tissues, such as adipose, that accumulate the drug.

For some drugs, the natural logarithm of the plasma concentration–time curve shows three distinct phases; such curves require three exponential rates and represent a *three-compartment model*. Although two- or three-compartment models may be necessary to give a mathematical description of the data, they are of limited practical value.

Extent of distribution

The extent of distribution of a drug from plasma into tissues is of clinical importance because it determines the relationship between plasma concentration and the total amount of drug in the body (body burden). In consequence, the extent of distribution determines the amount of a drug that has to be administered in order to produce a particular plasma concentration (see below).

The extent of distribution of a drug from blood or plasma into tissues can be determined in animals by measuring concentrations in both blood and all the

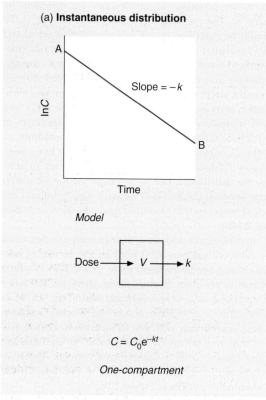

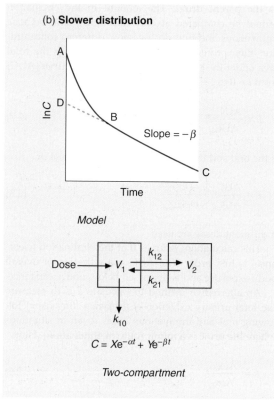

Fig. 2.17

Plasma concentration–time curves for the distribution of drugs into one- and two-compartment models. The terms k, α, β, k_{10}, k_{12}, k_{21}, are rate constants; α and β are composite rate constants which define the distribution and elimination rates. The terms α and β relate to distribution (k_{12} or k_{21} and elimination (k_{10}) processes and are determined by k_{10}, k_{12}, and k_{21}. V are volumes of distribution and X and Y are constants. (Note: the equation for a two-compartment system is usually written as $C = Ae^{-\alpha t} + Be^{-\beta t}$ where A and B are constants equivalent to X and Y; X and Y were used to avoid confusion with points A and B on the graph.)

tissues of the body. However, in humans only the concentration in blood or plasma can be measured, and therefore the extent of distribution has to be estimated from the amount remaining in blood, or more usually plasma, after completion of distribution.

The parameter that describes the extent of distribution is the *apparent volume of distribution* (V) where:

$$V = \frac{\text{Total amount of drug in the body}}{\text{Plasma concentration}} \quad (2.10)$$

The term V is a characteristic property of the drug that, like half-life, bioavailability and clearance, is independent of dose. In the simple example shown by Figure 2.17a, if a dose of 20 mg of a particular drug is injected this will mix instantaneously into the volume V. If the initial plasma concentration is $2\ \mu g\ ml^{-1}$ (equivalent to point A on Fig. 2.17a) then the apparent volume of distribution will be given by:

$$V = \frac{\text{Total amount (dose)}}{\text{Plasma concentration}} = \frac{20\,000\ \mu g}{2\ \mu g\ ml^{-1}} = 10\,000\ ml = 10\,l$$

In other words, after giving the dose it appears that the drug has been dissolved in $10\,l$ of plasma. However, plasma volume is only $3\,l$ and, therefore, some of the drug must have left the plasma and entered tissues, in order to give the low concentration present ($2\ \mu g\ ml^{-1}$). The clinical relevance of V is shown when a physician needs to calculate how much drug should be given to a patient to produce a specific desired plasma concentration. If an initial plasma concentration of $2.5\ \mu g\ ml^{-1}$ of the same drug were needed for a clinical effect, this would be produced by giving a dose of [plasma concentration $\times V$] or [$2.5\ \mu g\ ml^{-1} \times 10\,000\ ml$], that is $25\,000\ \mu g$ or 25 mg.

In the more complex example shown in Figure 2.17b, the dose of 20 mg will distribute instantaneously only into V_1, which is usually termed the central compartment. Measurement of the initial concentration (point A in Fig. 2.17b) will not represent distribution into V_2, and the volume calculated will under-represent the true extent of distribution (see Fig. 2.18). Distribution into V_2, which is usually termed the peripheral compartment, is not complete until point B in Figure 2.17b. However, by the time point B is reached there will have been consid-

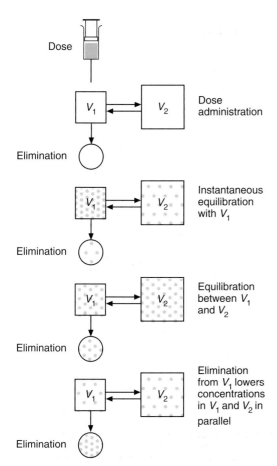

Dose

V_1 V_2 Dose administration

Elimination

V_1 V_2 Instantaneous equilibration with V_1

Elimination

V_1 V_2 Equilibration between V_1 and V_2

Elimination

V_1 V_2 Elimination from V_1 lowers concentrations in V_1 and V_2 in parallel

Elimination

Fig. 2.18
Schematic diagram of drug distribution. (Note at equilibrium the total concentrations in V_1 and V_2 may be different because of protein binding, etc.)

Table 2.10
The apparent volume of distribution (V) and plasma-protein binding of selected drugs

Drug	V (l kg⁻¹)	Binding (%)
Warfarin and furosemide (frusemide)	0.1	99
Aspirin	0.2	49
Gentamycin	0.3	<10
Propranolol	3.9	93
Nortriptyline	18.5	95
Chloroquine	185.7	61

Note: V is given in l/kg body weight; therefore, for chloroquine, the total volume of distribution will be 13 000 l per 70 kg patient.

The value of V is usually calculated using the total concentration in plasma, that is free (unbound) drug plus protein-bound drug. A low value for V can result if a drug is highly bound to plasma proteins but not to tissue proteins; if the drug shows an even higher affinity for tissue (lipid or protein; see Fig. 2.3), then it will have a high value for V. The term V reflects the relative affinity of plasma and tissues for a drug, and there is no simple relationship between plasma protein binding and V (Table 2.10).

If the tissues have a very high affinity for the drug, the value of V will be extremely high and may greatly exceed the body weight. Chloroquine is a good example of such a drug (Table 2.10) and the value illustrates clearly that V should be regarded as a mathematical ratio (not as an indication of physiological distribution to an actual volume of plasma!).

The term V is one of two physiological factors that determine the elimination half-life, because it represents the volume of plasma that has to be cleared of drug by the organs of elimination. It is independent of dose or concentration. Although it may seem a rather abstract (and possibly even irrelevant) parameter, it is important for two reasons. Firstly, it is the parameter that relates the total body drug load present at any time to the plasma concentration. Secondly, together with clearance, it determines the overall elimination rate constant (k) and therefore the half-life (see above). The half-life determines the duration of action of a single dose, the time interval between doses on repeated dosage and the potential for accumulation (see below).

erable elimination, and so the total amount of drug in the body is no longer known. This can be overcome by using the elimination phase (B–C in Fig. 2.17b) to back-extrapolate to the intercept (point D), which is the concentration that would have been obtained if distribution into V_2 had been instantaneous (see Equation 2.10):

$$V = \frac{\text{Dose}}{\text{Concentration at point D}} \qquad (2.11)$$

Alternative equations for the calculation of V are presented below.

V is simply a reflection of the amount of drug remaining in the blood or plasma after distribution and provides no information on where the drug has been taken up. Thus a high value for V could result from either reversible accumulation in adipose tissue (owing to dissolution in fat) or reversible accumulation in liver and lung (owing to high intracellular protein binding). The actual tissue distribution can be determined only by measurement of tissue concentrations.

Elimination

Elimination can also be described in terms of both *rate* and *extent*. The rate at which the drug is eliminated is important, since it can determine the duration of response, the time interval between doses and the time to reach equilibrium during repeated dosage. The extent of elimination is eventually 100%; the *route* of elimination is important because it can determine the effects of renal/liver disease, age and drug interactions.

Rate of elimination

The rate of elimination is usually indicated by the terminal half-life, that is the half-life for the final (slowest) rate (k in Fig. 2.17a; β in Fig. 2.17b). The elimination half-lives of drugs range from a few minutes to many days (and in rare cases, weeks). Precise knowledge about the half-life of every drug is not necessary and, therefore, in this book we have used the descriptive terms given in Table 2.11 to indicate the approximate half-life and the influence this would have on clinical use of the drug.

The rate at which a drug can be eliminated from the body, and therefore the half-life, is determined by two independent, physiologically based variables: the activity of the mechanisms metabolising/excreting the drug and the extent of movement of drug from the blood into tissues.

The activity of the metabolising enzymes or excretory mechanisms. The organs of elimination (usually liver and kidneys) remove drug that is brought to them via the blood. Providing that first-order kinetics apply (that is the process is not saturated), a constant proportion of the drug carried in the blood will be removed on each passage through the organ of elimination, independent of the concentration in the blood. In effect, this is equivalent to a constant proportion of the blood flow to the organ being cleared of drug. The more active the process (e.g. hepatic metabolism) the greater will be the proportion of the blood flow cleared of drug. For example, if 10% of the drug carried to the liver by the plasma (at a flow rate of 800 ml min⁻¹) is cleared, by uptake and metabolism, this is equivalent to a clearance of 10% of the plasma flow (80 ml min⁻¹); if 20% of the drug is cleared, this gives a clearance of 160 ml min⁻¹. The proportion of the blood flow cleared of drug will have units of volume per time (e.g. ml min⁻¹). The *plasma clearance* (CL) of the drug is the sum of all clearance processes and is the volume of plasma cleared of drug per unit time; it is the best indication of the activity of the eliminating processes.

$$CL = \frac{\text{Rate of elimination from the body}}{\text{Plasma concentration}} \quad (2.12)$$

For example $\dfrac{\mu g\ min^{-1}}{\mu g\ ml^{-1}} = ml\ min^{-1}$

The plasma clearance is a characteristic value for a particular drug (see Table 2.12) and is a constant for first-order (non-saturated) reactions and independent of dose or concentration. Because clearance is constant (Equation 2.12), a two-fold increase in plasma concentration will be accompanied by a two-fold increase in the rate of elimination. The greater the value of plasma clearance, the greater will be the rate at which the drug will be removed from the body, i.e. the elimination rate constant (k) is proportional to plasma clearance.

Passage of drug from the blood into tissues. The organs of elimination can only act on drug that is delivered to them via the blood supply. If, after equilibration with tissues, the blood or plasma concentration is very low, then V is very high. The low plasma concentration will result in a low rate of elimination from the body; in other words, the rate at which the drug can be eliminated will be limited by the extent of tissue distribution (which is inversely proportional to the apparent volume of distribution)

$$k \propto \frac{1}{V} \quad (2.13)$$

Plasma clearance

The overall rate of elimination is dependent on the two variables, the volume of plasma cleared per minute (CL), and the total apparent volume of plasma that has to be cleared (V):

$$k = \frac{CL}{V} \quad (2.14)$$

or

$$t_{1/2} = \frac{0.693\,V}{CL} \qquad \text{since } t_{1/2} = \frac{0.693}{k}$$

This is illustrated in Figure 2.19 and Table 2.12. The elimination rate constant (or half-life) is the best indica-

Table 2.11
Half-life descriptions

Description	Half-life (h)	Doses per day for chronic treatment	Comment
Very short	<1	–	A modified-release formulation may be preferred
Short	1–6	3–4	A modified-release formulation may be preferred
Intermediate	6–12	1–2	
Long	12–24	1	Once daily dosage may be adequate
Very long	>24	1	Potential for accumulation

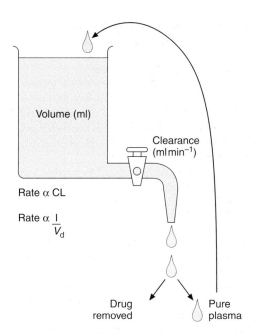

Fig. 2.19
The relationship between clearance, volume of distribution and overall elimination rate. The drug is eliminated by the clearance process, which removes a fixed volume of plasma per unit time. The drug is then separated and the pure plasma added back to the tank to maintain a constant volume (the apparent volume of distribution, V). The fluid, therefore, continuously recycles via the clearance process and the concentration of drug decreases exponentially. The time taken for one cycle is equal to the volume divided by the clearance (the greater the volume the greater the time needed, but the greater the clearance the shorter the time).

tion of changes in drug concentration with time, and for many drugs this will relate to changes in therapeutic activity following a *single dose*. Clearance is the best measurement of the ability of the organs of elimination to remove the drug and determines the average plasma

concentrations (and therefore therapeutic activity) at *steady state* (see below). Clearance is usually determined using a model-independent method, which uses the area under the concentration–time curve (AUC).

The rate of elimination from the body (dA_b/dt) is equivalent to the rate of change of the amount in the body (A_b) with time, that is:

$$CL = \frac{dA_b/dt}{C} \tag{2.15}$$

where C is plasma concentration. By rearranging

$$CL \times C = \frac{dA_b}{dt}$$

and

$$CL \times C dt = dA_b$$

If the equation is integrated between $t = 0$ and $t = \infty$, then the change in body load to infinity (dA_b) will equal the dose given:

$$CL \times C dt = \text{Dose} \tag{2.16}$$

The integral between $t = 0$ and $t = \infty$ of $C dt$ is the AUC to infinity:

$$CL \times \text{AUC} = \text{Dose} \tag{2.17}$$

or

$$CL = \frac{\text{Dose}}{\text{AUC}}$$

This simple equation is used to calculate clearance (one of the most important pharmacokinetic parameters) under the following conditions:

Table 2.12
Pharmacokinetic parameters of selected drugs

	Clearance (ml min⁻¹)	Apparent volume of distribution (l per 70 kg)	Half-life (h)
Warfarin	3	8	37
Digitoxin	4	38	161
Diazepam	27	77	43
Valproic acid	76	27	5.6
Digoxin	130	640	39
Ampicillin	270	20	1.3
Amlodipine	333	1470	36
Nifedipine	500	80	1.8
Lidocaine	640	77	1.8
Propranolol	840	270	3.9
Imipramine	1050	1600	18

Note: The drugs are arranged in order of increasing plasma clearance. A long half-life may result from a low clearance (e.g. digitoxin), a high apparent volume of distribution (e.g. imipramine) or both

1. The dose must be given intravenously so that it is all available to the organs of elimination (i.e. $CL = Dose/AUC_{iv}$). For the oral route, only a fraction (F; see above) may reach the general circulation and therefore the dose used in the calculation should be the corrected dose (the administered dose $\times F$, as applied in Equation 2.8).
2. The AUC should be the area under the concentration–time curve not the logarithm of the concentration–time curve.
3. The AUC should be extrapolated to infinity.

Equation 2.17 can be used to calculate V and is more reliable than the extrapolation method given in Figure 2.17b:

$$CL = \frac{Dose}{AUC} = kV$$

$$V = \frac{Dose}{AUC \times k} \quad \text{or} \quad \frac{Dose}{AUC \times \beta} \qquad (2.18)$$

The plasma clearance, as defined above, is the sum of all clearance processes, for example metabolic, renal, biliary, airways, etc. and is the best measure of the functional status of the total elimination processes. Measurement of specific processes such as metabolic clearance or renal clearance would require specific measurement of the rate of elimination by that process. In practice this is only really possible for *renal clearance* (CL_r).

Renal clearance can be calculated from the rate of excretion in urine (*as the parent drug*) during a urine collection and the mid-point plasma concentration:

$$CL_r = \frac{\text{Rate of excretion in urine (as the parent drug)}}{\text{Plasma concentration (mid-point)}} \qquad (2.19)$$

$$\frac{\mu g\ min^{-1}}{\mu g\ ml^{-1}} = ml\ min^{-1}$$

Alternatively, CL_r can be measured from the amount of parent drug excreted in urine over a known time interval (for example 48 h), divided by the AUC for the same time interval:

$$CL_r = \frac{\text{Total amount of parent drug in urine}_{(0-t)}}{AUC_{(0-t)}} \qquad (2.20)$$

Measurement of renal clearance can be useful in a number of ways:

- comparison of renal with plasma clearance will show the importance of the kidney in the overall elimination of the compound. This can be of value in predicting the potential impact of renal disease

- the difference between plasma and renal clearance is equivalent to **metabolic clearance** (for most drugs), and this can be of value in predicting the potential impact of liver disease
- comparison of renal clearance with the glomerular filtration rate (GFR), after allowance for protein binding, allows an estimate of the extent of either reabsorption (if clearance is less than filtration) or active secretion (if clearance is greater than filtration rate)
- renal clearance can be changed by altering kidney function, for example by changing the urine pH (see Ch. 53).

Biliary clearance of a drug can be measured using the above approach, but in practice is seldom done because of the difficulty of collecting bile samples.

Extent of elimination

The extent of elimination is of limited value since eventually all the drug will be removed from the body. Measurement of total elimination in urine, faeces and expired air as parent drug and metabolites can give useful insights into the extent of absorption, metabolism and renal and biliary elimination.

Chronic administration

Long-term or chronic drug therapy is designed to maintain a constant concentration of the drug in blood, with an equilibrium (steady state) established between blood and all tissues of the body, including the site of action. In practice a constant concentration can only be achieved by an intravenous infusion that has continued long enough to reach steady state (Fig. 2.20).

Time to reach steady state

During constant infusion, the time to reach steady state is dependent on the elimination half-life, and steady state is approached after four or five half-lives. Intuitively it may seem peculiar that the elimination half-life determines the time required to reach equilibrium during constant input. The relationship is more readily understood if plasma concentrations following both increases and decreases in dose rate are considered (Table 2.13). The plasma concentration at steady state (C_{ss}), is directly proportional to the infusion rate; plasma concentrations reach 95% of the new steady-state conditions by four or five half-lives after a change in infusion rate.

Since the elimination half-life is dependent on both clearance and V, each of these can contribute to the delay in achieving steady state. A drug with a large V

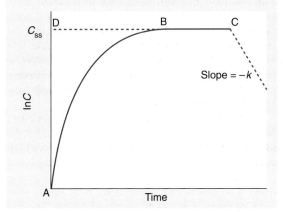

Fig. 2.20
Constant intravenous infusion (between points A and C). Steady state is reached at point B and the steady-state concentration (C_{ss}; given by D) can be used to calculate clearance: CL = rate of infusion/C_{ss} (see text). Clearance can also be calculated from the area under the total curve (AUC) and the total dose infused between A and C. The slope on cessation of infusion is the terminal elimination phase (k or β). The distribution phase is not usually detected because distribution is occurring throughout the period A to C. The apparent volume of distribution can be calculated as: V = Dose/(AUC × k). The *increase* to steady state is determined by the *elimination* rate constant and it takes approximately four to five half-lives to reach steady state.

will have a long half-life and, therefore, it will take a longer time to reach steady state. It is easy to envisage the slow filling of such a high volume of distribution during regular administration.

Plasma concentration at steady state

Once steady state has been reached, the plasma and tissues are in equilibrium, and the distribution rate con-

stant and V will not affect the plasma concentration. The value of C_{ss} is determined solely by the balance between the rate of infusion and the rate of elimination (or clearance):

$$C_{ss} = \frac{\text{Rate of infusion}}{\text{CL}} \qquad (2.21)$$

This relationship for an intravenous infusion can be used to calculate plasma clearance. At steady state, the rate of infusion is exactly balanced by the rate of elimination from the body. From Equation 2.12, the rate of elimination will be given by CL × C_{ss} and, consequently;

$$\text{CL} = \frac{\text{Rate of infusion}}{C_{ss}} \qquad (2.22)$$

Clearance and volume of distribution can also be calculated using the AUC between zero and infinity and the terminal slope after cessation of the infusion (see Fig. 2.20).

Oral administration

Most chronic administration is via the oral route, and the rate and extent of absorption need to be considered. Also oral therapy is by intermittent doses and therefore there will be a series of peaks and troughs between doses (Fig. 2.21).

The *rate of absorption* will influence the interdose profile since very rapid absorption will exaggerate fluctuations, while slow absorption will dampen down the peak.

The *extent of absorption*, or bioavailability (F), will influence the average steady-state concentration

Table 2.13
Plasma concentrations following a change in dosage[a]

	Drug concentration in plasma (ng ml⁻¹) after a change in dose rate (mg h⁻¹)					Percentage change A–E
	A	B	C	D	E	
	(1 to 0)	(1 to 0.5)	(1 to 2)	(0 to 1)	(0 to 2)	
Initial concentration	100	100	100	0	0	0
After 1 half-life	50	75	150	50	100	50
After 2 half-lives	25	62.5	175	75	150	75
After 3 half-lives	12.5	56.25	187.5	87.5	175	87.5
After 4 half-lives	6.25	53.125	193.75	93.75	187.5	93.75
After 5 half-lives	3.125	51.5625	196.875	96.875	193.75	96.875
At infinity	0	50	200	100	200	100.0

[a]Theoretical changes in plasma concentrations of a drug that has been given by continuous intravenous infusion.
Notes:
The steady-state concentrations (initial and infinity) are directly proportional to the infusion rate.
The percentage changes (from initial conditions to infinity) are identical and independent of the rate of infusion
After four or five half-lives, the change in concentration represents about 95% of the overall change to infinity (the new steady state).
Clearance = *rate of infusion*/C_{ss} = 1 000 000 ng h⁻¹/100 ng ml⁻¹ = 10 000 ml h⁻¹ = 167 ml min⁻¹.

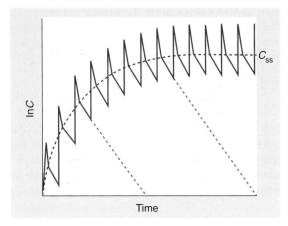

Fig. 2.21
Chronic oral therapy (———) compared with intravenous (- - - - -) infusion at the same dosage rate. The oral dose shows very rapid absorption and distribution followed by a more slow elimination phase within each dose interval. Cessation of therapy after any dose would produce the line shown in blue.

because it determines the dose entering the circulation. The rate of input during chronic oral therapy is given by:

$$\frac{D \times F}{t} \tag{2.23}$$

where D is administered dose, F is bioavailability and t is interval between doses. At steady state, the rate of input is balanced by the rate of elimination, that is:

$$\frac{D \times F}{t} = CL \times C_{ss} \tag{2.24}$$

Therefore:

$$C_{ss} = \frac{D \times F}{t \times CL} \tag{2.25}$$

The balance between input and output is in reality a balance between the doctor and the patient:

- the input of drug is determined by the doctor, who can change C_{ss} by altering either the dose or the dose interval (and sometimes the bioavailability of the drug formulation)
- the removal of drug is determined by patient characteristics: metabolism/renal function can change C_{ss} by altering bioavailability and/or clearance.

Loading dose

A therapeutic problem may arise when a rapid effect is required for a drug that has a long or very long half-life; for example, the steady-state conditions will not be reached until 2–4 days if the half-life is 12–24 h, or over

4 or 5 days if the half-life is over 24 h (Table 2.13). Increasing the dose rate (for example column E compared with column D in Table 2.13) does not reduce the time to reach steady state. A higher dose rate will reduce the time taken to reach any particular concentration, but plasma concentrations will continue to increase to give a higher steady-state level (after the same time interval of about four or five half-lives).

Any delay between the initiation of treatment and the attainment of steady state may be avoided by the administration of a *loading dose*. A loading dose is a high initial or first dose that, as the name implies, is designed to 'load up' the body. In principle, this is done by giving a first dose that is equivalent to the total steady-state body load which would be produced by the intended chronic dosage regimen. This will avoid the slow build up to steady state, and the steady-state body load can then be maintained by giving the dosage regimen that would eventually have resulted in the same steady-state concentration.

$$\text{Loading dose} = C_{ss} \times V \tag{2.26}$$

The amount of drug equivalent to the steady-state body load is the target C_{ss} multiplied by V. In cases where C_{ss} or V are not known, the loading dose can be calculated based on the proposed maintenance regimen by replacing C_{ss} with Equation 2.26 and V by CL/k (Equation 2.14):

$$
\begin{aligned}
\text{Loading dose} &= \frac{D \times F}{t \times CL} \times \frac{CL}{k} \\[2mm]
&= \frac{D \times F}{t \times k} \\[2mm]
&= \frac{D \times F \times 1.44 \times t_{1/2}}{t}
\end{aligned}
\tag{2.27}
$$

It is clear from this last equation that the magnitude of any loading dose compared with the maintenance dose is proportional to the half-life.

Good examples of drugs that may require a loading dose are the cardiac glycosides digoxin and digitoxin, which are compared in Table 2.14. The values given in Table 2.14 are to illustrate the concept of a loading dose: the doses used clinically should take into account body weight, age and the presence of severe renal or liver impairment.

Loading doses may need to be given in two or three fractions over a period of about 24–36 h. The reason is that during distribution of the loading dose, there are higher (non-steady-state) concentrations in the blood and rapidly equilibrating tissues and lower (non-steady-state) concentrations in the slowly equilibrating tissues (see Fig. 2.6). The excessive concentrations in rapidly equilibrating tissues may give rise to toxicity. This can be min-

Table 2.14
Pharmacokinetics and dosage for digoxin and digitoxin

	Digoxin	Digitoxin
Elimination half-life (days)	1.6	7
Time to steady state (days; $4 \times t_{1/2}$)	6	28
'Therapeutic' plasma concentrations (ng ml^{-1} or μg l^{-1})	0.5–2.0	10–35
Volume of distribution (l/70 kg)	600	40
Typical loading dose ($C_{ss} \times V$) (mg)	up to 1.2	up to 1.4
Bioavailability (F)	0.75	>0.9
Normal oral maintenance dose (Dose $\times F/t$; mg per day)	0.125–0.5	0.05–0.2
Typical loading dose (maintenance dose $\times 1.44 \times t_{1/2}$) (mg)	0.3–1.2	0.5–2.0

imised by giving the loading dose in fractions, which would allow distribution of one fraction before the next was given. The fractional loading doses should be given within the period of the normal dose interval.

Factors affecting pharmacokinetics

A number of factors can affect the physiological processes of absorption, distribution and elimination.

Aspects such as pregnancy, age and diseases of the organs of elimination are discussed in Chapter 56. Clinically important variability arises from differences in bioavailability, V and clearance:

- **drug interactions**: see Chapter 56, and the induction and inhibition of P450 discussed above
- **age**: see Chapter 56
- **diseases**, especially of the liver and kidneys: see Chapter 56.
- **environmental factors**, for example alcohol and smoking.
- **genetics**: see factors affecting drug metabolism (above).

FURTHER READING

Cholerton S, Daly AK, Idle JR (1992) The role of individual human cytochromes P450 in drug metabolism and clinical response. *Trends Pharmacol Sci*, **13**, 434–439.

Gonzalez TJ (1992) Human cytochromes P450: problems and prospects. *Trends Pharmacol Sci* **13**, 346–352

Self-assessment

1. The following statements describe drug pharmacokinetics. Are they true or false?

   a. The plasma clearance of a drug usually decreases with increase in the dose prescribed.

   b. First-pass metabolism may limit the bioavailability of orally administered drugs.

   c. Drugs that show high first-pass metabolism in the liver also have a high systemic clearance.

   d. The half-life of many drugs is longer in infants than in children or adults.

   e. A decrease in renal function may affect both systemic clearance and oral bioavailability.

   f. Benzathine benzylpenicillin has a prolonged half-life because the renal extraction of penicillin is reduced.

   g. Nifedipine is eliminated more rapidly in cigarette smokers.

   h. Chronic treatment with phenobarbital can increase the systemic clearance and oral bioavailability of co-administered drugs.

   i. A loading dose is not necessary for drugs that have short half-lives.

   j. An obese patient is likely to show an increased volume of distribution and decreased clearance of prescribed drugs.

   k. Drugs are always taken with meals in order to reduce side effects.

2. Figure 2.22 shows the changes in plasma levels of two drugs, A and B, given as 10 mg doses by oral and intravenous routes. From the plasma concentration–time curves compare the two drugs for the following properties (do not perform detailed calculations):

   a. Absorption from the gut

   b. Oral bioavailability

   c. Distribution to tissues

   d. Elimination half-life

   e. Extent of accumulation during daily administration of each drug

3. The pharmacokinetics of three drugs, A, B and C, were studied in the blood and urine of a healthy adult male volunteer (70 kg) following both oral and intravenous administration of 20 mg doses (Table 2.15). From the data given compare:

   a. The extent of absorption (bioavailability, F) (you cannot calculate the rate of absorption from these data)

   b. The apparent volume of distribution (V) (you cannot calculate the rate of distribution from these data)

   c. The elimination of these drugs (half-life, $t_{1/2}$) and clearance (CL, and route)

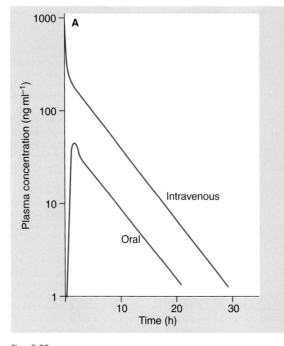

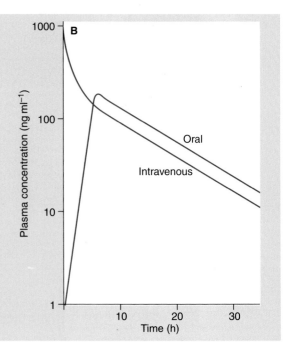

Fig. 2.22
Plasma concentration–time curves for two drugs.

Table 2.15
Data for question 3

Parameter	A		B		C	
	Intravenous	Oral	Intravenous	Oral	Intravenous	Oral
AUC (μg ml^{-1} min)	16	2	1000	995	40	26
Terminal slope (min^{-1})	0.0063	0.0063	0.00022	0.00022	0.014	0.003
Percentage of dose in urine (unchanged)	0		5		98	
Percentage of dose in urine as metabolites	100		95		0	

AUC, total area under the plasma concentration–time curve.

d. Their potential for accumulation during chronic dosage (related to half-life and interval between doses)

e. Discuss genetic and environmental factors that may affect the disposition of these drugs (A, B, C,) in patients

The answers are provided on pages 597–600.

3

Drug discovery, evaluation and safety

> One of the features which is thought to distinguish man from other animals is his desire to take medicines
>
> (Sir William Osler, 1849–1919)

Initially, most medicines were of botanical or zoological origin; however, since the 1950s, there has been an enormous increase in the use of synthetic organic chemicals. The recent introduction of molecules produced by recombinant DNA technology has extended this to agents identical to those of human origin: examples include epoetin (recombinant erythropoietin) and human insulins. The major benefit of drugs for the treatment of disease is illustrated most dramatically with antimicrobial chemotherapy. Antimicrobial chemotherapy has revolutionised the chances of patients surviving severe infections such as lobar pneumonia, the mortality of which was 27% in the pre-antibiotic era but fell to 8% (and subsequently less) following the introduction of sulfonamides and, later, penicillins.

Early agents were often naturally occurring inorganic salts such as mercury compounds or plant extracts containing one or more complex organic compounds. The active component of many plant-derived preparations was a nitrogen-containing organic molecule or alkaloid; laudanum, for example, is an alcohol extract of opium which contains high concentrations of the alkaloid morphine. Early therapeutic successes included the use of foxgloves (which contain cardiac glycosides) for the treatment of 'dropsy' (fluid retention); however, there was also considerable toxicity since the plant preparations contained variable amounts of the active glycoside and such compounds have a narrow therapeutic index.

A major advance in the safe use of naturally derived agents was the isolation, purification and chemical characterisation of the active component. This had three main advantages:

1. The administration of controlled amounts of the active agent removed any biological variability in potency of the plant preparation, for example due to climatic or soil conditions when the plant grew.
2. The active component with the desired effect could be prescribed without having to give a cocktail of other unnecessary natural components. Other components may have interfered with therapy by producing unrelated and unwanted effects or possibly reduced the desired effect by blocking the mechanism of action.

47

3. The identification and isolation of the active component allowed the mechanism of action to be defined leading to the synthesis and development of improved agents with the same action but with greater potency, greater selectivity, fewer side-effects, altered duration of action, greater absorption, etc.

Thus, although drug therapy has natural and humble origins, it is the application of scientific principles which has given rise to the clinical safety and efficacy of modern medicines. The aim of this book is to give the principles of clinical pharmacology and to show their relationship to the clinical use of modern therapeutic drugs.

A major advantage of modern drugs is their ability to act selectively, that is, to affect only certain specific body systems or processes. For example, a drug which lowered blood glucose but also reduced blood pressure would not be suitable for the treatment of patients with diabetes or patients with hypertension or even patients with both conditions (because different doses may be needed for each effect).

Drug discovery

The discovery of a new drug can be achieved in several different ways (Fig. 3.1). The simplest and crudest method is to subject new chemical entities to a battery of screening tests that are designed to detect particular types of biological activity. These include studies of animal behaviour, as well as work on isolated tissues. Chemicals for screening may be produced by direct chemical synthesis or may be isolated from biological sources, such as plants, and then purified and characterised. In general, this is not an efficient type of research since several thousand chemicals may need to be screened to identify a compound that eventually can be marketed as a medicine.

A second approach involves the synthesis and testing of chemical analogues of existing medicines, but the products of this research usually show only minor

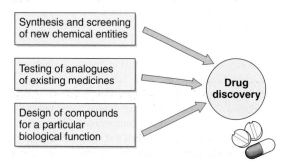

Fig. 3.1
Approaches to drug discovery.

advances in absorption, potency or a more selective action. However, unexpected additional properties may become evident when the compound is tried in humans; for example, minor modifications of the sulfanilamide antibiotic molecule gave rise to the thiazide diuretics and the sulfonylurea type of oral hypoglycaemics.

More recently, attempts have been made to design substances to fulfil a particular biological role, which may entail the synthesis of a naturally occurring substance (or a structural analogue), its precursor or an antagonist. Good examples include levodopa, used in the treatment of Parkinson's disease, the histamine H_2 receptor antagonists, and omeprazole, the first proton pump inhibitor. Logical drug development of this type depends, however, on a detailed understanding of human physiology both in health and disease. Most recently, the modelling of receptor-binding sites has facilitated the development of ligands with high binding affinities and often high selectivity.

Drug approval

Each year, a vast number of synthetic novel compounds (new chemical entities) and pure compounds isolated from plant sources are screened for useful and/or novel pharmacological activities. Potentially valuable compounds are then subjected to a sequence of in vitro and in vivo animal studies and clinical trials, which provide essential information on safety and therapeutic benefit (Fig. 3.2).

All drugs and formulations licensed for sale in the UK have to pass a rigorous evaluation of three principal aspects:

● safety
● quality
● efficacy.

The UK Committee on Safety of Medicines (CSM) is one of a number of committees established under the Medicines Act (1968) to advise the Secretary of State for Health *via* the Medicines Control Agency on the quality, safety and efficacy of all products licensed for medicinal use in the UK.

Harmonisation of drug regulation in the European Union has resulted in the establishment of a central organisation, in addition to national bodies. The European Agency for the Evaluation of Medicinal Products (EMEA) is responsible for medicines in the European Union and receives advice from the Committee on Proprietary Medical Products (CPMP), which is a body of international experts equivalent to the CSM. Under the current systems, new drugs are evaluated by the CPMP, and national advisory bodies, such as the CSM, have an opportunity to assess the data before a final CPMP conclusion is reached.

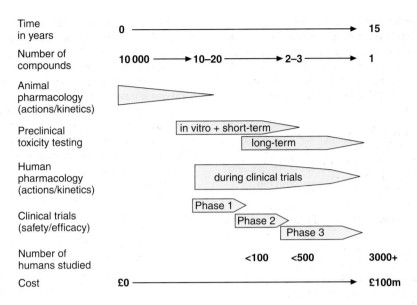

Fig. 3.2
The development of a new drug to the point at which a licence is approved. Postmarketing surveillance will continue to add data on safety and efficacy.

Safety

Historically, the introduction of new drugs has been bought at a price of significant toxicity, and regulatory systems have arisen as much to protect patients from toxicity, as to ensure benefit. The establishment of the Food and Drugs Administration (FDA) in the USA followed a dramatic incident in 1937 when 76 people died of renal failure after taking an elixir of sulfanilamide, which contained the solvent diethylene glycol. Similarly, some 30 years later, the occurrence of limb malformations (phocomelia) and cardiac defects in infants born to mothers who had taken thalidomide for the treatment of nausea in the first trimester of pregnancy led to the establishment of the precursor of the UK CSM.

Today, major tragedies are avoided by a combination of animal toxicity tests and careful observation during clinical studies on new drugs (see below). The development and continuing refinement of preclinical animal toxicity testing has increased the likelihood of identifying chemicals with direct organ toxicity. Such adverse actions can be revealed by clinical studies, which may also be able to detect immunologically mediated effects (see Ch. 53).

Quality

An important function of regulatory bodies is to ensure the consistency of prescribed medicines. Drugs have to comply with defined criteria for purity, and limits are set on the content of any potentially toxic impurities. The stability, and if necessary sterility, of the drug also has to be established. Similarly, licensed formulations have to contain a defined, and approved, amount of the active drug, which has to be released at a specified rate. There have been a number of cases in the past where a simple change to the manufactured formulation has affected tablet disintegration, the release of drug and the therapeutic response. The quality of drugs for human use is defined by the specifications in the British Pharmacopoeia and European Pharmacopoeia.

Efficacy

All medicines, apart from homeopathic products, must have evidence of efficacy for their licensed indications. Efficacy can be established only by trials in the patients for whom the medicine is intended, and therefore the demonstration of efficacy is a major aim of the later phases of clinical research (Fig. 3.2). A recently completed, systematic review of all 39 000 products that were licensed for use in the UK resulted in the withdrawal of thousands of products, many because of doubtful efficacy.

Establishing safety and efficacy

Regulatory bodies, such as the CSM and CPMP, require supporting data from animal studies and clinical investigations before a new drug is approved. Although there is some overlap, the aims and goals are:

preclinical studies: to establish the basic pharmacology, pharmacokinetics and toxicological profile of the drug, using animals and in vitro systems

phase I clinical studies: to establish the human pharmacology and pharmacokinetics, together with a simple safety profile

phase II clinical studies: to establish the dose reponse and develop the dosage protocol for clinical use, together with more extensive safety data

phase III clinical studies: to establish the efficacy and safety profile of the drug in patients with the proposed indications

pharmacovigilance: to monitor adverse events following approval and the more widespread use of the drug.

Preclinical studies

Preclinical studies must be carried out before a compound can be given to humans. These studies investigate three areas:

pharmacological effects: in vitro effects using isolated cells/organs; receptor-binding characteristics; in vivo effects in animals and/or animal models of human diseases; prediction of potential therapeutic use

pharmacokinetics: identification of metabolites (since these may be the active form of the compound); evidence of bioavailability (to assist with the design of both clinical trials and in vivo animal toxicity studies); establishment of principal route and rate of elimination

toxicological effects: a battery of in vitro and in vivo studies undertaken with the aim of identifying toxic compounds as early as possible, and before there is extensive in vivo exposure of animals or, subsequently, of humans.

Toxicity testing

Toxicity testing has two primary goals: recognition of hazards and prediction of the likely risk of that hazard occurring in humans receiving therapeutic doses. A wide range of doses is studied, since high doses are required to increase the ability to detect hazards and lower doses are needed to predict the risk at the anticipated therapeutic doses for humans. Toxicity tests include:

- **Mutagenicity**: A variety of in vitro tests using bacteria and mammalian cell lines are employed at an early stage to define any potential effect on DNA that may be linked to carcinogenicity or teratogenicity.

- **Acute toxicity**: A single dose is given by the route proposed for human use; this may reveal a likely site for toxicity and is essential in defining the initial dose for human studies. Acute toxicity data are essential for safe manufacture; the LD_{50} (a precise estimate of the dose required to kill 50% of an animal population) has been replaced by simpler and more humane methods, which define the dose range associated with acute toxicity.

- **Subacute toxicity**: Repeated doses are given for 14 or 28 days; this will usually reveal the target for toxic effects, and comparison with single-dose data may indicate any potential for accumulation.

- **Chronic toxicity**: Repeated doses are given for up to 6 months; this reveals the target for toxicity (except cancer). The aim is to define dose regimens associated with adverse effects and a no-observed adverse effect level ('safe' dose).

- **Carcinogenicity**: Repeated doses are given throughout the lifetime of the animal (usually 2 years in a rodent bioassay).

- **Reproductive toxicity**: Repeated doses are given from prior to mating and throughout gestation to assess any effect on fertility, implantation, fetal growth, the production of fetal abnormalities (teratogenicity) and neonatal growth.

The extent of animal toxicity testing considered necessary prior to the first administration to humans is related to the proposed duration of human exposure, and the population to be treated. All drugs are subjected to an initial in vitro screen for mutagenic potential: if satisfactory this is followed by acute and subacute studies for up to 14 days of administration to two animal species.

Currently, there is an international review of the extent of in vivo animal testing necessary prior to clinical trials. It has been proposed that the duration of animal toxicity tests should be the same as the proposed human exposure, i.e. a 3-month toxicity study in animals prior to a 3-month study in humans. The recently proposed European Union guidelines require a more prolonged duration of in vivo animal studies than the intended human exposure (Table 3.1).

Teratogenicity and reproductive toxicity studies are required if the drug is to be given to women of child-bearing age. Carcinogenicity testing is necessary for

Table 3.1

European Union guidelines for the length of animal toxicity studies prior to studies in humans

Intended human exposure (days)	Duration of animal study (days)
1	14
2–10	28
10–30	90
>30	180

drugs that may be used for long periods, for example over 1 year.

The use of animals for the establishment of chemical safety is an emotive issue, and there is extensive current research to replace in vivo animal studies with in vitro tests based on known mechanisms of toxicity. Despite these advances, toxicology as a predictive science is still in its infancy, and at present it is impossible to replicate the complexity of mammalian physiology and biochemistry by in vitro systems. In vivo studies remain essential to investigate both interference with integrative functions and complex homeostatic mechanisms. Carefully controlled safety studies in animals are an essential part of the current procedures adopted to prevent extensive human toxicity, which would inevitably result from the use of untested compounds. Although toxicology has failed in the past to prevent some tragedies (see above), these have led to improvements in methods; for example rabbits, which are sensitive to thalidomide, are now used as the second species for teratology studies.

Although toxicity studies are not infallible, they have provided an effective predictive screen. It is worth noting that, in recent years, the few cases where drugs have been withdrawn after initial approval have mostly been because of rare, idiosyncratic reactions, which may have an immunological mechanism (see Ch. 53) and which are not detected adequately in preclinical studies.

Students should be aware that not all hazards detected at very high doses in experimental animals are of relevance to human health. An important function of expert advisory bodies such as the CSM (and other advisory bodies for food additives, environmental chemicals, pesticides, etc.) is to assess the relevance to human health of effects detected in experimental animals at doses that may be two orders of magnitude (or more) above human exposures. Many 'chemical scare' stories in the media are based on a hazard detected at high experimental doses in animals rather than the relevant risk estimated for human exposures.

Premarketing clinical studies: phases I–III

The purposes of premarketing clinical studies are:

- to establish that the drug has a useful action in humans
- to define any toxicity at therapeutic doses in humans
- to establish the nature of common (type A) unwanted effects (see Ch. 53).

Traditionally, premarketing clinical studies have been subdivided into three phases, but the distinction between these is blurred and there are differences of opinion about the classification system that follows.

Phase I studies

Phase I is the term used to describe the first few administrations of a new drug to humans. A principal aim of these studies is to define basic properties, such as route of administration, pharmacokinetics and metabolism and tolerability. The studies may be carried out either by pharmaceutical companies or units associated with major hospitals. Subjects taking part in phase I studies are often healthy volunteers recruited by open advertisement, especially when the compound is of low toxicity and has wide potential use, for example an antihistamine. In some cases, patients suffering from the condition in which the drug will be used may be studied, for example cytotoxic agents used for cancer chemotherapy.

The first few administrations are usually by mouth in a dose that (after scaling for body weight) may be as low as one-fiftieth of the minimum required to produce a pharmacological effect in animals. Depending upon what is found, the dose may be then built up either in small increments or by doubling until a pharmacological effect is observed or an unwanted action occurs. During these studies, toxic effects are looked for by means of routine haematology and biochemical investigations of liver and renal function; other tests including an electrocardiogram will be performed as appropriate. It is also usual to study the disposition, metabolism and main pathways of elimination of the new drug at this stage. Such studies help to identify not only the most suitable dose and route of administration for future clinical studies but also the choice of appropriate animal species for further toxicity studies. Investigations of drug metabolism and pharmacokinetics often necessitate the use of isotopically labelled beta-emitting compounds containing carbon-14 or tritium (^{3}H).

Phase II studies

During phase II studies, the detailed clinical pharmacology of the new compound is determined by skilled investigators in patients with the intended clinical condition. A principal aim of these studies is to define the relationship between dose and pharmacological and/or therapeutic response in humans. During phase II studies, some evidence of a beneficial effect may emerge. However, the large subjective element in human illness may make it difficult to distinguish between pharmacological and placebo effects. Additional studies may be undertaken at this stage in special groups: for example elderly people if it is intended that the drug will be used in that population. Other studies may include investigation of the mechanism of action and tests for potential interactions with other drugs. The optimum dosage regimen should be defined in the phase II studies, and this is then used in large clinical trials, which aim to demonstrate the efficacy and safety of the drug.

Phase III studies

The phase III studies are the main clinical trials and usually involve comparison with a placebo that looks (and tastes) similar to the active compound. Additionally, it is normal to establish the advantages and disadvantages of the new compound by comparison with the best available treatment or the leading drug in the class. For example, new antihypertensive drugs might be compared with a diuretic, a β-adrenoceptor antagonist, a calcium channel antagonist or an angiotensin-converting enzyme (ACE) inhibitor. In these trials, the drug under evaluation may be used alone or given with other established treatment for the disease being treated. In some circumstances, (e.g. cancer chemotherapy), the new agent or placebo is added to the best available current treatment.

Clinical trials are of two main types (Fig. 3.3): within patient and between patient comparisons. In within-patient trials, a patient is randomly allocated to commence treatment with either the new compound or its comparator before 'crossing-over' to the alternative therapy. By contrast, between-patient comparisons involve randomization to receive one or other of two (or more) treatments.

Within-patient comparisons can usually be performed on a smaller number of patients (about half that required for between-patient studies), since the patient acts as his or her own control and most other variables are, therefore, eliminated. However, such studies often take longer for the individual patient and there may be carry-over effects from one treatment that affect the apparent efficacy of the alternative therapy. Studies of this type may be difficult to interpret when there is a pronounced seasonal variation in the severity of a condition, such as Raynaud's phenomenon or hay fever. Cross-over studies (Fig. 3.3) cannot be used if the treatment is curative, for example an antibiotic for treating acute infections.

Between-patient comparisons require roughly twice as many participants but have the advantages that each

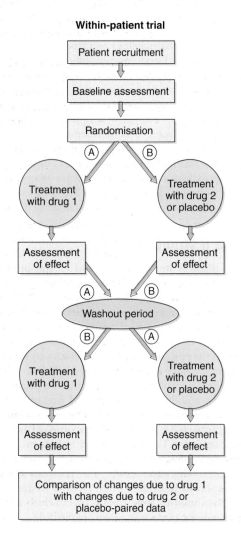

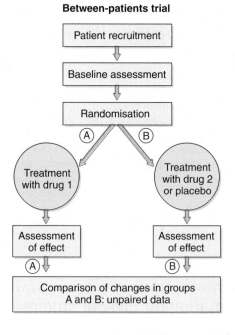

Fig. 3.3
The design of clinical trials. Subjects are randomly allocated to group A or group B.

Table 3.2
Examples of response measurements during clinical trials

New drug type	Measurement techniques	
	Objective	Subjective[a]
Anti-anginal	Exercise tolerance	Fatigue
	Blood pressure	Frequency of anginal
	Heart rate	attacks
	GTN use	Pain intensity
Anti-arthritic	Grip strength	Duration of morning
	Joint size	stiffness
	Paracetamol use	Pain intensity

[a]Subjective effects are often quantified by the use of a 10 cm visual analogue scale, e.g. 0 cm = no pain at all; 10 cm = the worst pain I have ever had.

patient will usually be studied for shorter periods of time and carry-over effects are avoided. Although it is not possible to provide a perfect match between patients entering the two or more different treatment groups, this approach to the evaluation of new drugs is preferred by many drug regulatory authorities.

Whichever form of comparison is made, measurements of benefit (and adverse effects) are made at regular intervals using a combination of objective and subjective techniques (Table 3.2). Throughout these studies, careful attention is paid to the detection and reporting of both unwanted effects (type A reactions) and other unpredictable type B reactions (Ch. 53). However, the majority of the latter are not seen prior to the marketing of a new drug because they may occur only once in every 1000–10 000 or more patients treated with the drug. It is salutory to note that, by the time that a new medicine is marketed, only 2000–3000 people may have taken the drug, usually for short periods. Only a few hundred people may have 6 months or more of exposure to the new compound and the total experience may amount to no more than 500 patient-years (1000 patients taking the drug for 6 months is 500 patient-years).

Postmarketing surveillance: phase IV

Phase IV studies involve pharmacovigilance (postmarketing surveillance) and further studies of efficacy. The full spectrum of benefits and risks of medicines may not become clear until after marketing. Reasons for this include the low frequency of certain adverse drug reactions, and the tendency to avoid the inclusion of children, the elderly and women of child-bearing age in premarketing clinical studies. Another factor is the widespread use of other medicines in normal clinical practice, which could produce an unexpected interaction with the new drug.

Two main systems of pharmacovigilance, or postmarketing surveillance, are in use in the UK. The first and most important is known as the yellow card system; it depends upon doctors reporting suspected serious adverse reactions directly to the Medicines Control Agency using postage prepaid cards (available in the British National Formulary (BNF), GP prescribing pads and the Monthly Index of Medical Specialties (MIMS)). In some health regions (Mersey, West Midlands, Northern and Wales) yellow cards are sent initially to centres located in Liverpool, Birmingham, Newcastle-upon-Tyne and Cardiff. In addition to reporting suspected serious adverse effects of established drugs, doctors are asked to supply information about all unwanted effects of medicines that have been marketed recently. These products are identified by the use of inverted black triangles in the BNF, MIMS and drug data sheets. Each year, the Medicines Control Agency receives some 20 000 yellow cards/slips. In return for their efforts, doctors are supplied at regular intervals with an information circular about current drug-related problems.

The second form of pharmacovigilance involves systematic postmarketing surveillance of recently marketed medicines. This may be organized by the pharmaceutical company responsible for the manufacture of the new drug (companies also receive information via their representatives).

Prescription event monitoring (PEM) provides a method for the detailed further study of observations or possible associations provided by pharmacovigilance programmes. This involves the identification by the Prescription Pricing Authority of individual patients prescribed a drug of interest, and the subsequent distribution of 'green cards' to the patients' general practitioners with a request that they complete all details about the patient and events that occurred. The cards are then returned to the coordinating unit in Southampton, where the data are analysed. PEM has the advantage that it does not require doctors to make a value judgement concerning a link between the prescription of a drug and any medical event that occurs in the patient while receiving the drug. At first sight, a broken leg may be thought an unlikely drug side-effect, but it could be the result of drug-related hypotension, ataxia or metabolic bone disease. In a recent PEM study, broken limbs were found to be more common amongst patients receiving terodiline for urinary incontinence. Subsequent analysis has suggested that these fractures were linked to syncope associated with a rare form of drug-induced ventricular tachycardia known as torsade de pointes.

Finally, detailed monitoring of adverse reactions to drug therapy takes place in certain hospitals. These data contribute further to our overall knowledge. The future computerisation of medical records, including drug prescribing, offers the promise of more rapid identification of adverse events and a greater ability to investigate possible associations between prescription and adverse events.

4

The nervous system, neurotransmission and the peripheral autonomic nervous system

There are two principal, inter-related neuronal systems in the body:

- the central nervous system (CNS), which comprises the brain and spinal cord
- the peripheral nervous system, which connects the CNS to the organs of the body; it includes afferent nerves from the peripheral tissues to the CNS, efferent nerves from the CNS to voluntary muscles via the neuromuscular junction (see Ch. 27) and efferent nerves to involuntary muscles (the autonomic nervous system (ANS)).

The CNS, therefore, has an integrating role, receiving information via visceral afferents (from viscera, smooth muscle and cardiac muscle) and somatic afferents (from skeletal muscle joints and skin) and sending instructions via the autonomic efferents (to glands, smooth muscle and cardiac muscle) and motor efferents (to skeletal muscle) (Fig. 4.1).

The basic unit of the nervous system is the neuron, which usually consists of a cell body (or soma), an axon (which transmits the impulse to another nerve or an effector organ) and dendrites (which receive impulses from other nerves). Both axons and dendrites may show numerous branches. The interconnections between neurons are known as synapses.

The human brain contains approximately 10^{-12} neurons, each of which may connect via synapses with hundreds or even thousands of other neurons. The neurons and interconnections may occur in well-defined

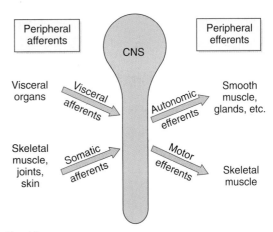

Fig. 4.1
The major neuronal connections of the central nervous system (CNS).

areas or tracts and control specific functions or activities, but some areas of the brain represent a more diffuse network, for example the cerebral cortex. In the peripheral nervous system, the axons tend to be longer and less branched.

There are three main types of neuron–neuron synapse (Fig. 4.2):

- axo-dendritic: the axon of the transmitting (innervating) cell forms a synaptic knob with the dendrite of the receiving (innervated) cell; this type accounts for 98% of synapses in the cortex
- axo-somatic: the axon of the innervating cell makes a synapse on the cell body of the innervated cell
- axo-axonal: the synapse with the axon of the innervating cell is on the axon of the innervated cell; this type usually serves to alter the local release of neurotransmitter from the receiving cell (for example see opioid analgesics, Ch. 19).

Synapses and interconnections are so numerous in the brain that about 50% of the total surface area of neuronal cells, and their processes, is covered by synapses. The CNS shows a far greater range of types of interneuronal junction compared with the peripheral nervous systems.

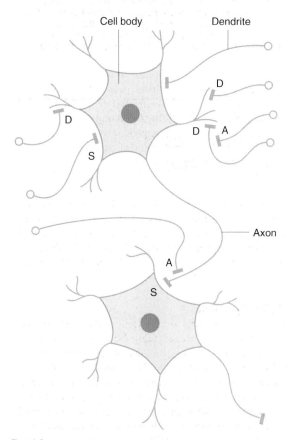

Fig. 4.2
Types of interneuronal synapses in the central nervous system.
D, axo-dendritic; S, axo-somatic; A, axo-axonal.

Neurotransmission

The synapse

The action potential in a nerve represents a wave of depolarisation in which the normally electronegative cytosol becomes positive owing to the opening of voltage-gated Na^+ channels and the influx of Na^+. This influx causes slight depolarisation further along the axon, and the adjacent Na^+ channels open causing full depolarisation, thereby propagating or conducting the action potential along the axon. The propagation along nerves is fast and conduction velocities range from 1 to 100 m s^{-1}, depending on the type of nerve fibre (see Ch. 18). Depolarisation is propagated along the axon to its end, until the synaptic knob is reached.

The synapse is responsible for transfer of the signal, represented by the action potential, to the adjoining innervated nerve (via one of the connections shown in Fig. 4.2). In mammals, the signal is transferred in the form of a 'chemical message'; the chemical that is released is called a *neurotransmitter*. There are a large number of different neurotransmitters, and each transmitter has its own specific processes for synthesis, storage, release, reuptake and inactivation as well as its own family of receptors. In consequence, neurotransmission is a particularly fertile area for drug action, affecting the CNS and the peripheral somatic and autonomic systems. A schematic for 'typical' neurotransmission is given in Figure 4.3.

The typical neurotransmitter is either synthesised in the soma and transferred to the nerve terminal (for example peptides), or synthesised locally in the presynaptic nerve terminal by enzymes that are produced by protein synthesis in the cell soma and transported along the axon to the nerve terminal (for example acetylcholine and noradrenaline).

The neurotransmitter is taken up from the cytosol (by a specific transporter) and enclosed within membrane vesicles. This results in a low concentration of neurotransmitter free in the cytoplasm, allowing the synthesis of large amounts (by the prevention of end-product inhibition). The concentration of free transmitter within the vesicle may be reduced by the formation of a complex (for example noradrenaline with adenosine trisphosphate (ATP)). When the action potential, associated with the opening of Na^+ channels, reaches the presynaptic nerve terminal it causes the opening of voltage-dependent Ca^{2+} channels. The influx of Ca^{2+} causes the membranes of the vesicles to fuse with the presynaptic cell membrane and release the neurotransmitter into the synapse. The membrane of the vesicle is recovered by endocytosis and 'refilled' for later use. The neurotransmitter binds to the receptors on the postsynaptic mem-

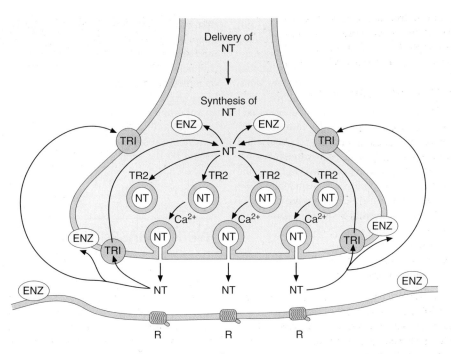

Fig. 4.3
Generalised scheme for synaptic transmission. NT, neurotransmitter (which is either synthesised in the soma and delivered to the nerve terminal (e.g. peptides) or synthesised locally in the nerve terminal (e.g. catecholamines and acetylcholine)); ENZ, enzyme that metabolises NT to inactive products; TR1, specific transporter that carries NT from the synaptic cleft into the cytoplasm of the presynaptic axon; TR2, specific transporter that carries NT from the cytoplasm into the vesicles; R, receptor on postsynaptic membrane, which binds NT and produces the appropriate change in the postsynaptic cell (there are also presynaptic receptors; see text for details). Ca^{2+}, involved in transmitting the signal (see text for details).

brane and thereby transmits the signal to the innervated cell, via its action on the receptor (see Ch. 1).

The association of the neurotransmitter and the postsynaptic receptor is only transient because the concentration of transmitter within the synapse decreases very rapidly. There is an equilibrium established between neurotransmitter (NT) free in the synapse, the receptors (R) and the neurotransmitter–receptor complex (NT–R).

$$[NT] + [R] \rightleftharpoons [NTR]$$

Two main processes can be involved in lowering the concentration of neurotransmitter:

- specific carriers can transport the neurotransmitter back into the presynaptic nerve ending
- inactivating enzymes around the synapse can metabolise the neurotransmitter.

As the concentration of neurotransmitter decreases, so the complex NT–R will dissociate to re-establish the equilibrium, thereby reducing receptor occupancy and stopping the signal on the postsynaptic cell.

The release of the neurotransmitter can be 'fine-tuned' by axo-axonic connection and by presynaptic receptors (which are discussed below).

Electrophysiological consequences of neurotransmission

Binding of the neurotransmitter to the receptor on the postsynaptic membrane may result in a range of possible effects, depending on the type of the receptor and the system to which it is coupled (see Ch. 1). Receptor binding can either activate (excite) or inhibit the innervated neuron or cell.

Excitatory effects
Binding of the neurotransmitter to the postsynaptic membrane receptors causes depolarisation of the membrane, giving rise to an excitatory postsynaptic potential (EPSP). The current inflow from the release of small numbers of synaptic vesicles is insufficient to cause generalised depolarisation, which only occurs when a threshold potential is reached (Ch. 8); the release of small numbers of vesicles serves to increase the excitability of the innervated neuron. EPSPs decay rapidly because the resting potential is maintained by the activity of a range of ion channels and Na^+/K^+-ATPase, which maintains the

concentration gradients of Na⁺ (high outside the cell) and K⁺ (high inside cell) (Fig. 4.4). These homeostatic processes reverse small changes in ion concentrations. Summation of the effects of the release of a large number of synaptic vesicles within a short time (a few milliseconds) is necessary to reach the threshold, above which the action potential will be transmitted to the innervated neuron. Nicotinic acetylcholine (ACh) receptors, for example, are associated directly with Na⁺ channels, and the binding of two molecules of ACh causes channel opening, thereby initiating a wave of depolarisation in the innervated nerve. The main ionic mechanism for an EPSP is the opening of a Na⁺ channel (Ch. 1) but the closing of a K⁺ channel will also cause an EPSP (see Fig. 4.4).

Inhibitory effects

Binding of the neurotransmitter to the postsynaptic receptor hyperpolarises the innervated neuron and thereby reduces its excitability, i.e. it causes an inhibitory postsynaptic potential (IPSP). The main ionic mechanism for an IPSP is the opening of chloride (Cl⁻) channels so that Cl⁻ diffuse down its concentration gradient into the cell; the opening of a K⁺ channel will also cause an IPSP. Enhancing the opening of Cl⁻ channels is an important mechanism of action of a number of anxiolytics (Ch. 20) and anti-epilepsy drugs (Ch. 23). Axoaxonal synapses frequently inhibit neurotransmitter release by the generation of an IPSP (see opioid analgesics, Ch. 19).

Neurotransmitters

There are numerous neurotransmitters, and modulators of neurotransmission; these may be divided into five major classes based on their chemical structure:

- **esters**, e.g. ACh
- **amines**, e.g. noradrenaline, dopamine, histamine, 5-hydroxytryptamine (5HT)
- **amino acids**, e.g. glutamate, glycine, gamma-aminobutyric acid (GABA)
- **peptides**, e.g. opioids, substance P
- **purines**, e.g. ATP:

The principal neurotransmitters within the central and peripheral nervous systems are described based on the processes given in schematic form in Figure 4.3.

Esters

Acetylcholine

Synthesis

ACh ($(CH_3)_3N^+CH_2CH_2OCOCH_3$) is synthesised within the cytosol of the neuron from choline ($(CH_3)_3N^+CH_2CH_2OH$) and acetyl-CoA. Choline is a highly polar, quaternary amino compound that is also present in phospholipids (e.g. phosphatidylcholine) and which is obtained largely from the diet. Because of its fixed positive charge, it does not really cross membranes and there are specific transporters to allow uptake from the gastrointestinal tract and across the blood–brain barrier (Ch. 2), as well as across the neuronal membrane (TR1 in Fig. 4.3, which transports choline rather than ACh; see below). Acetylation of the hydroxyl group of choline is catalysed by the enzyme choline acetyltransferase. The rate of synthesis of ACh is controlled closely and related to ACh turnover, so that rapid release of ACh stores is associated with enhanced synthesis.

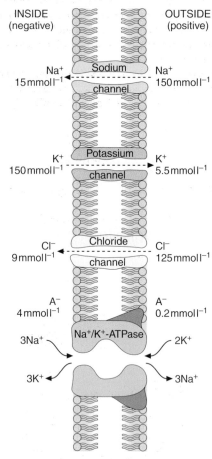

Fig. 4.4
Factors influencing the resting potential. The inside of the cell membrane is negative with respect to the outside because the diffusion of K⁺ down its concentration gradient (out of the cell) exceeds that of Na⁺ (into the cell). The concentration gradients are maintained by the Na⁺/K⁺-ATPase. Hyperpolarisation of the cell may arise from the opening of K⁺ or Cl⁻ channels or from the activation of the Na⁺/K⁺-ATPase. A, a protein anion.

Storage

The cytosolic ACh is taken up into membrane vesicles by a specific transmembrane transporter and is stored in the vesicles in association with ATP and acidic proteoglycans (which are also released on exocytosis of the vesicles). Each vesicle contains 1000 to 50 000 ACh molecules, and neuromuscular junctions contain about 300 000 vesicles.

Release

Release occurs by Ca^{2+}-mediated fusion of the vesicle membrane with the cytoplasmic membrane and exocytosis. This process can be inhibited by botulinum toxin and stimulated by the toxin from the black widow spider. The numbers of vesicles released depends on the site of the synapse, with between 30 and 300 vesicles undergoing exocytosis giving a range from 30 000 to over 3 million ACh molecules released into the synaptic cleft. Neurons within the CNS are more sensitive to ACh release and require fewer ACh molecules to cause an EPSP, whereas the neuromuscular junction is less sensitive and requires millions of molecules to be released. The drug carbachol can release stored ACh.

Removal of activity

Released ACh is very rapidly hydrolysed within the synaptic cleft to give choline and acetate, neither of which binds to the postsynaptic receptors. Both pre-synaptic and postsynaptic membranes are rich in *acetylcholine esterase* (AChE), and the released ACh is hydrolysed very rapidly (usually <1 ms). This rapid hydrolysis, and the rapid equilibration between ACh bound to the receptor and free in the synapse, means that the 'receptor phase' of the transmission process only lasts for 1–2 ms (the postsynaptic changes may be more prolonged; see below).

The active site of the esterase enzyme has two critical features (Fig. 4.5).

- an anionic site, which forms an ionic bond to the quaternary nitrogen of the choline part of ACh
- a hydrolytic site, which contains a serine moiety; the hydroxyl group of the serine accepts the acetyl group (CH_3CO-) from ACh and very rapidly transfers it to water to complete the hydrolysis reaction.

Inhibition of AChE will prevent the breakdown of ACh and lead to prolonged receptor occupancy, the consequences of which depend on the nature of the receptor and the innervated cell/tissue. AChE inhibitors can be divided into three types.

Inhibitors binding to the anionic site. The enzyme can be inhibited by an agent binding reversibly to the anionic site, for example edrophonium (Ch. 28).

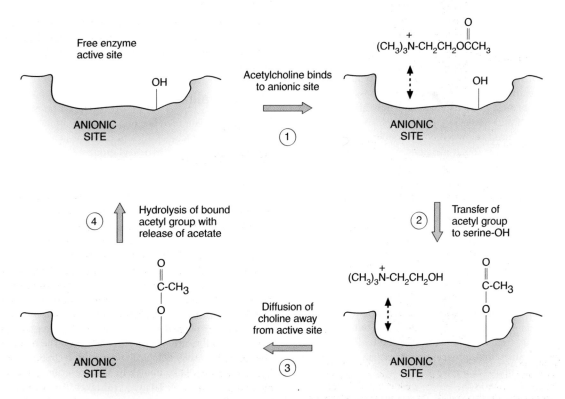

Fig. 4.5
The hydrolysis of acetylcholine by acetylcholine esterase. (Steps 3 and 4 would occur simultaneously.)

Inhibitors carbamylating the serine group. Some inhibitors bind to the anionic site and transfer a carbamoyl group ($(CH_3)_2NCO-$) instead of an acetyl group (CH_3CO-) from the drug to the serine hydroxyl group. The carbamoyl group is hydrolysed more slowly from the serine than is an acetyl group and, as a result, prolonged and profound (but reversible) inhibition of the enzyme occurs; this occurs, for example, with neostigmine and pyridostigmine These are used in treating myasthenia gravis and reversing neuromuscular block by non-depolarising blockers (Chs 27 and 28).

Inhibitors phosphorylating the serine hydroxyl group. Some inhibitors react with the serine hydroxyl group (with or without binding to the anionic site) to produce a phosphorylated enzyme. The phosphorylated enzyme is stable to hydrolysis and, therefore, inhibitors such as the organophosphates, which inhibit AChE in this way, cause irreversible inhibition of the enzyme (or very slowly and only partially reversible inhibition). Such permanent changes in enzyme activity are of limited clinical use. Compounds in this group may be encountered clinically in patients suffering accidental or intentional poisoning. They form an important group of environmental chemicals – the organophosphate pesticides – and there has been concern in recent years over the exposure of agricultural workers to such compounds, for example in sheep dips. Organophosphates have also been used as nerve gases for chemical warfare. The active serine hydroxyl group may be regenerated by administration of pralidoxime, which is an antidote to organophosphate poisoning. The drug ecothiopate acts via phosphorylation of AChE and has limited clinical use in ophthalmology. It should be appreciated that AChE inhibitors produce diverse effects because they increase the concentrations of ACh at all nicotinic and muscarinic receptor sites (Ch. 1 and see below). For example, when an AChE inhibitor is used to overcome reversible neuromuscular blockade (see Ch. 27), it increases ACh-mediated effects on the gastrointestinal tract and heart; these unwanted effects of ACh can be blocked by co-administration of an antimuscarinic agent (see the drug receptor table).

Unlike many other neurotransmitters, ACh is not inactivated by a specific reuptake process (TR1 in Fig. 4.3), but because choline is a limited resource there is a specific reuptake mechanism to allow choline to re-enter the presynaptic neuron rather than simply diffuse away. No such process occurs for acetate because it is readily available from intermediary metabolism. Presynaptic uptake of choline can be inhibited by structural analogues, such as hemicholinium, but such drugs are not useful clinically because of the widespread and non-specific consequences of impairment of ACh uptake, synthesis and release.

Acetylcholine receptors

There are three main types of ACh receptors (see drug receptor table), which show different distribution and agonist/antagonist specificities. The receptors were named after a nitrogen-containing basic compound (alkaloid) present in plants (nicotine) or fungae (muscarine).

Nicotinic (N_1) receptors. These occur within the CNS and on the postsynaptic membranes of all ganglia of both the sympathetic and parasympathetic branches of the ANS.

Nicotinic (N_2) receptors. These occur at the junction between the somatic motor nerves and somatic muscles (the neuromuscular junction; see Ch. 27). The differences between N_2 and N_1 receptors in their agonist/antagonist ligand-binding characteristics are clinically very important, because they allow neuromuscular blockade (paralysis) without major effects on the ANS.

Muscarinic (M) receptors. These occur within the CNS and postganglionic fibre/effector organ junctions of the parasympathetic branch of the ANS. These receptors are also present on most sweat glands (but not on the palms of the hands), which are innervated by the sympathetic branch of the ANS. Application of molecular biology has identified five subtypes of muscarinic receptor. Experimental studies have demonstrated that at least three of these show different antagonist specificities and, as a result, there is the potential for selective drug activity (see drug receptor table).

In addition to occurring on postsynaptic sites, N_1 and M receptors are also found presynaptically (see below).

··

Amines

Noradrenaline

Noradrenaline is a member of a group of amine transmitters called catecholamines (a catechol is a benzene ring with two-adjacent hydroxyl groups; Fig. 4.6a).

Both the catechol and amine groups are important for receptor binding and the catecholamines in Figure 4.6a are inter-related metabolically. Noradrenaline, adrenaline and dopamine may be used therapeutically. The approved names of noradrenaline and adrenaline *when used as medicines* are norepinephrine and epinephrine. In the USA, these alternative 'epinephric' names are used also to describe their neurotransmitter roles, but the receptors are still described by the 'adrenal' nomenclature; hence US texts describe epinephrine activity on adrenergic receptors. To avoid this confusion (and to avoid the term 'norepinephrinergic receptors'), we have kept the 'adrenal' nomenclature for the neurotransmitter and physiological roles and restricted the approved, epinephric, names to the prescribed drugs and their clinical uses. To avoid mistakes, the BNF and medicines packaging and information should include both names (adrenaline/epinephrine) for at least the next five years.

(a)

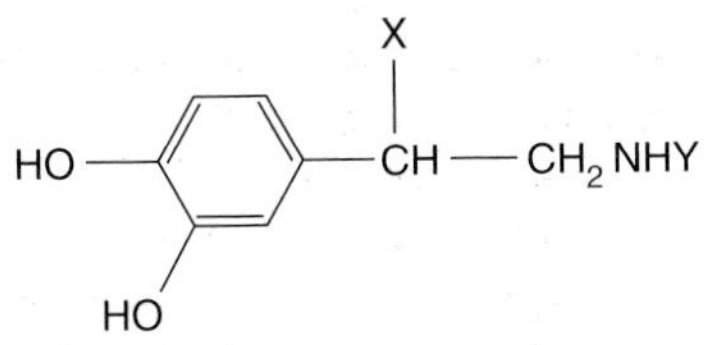
X
HO
CH
CH_2NHY
HO

	X	Y
Dopamine	H	H
Noradrenaline	OH	H
Adrenaline	OH	CH_3

(b)

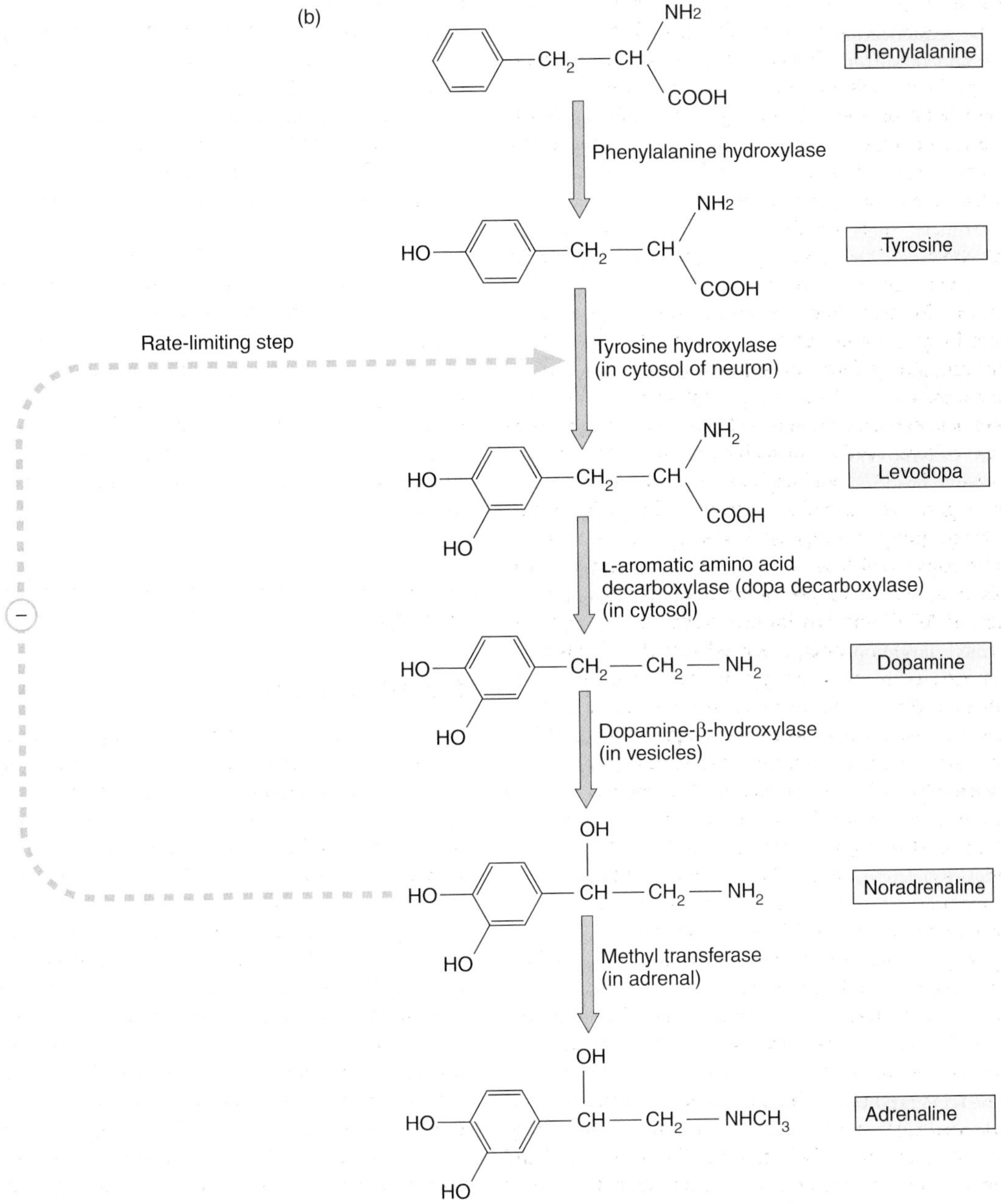
Phenylalanine
Phenylalanine hydroxylase
Tyrosine
Rate-limiting step
Tyrosine hydroxylase
(in cytosol of neuron)
Levodopa
L-aromatic amino acid
decarboxylase (dopa decarboxylase)
(in cytosol)
Dopamine
Dopamine-β-hydroxylase
(in vesicles)
Noradrenaline
Methyl transferase
(in adrenal)
Adrenaline

Fig. 4.6
The structure of the main physiological catecholamines (a) and their synthesis from amino acid precursors (b).

Synthesis

Catecholamine neurotransmitters are synthesised from inactive precursors (Fig. 4.6b). The basic carbon skeleton of catecholamines is derived from phenylalanine or tyrosine, which are aromatic amino acids. Phenylalanine has an unsubstituted benzene ring, while tyrosine has a 4-hydroxyl (phenolic) group. Both phenylalanine and tyrosine are used in protein synthesis. To convert tyrosine to a catecholamine requires oxidation at the aromatic ring (to produce a catechol) and decarboxylation at the amino acid end to produce an amine.

The sequence of synthesis of adrenaline (via dopamine and noradrenaline) is given in Figure 4.6b. The oxidation of tyrosine to levodopa by *tyrosine hydroxylase* commits the molecule to become a neurotransmitter, because levodopa is not used in protein synthesis (there is no t-RNA). This is the rate-limiting step, and it is subject to negative feedback by the subsequent catecholamines, thereby regulating supply. Tyrosine hydroxylase is activated by cyclic AMP (cAMP) dependent protein kinases, and this may be involved in the presynaptic regulation of transmitter synthesis (via presynaptic receptors; see below).

Conversion of levodopa to dopamine is catalysed by a cytosolic enzyme, *L-aromatic amino acid decarboxylase* (usually abbreviated to dopa decarboxylase), which is able to decarboxylate a range of aromatic amino acids. The amine product, dopamine, is then taken up by vesicles via a specific transporter. In dopaminergic neurons, this is the end of the synthetic pathway.

The vesicles of noradrenergic neurons contain the enzyme *dopamine-β-hydroxylase*, which oxidises the β-carbon (i.e. that next to the CH_2NH_2 group). This enzyme is largely present in the membranes of the vesicles, but on exocytosis some is lost into the synapse, following which it diffuses into the blood stream and is slowly cleared. Dopamine-β-hydroxylase in blood is a reflection of peripheral noradrenaline release. In noradrenergic neurons, this is the end of the synthetic pathway.

The adrenal medulla contains an additional enzyme (*phenylethanolamine-N-methyl transferase*), which converts noradrenaline to adrenaline.

Administration of levodopa directly (see Parkinson's disease; Ch. 24) bypasses the rate-limiting step and, therefore, results in increased formation of dopamine. This treatment can remain effective so long as there is sufficient dopa decarboxylase to convert the catechol amino acid to the catecholamine.

The recognition of this synthetic sequence led to the development of α-methyldopa (an analogue of levodopa with a –CH$_3$ group in addition to the –NH$_2$ and –COOH groups on the α-carbon) as an inhibitor of dopa decarboxylase. For many years, it was thought that the hypotensive effect of α-methyldopa was a result of inhibition of noradrenaline synthesis. It is now realised that it is a substrate for dopa decarboxylase and that the products (α-methyldopamine and α-methylnoradrenaline) act presynaptically within the CNS to reduce sympathetic output (Ch. 6).

Storage

Noradrenaline (or dopamine) is stored in the vesicles as a complex with ATP and proteoglycans. Formation of the complex reduces the osmotic pressure that would result from a similar amount of noradrenaline in solution. There is a specific catecholamine transporter (TR2 in Fig. 4.3) that takes up noradrenaline (or dopamine) from the cytoplasm into the vesicles. The transporter can be inhibited by the drug reserpine, which was used to lower blood pressure but is no longer used because of unacceptable side-effects arising from its non-specificity.

Release

Release, in response to a nerve impulse, occurs by Ca^{2+}-mediated fusion of the noradrenaline vesicle with the cytoplasmic membrane.

Noradrenaline present in the cytoplasm may be released by certain low-molecular-weight basic compounds, for example food constituents (such as tyramine), therapeutic drugs (such as ephedrine) and some drugs of abuse (such as amphetamines and metamphetamine). Such compounds are taken into the synapse cytosol by uptake 1 (see below) and into the vesicles, from which they displace noradrenaline. The increased noradrenaline in the cytoplasm is either degraded by monoamine oxidase (MAO; see below) or exchanges with amphetamine via the uptake 1 transporter (TR1 in Fig. 4.3) and is transported out of the cell into the synapse. This releases noradrenaline into the synapse and is responsible for the effects produced by compounds like tyramine. Such compounds are, therefore, called 'indirectly acting sympathomimetic amines'.

Adrenergic neuron-blocking drugs also exert their principal action presynaptically on noradrenaline release. Drugs such as bretylium, bethanidine, guanethidine and debrisoquine are taken into the neuron by uptake 1 (see below; TR1 in Fig. 4.3) and then bind to the vesicle and block its exocytosis in response to a nerve stimulation. Such drugs lower blood pressure but are of little clinical use because of side-effects, which can include an initial hypertension as the drug enters the cytoplasm and displaces noradrenaline. Guanethidine results in depletion of noradrenaline and is more toxic than the other drugs in this class.

Removal of activity

The principal mechanism for the removal of noradrenaline from the synapse is reuptake into the presynaptic neuron via a specific carrier called uptake 1 (TR1 in Fig. 4.3) (uptake 2 is a low-affinity transporter into non-neuronal tissue, but this process does not seem to be critical). The uptake 1 transporter protein varies with the neurotransmitter type released from the neuron, for example noradrenaline, dopamine and 5HT. Newer therapeutic agents are able to exploit the differences between transporters. Blockade of noradrenaline re-uptake, by drugs such as tricyclic antidepressants (Ch. 22) and cocaine (Ch. 18), increases the concentrations of noradrenaline in the synapse and, therefore, increases the activity at the postsynaptic receptor.

Metabolism is important in the elimination of noradrenaline but plays only a minor role in the termination of action in the synapse. There are two main enzymes involved in noradrenaline metabolism: MAO and catechol-*O*-methyltransferase (COMT).

Monoamine oxidase. MAO is present inside the cell on the surface of the mitochondria and is primarily responsible for degradation of intracellular noradrenaline. Oxidation via MAO is the major pathway of metabolism of noradrenaline and other aminergic neuro-transmitters, and converts the primary amino group ($-CH_2NH_2$) into an aldehyde (-CHO). In the periphery, the aldehyde is oxidised to an acid (-COOH), which is excreted in the urine, whereas in the CNS the aldehyde is reduced to an alcohol ($-CH_2OH$), which is conjugated with sulfate (see Ch. 2) before being excreted in the urine. There are two main forms of MAO (Table 4.1), which differ in their organ distribution and substrate affinities. MAO inhibitors that are selective for one of the isoenzymes are able to exploit these differences and minimise unwanted effects. MAO inhibitors are used mainly for their effects on aminergic transmitters within the CNS rather than the peripheral sympathetic nervous system and are discussed in the sections on antidepressants (Ch. 22) and Parkinson's disease (Ch. 24).

Catechol-*O*-methyltransferase. COMT is a membrane-bound enzyme present around the synapse and within the presynaptic neuron. The enzyme catalyses the transfer of a methyl group onto the phenolic group at position 3 of the aromatic ring. This removes the cat-echol centre and prevents binding to the postsynaptic receptor. COMT is a minor route of inactivation of both dopamine and noradrenaline. Inhibitors of COMT are used as an adjunct to levodopa therapy for Parkinson's disease (Ch. 24).

Metabolites of noradrenaline. These two metabolic pathways permanently remove the receptor affinity from the molecule. The main metabolites of noradrenaline include:

- 3,4-dihydroxymandelic acid (formed by replacement of $-CH_2NH_2$ by -COOH) and vanillylmandelic acid (its 3-methyl analogue)
- 3,4-dihydroxyphenylglycol (formed by replacement of $-CH_2NH_2$ by CH_2OH), 3-methoxy-4-hydroxyphenylglycol (its 3-methyl analogue) and their sulfate conjugates.

Receptors

Noradrenaline receptors were originally divided into two types, α and β, based on pharmacological responses, but it was soon recognised that there were two main α-subtypes and three main β-subtypes (see the drug receptor table). Noradrenaline receptors occur in the CNS and in the periphery, particularly at the junction between the postganglionic nerve and the effector organ of the sympathetic branch of the ANS. The clinical uses of drugs that act on these receptors are discussed in later chapters. In addition, it is now realised that there are multiple forms of some of these subtypes (especially α_2-adrenoceptors). The different receptor subtypes show different affinities for the endogenous catecholamines noradrenaline and adrenaline:

α_1, α_{2a}, α_{2c}, β_2:	adrenaline > noradrenaline
β_1:	adrenaline = noradrenaline
α_{2b}, β_3:	noradrenaline > adrenaline.

Table 4.1
Monoamine oxidase (MAO) and its inhibitors

Isoenzyme	Location in human tissues	Main substrates	Inhibitors	
			Irreversible	Reversible
MAO-A	Gastrointestinal tract, placenta	5-hydroxytryptamine, noradrenaline	Clorgiline	Moclobemide
MAO-B	Brain,[a] liver,[a] platelets	Phenylethylamine, tyramine	Selegiline	Lazabemide
MAO-A or MAO-B		Tyramine, dopamine, adrenaline	Iproniazid, tranylcypromine, pargyline, phenelzine	

[a]Both isoenzymes are present, but in humans the amount of MAO-B exceeds that of MAO-A.

Dopamine

Dopamine is a neurotransmitter in its own right both within the CNS and in the periphery (Fig. 4.6a).

Synthesis

Synthesis is described with noradrenaline.

Storage

Storage is described with noradrenaline.

Release

Nerve stimulation causes release of dopamine present in vesicles (see noradrenaline). Dopaminergic neurons are not important in the clinical responses to indirectly acting sympathomimetics and adrenergic neuron-blocking drugs (see above), although certain behavioural responses to amphetamines in rats are linked to dopamine D_2 receptor activity. The antiviral drug amantadine, which is of some value in Parkinson's disease, causes release of dopamine.

Removal of activity

Dopamine is removed by similar mechanisms to those seen with noradrenaline, with reuptake representing the major pathway. Metabolism yields primarily 3,4-dihydroxyphenylacetic acid and its 3-methyl analogue (homovanillic acid).

Receptors

It is now recognised that there are a number of dopamine receptors, although selective therapeutic agents are not available for some of these (see drug receptor table). The original classification was into D_1 (which increase cAMP) and D_2 (which decrease cAMP). The latter are more closely linked to schizophrenia. This subdivision has now been revised into (D_1 and D_5) (which increase cAMP) and (D_2, D_3 and D_4) (which decrease cAMP). The D_4 receptor shows polymorphic expression; hopes that this subtype may be the key to schizophrenia have not been fulfilled, although clozapine, a selective D_4 receptor antagonist, is a valuable antipsychotic drug.

5-Hydroxytryptamine

5HT (or serotonin; Fig. 4.7a) is a neurotransmitter in the CNS and periphery that shows characteristics similar to the catecholamines.

Synthesis

5HT is synthesised from the amino acid tryptophan, by two reactions that are similar to those used in the conversion of tyrosine to dopamine. The first reaction is oxidation of the benzene ring of tryptophan to form 5-hydroxytryptophan, which is catalysed by the enzyme *tryptophan hydroxylase* (which is the rate-limiting step and is only found in 5HT-producing cells). Conversion

(a)

(b)

(c)

(d)

(e)

(f)

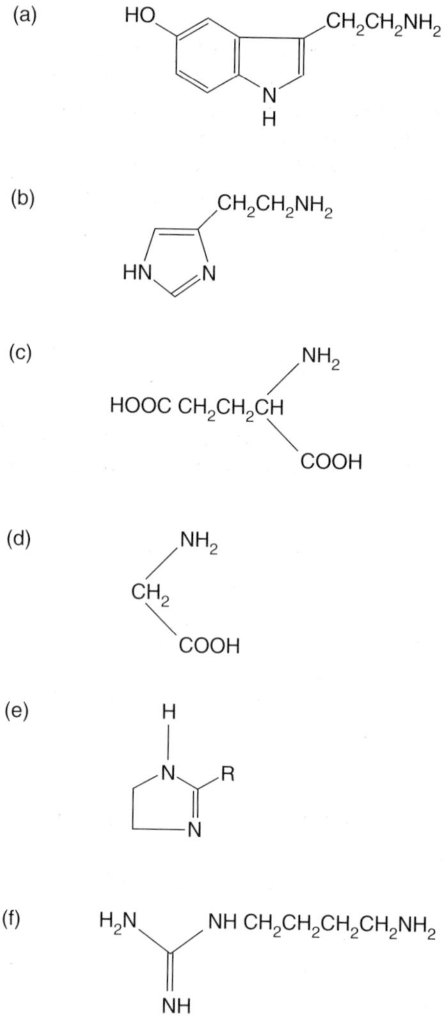

Fig. 4.7
The structure of (a) 5-hydroxytryptamine, (b) histamine, (c) glutamate (aspartate is similar but has only one CH_2 group), (d) glycine, (e) the imidazoline structure and agmatine

of the amino acid function to an amine is catalysed by aromatic amino acid decarboxylase (see noradrenaline synthesis).

5HT is present in the diet but undergoes essentially complete first-pass metabolism by MAO in the gut wall and liver. 5HT is not synthesised by blood platelets, but they have a very efficient transporter, which allows them to accumulate high concentrations of 5HT from the circulation.

Storage

The major sites of 5HT storage in the body are the enterochromaffin cells of the gastrointestinal tract and platelets, with less than 10% in the brain. 5HT is stored in vesicles as a complex with ATP. There is an active uptake process, which is similar to that in adrenergic neurons and which can be inhibited by reserpine.

Release

The release of 5HT vesicles is by Ca^{2+}-mediated exocytosis. A rise in intraluminal pressure in the gastrointestinal tract stimulates the release of 5HT from the chromaffin cells. Release of 5HT from chromaffin cells contributes to nausea following cancer chemotherapy with cytotoxic drugs, both locally and via an action on the chemoreceptor trigger zone. There is a significant release of platelet 5HT in migraine.

Removal of activity

The principal mechanism of inactivation of released 5HT is via its reuptake into the presynaptic nerve. The process shows a high affinity for 5HT and is different from that on adrenergic neurons, which has allowed selective inhibitors to be developed. Selective serotonin (5HT) reuptake inhibitors (SSRIs) are useful antidepressants (Ch. 22).

Metabolism within the neuron is by MAO, which converts the $-CH_2NH_2$ group to an aldehyde (-CHO), which is then oxidised to a carboxylic acid (-COOH), producing the excretory product 5-hydroxyindoleacetic acid (5-HIAA). There is a considerable turnover of 5HT in the chromaffin and nerve cells, and 5-HIAA is a normal constituent of human urine.

Receptors

There is a family of 5HT receptors, which has allowed the development of selective drugs (see drug receptor table). Not all of the subtypes of receptors have recognised physiological roles. The $5HT_1$ group are mostly presynaptic and inhibit adenylate cyclase, whereas the $5HT_2$ group are mostly postsynaptic in the periphery and activate phospholipase C.

Histamine

Histamine (Fig. 4.7b) is an important transmitter both in the CNS and in the periphery, as well as being a mediator released from mast cells and basophils.

Synthesis

The amino acid histidine is converted to histamine through decarboxylation by *histidine decarboxylase*. In addition to the synthesis and storage of histamine by mast cells and basophils, there is continual synthesis, release and metabolic inactivation by growing tissues and in wound healing.

Storage

Most attention has focused on the storage of histamine in mediator-releasing cells, such as mast cells and basophils. In such cells, it is present in granules, associated with heparin. The presence of histidine decarboxylase and the storage of histamine in neurons in the CNS and periphery have not been clearly demonstrated.

Release

The release of histamine from mast cells and basophils has been studied extensively in relation to allergic reactions (see Chs. 12 and 38). The release of histamine from neurons may be similar to the release of other amine neurotransmitters, but this has not been demonstrated unequivocally.

Removal of activity

Histamine is rapidly inactivated by oxidation of the amino group ($-CH_2NH_2$) to an aldehyde and then an acid (-COOH), imidazoleacetic acid. Histamine is not a substrate for MAO and the oxidation is catalysed by *diamine oxidase* (or histaminase). A second, minor route of metabolism is methylation of the cyclic -NH group by *histamine-N-methyltransferase*, and the product is then a substrate for MAO, producing *N*-methylimidazoleacetic acid. Histamine is also eliminated as an *N*-acetyl conjugate.

Receptors

There are three receptors for histamine (see drug receptor table). H_1 receptors have been studied extensively in relation to inflammation and allergy (Chs. 12 and 38). The discovery of H_2 receptors affecting the release of gastric acid led to the development of an important treatment for peptic ulcer disease (Ch. 33). Histamine-containing neurons are found in the brain, particularly in the brainstem, with pathways projecting into the cerebral cortex. H_1 receptors are probably important in these pathways, because sedation is a serious problem with H_1 receptor antagonists (Ch. 38), which are able to cross the blood-brain barrier (Ch. 2). The so-called second-generation antihistamines produce less sedation. H_1 receptors are also involved in emesis (Ch. 32). H_2 receptors are present in the brain and are probably responsible for the confusional state associated with the use of the H_2 receptor antagonist cimetidine (Ch. 33).

Amino acids

Gamma-aminobutyric acid

GABA ($HOOCCH_2CH_2CH_2NH_2$) is an important inhibitory neurotransmitter within the brain responsible for about 40% of all inhibitory activity in the CNS.

Synthesis

GABA is formed by the decarboxylation of glutamate via the enzyme *glutamate decarboxylase*, which is present in GABAergic neurons.

Storage

GABA is stored in membrane vesicles in the brain and in interneurons within the spinal cord (particularly laminae II and III).

Release

GABA is released by Ca^{2+}-mediated exocytosis. Cotransmitters, such as glycine, met-enkephalin and neuropeptide Y, are stored in GABA vesicles and released with GABA.

Removal of activity

Uptake is the principal mechanism for the removal of GABA from the synaptic cleft. The anti-epilepsy drug tiagabine may act as a specific inhibitor of GABA uptake.

GABA is metabolised by transamination with α-ketoglutarate, which forms the corresponding aldehyde (succinic semialdehyde) and amino acid (glutamic acid). The anti-epileptic drug vigabatrine inhibits GABA transamination.

Receptors

There are two main GABA receptors with different mechanisms of action (see drug receptor table). Both mechanisms inhibit depolarisation, with $GABA_A$ causing rapid inhibition and $GABA_B$ giving a slower and more prolonged response. The $GABA_A$ receptor comprises four subunits (α, β, γ and δ). There are multiple forms of each subunit and numerous possible combinations; consequently, the $GABA_A$ receptor should be regarded as a family of receptors. $GABA_B$ receptors are G-protein-linked receptors that hyperpolarise the cell by closing Ca^{2+} channels and opening K^+ channels. In addition, there is a third receptor, $GABA_C$, which is linked to rapid changes in Cl^- conductance, but its physiological and clinical significance remains unclear. Both $GABA_A$ and $GABA_B$ receptors are found presynaptically and inhibit neurotransmitter release by hyperpolarising the cell (via opening Cl^- or K^+ channels) and reducing release of the vesicles of the innervated cell (via closing Ca^{2+} channels). Many important drugs act by altering GABA breakdown or by enhancing GABA activity at its receptor (Chs. 20 and 23).

Glutamate

Glutamate (Fig. 4.7c) is an important excitatory amino acid neurotransmitter that acts on receptors in the CNS. Aspartate (which is similar to glutamate but has only one CH_2 group) acts at the same receptors. Administration of glutamate or aspartate causes CNS excitation, tachycardia, nausea and headache and convulsions at very high doses. Hyperactivity at glutamate receptors has been proposed as a factor in the generation of epilepsy (Ch. 23).

Synthesis

Glutamate (glutamic acid) is a normal endogenous amino acid that is formed in most cells and is widely distributed within the CNS.

Storage

Glutamate is stored in presynaptic vesicles in the neurons.

Release

Exocytosis of vesicles is mediated via the influx of Ca^{2+} into the presynaptic nerve terminal, as occurs for other neurotransmitters. Some anti-epilepsy drugs, for example lamotrigine and valproate (Ch. 23), inhibit glutamate release.

Removal of activity

The action of glutamate in the synapse is terminated by a specific carrier, which transports glutamate into the neuron and surrounding glial cells.

Receptors

Glutamate receptors are described by names rather than symbols such as G_1, G_2 etc. (see drug receptor table).

Glycine

Glycine (Fig. 4.7d) is a widely available amino acid that acts as an inhibitory neurotransmitter. It is released in response to nerve stimulation and acts in the spine, lower brainstem and retina.

Synthesis

Glycine is present in all cells and is accumulated by neurons.

Storage

Glycine is stored within neurons in vesicles; few details are available.

Release

Vesicle release accompanies an action potential, as described above for other neurotransmitters. Tetanus toxin prevents glycine release, and the decrease in glycine-mediated inhibition results in reflex hyperexcitability.

Removal of activity

Released glycine is inactivated by a high-affinity uptake process.

Receptors

Glycine receptors are ligand-gated Cl^- channels similar in structure to $GABA_A$ channels: they are present mainly on interneurons in the spinal cord. Strychnine produces convulsions through the blockade of glycine receptors. (Glycine is important for the activity of NMDA (N-methyl-D-aspartate) receptors; see drug receptor table).

Peptides

The importance of peptides as neurotransmitters has been appreciated in recent years, largely because of the development of highly specific and sensitive probes, combined with histochemical techniques, that allow their detection and measurement. Unlike other classes of neurotransmitter, peptides are synthesised in the cell body as a precursor, which is transported down the axon to its site of storage. An action potential causes the release of the peptide from its precursor; inactivation is probably via hydrolysis by a local peptidase.

Peptide neurotransmitters are often found stored in the same nerve endings as other transmitters (described above) and undergo simultaneous release (cotransmission).

Peptides do not cross the blood–brain barrier readily. A major problem for exploiting our increasing knowledge of the importance of peptides is delivering the novel products of molecular biology to the sites within the brain where they can have an effect.

Substance P is released from C-fibres (Ch. 19) by a Ca^{2+}-linked mechanism and is the principal neurotransmitter for sensory afferents in the dorsal horn. It is also present in the substantia nigra associated with dopaminergic neurons and may be involved in the control of movement.

Opioid peptides are a range of peptides that are the natural ligands for what used to be known as the morphine receptor; the receptor was recognised in the brain and gastrointestinal tract for many years before the natural ligand was identified. These are discussed in Chapter 19.

A number of other peptides are detectable in the CNS and produce physiological effects if given by intrathecal injection. A number of these peptides in the brain are also present in high concentrations in the hypothalamus and/or pituitary gland (e.g. neurotensin, oxytocin, somatostatin, vasopressin; see Chs 43, 45) or in the gastrointestinal tract (e.g. cholecystokinin and vasoactive intestinal peptide).

Low-molecular-weight peptides frequently act via G-protein-linked receptors. The principal peptide receptors and their effects are given in the drug receptor table.

Purines

Adenosine and guanosine are endogenous purines and exist in the body as such, attached to ribose or deoxyribose (as nucleosides) and as mono-, bi- or triphosphorylated nucleotides. The nucleotides are the usual intracellular form and are involved in the energetics of biochemical processes (for example ATP) and as intracellular signals (cAMP and cGMP) as well as being involved in the synthesis of RNA and DNA. ATP is present in the presynaptic vesicles of some other neurotransmitters and is released along with the primary neurotransmitter, following which it may act on postsynaptic receptors (cotransmission). Extracellular ATP is rapidly hydrolysed via ADP to form adenosine. Adenosine itself is very rapidly metabolised and inactivated.

There is a family of purine receptors that show high selectivity (almost specificity) for different purines and give different responses (see the drug receptor table). The adenosine receptors (A_1–A_3) show very high selectivity for adenosine and are specific under physiological conditions. In contrast P_2 receptors are specific for the triphosphates, such as ATP.

Imidazolines

The realisation that there may be an additional unrecognised group of neurotransmitters/receptors involved in the control of blood pressure arose from studies on α_2-adrenoceptor agonists. The side-effects produced by the drug clonidine, an early imidazoline α_2-adrenoceptor agonist, led to the development of moxonidine and rilmenidine. These imidazolines possessed fewer side-effects, but not all of their actions could be interpreted in relation to the α_2-adrenoceptor. A specific imidazoline-binding site was identified in the rostral ventrolateral medulla, and an endogenous 'ligand' that would displace clonidine from this site was proposed (see Ch. 6).

This led to the suggestion that there is an imidazoline receptor that has a high affinity for imidazoline compounds (Fig. 4.7e). It was subsequently suggested that there are three imidazoline receptors (I_1, I_2 and I_3) and that agmatine (Fig. 4.7f) is an endogenous ligand. This compound occurs in synaptosomes and is a postulated natural transmitter.

Binding sites of the I_1 type are present in the brainstem and kidney, liver and prostate. However, there are still considerable doubts about the validity of these binding sites as receptors for neurotransmission. The role of the I_1 receptor in controlling blood pressure is not clearly established; a receptor protein has not been identified, and most I_1-binding agents also bind to the α_{2A}-adrenoceptor. In contrast to these uncertainties about the I_1 site, the I_2-binding site has been established as being associated with MAO and is an allosteric modulating region on the enzyme not a neurotransmitter receptor. The I_3 site appears to modulate the action of K^+_{ATP} channels and to be linked to insulin release from the pancreas. Finally, the role of agmatine is questioned because although it shows appropriate binding characteristics, it does not appear to exhibit any activity.

Presynaptic receptors

An important characteristic complementary to the schematic for synaptic neurotransmission (Fig. 4.3) is the presence of presynaptic receptors. Presynaptic receptors may either increase or decrease the release of the

Table 4.2
Presynaptic receptors and the release of neurotransmitters

Neurotransmitter	Autoreceptor		Heteroreceptor	
	Inhibitory	Facilitatory	Inhibitory	Facilitatory
Acetylcholine	M_2	N_1	α_2, D_2/D_3, $5HT_3$	NMDA
Dopamine	D_2/D_3	–	M_2	N_1, NMDA
Gamma-aminobutyric acid (GABA)	$GABA_B$	–	–	–
Histamine	H_3	–	–	–
5-Hydroxytryptamine (5HT)	$5HT_{1D}$	$5HT_3$	α_2	–
Noradrenaline	α_2	β_2	H_3, M_2, D_2, opioid	N_1, angiotensin II

NMDA, N-methyl-D-aspartate.

neurotransmitter and are described as facilitatory and inhibitory, respectively. There are two main sources of ligands for pre-synaptic receptors:

- neurotransmitter released from the vesicles that can act presynaptically (autoreceptors)
- neurotransmitter released from other neurons, usually by axo-axonal synapses, involving a different neurotransmitter to that released by the neuron itself (heteroreceptors).

The first recognition of a clinically important pre-synaptic receptor was the discovery that the α-agonist clonidine decreased blood pressure (rather than increasing it via α_1-adrenoceptors) and it was shown to act via presynaptic α_2-adrenoceptors, which inhibit the release of noradrenaline. Presynaptic receptors (Table 4.2) are increasingly being recognised as having important roles in the clinical effects produced by many drugs.

The central nervous system

The CNS is the site of action for the drugs discussed in many later chapters. The CNS contains large numbers of neurotransmitters, which produce different effects in different brain regions. The greatest opportunities for selective therapeutic intervention occur when specific activities or functions are associated with a specific neurotransmitter. However, this is rare, and modification of the activity of a neurotransmitter within the CNS will usually affect a number of functions either directly controlled by that neurotransmitter or indirectly linked to its activity.

In many cases, the side-effects of a drug can be anticipated from the roles of the neurotransmitter affected. Selectivity of therapeutic effect, within a spectrum of possible actions mediated by the 'target' neurotransmitter, may be possible if the dose is adjusted carefully to correct an underlying pathophysiological imbalance in one part of the brain, while at the same time not creating an imbalance elsewhere within normally functioning tracts. However, in many cases, the dose–response relationships for therapeutic and unwanted effects are very close and toxicity is inevitable to some degree, in at least a proportion of patients (see Ch. 53). These concepts are illustrated well by the example of dopamine, because psychotic changes and nausea may accompany attempts to increase dopaminergic activity to treat Parkinson's disease (Ch. 24), while parkinsonism-like side-effects are frequently encountered when dopamine antagonists are used in the treatment of psychotic disorders (Ch. 21) or given as anti-emetics (Ch. 32).

The composition of the 'internal environment' of the brain is controlled by the blood–brain barrier (Ch. 2), which limits the entry of potentially neuroactive, polar compounds such as catecholamines, amino acids and peptides, as well as polar therapeutic drugs.

The peripheral autonomic nervous system

The ANS is an important site for drug action because:

- the ANS either controls or contributes to the control of the functioning of nearly all of the major organ systems of the body
- ANS dysfunction is present in many diseases
- the ANS utilises two major different neurotransmitters and a number of receptor subtypes, providing a number of sites for drug action (Box 4.1), which allows the activity of different organs to be modified selectively and independently.

The peripheral ANS is subdivided into two main branches:

- *parasympathetic nervous system*, which utilises ACh as the final transmitter at muscarinic receptors on the effector organs

- *sympathetic nervous system*, which utilises noradrenaline as the transmitter at adrenoceptors on most but not all effector organs.

Anatomically, in both branches of the ANS, the efferent neurons innervating effector organs are linked to neurons in the CNS via ganglia (Figs 4.8 and Box 4.2). The distribution and neuronal interconnections differ between the two branches.

- The parasympathetic efferents give discrete innervations of organs and the ganglia are close to the innervated organs; there are few or no interconnections between ganglia; consequently, organs can be affected individually and independently.
- The sympathetic efferents are involved in the 'flight or fight' response and affect multiorgan systems simultaneously. Many of the ganglia are close to the spinal column, lying in the paravertebral sympathetic ganglion chain, and have broad interconnections. The whole system can be activated simultaneously because the nerve fibres leaving the spinal column interconnect with more than one ganglion and because a preganglionic nerve can give

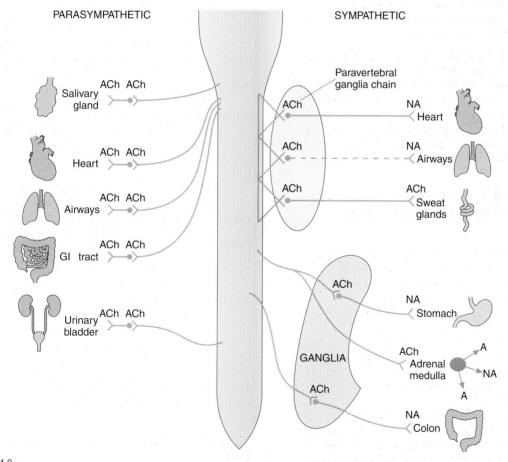

Fig. 4.8
Schematic diagram of the autonomic nervous system illustrating the types of organisation occurring. ACh, acetylcholine; NA, noradrenaline; A, adrenaline; GI, gastrointestinal. The ganglia innervating some organs are not part of the paravertebral chain but are grouped together to form the coeliac, superior mesenteric and inferior mesenteric ganglia. Airways have sparse innervation and dilation is mainly a result of circulating adrenaline.

Box 4.2

Organisation of the autonomic nervous system (ANS)

Both parasympathetic and sympathetic efferent nerves are connected to CNS via ganglia
Acetylcholine and noradrenaline are the principal neurotransmitters in the ANS
The neurotransmitters are synthesised in the presynaptic neuron, stored and released into the synapse in response to depolarisation
Ganglia have nicotinic N_1 acetylcholine receptors
Parasympathetic efferents have muscarinic receptors at neuroeffector synapses
Most sympathetic efferents have noradrenergic receptors at neuroeffector synapses

---

Table 4.3
Autonomic nervous system innervation of the major organ systems

Organ system	Parasympathetic NS		Sympathetic NS	
	Effect	Receptor type[a]	Effect	Receptor type[a]
Heart				
Rate	↓	M	↑	β_1, β_2
Contractility	↓ in atria	M	↑	β_1
Vascular smooth muscle				
In skin/gut	(Dilate)	(M)	Constrict	α_1
In skeletal muscle	(Dilate)	(M)	Dilate	β_2[b]
Bronchial smooth muscle	Constrict	M	Dilate	β_2[b]
Gastrointestinal tract				
Motility	↑	M	↓	α_1, β_2
Sphincter tone	↓	M	↑	α_1
Secretions	↑	M	(↓)	?
Uterine smooth muscle	–	–	↑	α_1
tone in pregnancy	–	–	↓	β_2
Urinary bladder				
Detrusor	↑	M	(↓)	β_2
Sphincter	↓	M	↑	α_1
Penis	Erection	M	Ejaculation	α_1
Skin				
Pilomotor muscles	–	–	↑	α_1
Sweat glands	–	–	Secretion	M
			Local secretion	α_1
Eye				
Radial muscle	–	–	↑	α_1
Sphincter muscle	↑	M	–	–
Ciliary muscle	↑ near vision	M	(↓ far vision)	β_2
Metabolic functions				
Hepatic glycogenolysis	–	–	↑	β_2; α
Skeletal muscle glycogenolysis	–	–	↑	β_2[b]
Fat cell lipolysis	–	–	↑	β_1; α; β_3[b]
Pancreas insulin secretion	↑	M	↓	α

Functions in parentheses are of doubtful physiological significance. M, muscarinic receptor; α and β, adrenoceptors; ↑ *or* ↓ increase *or* decrease: contraction *or* relaxation.
[a] Only the principal receptor types are shown.
[b] Respond to circulating adrenaline; no noradrenergic innervation.

rise to a large number of postganglionic fibres. Some sympathetic nerves (e.g. those involved in the emptying of the bladder or rectum) have long preganglionic sympathetic fibres and the ganglia are not part of a paravertebral chain but occur in more distal sites, such as the coeliac ganglia (Fig. 4.8).

The ANS is important in pharmacology because of its potential to be modulated by therapeutic drugs and the ability of receptor subtypes to produce specific effects. The structures of the transmembrane ACh and noradrenaline receptors, together with their related second messenger systems, have been described above and in Chapter 1.

Many organs are innervated by both the parasympathetic and sympathetic nervous systems, which frequently have opposite effects on the organ function; this has given rise to the concept of *physiological antagonism* between the two branches of the ANS. Table 4.3 shows the principal organ systems, their efferent ANS innervation, their response to parasympathetic and sympathetic stimulation and the principal neurotransmitter released at postganglionic fibre/effector organ junctions.

ACh is the neurotransmitter at all ANS ganglia. The postsynaptic ACh receptors of ganglia are nicotinic N_1 receptors (Ch. 1), which cause a fast EPSP mediated by the opening of Na^+ channels. In addition, ganglia contain M_2 receptors, which inhibit depolarisation (IPSP) through an increase in K^+ conductance; in addition, a more prolonged EPSP may be produced via M_3

receptors (up to 10 s), which close K^+ channels, and this EPSP may be extended via a peptide-mediated action.

Ganglion-blocking drugs were one of the earliest class of drug found to affect the ANS. As their name implies, they are able to block selectively the ACh receptors in the postsynaptic membrane of the ganglia of both branches of the ANS. Because they produce both sympathetic effects (lowering blood pressure) and parasympathetic effects (producing side-effects), they have very restricted clinical use. Antagonists acting at nicotinic N_1 receptors on autonomic ganglia (ganglion-blocking drugs) may produce either a simple competitive blockade (mecamylamine) or a depolarising blockade (hexamethonium; not used clinically).

The effects of ganglion-blocking drugs under resting conditions are given in Table 4.4. Under resting conditions, most organs are under a parasympathetic drive, but this will be affected by activities that produce an increase in sympathetic drive, for example exercise or a flight or fight response, which releases adrenaline from the adrenal medulla.

Physiological functions may require coordination of sympathetic and parasympathetic activities; for example, urination is brought about by a decreased adrenergic drive to the sphincter muscle and increased muscarinic drive to the detrusor muscle (see urinary bladder; Table 4.3).

Students should familiarise themselves with the ANS and the possible sites of drug action (Table 4.3). Such knowledge is fundamental to understanding both the principal mechanisms of action for some drugs and the source of unwanted effects for others.

Table 4.4
The effects of ganglion blockade in a resting subject

Organ	Effect of ganglion blockade	Predominant system
Heart	Increased rate	PNS
Vascular smooth muscle	Decreased tone/dilation	SNS
Bronchial smooth muscle	Little effect/slight dilation	PNS
Gastrointestinal tract	Decreased motility	PNS
Urinary bladder	Urinary retention	PNS
Penis	Blocked erection and ejaculation	PNS/SNS
Sweat glands	Blocked secretion	SNS
Eye	Dilation of pupil	PNS
	Loss of accommodation	PNS

PNS and SNS, parasympathetic and sympathetic nervous systems, respectively.

FURTHER READING

Barnes NM, Sharp T (1999) A review of central 5-HT receptors and their function. *Neuropharmacology* 38, 1083–1152

Berg KA, Maayani S, Clarke WP (1998) Interactions between effectors linked to serotonin receptors. *Ann NY Acad Sci* 861, 111–120

Bloom FE, Morales M (1998) The central 5-HT₃ receptor in CNS disorders. *Neurochem Res* 23, 653–659

Bousquet P, Monassier L, Feldman J (1998) Autonomic nervous system as a target for cardiovascular drugs. *Clin Exp Pharmacol Physiol* 25, 446–448

Bousquet P, Dontenwill M, Greney H, Feldman J (1998) Il-Imidazoline receptors: an update. *J Hypertens* 16 (suppl), S1–S5

Buckley NJ, Bachfischer U, Canut M et al. (1999) Repression and activation of muscarinic receptor genes. *Life Sci* 64, 495–499

Burgen AS (2000) Targets of drug action. *Annu Rev Pharmacol Toxicol* 40, 1–16

Buscher R, Herrmann V, Insel PA (1999) Human adrenoceptor polymorphisms: evolving recognition of clinical importance. *Trends Pharmacol Sci* 20, 94–99

Cartmell J, Schoepp DD (2000) Regulation of neurotransmitter release by metabotropic glutamate receptors. *J Neurochem* 75, 889–907

Docherty JR (1998) Subtypes of functional alpha1- and alpha2-adrenoceptors. *Eur J Pharmacol* 361, 1–15

Eglen RM, Reddy H, Watson N, Challiss RAJ (1994) Muscarinic acetylcholine receptor subtypes in smooth muscle. *Trends Pharmacol Sci* 15, 114–119

Eglen RM, Choppin A, Dillon MP, Hegde S (1999) Muscarinic receptor ligands and their therapeutic potential. *Curr Opin Chem Biol* 3, 426–432

Frishman WH, Kotob F (1999) Alpha-adrenergic blocking drugs in clinical medicine. *J Clin Pharmacol* 39, 7–16

Grace AA, Gerfen CR, Aston-Jones G (1998) Catecholamines in the central nervous system. Overview. *Adv Pharmacol* 42, 655–670

Green AR, Hainsworth AH, Jackson DM (2000) GABA potentiation: a logical pharmacological approach for the treatment of acute ischaemic stroke. *Neuropharmacology* 39, 1483–1494

Hieble JP (2000) Adrenoceptor subclassification: an approach to improved cardiovascular therapeutics. *Pharm Acta Helv* 74, 163–171

Insel PA (1996) Adrenergic receptors – evolving concepts and clinical implications. *N Engl Med J* 334, 580–585

Mackinnon AC, Spedding M, Brown CM (1994) α₂-Adrenoceptors: more subtypes but fewer functional differences. *Trends Pharmacol Sci* 15, 119–123

Mayersohn M, Guentert TW (1995) Clinical pharmacokinetics of the monoamine oxidase-A inhibitor moclobenide. *Clin Pharmacokinet* 29, 292–332

Minneman KP, Esbenshade TA (1994) α₁-Adrenergic receptor subtypes. *Annu Rev Pharmacol Toxicol* 34, 117–133

Noll G, Wenzel RR, Binggeli C, Corti C, Luscher TF (1998) Role of sympathetic nervous system in hypertension and effects of cardiovascular drugs. *Eur Heart J* 19(suppl), F32–F38

Rangachari PK (1998) The fate of released histamine: reception, response and termination. *Yale J Biol Med* 71, 173–182

Satchell D (2000) Purinergic nerves and purinoceptors: early perspectives. *J Auton Nerv Syst* 81, 212–217

Sherwin AL (1999) Neuroactive amino acids in focally epileptic human brain: a review. *Neurochem Res* 24, 1387–1395

Simons FE, Simons KJ (1999) Clinical pharmacology of new histamine H₁ receptor antagonists. *Clin Pharmacokinet* 36, 329–352

Strosberg AD, Pietri-Rouxel F (1996) Function and regulation of the β₃-adrenoceptor. *Trends Pharmacol Sci* 17, 373–381

Takana K (2000) Functions of glutamate transporters in the brain. *Neurosci Res* 37, 15–19

Torphy TJ (1994) β-Adrenoceptors, cAMP and airway smooth muscle relaxation: challenges to dogma. *Trends Pharmacol Sci* 15, 370–374

Vanden Broeck J, Torfs H, Poels J, van Poyer W, Swinnen E, Ferket K, de Loof A (1999) Tachykinin-like peptides and their receptors. A review. *Ann NY Acad Sci* 897, 374–387

Waagepetersen HS, Sonnewald U, Schousboe A (1999) The GABA paradox: multiple roles as metabolite, neurotransmitter, and neurodifferentiative agent. *J Neurochem* 73, 1335–1342

Williams M (2000) Purines: from premise to promise. *J Auton Nerv Syst* 81, 285–288

Self-assessment

In the following questions the first statement, in italics, is true. Is the accompanying statement also true?

1. *The autonomic nervous system (ANS) is only one of the neuronal systems controlling bodily functions.* The sympathetic division of the ANS utilises adrenaline as its primary transmitter substance.

2. *Drugs acting at the ganglia affect both sympathetic and parasympathetic nervous systems.* Ganglion-blocking drugs also block the neuromuscular junction.

3. *Acetylcholine is metabolised with extreme rapidity by acetylcholinesterase in the synaptic cleft.* Acetylcholine esterase is not the only enzyme in the body that breaks down acetylcholine.

4. *Dopamine and noradrenaline are synthesised from the intermediate precursor levodopa.* Dopamine is a transmitter in the peripheral autonomic nervous system.

5. *There are two major monoamine oxidase isoenzymes, MAO-A and MAO-B.* Both isoenzymes metabolise tyramine.

6. *The differentiation of adrenergic receptors into several subtypes is of clinical importance.* Both α_1 and α_2 adrenoceptor-blocking drugs can be used to lower blood pressure.

7. *Botulism periodically causes fatalities and is caused by poisoning by the bacterial toxin from* Clostridium botulinum. Botulinum toxin enhances acetylcholine release from cholinergic neurons.

8. *There are three major types of β-adrenoceptor: β_1, β_2 and β_3.* The β_3-adrenoceptor is most widespread.

9. *Stimulation of presynaptic adrenoceptors controls noradrenaline release.* Propranolol inhibits noradrenaline release.

10. *The major route by which the action of synaptic noradrenaline and 5-hydroxytryptamine (5HT) is curtailed is by reuptake into presynaptic neurons by an uptake mechanism.* The reuptake of noradrenaline and 5HT can be selectively controlled.

11. *The parasympathetic and sympathetic nervous systems often have opposite effects in an organ.* Sympathetic nervous stimulation to the gut inhibits gut motility and sphincter tone.

12. *The vagal cranial nerve to the eye decreases pupil size and limits accommodation to near vision.* Epinephrine decreases pupil size.

The answers are provided on pages 600–601.

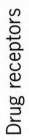

Drug receptors

Types of receptors and examples of agonists and antagonists

Receptor type	Principal location(s)	Mechanism	Main effects	Agonists	Antagonists
Acetylcholine					
Muscarinic[a]					
M_1	CNS and autonomic ganglia (minor role)	G_q: ↑ phospholipase C	Neurotransmission in CNS	Oxtremorine	Pirenzepine
M_2	Heart	G_i: ↓ adenylate cyclase	Bradycardia		
M_3	Smooth muscles, secretory glands	G_q: ↑ phospholipase C	Contraction, secretion	Ipratropium	
$M_1 + M_2 + M_3$				Bethanecol, pilocarpine, carbachol	Atropine, hyoscine, propantheline
Nicotinic					
N_1	Autonomic ganglia	Ligand-gated ion channel	Postganglionic activation	Carbachol, nicotine	Trimetaphan, mecamylamine
N_2	Neuromuscular junction	Ligand-gated ion channel	Muscle contraction	Nicotine	Gallamine, vecuronium
Adrenergic					
α-Adrenoceptors[b]					
α_1	CNS and postsynaptic in sympathetic nervous system	G_q: ↑ phospholipase C	Contraction of arterial smooth muscle, decrease in contractions of gut	Phenylephrine, oxymetazoline	Prazosin, indoramin
α_2	Presynaptic (in both α- and β-adrenergic neurons)	G_i: ↓ adenylate cyclase	Decreased noradrenaline release	Clonidine	Yohimbine
$\alpha_1 + \alpha_2$				Noradrenaline, adrenaline	Phenoxybenzamine, phentolamine
β-Adrenoceptors[c]					
β_1	CNS and heart (nodes and myocardium)	G_s: ↑ adenylate cyclase	Increased force and rate of cardiac contraction	Dobutamine	Atenolol, metoprolol
β_2	Widespread	G_s: ↑ adenylate cyclase	Bronchial dilatation, decrease in contraction of gut, metabolic effects	Salbutamol, terbutaline	Butoxamine
β_3	Adipocytes	G_s: ↑ adenylate cyclase	Mobilisation of fat stores	–	–
				Adrenaline, isoprenaline	Propranolol, oxprenolol

	Location	Transduction	Notes	Agonist	Antagonist
D2	CNS (C, N, O, SN), pituitary gland, chemoreceptor trigger zone gastrointestinal tract heart[d]	G; ↓ adenylate cyclase, ↑ K+ channels, ↓ Ca^{2+} channels	Linked to schizophrenia, prolactin secretion, movement control, memory	Bromocriptine, pergolide	Butyrophenones, sulpiride, renoxipride
D3	CNS (F, Me, Ml) (limbic system)	G; ↓ adenylate cyclase	Cognition, emotion		Sulpiride
D4	CNS, heart	G; ↓ adenylate cyclase	Linked to schizophrenia		Clozapine
D5	CNS (Hi, Hy)	G$_s$; ↑ adenylate cyclase			
D1 + D2					Phenothiazines

5-Hydroxytryptamine (5HT, serotonin)[e]

	Location	Transduction	Notes	Agonist	Antagonist
5HT$_{1A}$	CNS (Hi,R)	G; ↓ cAMP	Autoregulation	Buspirone	
5HT$_{1B}$	CNS (B, G, S), blood vessels	G; ↓cAMP	Autoregulation, vasoconstriction		
5HT$_{1D}$	CNS, blood vessels	G; ↓ cAMP	Vasoconstriction	Sumatriptan	Metergoline
5HT$_{1E}$	CNS (Co, P)	G; ↓cAMP			
5HT$_{1F}$	CNS (Co, Hi)	G; ↓cAMP		Sumatriptan	
5HT$_{2A}$	CNS (Co), platelets, smooth muscle	G$_q$; ↑IP$_3$	Schizophrenia, platelet aggregation, vasodilation		Ketanserin, trazodone, mianserin, clozapine
5HT$_{2B}$	Stomach	G$_q$; ↑ IP$_3$	Contraction, morphogenesis		
5HT$_{2C}$	CNS (Ch, Hi, SN)	G$_q$; ↑IP$_3$	Satiety		
5HT$_3$	CNS (A), enteric nerves, sensory nerves	Ligand-gated Na+/K+ channels	Emesis		Granisetron, ondansetron
5HT$_4$	CNS, myenteric plexus, smooth muscle	G$_s$; ↑ cAMP	Anxiety, memory	Metoclopramide, renzapride, cisapride	
5HT$_5$	CNS	?			
5HT$_6$	CNS	G$_s$; ↑cAMP			
5HT$_7$	CNS	G$_s$; ↑cAMP			Clozapine

continued

Drug receptors

Types of receptors and examples of agonists and antagonists *(continued)*

Receptor type	Principal location(s)	Mechanism	Main effects	Agonists	Antagonists
Histamine					
H_1	CNS, endothelium, smooth muscle	G_q: ↑ phospholipase C, ↑ IP_3	Sedation, sleep		Mepyramine
H_2	CNS, cardiac muscle, stomach	G_s: ↑ cAMP	Gastric acid secretion	Dimaprit	Cimetidine, ranitidine
H_3	CNS (presynaptic), myenteric plexus	?	Appetite, cognition		Thioperamide
Gamma-aminobutyric acid (GABA)[f]					
$GABA_A$	Brain neurons, spinal motor neurons and interneurons	Ligand gated Cl⁻ channel (opens)[g]	Widespread reduction of impulse transmission in CNS, inhibition of sensory signals at spinal level	Muscimol (benzodiazepines) (zolpidem)	(Picrotoxin) (flumazenil)
$GABA_B$	Brain neurons, glial cells, spinal motor neurons and interneurons	G-protein effects on Ca^{2+} channel (closes) and K⁺ channel (opens)	Widespread reduction of impulse transmission in CNS, suppression of polysynaptic reflexes in spine, generation of spike and wave discharges in absence epilepsy	Baclofen	
Glutamate[h]					
N-Methyl D-aspartate (NMDA)[i]	CNS (B, C, sensory pathways)	Ligand-gated Ca^{2+} channel (slow)	Learning		Ketamine, phencyclidine (inhibit Ca^{2+} flux)
Kainate	CNS (Hi)	Ligand-gated Ca^{2+} channel (fast)		Kainate	
AMPA	CNS (similar to NMDA receptors)	Ligand-gated Ca^{2+} channel (fast)			
Metabotropic	CNS (Hi, S, T)	G_q: ↑ phospholipase C ↑ IP_3	Increased attentiveness		
Group I (mglu₁ and mglu₅)					
Group II (mglu₂ and mglu₃)		G_i: ↓cAMP G_i: ↓cAMP			
Group III (mglu₄, mglu₆, mglu₇					

	Mechanism	Function
Angiotensin		
AT$_1$	G$_q$: ↑ phospholipases C G$_i$: ↓cAMP	Vasoconstriction, salt retention
AT$_2$	G$_i$: ↓cAMP	Weak vasodilatation, fetal development, vascular growth
Bradykinin		
B$_1$	G$_q$: ↑ phospholipase C	Inflammation
B$_2$	G-protein; multiple signals, may be multiple receptors	Most actions of kinins, relaxation of blood vessels, pain response
Endothelins		
ET$_A$	G$_q$: ↑ phospholipase C: ↑ Ca^{2+} via IP$_3$	Vasoconstriction
ET$_B$	G$_q$: ↑ phospholipase C	Release of nitric oxide, vasodilation
Natriuretic peptide		
ANP$_A$	G-protein, guanylate cyclase	
ANP$_B$	G-protein, guanylate cyclase	
Neurokinins (tachykinins)		
NK$_1$	G$_q$: slow build-up of response	Nociception (substance P)
NK$_2$	G$_q$: slow build-up of response	Nociception (neurokinin A)
NK$_3$	G$_q$	(Neurokinin B)
Opioids		
δ, κ, μ	G$_i$: ↓ cAMP	See Chapter 19 for details
Vasopressin		
V$_1$	G$_q$: ↑ phospholipase C, ↑ IP$_3$, ↑ Ca^{2+}	Vasoconstriction
V$_2$	G$_s$: ↑ adenylate cyclase	Antidiuretic effect on collecting duct and ascending limb of loop of Henle

continued

Drug receptors

Drug receptors

Types of receptors and examples of agonists and antagonists *(continued)*

Receptor type	Principal location(s)	Mechanism	Main effects	Agonists	Antagonists
Purines					
Adenosine[j]					
A_1		G_i; ↓ adenylate cyclase, ↑ K^+ conduction in heart	Decreased glomerular filtration rate, cardiac depression, vasoconstriction, decreased CNS activity, bronchoconstriction	—	Methylxanthines[k]
Adenosine[j]					
A_{2A}		G_s; ↑ adenylate cyclase	Vasodilation, decreased CNS activity, inhibition of platelet aggregation, bronchodilation		
A_{2B}		G_q; ↑ phospholipase C G_s; ↑ cAMP: Ca^{2+} influx	Action on intestine and bladder Release of mediators from mast cells?		Enprofylline[l]
A_3		G_q; ↑ phospholipase C	Wide tissue distribution; release of mediators from mast cells?		
ATP					
P2X (P2Y$_\alpha$ in brain)		ligand-gated ion channels (Na^+, Ca^{2+} and K^+)	Neuronal depolarisation, influx of Na^+ and Ca^{2+} > efflux of K^+		
P2Y$_\beta$ in brain		G-protein, closes K^+ channel			
ADP					
P2Y$_1$		G_q; ↑ phospholipase C	Change of platelet shape,[m] activation of nitric oxide synthetase[m]		
P2$_{ADP}$		G_i; ↓ cAMP	Platelet aggregation[m]		
UTP or ATP					
P2Y$_2$		G_q; ↑ phospholipase C	Vasoconstriction[m]		

[a] Additional muscarinic receptors (M_4 (G_i) and M_5 (G_q)) have been identified recently but their physiological importance is not defined.

[b] Three α_1-adrenoceptors have been identified (α_{1A}, α_{1B}, α_{1C}) all of which act via G_q proteins: α_{1A} adrenoceptors have a higher affinity for noradrenaline than for adrenaline, α_{1B} and α_{1C}-adrenoceptors do not show selectivity.

[c] The β-adrenoceptors differ in their affinities for noradrenaline (NA) and adrenaline (A): β_1, A ≥ NA; β_2, A > NA; β_3, NA = A.

[d] The mRNA for D_5 receptors has not been found in heart and kidneys and, therefore, the type of receptor in these organs remains questionable (it could be D_4). CNS areas: A, area postrema; B, basal ganglia; C, caudate putamen; Ch, choroid; Co, cortex; F, frontal cortex; G, globus pallidus; Hi, hippocampus; Hy, hypothalamus; Me, medulla; Mi, midbrain; N, nucleus accumbens; O, olfactory tubercle; P, putamen; R, raphe nucleus; S, striatum; SN, substantia nigra; T, thalamus; IP_3 inositol triphosphate.

[e] There are many experimental drugs that are selective agonists and antagonists for receptor subtypes and some are undergoing clinical trials for various conditions. Only clinically useful examples are given. The identification and classification of 5HT receptors is a complex and rapidly changed field (for example four variants of the $5HT_2$ have been recognised, three of which occur in humans). $5HT_{1C}$ was the first 5HT receptor sequence to be cloned but was reclassified as $5HT_{2C}$ when it was found to alter inositol trisphosphate not cAMP. 5HT is involved in numerous pathways within the CNS and the roles of the different receptor types has not been characterised. Effects associated with the different receptors are not well established, with the exception of $5HT_3$ and emesis. Ergotamine is a selective antagonist (and partial agonist) for $5HT_1$ subgroup; methysergide is a selective antagonist (and partial agonist) for $5HT_2$ subgroup.

[f] GABA produces inhibition of neurotransmission widely throughout the brain.

[g] The $GABA_A$ receptor Cl^- channel has a binding site for GABA and also adjacent binding sites for benzodiazepines (which affect the response to GABA), barbiturates, picrotoxin and steroids.

[h] Glutamate produces increased neuronal activity in many regions of the CNS; the different receptors are formed from subunits that can exist in different isoforms; a number of variants have been demonstrated for each.

[i] A low concentration of glycine (below endogenous levels) is necessary for NMDA receptors to open; endogenous amines such as spermidine also facilitate opening. Alcohol inhibits NMDA receptors and tolerance to alcohol is linked to upregulation of NMDA receptors associated with hyperexcitability on withdrawal (see Ch. 54).

[j] A_1–A_3 receptors used to be called P_1 receptors; A_3 receptors have been identified on rat mast cells and A_{2B} on human mast cells.

[k] Methylxanthines increase alertness by blocking A_1/A_2 receptors.

THE CARDIOVASCULAR SYSTEM

5

Ischaemic heart disease

Ischaemic heart disease most frequently occurs as a result of atheroma in large epicardial coronary arteries. Atheromatous plaques tend to form in areas of flow disturbance, such as bends in the vessels or near branching vessels. The plaques are often localised, but atheroma can diffusely involve a long segment of the vessel. When localised, plaques are frequently eccentric, leaving a portion of the arterial wall free of significant disease and still able to respond to vasoconstrictor and vasodilator influences. These segments of artery are particularly prone to vasospasm, since endothelial function is impaired in areas affected by atheroma, and local generation of the vasodilator substance nitric oxide (EDRF, endothelium-derived relaxing factor) is reduced. In some patients, particularly those with long-standing ischaemic heart disease, smaller collateral vessels open up and improve perfusion beyond the obstruction.

Coronary artery atheroma, in common with atheroma in other parts of the vascular tree, occurs at a younger age and more extensively in smokers and individuals with hypertension or hypercholesterolaemia. Some atheromatous plaques are lipid rich, with substantial inflammatory infiltrate and a thin fibromuscular cap. Such plaques are relatively unstable; other plaques are more fibrotic with a thick fibromuscular cap and are stable (Ch. 48). These properties are important in determining which patients develop unstable angina or acute myocardial infarction, since unstable plaques are more prone to disruption (see below)

Angina

Stable angina

Angina pectoris is a symptom of reversible myocardial ischaemia and is most frequently experienced as chest pain on exertion that is relieved by rest. The pain is the consequence of an imbalance between oxygen supply and oxygen demand in the ischaemic area of myocardium (Fig. 5.1). This results from an inability of the coronary blood flow to meet the metabolic demands of the heart, usually because of a fixed atheromatous narrowing of a coronary artery. Coronary artery spasm often accentuates the reduction in flow produced by fixed obstructions, and when vasospasm is present angina occurs at a lower work load. Vasospasm occasionally

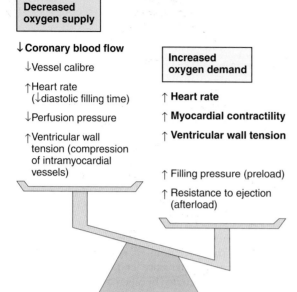

Decreased oxygen supply

↓ **Coronary blood flow**

↓ Vessel calibre

↑ Heart rate (↓diastolic filling time)

↓ Perfusion pressure

↑ Ventricular wall tension (compression of intramyocardial vessels)

Increased oxygen demand

↑ **Heart rate**

↑ **Myocardial contractility**

↑ **Ventricular wall tension**

↑ Filling pressure (preload)

↑ Resistance to ejection (afterload)

Fig. 5.1
Factors affecting the balance of oxygen supply and demand in angina.

leads to angina in patients with otherwise healthy coronary arteries (Printzmetal's variant angina).

Unstable angina

Disruption of unstable atheromatous plaques can be precipitated by sudden stresses on the fibrous cap of the plaque, produced by local disturbance of blood flow or by vasospasm. The resultant fissuring or ulceration of the surface of the plaque promotes platelet aggregation, thrombus formation and local vasospasm.

If vessel occlusion is incomplete, angina occurs on minimal exertion; if the vessel is almost completely occluded then angina occurs at rest. In unstable angina, spontaneous lysis of thrombosis and reduction in local vasospasm takes place within about 20 min; reperfusion of the ischaemic tissue then occurs without lasting damage. More prolonged occlusion leads to myocardial infarction.

Myocardial infarction and sudden cardiac death

Myocardial infarction most commonly arises from complete coronary artery occlusion, following disruption of an unstable atheromatous plaque (see unstable angina above). Occlusion often occurs at the site of an atheromatous lesion that previously was only mildly or moderately stenotic, and may not have caused symptoms prior to disruption. If the occlusion lasts for longer than 20–30 min, muscle necrosis begins subendocardially and then extends transmurally over the next few hours.

If early reperfusion occurs this results in a subendocardial infarction (more usually called a non-Q wave infarction because of the absence of pathological Q waves on the electrocardiograph (ECG)). More prolonged occlusion produces a Q-wave (full-thickness) infarction. Activation of endogenous thrombolysis (Ch. 11), or the presence of a good collateral circulation, are factors that naturally limit the size of the infarct.

Sudden cardiac death results when fatal ventricular arrhythmias arise from ischaemic tissue, often following complete coronary artery occlusion.

Drug treatment of angina

Drug treatment for angina is directed either to increasing oxygen supply by improving coronary blood flow or to reducing oxygen demand by decreasing cardiac work. Drugs can be taken to relieve the ischaemia rapidly during an acute attack or as regular prophylaxis to reduce the risk of subsequent episodes. Four major classes of drug are used to treat angina:

● nitrovasodilators (especially organic nitrates)
● β-adrenoceptor antagonists (β-blockers)
● calcium channel antagonists (Ca^{2+} antagonists)
● potassium channel openers.

Organic nitrates

Examples: glyceryl trinitrate (nitroglycerin), isosorbide dinitrate, isosorbide mononitrate.

Mechanism of action and effects
The organic nitrates are vasodilators that relax vascular smooth muscle by mimicking the effects of endogenous nitric oxide. Enzymatic degradation of the nitrate releases nitric oxide, which combines with thiol groups in vascular endothelium to form nitrosothiols. Nitric oxide and nitrosothiols activate guanylate cyclase and lead to generation of cyclic guanosine monophosphate (cGMP, Fig. 5.2). This, in turn, reduces the availability of intracellular Ca^{2+} to the contractile mechanism of vascular smooth muscle and may have other effects on the muscle. Vasodilation is produced in three main vascular beds.

● **Venous capacitance vessels**, leading to peripheral pooling of blood and reduced venous return to the heart. This lowers left ventricular filling pressure (preload), decreases ventricular wall tension and, therefore, reduces myocardial oxygen demand. Venous dilatation is produced at moderate plasma

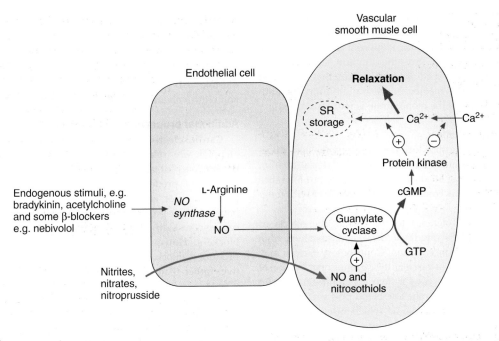

Fig. 5.2
Actions of endogenous and exogenous nitric oxide (NO). Endogenous NO from endothelial cells (EDRF) relaxes smooth muscle via generation of cGMP. Organic nitrates react with tissue thiols generating NO or nitrosothiols, which then activate guanylate cyclase and increase cGMP. The steps involved in muscle relaxation are not yet certain but may include reduced Ca^{2+} influx, increased Ca^{2+} sequestering in sarcoplasmic reticulum (SR) and myosin light chain dephosphorylation.

nitrate concentrations, and tolerance to this action occurs rapidly during continued treatment.

- **Arterial resistance vessels (mainly large arteries)**, leading to reduced resistance to ventricular emptying (afterload). This lowers blood pressure, decreases cardiac work and contributes to a reduced myocardial oxygen demand. Arterial dilatation requires higher plasma nitrate concentrations; tolerance occurs less readily during long-term treatment.
- **Coronary arteries**: nitrates have little effect on total coronary blood flow in angina; indeed flow may be reduced owing to a decrease in perfusion pressure. However, blood flow through collateral vessels may be improved, and nitrates also relieve coronary artery spasm. The net effect is increased blood supply to ischaemic areas of myocardium. Coronary artery dilatation occurs at low plasma nitrate concentrations, and tolerance is slow to develop.

Pharmacokinetics

Glyceryl trinitrate is the most widely used organic nitrate. It is well absorbed from the gut but extensive first-pass metabolism in the liver generates inactive metabolites. To increase its bioavailability, glyceryl trinitrate is given by one of four routes that avoid first-pass metabolism.

- **Sublingual:** the tablet is placed under the tongue and rapid absorption occurs from the buccal

mucosa. The very short half-life of glyceryl trinitrate (less than 5 min) limits the duration of action to approximately 30 min. Tablets lose their potency with prolonged storage; a metered-dose aerosol spray is a more stable delivery mechanism.
- **Buccal:** a tablet containing glyceryl trinitrate in an inert polymer matrix is held between the upper lip and gum, which permits slow release of drug to prolong the duration of action.
- **Transdermal:** glyceryl trinitrate is absorbed well through the skin and can be delivered from an adhesive patch via a rate-limiting membrane or matrix. Steady release of the drug maintains a stable blood concentration for at least 24 h after application of the patch.
- **Intravenous:** the short duration of action of glyceryl trinitrate is an advantage for intravenous dose titration.

Isosorbide dinitrate is well absorbed orally but undergoes extensive first-pass metabolism, which produces both active and inactive metabolites. The majority of the sustained clinical effect results from the formation of isosorbide 5-mononitrate. Isosorbide dinitrate is longer acting than glyceryl trinitrate but still has a short half-life; therefore sustained release formulations are often used. It is also used as a chewable tablet for buccal absorption and a rapid onset of action, or by intravenous infusion.

Isosorbide 5-mononitrate is not subject to first-pass metabolism and can be used orally as an alternative to isosorbide dinitrate, when it gives a more predictable clinical response. Since the amount of isosorbide mononitrate absorbed is greater than that generated during first-pass metabolism of the dinitrate, the anti-anginal action of the mononitrate is more sustained.

Unwanted effects

Venodilation can produce postural hypotension, dizziness, syncope and reflex tachycardia. Arterial dilation causes throbbing headaches and flushing, but tolerance to these effects is common during treatment with long-acting nitrates.

Tolerance. Tolerance to the therapeutic effects of nitrates develops rapidly if there is a sustained high plasma nitrate concentration. Contributory factors may include depletion of vascular thiol groups or activation of the sympathetic nervous system and renin–angiotensin system in response to the low blood pressure; this leads to expansion of blood volume, which offsets the reduced preload. Recent evidence suggests, however, that tolerance is caused by superoxide production within the target cells, leading to reduced generation of nitric oxide or to rapid degradation of the nitric oxide after it is produced by the drug. Tolerance can be avoided by a 'nitrate-low' period of several hours in each 24 h. This is preferable to a 'nitrate-free' period, which carries a risk of rebound angina. In practice, a nitrate-low period is achieved by asymmetric dosing with conventional formulations of isosorbide mononitrate or dinitrate (for example 8 a.m., 1 p.m.) or by using a once daily formulation of isosorbide mononitrate that allows nitrate plasma concentrations to fall overnight. Transdermal nitrate patches have to be removed for part of each 24 h (e.g. overnight) to prevent tolerance, creating a nitrate-free period. There is limited evidence that co-administration of an angiotensin-converting enzyme (ACE) inhibitor, angiotensin receptor antagonist or hydralazine (Ch. 6) may reduce nitrate tolerance by impairing superoxide formation.

Beta-adrenoceptor antagonists (beta-blockers)

Examples: atenolol, propranolol, pindolol, nebivolol, labetalol

Mechanism of action and effects in angina

All β-blockers act as competitive antagonists of catecholamines at β-adrenoceptors. They achieve their therapeutic effect in angina by blockade at the cardiac β_1-adrenoceptor and thereby:

- decrease heart rate

- reduce the force of cardiac contraction
- lower blood pressure.

These effects are most marked during exercise and reduce myocardial oxygen demand. The lengthening of diastole also gives more time for coronary perfusion and effectively improves oxygen supply.

Additional properties of β-blockers

Cardioselectivity. Some β-blockers, for example atenolol, are relatively selective antagonists at the β_1-adrenoceptor, a property known as 'cardioselectivity' because of predominant effects on the heart. Other β-adrenoceptor antagonists, for example propranolol, have equal or greater antagonist activity at β_2-adrenoceptors; these drugs are referred to as 'non-selective' β-blockers. However, even cardioselective β-blockers produce β_2-blockade at higher doses, so they are 'selective' rather than truly specific for the β_1-adrenoceptor (Ch. 1).

Partial agonist activity. Some β-adrenoceptor antagonists such as pindolol also possess partial agonist activity (Ch. 1) at the β-adrenoceptor. Such drugs weakly stimulate the receptor at rest. When the concentration of endogenous catecholamines rises, the drug becomes a competitive antagonist while retaining its mild stimulant activity. The rise in heart rate and force of cardiac contraction produced by catecholamines is, therefore, reduced to a lesser extent by a partial agonist than by a full antagonist, and myocardial oxygen demand remains higher. For this reason, β-blockers with partial agonist activity may be less effective than full antagonists in patients with severe angina. Partial agonists are less likely to cause a resting bradycardia. If the drug is a partial agonist at the β_2-adrenoceptor, it will produce vasodilation in some vascular beds (Fig. 6.8).

Vasodilator activity. Pure β-blockers do not cause vasodilation. However β-blockers that also have β_2-adrenoceptor partial agonist activity (e.g. pindolol) also produce vasodilation. Other β-adrenoceptor antagonists have a hybrid action and produce vasodilation by α-blockade (e.g. labetalol, see Fig. 6.8, p. 101) by increasing vascular nitric oxide concentrations (nebivolol) or by other direct actions on blood vessels (e.g. celiprolol). Vasodilation does not have any proven advantage for the treatment of angina but may be useful in the treatment of hypertension (Ch. 6). Nebivolol causes the release of nitric oxide via stimulation of a 5-hydroxy-tryptamine (5HT) $5HT_{1A}$ receptor subtype on the vascular endothelium. Of interest for future pharmacological developments is that nebivolol, like sotalol and propranolol is a racemic mixture. The D-isomer is responsible for both β-blockade and vasodilation but the L-isomer has only vasodilator properties.

Pharmacokinetics

Lipophilic β-blockers, such as propranolol, are well absorbed from the gut but undergo extensive first-pass metabolism in the liver, with considerable variability among individuals. Reduction in exercise heart rate is closely related to the plasma concentration of β-blocker. Consequently, dose titration of lipophilic β-blockers is particularly necessary to achieve the optimum clinical response in angina. Most lipophilic β-blockers have short half-lives.

Hydrophilic β-adrenoceptor antagonists, such as atenolol, are absorbed less completely from the gut and are eliminated unchanged by the kidney. The dose range to maintain effective plasma concentrations is narrower than for those drugs that undergo metabolism. The half-lives of hydrophilic drugs are usually intermediate.

Unwanted effects

The β-blockers have a number of unwanted effects.

Blockade of β_1-adrenoceptors. Since cardiac output is reduced, β-adrenoceptor antagonists can precipitate heart failure in patients with poor left ventricular function, who rely on high sympathetic nervous activity to maintain their cardiac output. However, used with great care, they can be given as part of the therapy of heart failure (Ch. 7). Reduction in cardiac output can also impair blood supply to peripheral tissues, which can increase symptoms of intermittent claudication when used with vasodilators or can provoke Raynaud's phenomenon (Ch. 10). Excessive bradycardia occasionally occurs, and β-adrenoceptor antagonists should be avoided in the presence of an atrioventricular conduction defect (heart block). Drugs with partial agonist activity are less likely to cause bradycardia or to reduce cardiac output.

Blockade of β_2-adrenoceptors. Bronchospasm can be precipitated in asthmatics or those with chronic pulmonary disease and even cardioselective drugs are not completely safe. Impaired vasodilation in skeletal muscle, which is mediated by β_2-adrenoceptors, can exacerbate intermittent claudication (Ch. 10). Insulin-requiring diabetics are prone to prolonged hypoglycaemic episodes while taking non-selective β-blockers. Gluconeogenesis, a component of the metabolic response to hypoglycaemia, is dependent on β_2-adrenoceptor stimulation in the liver. Beta-blockers also blunt the autonomic response, which alerts the patient to the onset of hypoglycaemia.

Effects on blood lipid levels. Most β-blockers raise the plasma concentration of triglycerides and lower the concentration of high density lipoprotein cholesterol (Ch. 48). These changes are potentially atherogenic. They are most marked with non-selective β-blockers and do not occur if the drug has partial agonist activity.

Central nervous system effects. These include sleep disturbance, vivid dreams and hallucinations. They are more common with lipophilic drugs, which readily cross the blood–brain barrier. Fatigue and more subtle psychomotor effects, for example lack of concentration, are also common.

Sudden withdrawal syndrome. Upregulation of β-adrenoceptors (Ch. 1) during long-term treatment makes the heart more sensitive to catecholamines. Beta-blockers should be stopped gradually in patients with ischaemic heart disease to avoid precipitating unstable angina or myocardial infarction.

Drug interactions. The Ca^{2+} channel antagonist verapamil (see below) has potentially hazardous additive effects with β-blockers, reducing the force of cardiac contraction and slowing heart rate. This is particularly marked if they are both given intravenously with a short interval between them. Similarly, diltiazem can cause excessive bradycardia when used with a β-blocker.

Calcium channel antagonists (calcium antagonists)

Examples: nifedipine, amlodipine, verapamil, diltiazem

Mechanism of action and effects

Calcium is essential for excitation–contraction coupling in muscle cells. Free Ca^{2+} must either enter the cell through transmembrane channels or be released from intracellular stores for contraction to occur. As myofilaments relax, Ca^{2+} is then either taken up by the sarcoplasmic reticulum or translocated out of the cell. In striated muscle, Ca^{2+} is almost entirely recycled intracellularly via the sarcoplasmic reticulum. However, in smooth muscle (such as that surrounding arteriolar resistance vessels) and to a lesser extent in cardiac muscle, intracellular Ca^{2+} recycling is poorly developed. Reduced Ca^{2+} entry into these cells will, therefore, inhibit muscle contraction.

Calcium channel antagonists (often referred to simply as Ca^{2+} antagonists) have widely different chemical structures but act principally by reducing Ca^{2+} influx through voltage-operated L-type (long-acting) slow Ca^{2+} channels. Voltage-operated T-type (transient) channels are also found at high concentrations in pacemaker cells of the sinoatrial and atrioventricular nodes, while L-type channels predominate in myocardial cells. Both types are found in vascular smooth muscle. T-type channels are activated by lower voltages than L-type channels and produce more transient depolarisation. None of the currently available Ca^{2+} antagonists affect T-type channels to any important extent, or influence receptor-operated Ca^{2+} channels, which respond to endogenous agonists such as noradrenaline (Fig. 5.3).

A number of effects of Ca^{2+} channel antagonists may be important in angina.

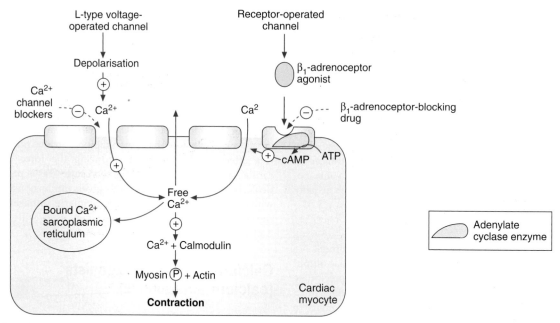

Fig. 5.3
Contraction of the cardiac myocyte by receptor and voltage-operated mechanisms. In the cardiac myocyte, depolarisation during the action potential activates the L-type voltage-operated channel. The influx of Ca^{2+} results in myosin phosphorylation and contraction. The Ca^{2+} influx is blocked by Ca^{2+} channel blockers. Adrenaline also causes contraction but acts via the β_1-adrenoreceptor to activate adenylate cyclase and increased intracellular cAMP. This results in phosphorylation of Ca^{2+} channels causing Ca^{2+} influx. The receptor-operated Ca^{2+} channel is not blocked by Ca^{2+} channel antagonists. +, stimulates activity; −, inhibits activity.

Arteriolar dilation. Dihydropyridine derivatives such as nifedipine or amlodipine are the most potent. Arterial dilation reduces peripheral resistance, lowers the blood pressure and, therefore, reduces the work of the left ventricle and myocardial oxygen demand. Short-acting dihydropyridines produce a rapid drop in blood pressure, and reflex sympathetic nervous system activation leads to tachycardia (Fig. 5.4). Longer-acting compounds or modified-release formulations of short-acting drugs gradually reduce blood pressure and cause little tachycardia.

Coronary artery dilation. Prevention or relief of vasospasm will improve myocardial blood flow.

Negative chronotropic effect. Verapamil and diltiazem (but not the dihydropyridines such as nifedipine or amlodipine) slow the rate of firing of the sinoatrial node and slow impulse conduction through the atrioventricular node, thus reflex tachycardia is not seen with these drugs (Ch. 8). They slow the rate of rise in heart rate during exercise.

Reduced cardiac contractility. Many Ca^{2+} antagonists (particulary verapamil) have a negative inotropic effect. Amlodipine does do not impair myocardial contractility.

There are clinically important differences among the Ca^{2+} antagonists. A comparison of the cardiovascular effects of the different classes of Ca^{2+} antagonist is shown in the drug compendium table.

Pharmacokinetics

Most Ca^{2+} antagonists are lipophilic compounds with similar pharmacokinetic properties. They are almost completely absorbed from the gut, undergo extensive and variable first-pass metabolism in the liver and have short half-lives. Modified-release formulations are widely used to prolong the duration of action. Nifedipine is also available in a liquid-containing capsule formulation; biting the capsule and swallowing the contents leads to a rapid onset of action.

Nifedipine is inactivated by metabolism while verapamil and diltiazem have active, although less potent, metabolites. Verapamil can be given intravenously, a route that is usually reserved for the treatment of arrhythmias (Ch. 8).

Amlodipine differs from other Ca^{2+} antagonists in that it is slowly and incompletely absorbed and does not undergo first-pass metabolism. A high volume of distribution and slower metabolism by the liver give amlodipine a very long half-life of about 1–2 days.

Unwanted effects

Arterial dilation. Headache, flushing and dizziness may be troublesome, although tolerance often occurs with continued use. Ankle oedema, which is frequently resistant to diuretics, may be a consequence of increased transcapillary hydrostatic pressure. Tolerance to oedema

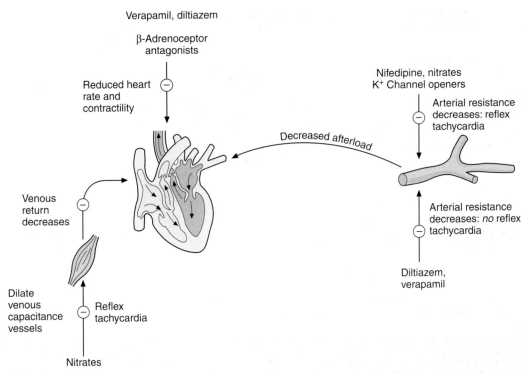

Fig. 5.4

The complementary major sites of action of some anti-anginal drugs and the reflex response of the heart to their actions. Reflex tachycardia results from the actions of nifedipine and K⁺ channel openers. This is not a problem with diltiazem and verapamil, which slow heart rate. Modified-release formulations of nifedipine or amlodipine do not cause tachycardia.

does not occur. These unwanted effects are most common with the dihydropyridines.

Reduced cardiac contractility. This can precipitate heart failure in susceptible patients with pre-existing poor left ventricular function, particularly with verapamil.

Bradycardia and heart block. Verapamil or diltiazem can excessively slow the heart, particularly if they are used in combination with other drugs that have similar effects on heart rate or atrioventricular nodal conduction, for example digoxin (Ch. 8) or β-blockers.

Altered gut motility. Constipation is most common with verapamil, less so with diltiazem. Nifedipine and related drugs can cause nausea and heartburn.

Potassium channel openers

Example: nicorandil

Mechanism of action

There are many different K⁺ channels in cell membranes (Table 5.1). Nicorandil opens the ATP-sensitive channel and hyperpolarises the cell membrane. ATP binding to these channels inhibits K⁺ conductance; but nicorandil opens the channels even in the presence of ATP. Hyperpolarisation of vascular smooth muscle cells inhibits opening of the L-type Ca²⁺ channels, which are voltage dependent (Fig 5.5). This produces vasodilation in systemic and coronary arteries.

Nicorandil also carries a nitrate moiety, and part of its vasodilator action is via generation of nitric oxide in vascular smooth muscle (see organic nitrates above). This may account for the venodilation produced by the drug.

Pharmacokinetics

Nicorandil is rapidly and almost completely absorbed from the gut. It is eliminated by liver metabolism and has a short half-life; however, the tissue effects correlate poorly with plasma concentrations, and the biological effect lasts up to 12 h.

Unwanted effects

Arterial dilation. Headache occurs in 25–50% of patients. Tolerance usually occurs with continued use. Palpitations (caused by reflex activation of the sympathetic nervous system) and flushing can also occur.

Dizziness, nausea, vomiting. These can also occur.

Table 5.1
Major potassium channel subtypes

Subtypes	Probable function
Superfamily 1	
A channel (K_A)	Regulation of action potential frequency by rapid repolarisation
Delayed rectifier (K_V)	Initiates repolarisation at the end of the plateau phase after a time delay
Large conductance calcium-sensitive (BK_{ca})	Regulation of action potential frequency; accelerates repolarisation when cytosolic calcium concentrations are high
Superfamily 2	
Inward rectifier (K_{IR})	Setting of resting potential; prolongs plateau of action potentials; involved in physiological regulation of heart rate
ATP-sensitive (K_{ATP})	Control of resting potential in glucoreceptive cells; may act as a tissue protector in hypoxic states; inhibited by ATP, therefore opens in energy-depleted state

Potassium channels act as electrical rectifiers, i.e. the ability of the channel to pass current varies according to the membrane potential. Potassium currents repolarise cells via the outward rectifiers. Inward rectifiers tend to close when the cell is depolarised to maintain the depolarised state.

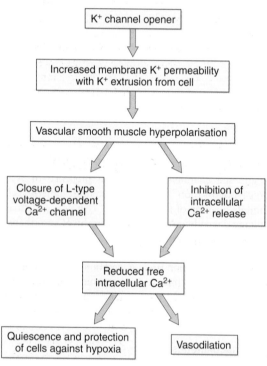

Fig. 5.5
The mechanism of action of K+ channel activators.

Management of stable angina

The principal aims of treatment in stable angina are to relieve symptoms and, secondly, to improve prognosis. Although patients with the greatest number of ischaemic episodes may be most likely to progress to myocardial infarction or sudden death, there is no convincing evi-dence that the extent of suppression of the ischaemia will affect survival, or the risk of myocardial infarction. Angina has a circadian rhythm and occurs most frequently in the hours after waking, so a drug given for prophylaxis should ideally provide cover at this time.

There are several important principles of management.

● Life style changes such as stopping smoking and weight loss if obese, and reduction of high blood pressure are important.
● Sublingual glyceryl trinitrate remains the treatment of choice for an acute anginal attack. It relieves symptoms within minutes but only gives short-lived protection for 20–30 min. Glyceryl trinitrate can also be taken for short-term prophylaxis before an activity that is likely to produce angina. For patients who cannot tolerate a nitrate, a capsule of immediate-release nifedipine can be bitten and the contents swallowed to achieve a rapid effect.
● If anginal attacks are frequent, a longer-acting prophylactic anti-anginal drug should be used. A β-blocker or a Ca^{2+} antagonist are the most effective treatments; nitrates are less suitable as first-line prophylactic agents because of the problems of tolerance. Since a rise in heart rate is one of the main precipitating factors for angina, a drug that lowers heart rate such as a β-blocker, verapamil or diltiazem, may be most effective for first-line treatment. If symptoms are not controlled by optimal doses of a single drug, then a combination of a β-blocker with a Ca^{2+} antagonist (not verapamil) or a β-blocker or Ca^{2+} antagonist with a long-acting nitrate can be given. The role of nicorandil is less well established; it is generally used in combination therapy. 'Triple therapy' (e.g. β-blocker, Ca^{2+} antagonist and a nitrate) has not been shown convincingly to be better than two agents but may benefit some patients.

- Low-dose aspirin reduces the risk of subsequent myocardial infarction by about 35% (see Ch. 11).
- Treatment of a raised plasma cholesterol is desirable, initially by diet but by drugs if the response is inadequate (Ch. 48). Lowering plasma cholesterol to <5.0 mmol l^{-1} reduces the risk of subsequent non-fatal myocardial infarction, cardiac death and the need for surgical or percutaneous coronary artery revascularisation by about 25–30%.
- Coronary artery bypass grafting (CABG) improves long-term prognosis compared with medical treatment in patients with left main stem coronary artery stenosis, and in those with 'triple vessel disease' (significant left anterior descending, left circumflex and right coronary artery stenoses) who have impaired left ventricular function. In other patients it is used for symptom relief. Percutaneous transluminal coronary angioplasty (PTCA) (often with insertion of a stent to maintain patency) is currently used for symptom relief only.

Symptoms and response to treatment are a poor guide to the severity of coronary artery disease, and exercise stress testing is a more accurate predictor. Patients who perform poorly during such testing, as well as those who fail to respond to two prophylactic drugs in adequate dosages, should be considered for coronary angiography, with a view to CABG or PTCA.

Management of unstable angina

Unstable angina usually presents with symptoms at rest, or a rapidly accelerating pattern of angina attacks that are produced by minimal exertion (accelerated or crescendo angina). It usually requires urgent treatment to reduce the 10% risk of subsequent myocardial infarction or death.

- Low-dose aspirin should be given (Ch. 11) after a loading dose if the patient is not already taking aspirin. Full anticoagulation with intravenous heparin or subcutaneous low-molecular-weight heparin (Ch. 11) produces additive benefit; the risk of myocardial infarction or death within 14 days is reduced by about 60% after the onset of combined treatment.
- A β-blocker is the first choice anti-anginal treatment, although a heart-rate-limiting Ca^{2+} antagonist such as verapamil or diltiazem can be used if a β-adrenoceptor antagonist is contraindicated or not tolerated. Dihydropyridine Ca^{2+} antagonists such as nifedipine do not improve outcome when used alone, but they can be used with a β-adrenoceptor antagonist if the symptoms do not settle. These regimens reduce the rate of myocardial infarction by about 15% compared with that with no anti-anginal treatment.

- Nitrates are widely used either sublingually or, for more prolonged effect, by the buccal or intravenous route. Nitrates relieve symptoms, but there is no evidence that they improve prognosis in unstable angina.
- Platelet inhibition with an intravenous glycoprotein IIb/IIIa antagonist such as tirofiban reduces myocardial infarction and death in high-risk patients. Those with a raised plasma concentration of the markers of myocardial damage, troponin I or T, benefit most (Ch. 11).
- In the acute phase of unstable angina, angiography, followed by CABG or PTCA, is usually reserved for the 10% of patients who are refractory to full medical treatment. If the unstable angina settles, patients who develop symptoms or ECG changes at an early stage during a standardised exercise test, and those who had evidence of myocardial damage during the acute episode (for example, an increase in the plasma concentration of sensitive markers of cardiac damage such as troponin T or I), should also be investigated with angiography.
- Cholesterol reduction to <5.0 mol l^{-1} should be initiated by diet, with addition of drugs if the response is inadequate (Ch. 48). This reduces long-term risk of myocardial infarction or cardiac death by 25–30%.

Management of myocardial infarction

Acute management

Myocardial infarction is usually (but not invariably) associated with intense, prolonged chest pain and sympathetic nervous stimulation, which increases cardiac work. Drug therapy is directed initially towards two principal goals: pain relief and thrombolysis. For pain relief, an intravenous opioid analgesic such as diamorphine (Ch. 19) is given together with an anti-emetic. Intramuscular injection should be avoided since a low cardiac output and poor tissue perfusion often delay absorption. A nitrate (sublingual or intravenous) can also reduce pain by relief of coronary artery spasm at the site of the occlusion, with restoration of some blood flow. An intravenous β-blocker can be given to reduce cardiac work, especially if the patient is hypertensive or tachycardic but does not have signs of heart failure.

Natural thrombolysis can be enhanced by intravenous thrombolytic therapy (Ch. 11) to limit the size of the infarct. Two agents are in wide clinical use: streptokinase and recombinant tissue plasminogen activator (rt-PA). rt-PA produces more rapid reperfusion and opens a greater percentage of occluded vessels than streptokinase, but the extent of myocardial salvage and consequent reduction in mortality are similar for the two agents. Streptokinase is most widely used but produces symptomatic hypotension in up to 10% of patients. rt-PA is less likely to lower blood pressure and is given to patients with severe symptomatic hypotension prior to thrombolysis. It is also given to those who have previously received streptokinase, who are likely to have high titres of streptokinase neutralising antibodies (Ch. 11). rt-PA must be followed by intravenous heparin for 48 h to reduce reocclusion; this is unnecessary with streptokinase because of its longer duration of action. A third agent, anistreplase, is sometimes used in primary care when access to hospital is delayed since it can be given conveniently by a 5-min infusion. Its efficacy is similar to streptokinase.

Thrombolytic therapy significantly reduces mortality if given within 12 h of the onset of pain, but the survival advantage is greater the earlier treatment is given. Treatment within 6 h of the onset of pain saves 30 lives per 1000 patients treated, whereas delay to 6–12 h after the onset of pain saves 20 lives per 1000 patients treated. Thrombolysis should only be given to patients with clear ECG changes of acute myocardial infarction (characteristic ST elevation in two or more leads) or to those with left bundle branch block on the ECG and a good history of acute myocardial infarction. In the latter patients, an acute myocardial infarction cannot be easily diagnosed from the ECG but mortality is high. The greatest reduction in mortality is derived by those patient groups at highest risk (i.e those with anterior infarcts rather than inferior), the elderly (>65 years of age) and those with a presenting systolic blood pressure below 100 mmHg.

Other therapy

PTCA is helpful for some patients in the acute phase of myocardial infarction. It can be considered if access to a catheter laboratory is rapid and the patient is at high risk and has contraindications to thrombolysis; this is known as 'primary' PTCA. 'Rescue' PTCA can be considered if thrombolysis has failed to re-perfuse the infarct-related vessel.

In addition to the management discussed above, complications of myocardial infarction may need specific treatment (Box 5.1).

....

Secondary prophylaxis after myocardial infarction

Secondary prophylaxis to reduce late mortality after myocardial infarction can be achieved with several approaches.

- Stopping smoking is of major benefit since it reduces the mortality after a myocardial infarction by 50%. Rehabilitation programmes, which include exercise, also reduce mortality by up to 25% and improve psychological recovery.
- Low-dose aspirin (Ch. 11) reduces mortality in the first few weeks when started within 24 h of the onset of pain and reduces later mortality if continued long term (saving 20 lives per 1000 patients treated). Initial benefits may result from reduced reocclusion of vessels that have undergone natural or therapeutic thrombolysis. A loading dose is required for a rapid onset of effect.
- Beta-blockers started orally soon after the infarct reduce later deaths and reinfarctions by about 25% each, although the mechanism is unknown. Greatest benefit is seen in patients at highest risk, for example following anterior infarction and in those who have had serious postinfarct arrhythmias or postinfarct angina or heart failure. The latter must be controlled before a β-blocker is given.
- An ACE inhibitor (Ch. 6) is of greater benefit in patients with clinical or radiological evidence of heart failure after their infarction, reducing mortality by about 25% over the subsequent year. A lesser survival advantage is gained in patients with significant left ventricular dysfunction after the infarction (ejection fraction of 40% or less) but who have not had clinical evidence of heart failure. In these patients, a 20% reduction in mortality over 3–5 years after the event is accompanied by a significant reduction in non-fatal reinfarctions (although the mechanism of this effect is unknown). Most recently , a reduction in both non-fatal infarction and death has been shown in those with

---

Box 5.1

Complications after myocardial infarction

Heart failure
Cardiogenic shock
Cardiac rupture
    Free wall rupture
    Ventricular septal defect
Arrhythmias
    Ventricular fibrillation
    Ventricular tachycardia
    Supraventricular tachycardias
    Sinus bradycardia and heart block
Pericarditis
Intracardiac thrombus

well-preserved left ventricular function. The benefits of an ACE inhibitor may be additional to those of a β-blocker.

- Verapamil and diltiazem produce a small reduction in late mortality after myocardial infarction but may be detrimental in patients who have had symptoms or signs of heart failure. These drugs should only be considered as an option for high-risk patients who cannot tolerate a β-adrenoceptor antagonist and who do not have significant left ventricular dysfunction. Nifedipine and similar Ca^{2+} antagonists do not improve prognosis after myocardial infarction.

- Prophylactic anticoagulation with subcutaneous heparin (Ch. 11) can prevent deep vein thrombosis, but most patients are mobilised quickly after a myocardial infarct and do not need this. Long-term anticoagulation with warfarin (Ch. 11) reduces mortality and reinfarction to a similar extent to low-dose aspirin. It is used for high-risk patients who are unable to tolerate aspirin.

- Cholesterol reduction to <5.0 mmol l^{-1} should be attempted in all patients initially by diet. If dietary measures are inadequate, cholesterol-lowering drugs, especially the statins (Ch. 48), reduce reinfarctions and cardiac deaths by 25–30%.

FURTHER READING

American College of Cardiology/American Heart Association (1999) Update: ACC/AHA guidelines for the management of patients with acute myocardial infarction: executive summary and recommendations. *Circulation* 100, 1016–1030.

Anthonio RL, van Veldhuisen DJ, van Gilst WH (1998) Left ventricular dilatation after myocardial infarction: ACE inhibitors, β-adrenoceptor antagonists, or both? *J Cardiovasc Pharmacol* 32(suppl 1), S1–58

Bhatt DL, Topol EJ (2000) Current role of platelet glycoprotein IIb/IIIa inhibitors in acute coronary syndromes. *JAMA* 284, 1549–1558

Boermsa E, Steyerberg EW, van der Vlugt MJ et al. (1998) Reperfusion therapy for acute myocardial infarctions. *Drugs* 56, 31–48

Collins R, Peto R, Baigent C et al. (1997) Aspirin, heparin and fibrinolytic therapy in suspected acute myocardial infarction. *N Engl J Med* 336, 847–860

Fibrinolytic Therapy Trialists Collaborative Group (1994) Indications for fibrinolytic therapy in suspected acute myocardial infarction: collaborative overview of early mortality and major morbidity results from all randomised trials of more than 1000 patients. *Lancet* 343, 311–322

Gottlieb SS, McCarter RJ, Vogel RA (1998) Effect of beta-blockade on mortality among high-risk and low-risk patients after myocardial infarction. *N Engl J Med* 339, 489–497

Maynard SJ, Scott GO, Riddell JW et al. (2000) Management of acute coronary syndromes. *Br Med J* 321, 220–223

Teo KK, Yusuf S, Furburg CD (1994) Effects of prophylactic antiarrhythmic drug therapy in acute myocardial infarction. An overview of results from randomised controlled trials. *JAMA* 270, 1589–1595

The Heart Outcomes Evaluation Study Investigators (2000) Effects of an angiotensin-converting enzyme inhibitor, ramipril, on cardiovascular events in high-risk patients. *N Engl J Med* 342, 145–153

The Task Force on the Management of Acute Myocardial Infarction of the European Society of Cardiology (1996) Acute myocardial infarction: pre-hospital and in-hospital management. *Eur Heart J* 17, 43–63.

Unstable angina

Eikelboom JW, Anand SS, Malmberg K (2000) Unfractionated heparin and low molecular weight heparin in acute coronary syndrome without ST elevation: meta analysis. *Lancet* 355, 1936–1942

Heeschen C, Hamm CW, Goldmann B et al. (1999) Troponin concentrations for stratification of patients with acute coronary syndromes in relation to therapeutic efficacy of tirofiban. *Lancet* 354, 1757–1762

Manhapra A, Borzak S (2000) Treatment possibilities for unstable angina. *Br Med J* 321, 1269–1275

Oler A, Whooley MA, Oler J, Grady D (1996) Adding heparin to aspirin reduces the incidence of myocardial infarction and death in patients with unstable angina: a meta-analysis. *JAMA* 276, 811–815

Steeds RP, Channer KS (1998) Recent advances in the management of unstable angina and non-Q-wave myocardial infarction. *Br J Clin Pharmacol* 46, 335–341

Yeghiazarians Y, Braunstein JB, Askari A, Stone PH (2000) Unstable angina pectoris. *N Engl J Med* 342, 101–114

Stable angina

North of England Stable Angina Guideline Development Group (1996) North of England evidence based guidelines development project: summary version of evidence based guideline for the primary care management of stable angina. *Br Med J* 312, 827–832

Glasser SP (1999) Prospects for therapy of nitrate tolerance. *Lancet* 353, 1545–1546

Heidenreich PA, McDonald KM, Haslie T et al. (1999) Meta-analysis of trials comparing β-blockers, calcium antagonists and nitrates for stable angina. *JAMA* 281, 1927–1936

Self-assessment

1. In the following questions the first statement, in italics, is true. Is the accompanying statement also true?

   a. *The mechanism by which glyceryl trinitrate causes vasodilation is through its ability to release nitric oxide.* Nitric oxide causes vasodilatation by increasing cAMP synthesis in vascular smooth muscle cells.

   b. *Glyceryl trinitrate has a more rapid onset of action when given sublingually than when given by a transdermal patch.* Transdermal absorption of glyceryl trinitrate from a patch avoids first-pass metabolism.

   c. *The increased oxygen demand of a rise in workload in the heart is met by an elevation in coronary blood flow.* In angina, glyceryl trinitrate increases total coronary blood flow.

   d. *Glyceryl trinitrate can be safely administered with a β-blocker.* The benefit of glyceryl trinitrate in angina is only a result of its effect on coronary arteries.

   e. *Tissue type plasminogen activator (rt-PA) is an endogenous fibrinolytic agent.* rt-PA inhibits the formation of plasmin.

2. Case history

   TK, a 45-year-old male, long-distance lorry driver, had been having episodes of chest pain that he likened to indigestion. They were brought on by moderately strenuous exercise and relieved by rest but were not relieved by antacids. They had been present for approximately 1 year but recently the frequency and intensity of the pains had become worse and they were now occurring several times a week. He was hypertensive and his serum cholesterol level was 6.6 mmol l^{-1}. He smoked 40 cigarettes/day and was overweight. He drank about 10 units of alcohol a week. He performed well on an exercise test but his exercise ECG showed anterolateral ST segment depression at peak exercise. There was no evidence of heart failure. A diagnosis of angina was made.

   a. How could his acute attacks of angina be treated?

   b. The frequency of his attacks required prophylactic treatment. What options are available to reduce the frequency of anginal attacks?

   c. What other drugs are likely to be useful to improve his prognosis?

   d. Are life-style changes likely to help in this patient?

   e. If TK was an 80 year old, what additional precautions should you consider when prescribing his medication?

   f. In unstable angina, which drug treatments are likely to reduce the progression of the episodes to myocardial infarction or sudden death?

   Despite continuing medication, 6 months later TK awoke with severe chest pains and dyspnoea that was not relieved by glyceryl trinitrate. Examination, biochemical tests and ECG recordings all led to the diagnosis of an acute myocardial infarction.

   g. What is the likely cause of the myocardial infarction?

   h. Why is it important to give thrombolytic therapy as quickly as possible?

   i. TK was given the thrombolytic agent recombinant tissue type plasminogen activator (rt-PA) because of fears that he would get an allergic response to streptokinase. Was this justified?

   j. He was given 150 mg aspirin orally. Does this have any benefit if thrombolytic therapy is also given?

   k. The normal therapeutic dose of aspirin for headache is about 650 mg. Why was the dose given to TK so small?

   l. Consideration was given to administering intravenous heparin to TK but this was considered unnecessary because he had been given rt-PA. Was this decision correct?

   m. Following his myocardial infarction, TK had clinical evidence of heart failure and the long-term prophylactic treatment of his condition was considered. Which of the following drugs are likely to be of benefit: low-dose aspirin, a β-blocker, an ACE inhibitor, verapamil or diltiazem, warfarin?

   The answers are provided on pages 601–602.

Drugs used to treat ischaemic heart disease

Drug	Half-life (h)	Elimination	Comments
Calcium channel antagonists			
Dihydropyridines			Metabolites are generally active
Amlodipine	30–60	Metabolism	No detrimental effect in heart failure; oral bioavailability is 60–80%; oxidised in liver
Felodipine	12–25 (only MR available)	Metabolism	No detrimental effect in heart failure; oral bioavailability is about 15% owing to first-pass metabolism; oxidised by CYP3A4
Isradapine	2–6	Metabolism	Oral bioavailability is 20% owing to first-pass metabolism
Lacidipine	7–8	Metabolism	Low and variable oral bioavailability (4–52%) (common to many dihydropyridines owing to variable intestinal and hepatic CYP3A4 activity)
Lercanidipine	2–5	Metabolism	Recent compound; few published data available; long duration of action despite short plasma half-life
Nicardipine	1–12 (MR available)	Metabolism	Bioavailability is dose dependent owing to first-pass metabolism (5–10% at low doses and 30–45% at high doses); metabolised in liver
Nifedipine	2–4 (MR available)	Metabolism	Oral bioavailability is about 40% owing to first-pass metabolism by CYP3A4 in gut wall and liver
Nimodipine	8–9	Metabolism	Selective for cerebral arteries; used for subarachnoid haemorrhage; given orally or by intravenous infusion; oral bioavailability is 5–10%; eliminated by oxidation in the liver
Nisoldipine	2–4 (only MR available)	Metabolism	Oral bioavailability is low (5–10%) and variable owing to intestinal and hepatic CYP3A4 metabolism; numerous metabolites
Non-dihydropyridines			
Diltiazem	2–5 (MR available)	Metabolism	Reduces heart rate; some negative inotropic effect; oral bioavailability is about 50% owing to first-pass metabolism; a number of metabolites, mostly inactive
Verapamil	2–5 (MR available)	Metabolism	Reduces heart rate; marked negative inotropic effect; given orally or by slow intravenous injection (over 2 min); oral bioavailability is about 20% owing to first-pass metabolism; oxidised by CYP3A4; metabolites retain activity but are rapidly eliminated by conjugation; half-life is longer after chronic dosing (5–12 h)
Nitrates			
Glyceryl trinitrate (nitroglycerin)	1–3 min	Metabolism	Given sublingually, bucally, topically or as an intravenous infusion; essentially complete first-pass metabolism if swallowed; the dinitrate metabolites have 10% of the activity but half-lives of about 40 min
Isosorbide dinitrate	0.5–2	Metabolism	Given sublingually, orally (as normal or MR tablets), topically or by intravenous infusion; low bioavailability from sublingual (30–60%) and topical (10–30%); the active mononitrate metabolite inhibits clearance of the dinitrate during chronic treatment
Isosorbide mononitrate	3–7	Metabolism	Given orally; bioavailability approaches 100%; metabolised by denitration and glucuronide conjugation
Potassium channel activators			
Nicorandil	1	Metabolism	Given orally; essentially complete bioavailability; oxidised and denitrated in the liver; tolerance not a problem. Biological effect much longer than predicted by half-life

Beta-blockers – see Drug compendium table in Chapter 8

MR, modified release.

[a]All calcium channel antagonists are given orally unless stated otherwise. Indications include angina, hypertension, Raynaud's phenomenon, arrhythmias and subarachnoid haemorrhage (see Chs 6, 8–10).

Hypertension

Circulatory reflexes and the control of blood pressure

Systemic blood pressure is determined by the cardiac output and by peripheral resistance. It is maintained within fairly narrow limits by a series of physiological reflexes that respond to both acute and chronic changes in blood pressure. The two most important regulatory systems are:

- the sympathetic nervous system
- the renin–angiotensin–aldosterone system

A sudden change in systemic blood pressure is detected by baroreceptors in the aorta and carotid arteries. Afferent impulses from baroreceptors are integrated in the vasomotor centres of the sympathetic nervous system (Fig. 6.1). A rise in blood pressure increases the input of impulses from the baroreceptors to the vasomotor centre, resulting in decreased output from the

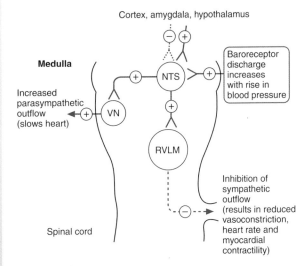

Fig. 6.1
The role of baroreceptors. Increased discharge from the baroreceptors results from stretch caused by increased blood pressure. This results both in a compensatory decrease in sympathetic outflow from the medulla and an increase in the vagal outflow. Both effects reduce peripheral resistance and are mimicked by centrally acting drugs that lower blood pressure (Fig. 6.10). NTS, nucleus of the tractus solitarius; VN, vagal nucleus (cardioinhibitory centre); RVLM, rostral ventrolateral medulla; +, stimulation; –, inhibition.

centre and a compensatory decrease in the efferent response of sympathetic nervous stimulation. Sympathetic efferents to the heart act mainly through β_1-adrenoceptors to increase myocardial contractility and heart rate, generating a greater cardiac output (Ch. 4). Efferents to arterial resistance vessels stimulate postsynaptic α_1-adrenoceptors, producing arteriolar vasoconstriction. This raises blood pressure and redistributes blood flow to specific vascular beds to maintain perfusion of vital organs. This redistribution is helped by β_2-adrenoceptor-mediated vasodilation in selected vascular beds, such as skeletal muscle. Arterial vasoconstriction produces an increase in afterload on the heart but cardiac output is maintained by an increase in cardiac contractility. Stimulation of postsynaptic venous α_1-adrenoceptors constricts venous capacitance vessels. This increases venous return to the heart (preload) and improves cardiac output (Fig. 6.2). If ventricular function is impaired cardiac output may fall (Fig. 7.1).

A slower compensatory mechanism to overcome reduction in blood pressure is initiated by release of renin from the juxtaglomerular apparatus of the kidney (Fig. 6.3). The major stimuli leading to renin release are reduced renal blood flow (often as a result of a decrease in blood pressure), excess Na^+ in the distal renal tubule and direct sympathetic stimulation via β_1-adrenoceptors at the juxtaglomerular apparatus.

Renin is a protease that acts on circulating renin substrate (angiotensinogen) to release the decapeptide angiotensin I. This in turn is cleaved by angiotensin-converting enzyme (ACE) to release the octapeptide angiotensin II. Angiotensin II is a potent vasoconstrictor that also enhances sympathetic nervous tone by an effect on presynaptic neurons. It has a number of additional properties, which can alter salt and water balance (Fig. 6.3). It also promotes the release of aldosterone from the adrenal cortex, which acts at the distal renal

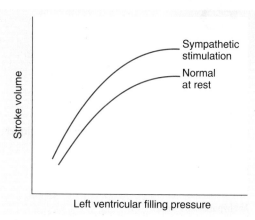

Fig. 6.2
The Frank–Starling phenomenon. The relationship between preload (left ventricular filling pressure) and stroke volume at different states of myocardial contractility.

tubule to conserve salt and water at the expense of K^+ loss (Ch. 14). Thus angiotensin II and aldosterone raise blood pressure by vasoconstriction and by increasing circulating blood volume.

The integration of the sympathetic nervous system and renin–angiotensin–aldosterone responses to a fall in blood pressure is shown in Figure 6.4. These mechanisms prevent hypotension due to peripheral pooling of blood on standing and during exercise.

Additional control mechanisms involved in the regulation of vascular tone and circulating blood volume include circulating or local hormones and metabolites such as atrial natriuretic peptide, prostaglandins, kinins, nitric oxide, endothelin and adenosine (Fig. 6.5). Their relative importance may differ in health and disease states.

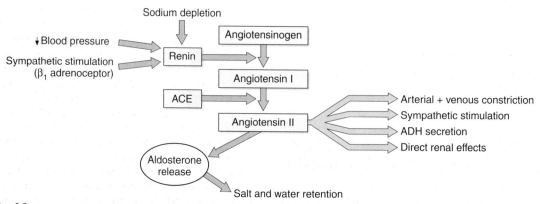

Fig. 6.3
Formation and actions of angiotensin II. ADH, antidiuretic hormone; ACE, angiotensin-converting enzyme.

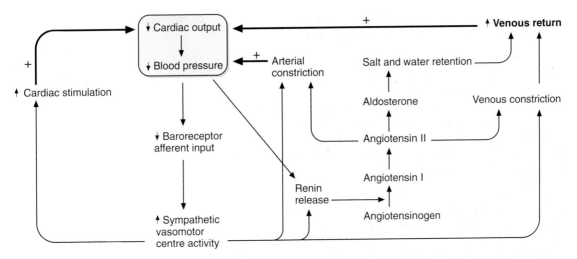

Fig. 6.4
The control of blood pressure via the sympathetic and angiotensin/aldosterone cascades. The integrated physiological compensatory mechanisms are shown in response to a fall in cardiac output or blood pressure. The sympathetic mediated responses on the left of the diagram are rapidly responding events whereas the angiotensin/aldosterone events are more slowly responding. The final outcomes are increased venous return, increased arterial constriction and increased cardiac stimulation. Events that may be important at the level of the endothelium are shown in Fig. 6.5.

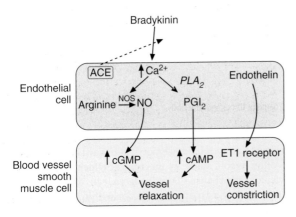

Fig. 6.5
The endothelial cell is an important site of production of vasoactive substances and enzymes that metabolise vasoactive substances. Both can be affected by many natural hormones and drugs, facilitating constriction or dilatation. An example with potential clinical importance is bradykinin, which generates increased endothelial nitric oxide (NO) and the prostaglandin (PGI$_2$, prostacyclin). The endothelial cell also contains angiotensin-converting enzyme (ACE), which breaks down bradykinin to inactive peptides. This is reduced by ACE inhibitor drugs, amplifying the effects of bradykinin on the synthesis of endothelial vasodilators. Endothelin is a potent vasoconstrictor of potential but as yet unrealised clinical importance. Other substances such as adenosine also cause vasodilatation. ET1, endothelin type 1 receptor; NOS, nitric oxide synthase; PLA$_2$, phospholipase A$_2$.

Hypertension

Hypertension is a common condition found in 20–30% of the population of the developed world. It is usually asymptomatic but produces progressive structural changes in the heart and circulation. These predispose to clinical complications that are often referred to as 'target organ damage'. The principal complications of hypertension are ischaemic heart disease, which is twice as frequent as in normotensives, and cerebrovascular disease, which usually presents as thromboembolic stroke or, less commonly, as cerebral haemorrhage. Such consequences are more common if hypertension is accompanied by hypercholesterolaemia and smoking. The underlying vascular lesions that occur in hypertension and their resulting complications, which together constitute target organ damage, are shown in Figure 6.6.

Sustained hypertension predisposes to hypertrophy of the muscle of the left ventricle (LVH). LVH is an independent risk factor for the complications of hypertension, particularly ischaemic heart disease (since the muscle outgrows its blood supply), diastolic heart failure (see Ch. 8) and arrhythmias leading to sudden death.

There is no absolute cut-off between normal and high blood pressure. Blood pressure in all populations is 'normally' distributed with a slight skew because of a small number of individuals with very high blood pressures. Defining a point at which blood pressure is 'high' is, therefore, somewhat arbitrary. A widely accepted view is that hypertension exists if the blood pressure is maintained at a level above which treatment has been shown to reduce the risk of developing complications. Using this criterion, hypertension exists in individuals below the age of 65 years if the diastolic blood pressure is sustained above 100 mmHg. Between the ages of 65 and 80 years, it exists if the diastolic blood pressure is above 90 mmHg and/or the systolic pressure is above 160 mmHg. The higher 'acceptable' blood pressure in younger people reflects the lower absolute risk of complication in this age

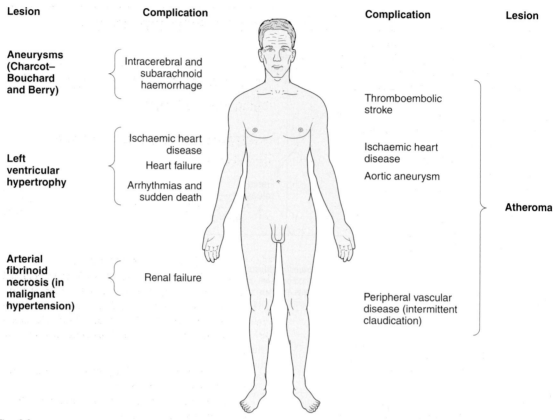

Lesion	Complication		Complication	Lesion

Aneurysms (Charcot–Bouchard and Berry) — Intracerebral and subarachnoid haemorrhage

Left ventricular hypertrophy — Ischaemic heart disease / Heart failure / Arrhythmias and sudden death

Arterial fibrinoid necrosis (in malignant hypertension) — Renal failure

Thromboembolic stroke

Ischaemic heart disease

Aortic aneurysm

Peripheral vascular disease (intermittent claudication)

Atheroma

Fig. 6.6
Complications of hypertension. Hypertension causes vascular lesions and damage throughout the body.

group. However, once complications are present, treatment at a lower level of blood pressure becomes desirable. In those over 80 years of age who develop high blood pressure for the first time without evidence of complications, a higher diastolic pressure, perhaps up to 110 mmHg, may be acceptable but this still requires evaluation in clinical trials.

The diagnosis of sustained hypertension requires at least three, and preferably more, blood pressure readings over several weeks, unless target organ damage gives a clear indication that treatment is necessary. Some patients are only hypertensive when the measurement is taken by a doctor or, to a lesser extent, by a nurse. This phenomenon is termed 'white coat' hypertension and appears to carry little risk of complications over the next few years. It can usually be detected either by repeated blood pressure readings (which gradually approach the normal range), by measuring the blood pressure at home, or with an ambulatory 24-h blood pressure recorder. 'White coat' hypertension often persists despite drug treatment, even though the patient can become quite hypotensive away from the surgery or clinic.

Malignant or accelerated hypertension is an infrequently encountered condition characterised by arterial fibrinoid necrosis. It is identified clinically by the presence of flame-shaped haemorrhages, hard exudates, and 'cotton wool' spots in the retina, which can lead to visual disturbance. Papilloedema can also occur. If untreated, most patients will die within 2 years from renal failure, heart failure or stroke.

Aetiology and pathogenesis of hypertension

In most hypertensive patients, the blood pressure is high as a result of increased peripheral arterial resistance, which arises from arteriolar smooth muscle constriction and hypertrophy of the arteriolar wall. The cause of the inappropriately raised peripheral resistance is unknown in the majority, who are said to have 'essential' hypertension. This condition probably has a polygenic inheritance, leading to several clinical subtypes with different underlying pathogenic mechanisms. It is believed that the genetic influences predispose to intracellular Ca^{2+} overload, which enhances vascular smooth muscle contractility. The genetic influence may be directly on Ca^{2+} transport or indirectly via disturbance of the movement of other ions across the cell membrane.

Environmental influences and factors such as diet, level of exercise, obesity and alcohol intake all interact with the genetic programming to determine the final level of blood pressure. A secondary underlying cause of the high blood pressure, often renal or endocrinological, can be identified in about 5% of hypertensive patients (Table 6.1).

Not surprisingly, since the cause of hypertension is unclear, treatment cannot be directed at the underlying mechanisms. Most antihypertensive drugs are vaso-dilators. They often modulate the natural hormonal or neuronal mechanisms responsible for blood pressure regulation, while others act directly on the blood vessel wall. Less commonly, the hypotensive action is achieved by reducing cardiac output. The principal classes of antihypertensive drug and their sites of action are shown in Table 6.2 and Figure 6.7.

Antihypertensive drugs

Drugs acting on the sympathetic nervous system

Beta-adrenoceptor antagonists (β-blockers)

Examples: atenolol, propranolol, pindolol

Mechanism of action in hypertension

The hypotensive action of the β-blockers is believed to have several components (Fig. 6.8). Selective β_1-adrenoceptor blockers are as effective as non-selective drugs, indicating that β_2-adrenoceptor blockade makes little contribution. The more important actions are probably:

- reduction of heart rate and myocardial contractility, which decrease cardiac output.
- blockade of renal juxtaglomerular β_1-adrenoceptors, which reduces renin secretion.
- peripheral vasodilatation, produced by compounds with β_2-adrenoceptor partial agonist activity, for example pindolol
- blockade of presynaptic β-adrenoceptors in sympathetic nerves supplying arteriolar resistance vessels may reduce the outflow of noradrenaline, but the importance of this is clinically uncertain.

Table 6.1
Principal causes of secondary hypertension

	Causes
Renal	Renal artery stenosis, glomerulonephritis, interstitial nephritis, arteritis, polycystic disease, chronic pyelonephritis
Endocrine	Conn's syndrome (aldosterone excess), Cushing's syndrome (glucocorticoid excess), phaeochromocytoma (catecholamine excess), acromegaly
Pregnancy	Pre-eclampsia and eclampsia
Drugs	Oestrogen, corticosteroids, non-steroidal anti-inflammatory drugs (NSAIDs), cyclosporin

Table 6.2
Principal classes of antihypertensive drugs and their sites of action

Sites of action	Drugs
Sympathetic nervous system	β-Adrenoceptor antagonists (β-blockers)
	α_1-Adrenoceptor antagonists (α_1-blockers)
	Selective imidazoline receptor agonists
	Centrally acting α_2-adrenoceptor agonists[a]
	Adrenergic neuron blockers[a]
	Ganglion blockers[a]
Hormonal control (renin–angiotensin system)	Angiotensin-converting enzyme (ACE) inhibitors
	Angiotensin II receptor antagonists
Vasodilation by other mechanisms	Diuretics
	Calcium channel antagonists
	Potassium channel activators
	Nitrovasodilators[a]

[a]Obsolescent drug or with limited use.

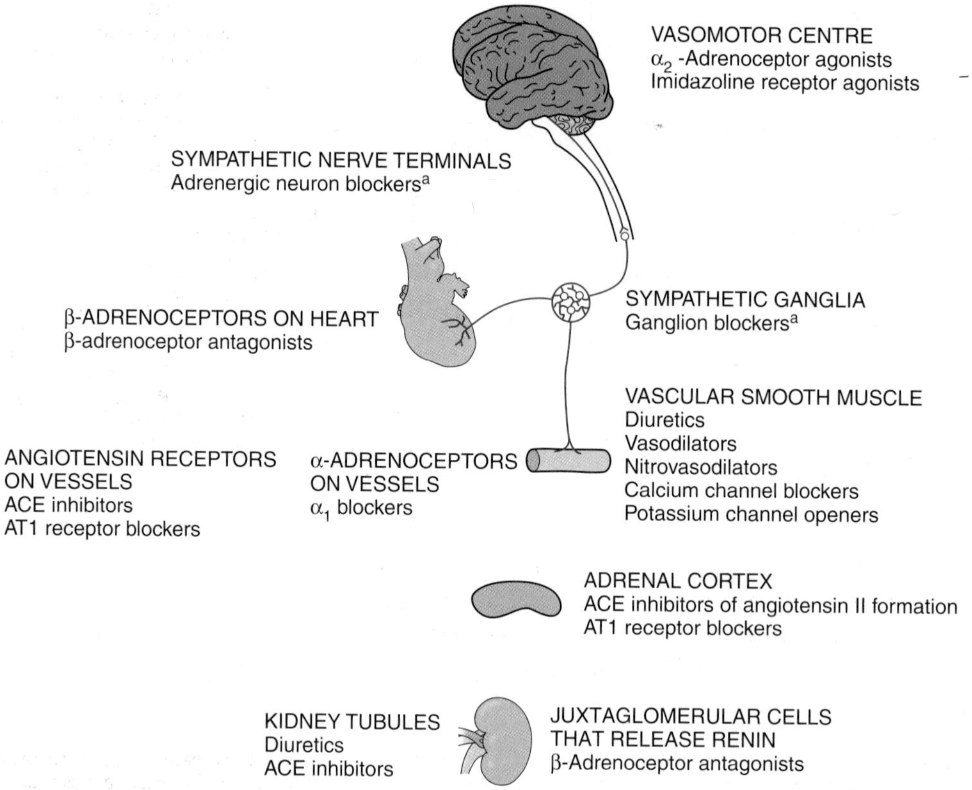

VASOMOTOR CENTRE
α_2-Adrenoceptor agonists
Imidazoline receptor agonists

SYMPATHETIC NERVE TERMINALS
Adrenergic neuron blockers[a]

SYMPATHETIC GANGLIA
Ganglion blockers[a]

β-ADRENOCEPTORS ON HEART
β-adrenoceptor antagonists

VASCULAR SMOOTH MUSCLE
Diuretics
Vasodilators
Nitrovasodilators
Calcium channel blockers
Potassium channel openers

ANGIOTENSIN RECEPTORS
ON VESSELS
ACE inhibitors
AT1 receptor blockers

α-ADRENOCEPTORS
ON VESSELS
α_1 blockers

ADRENAL CORTEX
ACE inhibitors of angiotensin II formation
AT1 receptor blockers

KIDNEY TUBULES
Diuretics
ACE inhibitors

JUXTAGLOMERULAR CELLS
THAT RELEASE RENIN
β-Adrenoceptor antagonists

Fig. 6.7
The classes of antihypertensive drug and their sites of action. [a]Classes of drug that are rarely used now; ACE, angiotensin-converting enzyme.

For further details about β-blockers, see Chapters 4 and 5 and Box 6.1.

Box 6.1

Clinical uses of β-blockers

Treatment of hypertension (this chapter)
Prophylaxis of angina (Ch. 5)
Secondary prevention after myocardial infarction (Ch. 5)
Prevention and treatment of arrhythmias (Ch. 8)
Control of symptoms in thyrotoxicosis (Ch. 41)
Alleviation of symptoms in anxiety (Ch. 20)
Prophylaxis of migraine (Ch. 26)
Topically for treatment of glaucoma (Ch. 50)

Alpha-adrenoceptor antagonists (α-blockers)

Examples:
α_1-selective: prazosin, doxazosin
non-selective: phenoxybenzamine

Mechanisms of action

Blockade of postsynaptic α_1-adrenoceptors lowers blood pressure by:

- reducing tone in arteriolar resistance vessels
- dilating venous capacitance vessels, which reduces venous return and, therefore, cardiac output.

The fall in blood pressure is detected by arterial baroreceptors, which initiate reflex sympathetic stimulation. Selective α_1-adrenoceptor antagonists do not block the inhibitory presynaptic α_2-adrenoceptors on sympathetic nerve terminals. Therefore, neurotransmitter released in response to this reflex sets up a negative feedback via these α_2-adrenoceptors to blunt the expected reflex tachycardia (Fig. 6.9).

Since non-selective α-blockers act at the presynaptic α_2-adrenoceptors and block this negative feedback, their use is accompanied by a marked reflex tachycardia. They now have little place in clinical practice except for the perioperative management of phaeochromocytoma.

Alpha-blockers produce a potentially beneficial effect on plasma lipids; they increase high density lipoprotein cholesterol and reduce triglycerides. The importance of this for the prevention of atheroma in hypertensive patients is uncertain (Ch. 48).

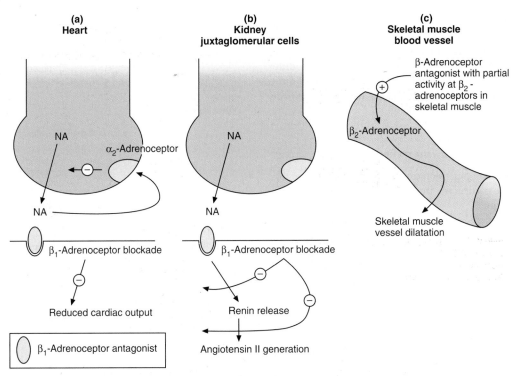

Fig. 6.8
Sites of action of the β-adrenoceptor antagonists (β-blockers) relevant to their use as antihypertensive agents. (a) In the heart, the β_1-adrenoceptor-blocking drugs reduce noradrenaline- and adrenaline-induced stimulation of the β_1-adrenoceptors. The presynaptic stimulation of α_2-adrenoceptors, which inhibit noradrenaline release, still functions normally. (b) In the kidney, β_1-adrenoceptor blockade reduces the activity of the angiotensin II system. (c) Some β-adrenoceptor blockers (e.g. pindolol) have partial agonist activity and stimulate the β_2-adrenoceptors in skeletal muscle blood vessels, which leads to vasodilatation and a lowering of peripheral resistance. These drugs reduce heart rate and cardiac output less than those without partial agonist properties. NA, noradrenaline.

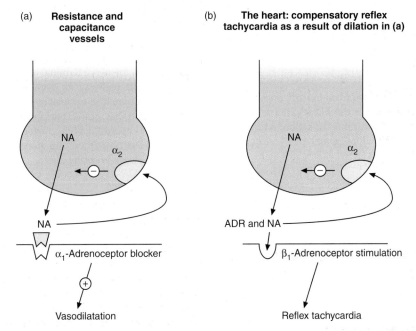

Fig. 6.9
Effect of α_1-adrenoceptor selective blockade and consequent reflex tachycardia. (a) Selective blockade of α_1-adrenoceptors in arteriolar resistance and venous capacitance vessels lowers blood pressure and results in reflex tachycardia. (b) The reflex tachycardia is blunted because the presynaptic α_2-adrenoceptors are free, reducing noradrenaline (NA) release.

Pharmacokinetics

Selective α_1-blockers are well absorbed from the gut and undergo extensive first-pass metabolism and subsequent elimination in the liver. The compounds differ principally in their plasma half-life and therefore duration of action, for example prazosin has a short half-life, while that of doxazosin is long.

Unwanted effects

There are several unwanted effects:

- postural hypotension caused by venous pooling; this can be particularly troublesome after the first dose
- lethargy
- palpitations owing to reflex cardiac stimulation; these occur more commonly with non-selective drugs.

Selective imidazoline receptor agonists

Example: moxonidine

Mechanism of action

Imidazoline I_1 receptors are important for regulation of sympathetic drive. They are concentrated in the rostral ventrolateral medulla, a part of the brainstem vasomotor centre. Increased neuronal activity in this area, either through baroreceptor stimulation or by direct stimulation of I_1 receptors, will decrease sympathetic outflow and increase vagal tone (Fig. 6.10). The result is a fall in blood pressure with no reflex tachycardia. Unlike other centrally acting drugs (clonidine and methyldopa), moxonidine has little affinity for α_2-adrenoceptors.

Pharmacokinetics

Moxonidine is well absorbed from the gut, and its principal route of elimination is the kidney. It has a short half-life but a prolonged duration of action, which may reflect its high affinity for I_1 receptors.

Unwanted effects

Unwanted effects include:

- dry mouth
- fatigue
- dizziness.

Centrally acting α_2-adrenoceptor agonists

Examples: methyldopa, clonidine

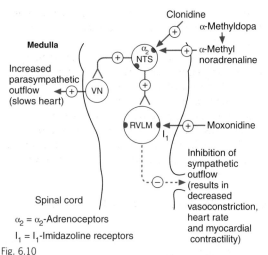

Fig. 6.10
Mechanisms of centrally acting drugs in the control of blood pressure. α-Methyldopa and moxonidine mimic the responses of the medulla to raised blood pressure by stimulating α_2-adrenoceptors in the nucleus of the tractus solitarius (NTS) or imidazoline receptors (perhaps also a subtype of α-adrenoceptor) in the rostral ventrolateral medulla (RVLM). VN, vagal nucleus (cardioinhibitory centre).

Unwanted effects limit the use of the centrally acting α_2-agonists, although methyldopa is a drug of choice in the treatment of hypertension in pregnancy (see below).

Mechanisms of action

The α_2-agonists reduce central sympathetic nervous outflow from the vasomotor centre (Fig. 6.10), which reduces both peripheral arterial and venous tone.

Methyldopa and clonidine stimulate central presynaptic α_2-adrenoceptors, which inhibits neurotransmitter release by negative feedback. Clonidine is a direct-acting α_2-adrenoceptor agonist, which also acts at imidazoline I_2 receptors (see above); methyldopa is first metabolised in the nerve terminal as a 'false substrate' in the biosynthetic pathway for noradrenaline to produce α-methylnoradrenaline, a potent α_2-adrenoceptor agonist. Clonidine also has some peripheral postsynaptic α-adrenoceptor agonist activity, which produces direct peripheral vasoconstriction; this initially offsets some of the blood pressure-lowering effect.

Pharmacokinetics

Methyldopa is incompletely absorbed from the gut and undergoes dose-dependent first-pass metabolism to an inactive sulfate conjugate. The half-life is short.

Clonidine is completely absorbed from the gut and is eliminated partly by the kidney and partly by liver metabolism. It has a long half-life.

Unwanted effects

Unwanted effects include:

- sympathetic blockade: failure of ejaculation and postural or exertional hypotension (unusual with clonidine owing to its direct peripheral action)

- unopposed parasympathetic action: nasal stuffiness (unusual with methyldopa), diarrhoea
- dry mouth
- central nervous system (CNS) effects: sedation and drowsiness occur in up to 50% of patients; depression is occasionally seen
- methyldopa induces a reversible positive Coombs' test, owing to IgG production, in up to 20% of patients; haemolytic anaemia, however, is rare
- sudden withdrawal of clonidine can produce severe rebound hypertension with tachycardia, sweating and anxiety.

Adrenergic neuron blockers

Example: debrisoquine

The adrenergic neuron blockers are rarely used because of their unwanted effects, but they are included for completeness.

Mechanism of action
Adrenergic neuron blockers use the active transport mechanism for monoamines (uptake 1) to accumulate in the adrenergic nerve terminal (Ch. 4). Inside the cell, they prevent the release of noradrenaline from vesicles by interfering with Ca^{2+} responses to the nerve action potential. The inhibition of adrenergic neuron activity produces arterial and venous dilatation and a relatively constant heart rate.

Pharmacokinetics
Debrisoquine is fairly well absorbed and undergoes extensive hepatic metabolism by hydroxylation through the enzyme CYP2D6. About 8% of the UK population have genetically determined low levels of CYP2D6 (Ch. 2) and show decreased metabolism of the drug, which greatly increases the clinical response. Platelet uptake leads to slow elimination and a long half-life.

Unwanted effects
Unwanted effects include:

- blockade of sympathetic neurons: venous pooling produces troublesome postural and exertional hypotension; inhibition of ejaculation
- unopposed parasympathetic actions: increased intestinal secretions with diarrhoea; nasal stuffiness
- fluid retention.

Ganglion blockers

Example: trimetaphan

Ganglion blockers are obsolete except for certain highly specialised indications such as during surgery.

Mechanism of action
Competitive blockade of nicotinic (N_1) receptors at autonomic ganglia reduces activity in both the sympathetic and parasympathetic nervous systems (Ch. 4). Arterial and venous dilatation both contribute to the hypotensive effects.

Pharmacokinetics
Trimetaphan is rapidly metabolised in the liver and has a duration of action of only a few minutes. It is given by intravenous infusion or intermittent injection for controlled hypotension during surgery.

Unwanted effects
Unwanted effects are of little importance during brief intravenous administration:

- blockade of sympathetic outflow: postural hypotension, inhibition of ejaculation
- blockade of parasympathetic outflow: dry mouth, constipation, urinary retention, blurred vision, impotence.

....

Drugs affecting the renin–angiotensin system

Angiotensin-converting enzyme (ACE) inhibitors

Examples: captopril, enalapril

Mechanisms of action
The ACE inhibitors act by several mechanisms.

- Competitive inhibition of ACE reduces generation of angiotensin II and consequently reduces the release of aldosterone (Fig. 6.11). Inhibition of tissue ACE in the vascular wall (rather than plasma ACE) is most important for the hypotensive effect of these drugs (Fig. 6.11). Reduced tissue concentrations of angiotensin II leads to arterial and, to a lesser extent, venous dilation.
- Lack of a reflex tachycardia may be because of stimulation of the vagus nerve or because of reduced potentiation of sympathetic nervous activity by angiotensin II (Fig. 6.3).
- Angiotensin II is also implicated in the development of arterial and left ventricular hypertrophy in

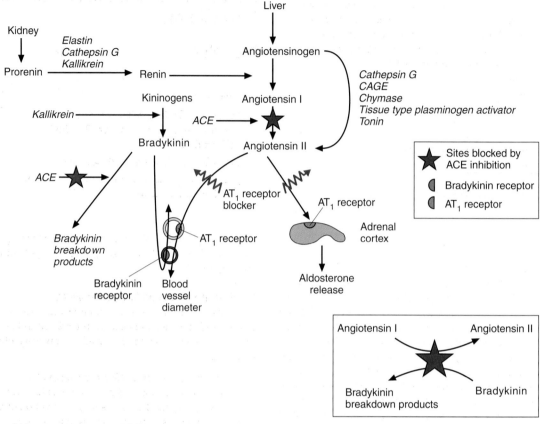

Fig. 6.11
The biological actions of bradykinin and angiotensin II and drugs that modify these actions. Bradykinin causes vasodilatation by acting on vascular smooth muscle and on the endothelial cell (Fig. 6.5). Angiotensin II causes vasoconstriction by stimulating AT$_1$ receptors in the blood vessels and causes Na$^+$ retention by stimulating AT$_1$ receptors in the adrenal cortex, which results in aldosterone release. Angiotensin-converting enzyme (ACE) inhibitors blocks angiotensin II formation from angiotensin I, but an alternative pathway still remains that can result in angiotensin II formation from angiotensinogen. Angiotensin II antagonists such as losartan act by inhibiting AT$_1$ receptors in blood vessels and on the adrenal cortex.

hypertension. The importance of ACE inhibitors compared with other antihypertensives in limiting these effects is uncertain.

● ACE also degrades vasodilator kinins (Fig. 6.11). Increased kinins or vasodilator prostaglandins and nitric oxide in the vascular wall may contribute to the hypotensive actions of ACE inhibitors.

Clinical uses of these drugs are given in Box 6.2.

Box 6.2

Clinical uses of ACE inhibitors

Treatment of hypertension (this chapter)
Treatment of heart failure (Ch. 7)
Secondary prevention after myocardial infarction (Ch. 5)
Diabetic nephropathy in insulin-dependent diabetes (Ch. 40 and this chapter)

Pharmacokinetics

Many ACE inhibitors are water soluble and poorly absorbed from the gut in the active form. These are given as prodrugs, which are converted in the liver to the active agent; for example enalapril is converted to the active compound enalaprilat. Others, for example captopril, are absorbed adequately as an active molecule. For most compounds, the active drug is excreted unchanged by the kidney. The half-life of captopril is short, while that of enalaprilat is intermediate.

Unwanted effects

ACE inhibitors have a number of unwanted effects:

● cough that is unproductive, not dose-related and may be caused by accumulation of kinins in the lung; it occurs in 10–30% of patients, is more common in women and can develop after many months of treatment
● postural hypotension, which is rare unless there is salt and water depletion, for example as a result of

therapy with diuretics; in such patients profound hypotension can occur, particularly after the first dose; this is rarely a problem in the treatment of hypertension, but can be in the treatment of patients with heart failure (Ch. 7)

- disturbance of taste
- rashes
- angioedema.

Angiotensin receptor antagonists

Example: losartan

Mechanism of action

The angiotensin receptor antagonists are selective for the AT_1 receptor subtype, which is found in the heart, blood vessels, kidney, adrenal cortex, lung and brain. They have less effect at a second receptor subtype, known as AT_2, which is believed to be involved in regulation of vascular growth in response to angiotensin II. Reduced generation of the intracellular second messengers diacylglycerol and inositol trisphosphate in target cells is responsible for the actions of these drugs. The effects show similarities to those produced by ACE inhibitors, except that kinin degradation is unaffected by angiotensin II antagonists, and inhibition of the effects of angiotensin II on the AT_1 receptor is more complete (Fig. 6.11).

Pharmacokinetics

Losartan is well absorbed from the gut but has a low oral bioavailability because of first-pass metabolism. It is partially converted to an active metabolite, which is believed to be responsible for most of the pharmacological effect, and to several inactive metabolites. The metabolites are excreted by the kidney. The half-life of losartan is short, while that of the active metabolite is intermediate. Losartan is a competitive AT_1 receptor antagonist, but the active metabolite is a non-competitive antagonist.

Unwanted effects

Drugs in this class are usually well tolerated. Their major advantage over ACE inhibitors is the low incidence of cough. Angioedema is also rare. Effects include:

- headache
- fatigue.

Vasodilators

Diuretics

Examples

thiazide and thiazide-like diuretics: bendroflumethiazide (bendrofluazide), chlortalidone

loop diuretic: furosemide (frusemide)

potassium-sparing diuretics: spironolactone, amiloride, triamterene

Three groups of diuretics are used to lower blood pressure: thiazide (and thiazide-like), loop and potassium-sparing diuretics.

Mechanism of action in hypertension

The sites and mechanisms of action of diuretics on the kidney and unwanted effects are considered in Ch. 14. There are several actions involved in lowering blood pressure.

- An initial hypotensive effect is produced by intravascular salt and water depletion. However, compensatory mechanisms such as activation of the renin–angiotensin–aldosterone system largely restore plasma and extracellular fluid volumes (see Fig. 6.4) (unless salt and water retention was a major component of the initial hypertension, e.g. in advanced renal failure or as a consequence of other antihypertensive treatment).
- Direct arterial dilation is responsible for the longer-term reduction in blood pressure. Vasodilation may result from reduced Ca^{2+} entry into the smooth muscle of the arteriolar resistance vessel walls (perhaps as a consequence of Na^+ depletion) and from synthesis of the vasodilator prostaglandins PGE_2 and PGI_2.

Thiazide and thiazide-like diuretics. These produce their maximum blood pressure-lowering effect at doses lower than those required for significant diuretic effects. This is an advantage since most unwanted effects are dose related.

Loop diuretics. Unless used in a modified-release formulation, loop diuretics are usually less effective hypotensive agents than thiazides in hypertension. Despite having a more powerful diuretic action, their duration of action is too short. However, hypertension with advanced renal impairment, or hypertension resistant to multiple drug treatment, is more likely to be associated with fluid retention and will respond better to a loop diuretic than to a thiazide.

Potassium-sparing diuretics. Spironolactone, a specific aldosterone antagonist, is reserved for hypertension caused by primary hyperaldosteronism (Conn's syndrome) because of concern about its long-term safety (see Ch. 14). Amiloride and triamterene are less effective than thiazides in essential hypertension.

Calcium channel antagonists

> Examples: nifedipine, verapamil, diltiazem

The Ca²⁺ channel antagonists (Ca²⁺ antagonists) lower blood pressure principally by arterial vasodilation. For clinical uses see Box 6.3. For further details see Chapter 5.

Box 6.3

Clinical uses of calcium antagonists

Treatment of hypertension (this chapter)
Prophylaxis of angina (Ch. 5)
Treatment of Raynaud's phenomenon (Ch. 10)
Prevention and treatment of supraventricular arrhythmias (Ch. 8)
Subarachnoid haemorrhage (Ch. 9)

Potassium channel activators

> Example: minoxidil

Mechanism of action
Minoxidil activates cell membrane potassium channels leading to potassium accumulation in the cell and hyperpolarisation of the cell membrane (see also potassium channel activators, Ch. 5). Minoxidil is one of the most powerful peripheral arterial dilators.

Pharmacokinetics
Minoxidil is well absorbed from the gut, and mainly metabolised in the liver. The half-life is short.

Unwanted effects
There are a number of unwanted effects:

- arterial vasodilation produces flushing and headache.
- the reflex sympathetic nervous system response to vasodilation causes tachycardia and palpitation (which can be blunted by concurrent use of β-blockers)
- increased transcapillary pressure can produce oedema, most marked in the ankles

- salt and water retention occur through stimulation of the renin–angiotensin–aldosterone system (Fig. 6.4); this can be reduced by the concurrent use of diuretics
- hirsutism; therefore rarely used for women.

Hydralazine

Mechanism of action
The mechanism of action of hydralazine is uncertain, but it may activate guanylate cyclase leading to the intracellular production of cGMP. This produces relaxation by a mechanism similar to that of organic nitrates (Fig. 6.5 and Ch. 5).

Pharmacokinetics
Hydralazine is well absorbed from the gut then undergoes extensive first-pass metabolism in the gut wall and liver, principally by N-acetylation. Some individuals, who are genetically determined slow acetylators (Ch. 2), require lower doses of hydralazine and are more susceptible to some of the unwanted effects. The half-life of hydralazine is short.

Unwanted effects
Unwanted effects include:

- arterial vasodilation and reflex sympathetic activation (see potassium channel activators above)
- a systemic lupus erythematosus-like syndrome, which usually occurs after several months of treatment, is dose-related and is more common in slow acetylators. It resembles the naturally occurring disease but does not produce renal or cerebral damage and is slowly reversed if treatment is stopped. A positive antinuclear antibody is found in many patients who do not develop the syndrome.

Nitrovasodilators

> Example: nitroprusside

Mechanism of action
Nitroprusside is a nitrovasodilator with a mechanism of action similar to that of organic nitrates (Ch. 5). It produces dilation of arterioles and veins, reducing both peripheral resistance and venous return. Its use is limited to the emergency management of some hypertensive states.

Pharmacokinetics
Nitroprusside is given by intravenous infusion and has a duration of action of less than 5 min. Metabolism to cyanide within red blood cells (by electron transfer from haemoglobin iron) terminates its effect. The cyanide is

partly bound in the erythrocyte and partly liberated, producing inhibition of cellular cytochrome oxidase. Free cyanide is converted in the liver to less toxic thiocyanate. This accumulates with prolonged infusion and, therefore, treatment is usually limited to a maximum of 3 days.

Unwanted effects

Unwanted effects include:

- confusion and psychosis
- metabolic acidosis owing to inhibition of aerobic metabolism in cells
- weakness and nausea caused by thiocyanate accumulation

Treatment of hypertension

The morbidity and premature deaths associated with untreated hypertension are considerable, and increase with advancing age. Treatment of the older hypertensive, therefore, prevents more events in the short term than treating a similar number of younger patients. However, early treatment will prevent vascular damage occurring in the younger hypertensive, an important consideration since the vascular changes are not completely reversible once established.

The optimal target blood pressure is a systolic pressure below 135 mmHg and diastolic pressure (phase V Korotkoff sound) below 85 mmHg. However, even if this cannot be achieved, the progressively greater morbidity associated with higher blood pressures means that any blood pressure reduction in the severely hypertensive patient will be beneficial. Treating isolated systolic hypertension (systolic >160 mmHg, diastolic <90 mmHg) in the elderly gives similar benefits to the treatment of diastolic hypertension in this age group.

It is rarely possible to correct the underlying cause of hypertension. Life-style modification, alone or combined with drug therapy, should be recommended initially to reduce blood pressure, although their effectiveness in preventing complications is unknown. Weight loss, restriction of alcohol and excess salt intake, and increasing exercise may be enough in some mildly hypertensive patients to lower the blood pressure satisfactorily. In more severely hypertensive individuals, these measures can produce a substantial reduction in blood pressure but rarely restore it to normotensive values. It is important to advise all patients not to smoke, since smoking doubles the risk of cardiovascular and cerebrovascular events at any level of blood pressure.

The decision to treat a hypertensive patient with drugs should be largely determined by an assessment of the overall risk of complications in that individual patient. Drug treatment is usually started if blood pressure remains above the levels discussed above despite non-pharmacological approaches. In patients with renal impairment, ischaemic heart disease, diabetes or previous stroke, there is a strong argument for treating patients with lower 'borderline' hypertensive readings to minimise the risk of progressive vascular disease.

Lowering blood pressure with drugs produces a substantial reduction in the risks of stroke, heart failure and kidney damage in patients in all age groups. Drug treatment also reduces coronary artery disease in the elderly, but the evidence for this is less convincing in the young. This may reflect either the short duration of the trials (up to 5 years) or a failure to treat coexisting risk factors such as smoking and hypercholesterolaemia. In most trials, the treatment regimens were based on β-blockers or diuretics. These have shown equal efficacy in younger patients for reducing events but diuretics are superior to β-blockers in the elderly. This may be because β-blockers are relatively poor for lowering blood pressure in the elderly, in whom high vascular resistance is the major pathophysiological cause. More recently, Ca^{2+} antagonists have been shown to have similar efficacy to diuretics, both in the young and in isolated systolic hypertension in the elderly. Many experts believe that evidence-based practice currently supports the use of β-blockers, thiazide diuretics and Ca^{2+} antagonists as first-choice drugs in essential hypertension unless

- they are poorly tolerated
- they are contraindicated
- there is concurrent disease that might benefit from another class of antihypertensive drug.

However, in all the long-term trials, drugs from various other classes were added if blood pressure control was inadequate with the first-choice drug. Therefore, there are advocates for the use of other classes of drug as first-line therapy, particularly ACE inhibitors. This argument is supported by the additional effects of these antihypertensive drugs, including:

- ACE inhibitors and Ca^{2+} antagonists may reverse left ventricular hypertrophy faster than the older agents
- potentially atherogenic changes in plasma lipids are produced by β-blockers and diuretics, but not by the newer drugs.

However, recently published trials have not supported these potential advantages of the newer drug classes in further reducing morbidity and mortality in hypertensive patients.

Drug regimens in hypertension

Treatment of hypertension usually follows a 'stepped care' approach. In mild or moderate hypertension, a single drug will achieve good blood pressure control in about 40% of patients. If the initial choice of drug fails to produce an adequate reduction in blood pressure, then a change in therapy to an alternative first-line drug may be recommended. However, if the fall in blood pressure with the first drug is substantial, but the target pressure is not reached, then the first drug should be continued and a second drug should be added. Examples of complementary drug combinations are

- β-blocker + diuretic
- β-blocker + Ca²⁺ antagonist (NB caution with verapamil)
- ACE inhibitor + diuretic
- ACE inhibitor + Ca²⁺ antagonist.

Most combinations of drugs from different classes will produce at least an additive response. There is some evidence, however, that an ACE inhibitor plus β-blocker, or dihydropyridine Ca²⁺ antagonist plus diuretic are less than additive.

If two drugs fail to control blood pressure, then a third can be added. If this is insufficient, then the patient is said to have 'resistant' hypertension.

Resistant hypertension

There are several possible causes of apparently resistant hypertension. These include:

- poor compliance with prescribed therapy (see Ch. 55)
- 'white coat' hypertension, which responds poorly to drug treatment
- secondary hypertension, usually caused by renal artery stenosis or Conn's syndrome
- other unidentified causes for poor response to drug treatments.

Some patients with resistant hypertension benefit from a loop diuretic, which will help if expansion of the

plasma volume is contributing to drug resistance. In male patients, minoxidil can prove a particularly powerful hypotensive agent, but excess hair growth limits its use for women. In a few individuals treatment with four or even five drugs may be necessary.

Malignant or accelerated hypertension

Early treatment is important for patients with retinal haemorrhages, exudates or papilloedema. Rapid blood pressure reduction is potentially dangerous, since it can lead to cerebral underperfusion and ischaemic damage. Oral atenolol or nifedipine are the most widely recommended treatments, which gradually reduce the blood pressure over 24 hours or more.

Hypertension in special patient groups

There are reasons for selecting particular classes of drugs under certain specific conditions or when concomitant illnesses are present (Table 6.3). Black patients respond less well to β-blockers and ACE inhibitors than Caucasians. Compared with younger patients, the elderly are less likely to achieve good blood pressure control with β-blockers (see above).

Renal artery stenosis

ACE inhibitors usually produce an excellent reduction in blood pressure in patients with renal artery stenosis but can produce a deterioration in renal function, especially if there are bilateral stenoses.

Table 6.3
Selection of antihypertensive drugs for patients with coexisting conditions

	Diuretic	β-Blocker	ACE inhibitor	Calcium antagonist	α₁-Blocker
Elderly	+	+/−	+	+	+/−
Black race	+	+/−	+/−	+	+
Angina	+/−	+	+/−	+	+/−
After myocardial infarction	+/−	+	+	−	+/−
Congestive heart failure	+	−	+	−	+/−
Diabetes mellitus (with or without nephropathy)	C	C	+	+/−	+/−
Raynaud's phenomenon	+/−	−	+	+	+
Gout	−	+/−	+/−	+/−	+/−
Prostatism	−	+/−	+/−	+/−	+
Supraventricular arrhythmias	+/−	+	+/−	+ᵃ	+/−
Dyslipidaemia	C	C	+/−	+/−	+/−
Migraine	+/−	+	+/−	+/−	+/−

ACE, angiotensin-converting enzyme. +, treatment of choice; +/−, no obvious advantages/not preferred; C, use with caution; −, usually contraindicated.
ᵃDiltiazem or verapamil only.

Diabetic nephropathy

ACE inhibitors (and possibly angiotensin receptor blockers) appear to protect the kidney more than other classes of antihypertensive drug. In particular, they reduce progression from microalbuminuria to overt nephropathy. The effect may be independent of blood pressure reduction and reflect a reduction in glomerular perfusion pressure. Other complications of hypertension in diabetics are prevented equally well by β-blockers.

Pregnancy

There are two issues peculiar to pregnant patients.

Pre-existing chronic hypertension. This may need treatment, but drugs given to the mother can carry a teratogenic risk for the fetus (Ch. 56). The drugs with the best safety record in this situation are methyldopa, nifedipine and labetalol. The risk of hypertension to mother and fetus is probably not great until the diastolic blood pressure reaches 110 mmHg and many obstetricians do not treat lower values in uncomplicated hypertension. In the second trimester, although the risk of teratogenesis is past, diuretics, β-blockers and ACE inhibitors are still contraindicated since they retard fetal growth.

Pre-eclampsia. This only occurs after 20 weeks of gestation. It presents as hypertension, with oedema and proteinuria or hyperuricaemia, in previously normotensive women. There is a risk to the mother of convulsions, cerebral haemorrhage, abruptio placentae, pulmonary oedema and renal failure if this condition is untreated. The fetal risk is of severe growth retardation or even death. Once the diagnosis is established, bed rest is supplemented by antihypertensive drugs as for pre-existing hypertension in pregnancy. Hydralazine, initially by intravenous bolus injection, is favoured in severe pre-eclampsia.

FURTHER READING

Black HR (1998) Individualized selection of antihypertensive drug therapy for older patients. *Am J Hypertens* 11, 62S–67S

Bousquet P, Dontenwill M, Greney H et al. (1998) I₁-Imidazoline receptors: an update. *J Hypertens* 16(suppl 3), S1–S5

Collins R, Peto R, MacMahon S et al. (1990) Blood pressure, stroke and coronary artery disease. Part 2. Short-term reductions in blood pressure: overview of randomised drug trials in their epidemiological context. *Lancet* 335, 827–838

Dickerson JEC, Hingorani AD, Ashby MJ et al. (1999) Optimisation of antihypertensive treatment by crossover rotation of four major classes. *Lancet* 353, 2008–2013

Girvin B, Johnston GD (1996) The implication of non compliance with antihypertensive medication. *Drugs* 52, 186–195

Hirshl MM (1995) Guidelines for the drug treatment of hypertensive crises. *Drugs* 50, 991–1000.

Howes IG, Lykas D, Rennie GC (1996) Effects of antihypertensive drugs on coronary artery disease risk: a meta-analysis. *Clin Exp Pharmacol Physiol* 23, 555–558

Ibrahim HAA, Vora JP (1999) Hypertension in diabetes: a good opportunity to practise evidence-based medicine? A commentary on the UKPDS. *J Hum Hypertens* 13, 221–223

Kapla NM, Gifford RWJ (1996) Choice of initial therapy for hypertension. *JAMA* 275, 1577–1580

Messerli FH, Grossman E, Goldbourt U (1998) Are β-blockers efficacious as a first-line therapy for hypertension in the elderly? A systematic review. *JAMA* 279, 1903–1909

Moser M (1998) Why are physicians not prescribing diuretics more frequently in the management of hypertension? *JAMA* 279, 1813–1816

Ramsay LE, Williams B, Johnston GD et al. (1999) British Hypertension Society guidelines for hypertension management 1999: summary. *Br Med J* 319, 630–635

Schlaich MP, Schmeider RE (1998) Left ventricular hypertrophy and its regression: pathophysiology and therapeutic approach. *Am J Hypertens* 11, 1394–1404

Sibai BM (1996) Treatment of hypertension in pregnant women. *N Engl J Med* 335, 257–265

Stroth U, Unger T (1999) The renin–angiotensin system and its receptors. *J Cardiovasc Pharmacol* 33(suppl 1), S21–S28

Tuomiehto J, Rastenyte D, Birkenhäger WH et al. (1999) Effects of calcium-channel blockade in older patients with diabetes and hypertension. *N Engl J Med* 340, 677–684

Self-assessment

1. In the following questions the first statement, in italics, is true. Is the accompanying statement true?

   a. *Thiazide diuretics reduce sodium and water reabsorption in the distal convoluted tubule.* They are the drugs of choice for treating pregnancy-related hypertension.

   b. *Nifedipine shows selectivity for vasodilatation over cardiac depression.* It does so principally by arterial vasodilation.

   c. *Moxonidine stimulates imidazoline receptors in the medulla.* This increases sympathetic outflow and decreases vagal tone, lowering blood pressure.

   d. *Propranolol lowers blood pressure.* It does so by (i) decreasing cardiac output, (ii) reducing renin secretion, and (iii) by peripheral vasodilatation.

e. *Amiloride and spironolactone are potassium-sparing diuretics.* Their diuretic action is through different mechanisms in the distal tubule and early collecting duct.

f. *Stretch of baroreceptors increases the afferent impulses to the vasomotor centre.* This results in enhanced afferent sympathetic nervous outflow and a rise in blood pressure.

g. *Stimulation of presynaptic α-adrenoceptors in arteriolar resistance vessels inhibits noradrenaline release.* Adrenergic α_1-adrenoceptor blockade by prazosin increases noradrenaline release.

h. *Thiazide diuretics initially lower blood pressure by depleting salt and water.* The long-term reduction in blood pressure by propranolol can be seen with doses that do not cause diuresis and natriuresis.

i. *Angiotensin-converting enzyme (ACE) inhibitors prevent the conversion of angiotensin I to the vasoconstrictor angiotensin II.* ACE inhibitors prevent the breakdown of the vasodilator bradykinin.

j. *Minoxidil opens K+ channels in smooth muscle membranes.* This K+ channel opening destabilises the cell membrane leading to vasoconstriction.

k. *The antihypertensive effect of nitroprusside is limited to emergency management of some hypertensive states.* It can be administered for up to 2 months.

2. Case history question

> A man aged 50, with non-insulin-dependent diabetes smokes 20 cigarettes a day. His plasma lipid levels are normal and there is no proteinuria. His height is 5'8" (1.70 m) and his weight 210 lb (95.5 kg). He has his blood pressure checked three times over a period of weeks and it is consistently 175/110 mmHg. He has no evidence of fluid retention or heart failure. His doctor prescribed propranolol, but the blood pressure was not fully controlled. Which of the following would be appropriate to prescribe to lower his blood pressure.

a. Bendrofluazide plus propranolol
b. Furosemide (frusemide) plus atenolol
c. Amiloride and ACE inhibitor
d. Calcium antagonist plus atenolol

> Following several months of treatment with your chosen regimen his blood pressure was still 165/100 mmHg and he then suffered a small myocardial infarction.

e. What changes in his therapy would you consider?

The answers are provided on page 602.

Drugs used in the control of hypertension

Drug	Half-life (h)	Elimination	Comments
β-blockers			See drug compendium tables in Chapter 8
α_1-selective adrenoceptor antagonists (all drugs given orally)			Indications include hypertension, benign prostatic hypertrophy, congestive heart failure, Raynaud's phenomenon
Doxazosin	9–12	Metabolism	Oral bioavailability is 65% owing to incomplete absorption; metabolised by oxidation
Indoramin	5	Metabolism	Oral bioavailability is 10–25%; eliminated by oxidation (CYP2D6) to an active hydroxymetabolite
Prazosin	3	Metabolism	Oral bioavailability is 60% owing to first-pass metabolism; high hepatic extraction and clearance by cytochrome P450
Terazosin	12	Metabolism	High oral bioavailability (>90%); mostly eliminated by hepatic metabolism but some eliminated unchanged in urine (5%) and faeces (25%)
Non-selective adrenoceptor antagonists[a]			Indications are severe hypertensive episodes associated with phaeochromocytoma (phenoxybenzamine) or as a short-acting compound, which is rarely used as a suppression test for phaeochromocytoma (phentolamine)
Phenoxybenzamine	24	Metabolism	Given orally or by intravenous infusion; low oral bioavailability (20–30%); metabolised in the liver
Phentolamine	1.5	Metabolism + renal	Given by intravenous injection; eliminated by poorly defined metabolism and unchanged by renal excretion (10%)
ACE inhibitors (all drugs given orally; many are prodrugs that undergo bioactivation by hepatic metabolism)			Indications include hypertension, congestive heart failure, postmyocardial infarction, diabetic nephropathy
Captopril	2	Renal + metabolism	Good absorption (70–80%) with limited first-pass metabolism (10%); eliminated by filtration plus secretion, and formation of inactive metabolites
Cilazapril	30 (cilazaprilat)[b]	Renal (cilazaprilat)	Prodrug, which is well absorbed (60%); converted in liver to cilazaprilat, which shows biphasic elimination with half-lives of 1–2 and 30–50 h
Enalapril	35 (enalaprilat)[b]	Renal (enalaprilat)	Prodrug, which is well absorbed (60%); converted in liver to enalaprilat; both enalapril and enalaprilat are eliminated in the urine
Fosinopril	12 (fosinoprilat)[b]	Renal (fosinoprilat)	Poorly absorbed prodrug of which about 30% is converted in the intestine and liver to fosinoprilat; fosinoprilat is eliminated unchanged in urine and faeces
Imidapril	8 (imidaprilat)[b]	Metabolism	Prodrug, which is well absorbed and rapidly hydrolysed (half-life 2 h) to the active imidaprilat (the fate of which has not been published)
Lisinopril	12	Renal	Incompletely absorbed from gut; excreted unchanged in urine (30%) and faeces (70%)
Moexipril	10 (moexiprilat)[b]	Renal (moexiprilat)	Poorly absorbed prodrug; converted in liver to moexiprilat; significant amounts (50%) are excreted in faeces as moexiprilat (possibly formed in gut lumen from unabsorbed compound)
Perindopril	29 (perindoprilat)[b]	Renal (perindoprilat)	Well-absorbed prodrug; about 20% is converted in liver to perindoprilat
Quinapril	2 (quinaprilat)[b]	Renal (quinaprilat)	Well-absorbed prodrug; converted in liver to quinaprilat, which is eliminated rapidly by renal tubular secretion
Ramipril	1–5 (ramiprilat)[b]	Renal (ramiprilat)	Well-absorbed prodrug; converted in liver to ramiprilat which is excreted in urine
Trandolapril	16–24 (trandolaprilat)[b]	Metabolism + renal	Well-absorbed prodrug; converted in liver to trandolaprilat and inactive metabolites; trandoprilat is eliminated in urine and by metabolism and has a slow minor terminal half-life 50–100 h (which is not clinically significant)

continued

Drug compendium

Drugs used in the control of hypertension *(continued)*

Drug	Half-life (h)	Elimination	Comments
Angiotensin II receptor antagonists (all drugs given orally)			Indications include hypertension
Candesartan	9–12	Renal + metabolism (?)	Highly selective blockade of AT$_1$ receptors; given as the prodrug candesartan cilextil, which is rapidly hydrolysed during absorption to the active candesartan (15%); candesartan is eliminated by renal excretion (26%) and in faeces (possibly as metabolites)
Irbesartan	11–15	Renal + metabolism	Highly selective blockade at AT$_1$ receptors; oral bioavailability is 60–80%; metabolised by oxidation (CYP2C9) and conjugation; parent drug plus conjugates eliminated in urine and bile
Losartan	2	Metabolism	Highly selective blockade at AT$_1$ receptors; extensive first-pass metabolism (50%) to inactive metabolites plus an active metabolite, which gives prolonged non-competitive selective blockade at AT$_1$ receptors
Telmisartan	16–23	Bile (+ metabolism)	Highly selective blockade at AT$_1$ receptors; good oral bioavailability (50%); eliminated unchanged in faeces possibly after biliary excretion of the glucuronide conjugate which is detected in blood
Valsartan	5–7	Metabolism	Highly selective blockade at AT$_1$ receptors; oral bioavailability is 25%; oxidised in liver to a hydroxy metabolite; duration of action is 24 h, allowing once daily dosing
Vasodilator antihypertensive drugs[a]			
Diazoxide	28	Renal (+ metabolism)	For severe hypertension associated with renal disease; given in emergencies by intravenous bolus injection; eliminated largely by glomerular filtration; long half-life is a result of high protein binding
Hydralazine	4	Metabolism	As an adjunct for treating moderate or severe hypertension; given orally, by slow intravenous injection or by intravenous infusion; undergoes first-pass metabolism by N-acetylation with a bioavailability of 10–15% in fast acetylators and 30–35% in slow acetylators; eliminated by acetylation and oxidation; slow acetylators have high circulating concentrations of hydralazine
Minoxidil	3–4	Metabolism + renal	For severe hypertension, in addition to a diuretic and β-blocker; given orally; complete oral bioavailability; mainly eliminated as a glucuronide conjugate
Sodium nitroprusside	Seconds	Decomposition + renal	For hypertensive crisis, for controlled hypertension in anaesthesia and for acute or chronic heart failure; decomposes to NO and CN which are eliminated largely in the urine as nitrite and thiocyanate ions; the clinical responses (owing to NO) are very rapid and short lived
Centrally acting antihypertensive drugs[a]			
Clonidine	20–25	Renal + metabolism	Given orally or by slow intravenous injection; sudden withdrawal may give hypertensive crisis; good oral bioavailability (70%+); eliminated unchanged in urine (60%) and as hydroxyl metabolites
Methyldopa	1–2	Renal + metabolism	Given orally or by intravenous infusion; oral bioavailability is 10–60% owing to conjugation with sulfate in the intestinal wall; eliminated by glomerular filtration and sulfate conjugation
Moxonidine	2–3	Renal + metabolism	Given orally; bioavailability is about 90%; eliminated largely in the urine unchanged

continued

Drugs used in the control of hypertension (continued)

Drug	Half-life (h)	Elimination	Comments
Adrenergic neuron-blocking drugs[a,c]			
Debrisoquine	3	Metabolism + renal	Given orally; eliminated by CYP2D6, which shows genetic polymorphism; higher blood concentrations in poor metabolisers after oral dosage; main interest is as a probe substrate for CYP2D6 activity since the ratio of the 4-hydroxy metabolite to parent drug in urine depends on CYP2D6 activity
Guanethidine	2 days	Renal	Given by injection for hypertensive crisis; eliminated by renal excretion and metabolism; very slow terminal phase (4–8 days) reported in some studies

[a]Drugs for hypertension and to control blood pressure under specified circumstances.
[b]The half-life and route of elimination relate to the active metabolite, which is named in parentheses.
[c]Adrenergic neuron-blocking drugs are rarely used because they do not control supine blood pressure and may cause postural hypotension.

Drug compendium

7

Heart failure

Maintenance of cardiac output

There are four major determinants of cardiac output:

- preload: this is governed by the ventricular end-diastolic volume, which in turn is related to ventricular filling pressure and, therefore, to venous return
- heart rate
- myocardial contractility
- afterload: the systolic wall tension in the ventricle; this reflects the resistance to ventricular emptying.

These factors normally balance the output from both sides of the heart. In the healthy heart, changes in cardiac output are achieved mainly by changes in heart rate and preload.

The relationship between preload and stroke volume (the amount of blood ejected from the ventricle during systole) is shown in Figure 7.1. The degree of stretch of the ventricular muscle (preload) determines the force of cardiac contraction (the Frank–Starling phenomenon). The curve describing this relationship is governed by intrinsic myocardial contractility: thus the curve is shifted downwards in the failing ventricle and upwards

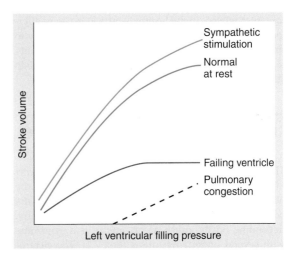

Fig. 7.1
The relationship between preload (left ventricular filling pressure) and stroke volume (the Frank–Starling phenomenon) in the healthy and failing heart. In the latter, if an increase in filling pressure and heart rate are insufficient to restore cardiac output, then pulmonary congestion will occur.

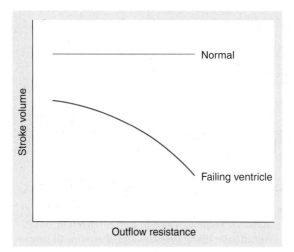

Fig. 7.2
The relationship between afterload (outflow resistance) and stroke volume in the presence of normal and reduced myocardial contractility.

when contractility is augmented, for example by sympathetic nervous stimulation. The left ventricular filling pressure in a healthy heart with normal contractility falls on the steep part of the curve, making stroke volume sensitive to changes in preload. In the failing ventricle, the curve is flatter, indicating that the cardiac output is less dependent on changes in preload.

The relationship between afterload and stroke volume is shown in Figure 7.2. Afterload is determined largely by peripheral resistance but also by the size of the ventricle. Enlargement of this chamber (e.g. as a result of increased venous return or preload) increases wall tension, and the heart must generate greater pressure both to initiate and to maintain contraction. Preload and afterload are therefore inter-related. In the healthy ventricle, a rise in afterload is met by an increase in myocardial contractility to maintain stroke volume. In the failing ventricle, inability to augment contraction leads to a progressive fall in stroke volume as afterload rises (Fig. 7.2).

Pathophysiology of heart failure

There is no universally accepted definition, but heart failure is usually said to exist when the output of the heart is insufficient to meet the metabolic needs of the body. It can arise suddenly or develop gradually, depending on the cause. Heart failure is a syndrome with several underlying causes (Box 7.1). The electrocardiograph (ECG) is almost always abnormal in patients with heart failure (arrhythmias, ischaemic changes, previous myocardial infarction, etc.), and a chest X-ray examination may reveal cardiomegaly or pulmonary congestion. One of the most useful investi-

gations is echocardiography. This may identify the cause of heart failure and establish the degree of left ventricular dysfunction, which is a guide to prognosis.

The syndrome of heart failure arises largely from neurohumoral counter-regulation in response to the low blood pressure and low renal perfusion pressure (Fig. 7.3). The consequences of these are vasoconstriction of both arteries and veins and excessive salt and water retention by the kidneys. These mechanisms are designed to increase the blood pressure, but in the setting of a failing heart can exacerbate the cardiac dysfunction and produce tissue oedema when the hydrostatic pressure in the veins exceeds the plasma oncotic pressure that holds fluid in the blood vessel.

Acute left ventricular failure

Acute left ventricular failure usually results from a sudden inability of the heart to maintain an adequate output and blood pressure. This leads to reflex arterial and venous constriction (Fig. 7.3). There is a rapid rise in filling pressure of the left ventricle as a result of increased venous return. If the heart is unable to expel the extra blood, the hydrostatic pressure in the pulmonary veins rises until it exceeds the plasma osmotic pressure and produces pulmonary oedema. The principal symptom is breathlessness, occurring on exertion in the early stages, then at rest with orthopnoea. Left ventricular failure can follow acute myocardial infarction, acute mitral or aortic valvular regurgitation, or arise from tachyarrhythmias in a patient with poor left ventricular function.

Cardiogenic shock

The syndrome of cardiogenic shock arises when the systolic function of the left ventricle is suddenly impaired

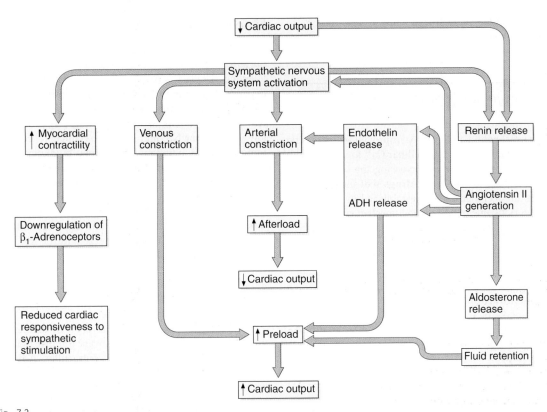

Fig. 7.3
Neurohumoral consequences of heart failure. The increase in preload can improve cardiac performance in the mildly impaired heart but will lead to oedema if cardiac function is significantly reduced, since the increased preload cannot restore a normal stroke volume (Fig. 7.1). The increased afterload will put additional strain on the failing heart and can further decrease cardiac output. These effects are compounded by downregulation of cardiac β_1-adrenoceptors. ADH, antidiuretic hormone.

to such a degree that there is insufficient blood flow to meet resting metabolic requirements of the tissues. This definition excludes shock caused by hypovolaemia. The clinical hallmarks are a low systolic blood pressure (usually <90 mgHg), with a reduced cardiac output and an elevated left ventricular filling pressure. Cardiogenic shock can follow acute myocardial infarction and in this situation usually indicates loss of at least 40% of the left ventricular myocardium. Other mechanical disturbances, such as acute mitral regurgitation or ventricular septal rupture, can produce cardiogenic shock in association with a lesser degree of myocardial damage. Less commonly, the syndrome is associated with right ventricular infarction.

Chronic heart failure

Myocardial damage from ischaemic heart disease is the most common cause of chronic heart failure, but potentially correctable causes such as valvular lesions, as well as treatable exacerbating factors such as anaemia or arrhythmias, may be identified. In most patients, there are signs of both right and left ventricular failure (con-

gestive heart failure). Chronic congestive heart failure is not a trivial complaint: even patients who have symptoms only on exertion have a 2-year mortality of about 20%, while if there are symptoms at rest the 1-year mortality is 80%. Death is either from progressive heart failure or from sudden arrhythmic death.

Symptoms in chronic heart failure are caused by a reduced cardiac output ('forward failure') or venous congestion ('backward failure'). The most common complaint is breathlessness, and many patients experience fatigue as a result of reduced cardiac output and impaired muscle perfusion. Biochemical changes also occur in muscle, which are not immediately reversed when peripheral blood flow is improved. Other symptoms, such as the discomfort of peripheral oedema and anorexia owing to bowel congestion, are attributable to a high systemic venous pressure.

Although the symptoms of chronic heart failure are often caused by reduced left ventricular systolic contractility (systolic heart failure), they can also arise from impaired diastolic relaxation (diastolic heart failure). If the left ventricle fails to relax adequately, it will not accommodate the venous return, leading to pulmonary venous congestion and a low cardiac output. Diastolic heart failure characteristically occurs in association with left ventricular hypertrophy, but it also occurs in ischaemic heart disease.

Positive inotropic drugs

Myocardial contractility can be improved by increasing the availability of free intracellular Ca^{2+} to interact with contractile proteins, or by increasing the sensitivity of the myofibrils to Ca^{2+}. Only drugs that increase myocardial intracellular Ca^{2+} are established in clinical use; they work by one of two distinct mechanisms:

- an action on the cell membrane Na^+/K^+-ATPase pump
- by increasing intracellular cAMP.

An advantage of positive inotropic drugs, which increase myocardial cAMP, is their ability to enhance the reuptake of Ca^{2+} by the sarcoplasmic reticulum in diastole. This improves diastolic relaxation in addition to augmenting systolic contractility.

Digitalis glycosides

Example: digoxin

Mechanism of action and effects

Digitalis glycosides are compounds with a steroid nucleus that were originally isolated from a species of foxglove (*Digitalis purpura*). They act on the energy-dependent Na^+ pump (Na^+/K^+-ATPase) in the myocyte membrane. This pump establishes and maintains the Na^+ and K^+ gradients across the cell (Fig. 7.4), producing low intracellular Na^+ and high intracellular K^+ concentrations. Partial inhibition of the pump by digitalis glycosides increases the intracellular Na^+ concentration and reduces the concentration gradient for Na^+ across the cell membrane. The effect on intracellular Ca^{2+} is a consequence of the change in Na^+ gradient; a separate passive transmembrane exchange of Na^+ and Ca^{2+} occurs down their concentration gradients; the activity of this ion-exchange mechanism is reduced by the increase in intracellular Na^+, and Ca^{2+} is retained in the cell. The excess intracellular Ca^{2+} is stored in the sarcoplasmic reticulum during diastole and released during membrane excitation, leading to enhanced contraction.

Digitalis glycosides have effects on the cardiac action potential and conduction of the cardiac impulse that are independent of their effects on contractility. Adverse direct actions of the drug can provoke arrhythmias by increasing myocardial excitability and automaticity (Ch. 8), by two mechanisms:

- reducing the resting membrane potential: the cell membrane Na^+/K^+- ATPase pump extrudes three Na^+ out of the cell for every two K^+ that enter, which increases the negative intracellular electrical

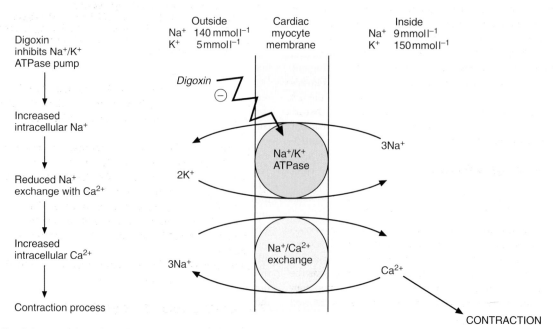

Fig. 7.4
The action of digoxin on the cardiac myocyte.

potential and hyperpolarises the cell; inhibition of this membrane pump by digoxin, therefore, leads to cell depolarisation and arrhythmias are more readily initiated

- triggering of spontaneous release of Ca^{2+} from the sarcoplasmic reticulum, which leads to transient depolarisation of the cell immediately following an action potential ('after potentials'); this is an important mechanism for initiating arrhythmias (Ch. 8).

Digitalis glycosides also have clinically useful indirect actions on the action potential via central stimulation of the vagus nerve and enhanced cardiac sensitivity to acetylcholine. The vagal stimulation is antiarrhythmic (Ch. 8) through:

- decreased automaticity of the sino-atrial node, which slightly slows sinus rate
- increased refractory period of the atrioventricular node, which decreases atrioventricular conduction. This is useful in the management of certain arrhythmias.

Digitalis glycosides produce distinctive changes on the ECG, which include non-specific T wave changes and sagging of the S–T segment ('reverse tick') (Fig. 7.5); these effects can be mistaken for those caused by myocardial ischaemia.

Pharmacokinetics

Digoxin is the most widely used of the digitalis glycosides in the UK. It is well absorbed from the gut; the kidney is the main route of elimination, partially by active tubular secretion. The half-life of digoxin is very long (about 1.5 days) and further lengthened when renal function is impaired. To achieve an early onset of action, initial loading doses should be given over 24–36 h (Ch. 2). If a rapid response is essential, digoxin can be given by slow intravenous injection.

Other digitalis glycosides are rarely used. Digitoxin is occasionally given in renal failure, since it is extensively metabolised and mainly excreted via the gut. However, it has a disadvantage of a very long half-life (approximately 8 days).

Unwanted effects

Digitalis glycosides have a narrow therapeutic index. Toxicity is mostly dose-related and includes:

- consequences of intracellular Ca^{2+} overload: increased automaticity of the atrioventricular node and Purkinje fibres produces junctional escape beats, junctional tachycardia, ventricular ectopic beats (including bigeminy or coupling of an ectopic after each normal beat) or (less commonly) ventricular tachycardia
- consequences of increased vagal activity: excessive atrioventricular nodal block can occur; when

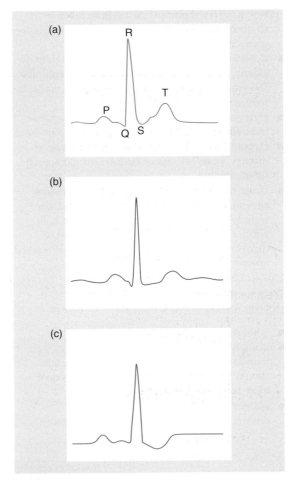

Fig. 7.5
The effect of digoxin on the S–T segment of an electrocardiograph (ECG). (a) Normal ECG trace. (b) Mild digoxin-induced changes with non-specific depression of the S–T segment and reduced T wave voltage. (c) Pronounced changes include a sagging S–T segment and a flat T wave.

associated with increased atrial automaticity this produces atrial tachycardia with 2:1 atrioventricular nodal block, a rhythm characteristic of digitalis toxicity

- gastrointestinal disturbances: anorexia, nausea and vomiting (largely a central effect at the chemoreceptor trigger zone; Ch. 32) and diarrhoea
- neurological disturbances: fatigue, malaise, confusion, vertigo, coloured vision (especially yellow halos around lights, possibly owing to inhibition of Na^+/K^+-ATPase in the cones of the retina)
- gynaecomastia or breast enlargement: caused by the oestrogen-like steroid structure.

Exacerbating factors for digitalis toxicity

- Hypokalaemia: a reduced extracellular K^+ concentration increases the effects of digitalis on the

Na$^+$/K$^+$-ATPase pump. Care must be taken if K$^+$- losing diuretics (Ch. 14) are used with digitalis glycosides.

- Renal impairment: this is not always obvious in the elderly, who may have a normal plasma creatinine concentration even when renal function is markedly reduced.
- Hypoxaemia: this sensitises the heart to digitalis-induced arrhythmias.
- Hypothyroidism: decreased renal elimination of digoxin occurs because of the lowered glomerular filtration rate.
- Drugs that displace digoxin from tissue-binding sites and interfere with its renal excretion: these include verapamil (Ch. 5) and quinidine (Ch. 8), which can double the plasma concentration of digoxin; amiodarone (Ch. 8) produces a less marked effect.

Treatment of digitalis toxicity

Digitalis toxicity can be treated by:

- withholding further drug
- using K$^+$ supplementation (Ch. 14) for hypokalaemia; this is usually given orally, but should be given by slow intravenous infusion if there are dangerous arrhythmias
- atropine (Ch. 8) for sinus bradycardia or atrioventricular block; temporary transvenous

pacing is used for marked bradycardia unresponsive to atropine
- digoxin-specific antibody fragments for serious toxicity (Ch. 53).

Sympathomimetic inotropes

Examples

non-selective β-adrenoceptor agonist: isoprenaline

selective β$_1$-adrenoceptor agonist: dobutamine

mixed non-selective β-adrenoceptor, α-adrenoceptor and dopaminergic agonist: dopamine

Mechanisms of action and effects

The mechanism of action of the sympathomimetic inotropes are also considered in Ch. 4.

Isoprenaline is a non-selective β-adrenoceptor agonist that increases both myocardial contractility (β$_1$-adrenoceptors) (Fig. 7.6) and heart rate (β$_1$- and β$_2$-adrenoceptors), and produces peripheral arterial vasodilation (β$_2$-adrenoceptors).

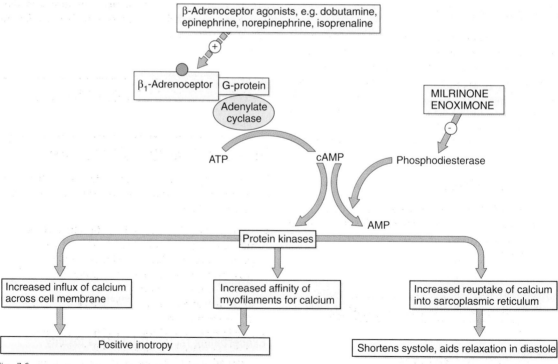

Fig. 7.6
Mechanisms by which sympathomimetics and phosphodiesterase inhibitors exert their positive inotropic effects.

Dobutamine, a synthetic dopamine analogue, is a selective β_1-adrenoceptor agonist that produces a powerful inotropic response, with relatively less increase in heart rate and little direct effect on vascular tone, even at high concentrations.

Dopamine has dose-related actions at several receptors.

- At low doses, it selectively stimulates peripheral dopamine (D) receptors, which are structurally distinct from those in the central nervous system (CNS) (Ch. 4). This produces renal arterial vasodilation and diuresis (D_1 receptors) and peripheral arterial vasodilation (D_2 presynaptic receptors, which inhibit noradrenaline release from sympathetic nerves).
- At moderate doses, non-selective β-adrenoceptor stimulation produces a positive inotropic response (Fig. 7.6). Tachycardia is more marked than with dobutamine, because of stimulation of cardiac β_1- and β_2-adrenoceptors and the reflex response to β_2-adrenoceptor-mediated peripheral arterial dilation.
- At high doses, α_1-adrenoceptor stimulation produces peripheral vasoconstriction, which also affects the renal arteries and overcomes D_1 receptor-mediated renal vasodilatation.

The doses that produce these different effects differ widely among individuals. It has been suggested that there is no dose that can be relied upon to act selectively at dopamine receptors without stimulating adrenoceptors.

Pharmacokinetics

Dobutamine, dopamine and isoprenaline are all administered by intravenous infusion because of their very short half-lives of about 2–10 min. Metabolic inactivation is by the same pathways as for noradrenaline (Ch. 4). Desensitisation and downregulation of β-adrenoceptors (Ch. 1) rapidly reduce the response to sustained infusions over 48–72 h. Owing to its vasoconstrictor actions, dopamine is usually given into a large central vein.

Unwanted effects

Unwanted effects can be predicted from agonist actions at adrenoceptors (Ch. 4) and mainly relate to excessive cardiac stimulation, with tachycardia, palpitations and arrhythmias.

Phosphodiesterase inhibitors

Examples: milrinone, enoximone

Mechanism of action and effects

Milrinone and enoximone are specific inhibitors of the isoenzyme of phosphodiesterase found in cardiac and smooth muscle (phosphodiesterase III). Their inotropic action on the heart results from the increase in intracellular cAMP with mobilisation of intracellular Ca^{2+} (Fig. 7.6). Unlike β-adrenoceptor agonists, their activity is not limited by desensitisation of cell surface receptors as they act at a site beyond the receptor. Because of their complementary sites of action, phosphodiesterase inhibitors and β-adrenoceptor agonists will have additive effects on the heart. Phosphodiesterase inhibition in vascular smooth muscle produces peripheral arterial vasodilatation.

Pharmacokinetics

These drugs are only given for short-term treatment by intravenous infusion because of doubts about long-term safety. They have short half-lives and are eliminated by the kidney or hepatic oxidation.

Unwanted effects

The unwanted effects are mainly those produced by excessive cardiac stimulation, including:

- tachycardia
- palpitation
- potentially serious arrhythmias.

Large trials of oral formulations have indicated that they increase mortality in patients with heart failure during long-term use.

Management of heart failure

Acute left ventricular failure

The immediate aim of treatment in acute left ventricular failure is to reduce the excessive venous return. Treatment includes:

- Intravenous injection of a loop diuretic such as furosemide (frusemide; Ch. 14). This initially produces venous dilation, which increases peripheral venous pooling. Symptoms are, therefore, improved even before the onset of a diuresis that reduces plasma volume and further decreases preload.
- Sublingual glyceryl trinitrate (Ch. 5). This dilates venous capacitance vessels and is a useful alternative or additional emergency treatment to diuretics.

- Intravenous opioid analgesic such as diamorphine (Ch. 19), often given to relieve distress and breathlessness.
- Oxygen in high concentration via a facemask.

Whenever possible a precipitating or exacerbating cause should be treated, for example arrhythmias, anaemia, thyrotoxicosis, acute mitral regurgitation or critical aortic stenosis. When this is not possible, patients will often require maintenance treatment with an oral diuretic.

Cardiogenic shock

The mortality of cardiogenic shock, even with intensive treatment, is in excess of 70%. The immediate aim of treatment is to resuscitate the patient, while looking for a remediable cause.

- Oxygen in high concentrations via a face mask.
- Correct any acid–base imbalance (especially acidosis) and electrolyte abnormalities (particularly hypokalaemia).
- Relieve pain, usually with an opioid analgesic such as diamorphine (Ch. 19).
- Correct any cardiac rhythm disturbance (Ch. 8).
- Ensure an adequate left ventricular filling pressure. This can be low after right ventricular infarction despite a high central venous pressure (right ventricular filling pressure). In this situation, monitoring of left heart function with a flow-guided balloon-tipped (Swan–Ganz) catheter is helpful to determine whether infusion of a colloid plasma expander is indicated.
- If intravenous volume is adequate but tissue perfusion remains impaired, dobutamine is the inotropic drug of choice. Dobutamine is often given in combination with low-dose dopamine with the intention that the dopamine will improve renal perfusion; however there is little evidence that dopamine is effective.
- Phosphodiesterase inhibitors are sometimes given to improve myocardial contractility and to give peripheral vasodilatation. They are usually reserved for patients who fail to improve with maximum tolerated doses of dobutamine.
- When there is profound hypotension, norepinephrine (Ch. 4) can be infused to produce peripheral vasoconstriction and maintain vital organ perfusion.
- Vasodilators can be given to 'offload' the heart once an adequate blood pressure has been established. This strategy is particularly helpful if there is significant mitral regurgitation since reduced resistance to left ventricular emptying will diminish the regurgitant volume. Either glyceryl trinitrate (Ch. 5) or nitroprusside (Ch. 6) is used.

- Intra-aortic balloon pumping can temporarily maintain intraaortic diastolic pressure and improve coronary perfusion. It is particularly useful for patients who can subsequently undergo surgery, for example to repair an incompetent mitral valve or an aquired ventricular septal defect.

Chronic heart failure

Much of the treatment of chronic heart failure is directed towards counteracting the compensatory mechanisms for the reduced cardiac output and low blood pressure generated by a failing heart, i.e. arterial and venous vasoconstriction and fluid retention. Treatment has two main aims: symptom relief and improved prognosis.

Non-pharmacological treatment

A number of life-style changes can be helpful:

- weight reduction should be encouraged in the obese
- bed rest may be appropriate to rest the heart during acute episodes of fluid retention
- modest salt restriction is desirable (severe salt restriction is unpleasant and unnecessary)
- fluid restriction is rarely required unless profound hyponatraemia accompanies severe oedema, a situation in which diuretics may be ineffective or even harmful unless the plasma Na^+ concentration is corrected
- if possible, drugs that exacerbate heart failure by producing myocardial depression (e.g. high-dose β-blockers, some Ca^{2+} antagonists) or by promoting fluid retention (e.g. non-steroidal anti-inflammatory drugs NSAIDs)) should be withdrawn.
- a graded exercise programme in stable patients has been shown to improve symptoms.

Diuretics

Diuretics remain the mainstay of treatment for chronic heart failure (Ch. 14). They are usually taken once daily, in the morning. A thiazide diuretic, such as bendro-flumethiazide (bendrofluazide) is only useful for mild symptoms. Most patients need a loop diuretic (usually furosemide, frusemide) for moderate or severe fluid retention. Modest doses of furosemide are usually sufficient, unless renal function is impaired, when additional diuresis can be produced by much larger doses. Bumetanide has few advantages over frusemide. Its more predictable absorption is sometimes useful, for example in marked right-sided heart failure with gut congestion. Hypokalaemia is unusual when loop diuretics are used alone in chronic heart failure, but use of a

K^+-sparing diuretic is advisable if the plasma K^+ falls below 3.5 mmol l^{-1} or if digoxin or antiarrhythmic therapy is given concurrently (because of an increased risk of generating rhythm disturbances. K^+-sparing diuretics are a more effective and more palatable treatment for hypokalaemia than K^+ supplements.

If fluid retention fails to respond to an oral loop diuretic, the addition of a distal tubular diuretic, such as bendroflumethiazide (bendrofluazide) or metolazone, for a few days often leads to profound natriuresis and diuresis. Care must be taken to avoid hyponatraemia, hypokalaemia, hypovolaemia and renal impairment with such combined diuretic regimens, and a K^+-sparing diuretic is almost always needed. Recent evidence supports the use of spironolactone in this situation. It can improve symptoms and prognosis if a low dose is added to maximal therapy with other drugs. In resistant patients, an intravenous infusion of furosemide (frusemide) can initiate a diuresis.

Angiotensin-converting enzyme inhibitors

Symptoms of heart failure often persist despite effective diuresis. Angiotensin-converting enzyme (ACE) inhibitors (Ch. 6) produce arterial and venous dilation, which improves peripheral haemodynamics and, therefore, cardiac function. Symptoms of breathlessness and fatigue are usually reduced, and exercise tolerance increases. The full symptomatic response is often delayed for 4 to 6 weeks after the start of treatment, despite early haemodynamic changes. A further benefit of ACE inhibitors is improved survival, which has been most clearly shown in patients with severe left ventricular systolic dysfunction (a left ventricular ejection fraction below 40%). With most ACE inhibitors, there is a small risk of severe hypotension after administration of the first dose to patients with heart failure. However, the risk is minimal if the patient is well hydrated; diuretics should be omitted on the first day of ACE inhibitor treatment, or for longer if there is evidence of dehydration (e.g. a postural fall in blood pressure). Use of a small initial dose of ACE inhibitor reduces the duration of any hypotension. K^+-sparing diuretics are usually unnecessary when an ACE inhibitor is used, since the combination can cause hyperkalaemia. However, with careful monitoring, the combination of an ACE inhibitor with spironolactone may be advantageous (see above). For patients unable to tolerate an ACE inhibitor (usually because of a cough), an angiotensin II receptor antagonist (Ch. 6) can be substituted. These agents appear to have similar efficacy to ACE inhibitors.

Digoxin

Digitalis glycosides are widely used when heart failure is associated with atrial fibrillation and a rapid ventricular rate. The use of digoxin in patients with heart failure who are in sinus rhythm has been more controversial, but there is now conclusive evidence that it is very effective as a supplement to diuretic and ACE inhibitor therapy in patients with severe left ventricular systolic dysfunction. Symptoms are improved and the need for hospitalisation reduced, but survival is unaffected. In sinus rhythm, the effective dose of digoxin is smaller than that required for control of atrial fibrillation. Hypokalaemia should be avoided to minimise the risk of digoxin toxicity.

Other vasodilators

Treatment with a combination of hydralazine (Ch. 6) and isosorbide dinitrate (or mononitrate) (Ch. 5), in addition to a diuretic and digoxin, provides balanced arterial and venous dilation. This combination improves exercise tolerance in heart failure but only produces a modest reduction in mortality.

Beta-blockers

Contrary to traditional teaching, β-blockers (Ch. 5) are effective for treatment of heart failure that has been stabilised with an ACE inhibitor and diuretic. Because of their negative inotropic properties, these drugs were once considered to be contraindicated. However, if introduced very gradually in small doses, they improve symptoms and survival. Possible explanations for this paradox are numerous (Box 7.2). Most patients with heart failure should now be treated with a β-blocker.

Box 7.2

Possible beneficial effects of β-blockers in heart failure

Reduced workload of the damaged myocardium
Suppression of the neurohumoral response to the low cardiac output
Antiarrhythmic effects
Inhibition of neutrophil-induced myocardial damage
Free radical scavenging in ischaemic myocardium

FURTHER READING

American College of Cardiology (1999) Consensus recommendation for the management of chronic heart failure. On behalf of the membership of the advisory council to improve outcomes nationwide in heart failure. *Am J Cardiol* 83(suppl 2A), 1A–38A.

Bonet S, Agusti A, Aman JM et al. (2000) β-adrenergic blocking agents in heart failure. Benefits of vasodilating and non-vasodilating agents according to patients' characteristics. A meta analysis of clinical trials. *Arch Intern Med* 160, 621–627

Califf RM, Bengtson JR (1994) Cardiogenic shock. *N Engl J Med* 330, 1724–1730

Denton MD, Chertow GM, Brady HR (1996) 'Renal-dose' dopamine for treatment of acute renal failure: scientific rationale, experimental studies and clinical trials. *Kidney Int* 49, 4–14

Dormans TPJ, Gerlag PGG, Russel FGM, Smits P (1998) Combination diuretic therapy in severe congestive heart failure. *Drugs* 55, 165–172.

Eccles M, Freemantle N, Mason J (1998) North of England evidence based development project: guideline for angiotensin converting enzyme inhibitors in primary care management of adults with symptomatic heart failure. *Br Med J* 316, 1369–1375

Flather MD, Yuisuf S, Kober L et al. (2000) Long term ACE-inhibitor therapy in patients with heart failure or left ventricular dysfunction: a systematic overview of data from individual patients. *Lancet* 355, 1578–1581

Gammage M (1998) Treatment of acute pulmonary oedema: diuresis or vasodilatation? *Lancet* 351, 382–383

Gheorghiade M, Cody RJ, Francis GS et al. (1998) Current radical therapy for advanced heart failure. *Am Heart J* 132, S231–S248

Hauptman PJ, Kelly RA (1999) Digitalis. *Circulation* 99, 1265–1270

Krämer BK, Schweda F, Riegger GAJ (1999) Diuretic treatment and diuretic resistance in heart failure. *Am J Med* 106, 90–96

Lonn E, Mckelvie RA (2000) Drug treatment in heart failure. *Br Med J* 320, 1188–1192

Mandinov L, Eberli FR, Seile C et al. (2000) Diastolic heart failure. *Cardiovasc Res* 45, 813–825

McKelvie RS, Benedict CR, Yusuf S (1999) Prevention of congestive heart failure and management of asymptomatic left ventricular dysfunction. *Br Med J* 318, 1400–1402

O'Connor CM, Gattis WA, Swedberg K (1998) Current and novel pharmacologic approaches in advanced heart failure. *Am Heart J* 135, S249–S263

Pepper GS, Lee RW (1999) Sympathetic activation in heart failure and its treatment with β-blockade. *Arch Intern Med* 159, 225–234

Rydén L, Remme WJ (1999) Treatment of congestive heart failure. Has the time come for decreased complexity. *Eur Heart J* 20, 867–871

Squire IB, Barnett DB (2000) The rational use of β-adrenoceptor blockers in the treatment of heart failure: the changing face of an old therapy. *Br J Clin Pharmacol* 49, 1–9.

van Veldhuisen DJ, Voors AA (2000) Blockade of the renin angiotensin system in heart failure: the potential place of angiotensin 2 receptor blockers. *Eur Heart J* 21, 14–16

Weber KT (1999) Aldosterone and spironolactone in heart failure. *N Engl J Med* 341, 753–754

Whorlow SL, Krum H (2000) Meta-analysis of effect of beta-blocker therapy on mortality in patients with New York Heart Association Class IV chronic congestive heart failure. *Am J Cardiol* 86, 886–889

Self-assessment

1. In the following questions, the first statement, in italics, is true. Is the accompanying statement true?

   a. *One of the determinants of cardiac output is afterload.* In healthy hearts, myocardial contractility increases following a rise in afterload.

   b. *In patients with pulmonary oedema, a principal symptom is breathlessness.* Oedema occurs when the pressure in the pulmonary veins is less than the plasma osmotic pressure.

   c. *Detrimental changes in body function in cardiac failure occur as a result of attempts by the body to compensate for the dysfunction.* In cardiac failure sympathetic outflow increases because of an increase in the sensory input from the baroreceptors in the carotid sinus.

   d. *Treatment of chronic heart failure is directed towards the compensatory mechanisms, i.e. vascular constriction and fluid retention.* Digoxin is the mainstay of treatment of the vascular constriction and fluid retention.

   e. *The positive inotropic action of digoxin on the cardiac myocyte is a result of inhibition of Na^+/K^+-ATPase pump on the myocyte membranes ultimately increasing intracellular Ca^{2+} concentrations.* Potassium ions and digoxin enhance the actions of each other at the Na/K^+- ATPase pump.

   f. *Digoxin has both direct and indirect effects on the electrical properties of the heart.* Digoxin inhibits the vagus, decreasing the refractory period of the atrioventricular node.

   g. *To improve tissue perfusion in cardiogenic shock, dobutamine or the phosphodiesterase inhibitor milrinone are given intravenously as their half-lives are very short.* Desensitisation of the response to dobutamine but not to milrinone can occur with sustained infusion.

h. *Dobutamine increases cardiac output and decreases ventricular filling pressure in heart failure.* Dobutamine produces peripheral vasodilation by its effect on β_2-adrenoceptors.

i. *Digoxin has a half-life of about 1.5 days.* The toxicity of digoxin increases in renal failure.

j. *In heart failure, drugs that do not have a direct action on the heart are very useful.* ACE (angiotensin-converting enzyme) inhibitors improve survival in chronic heart failure and have added benefit if given together with K^+-sparing diuretics such as spironolactone.

2. **Case history question**

> DY is 78 years of age and had a large anterior myocardial infarction 3 years ago. Echocardiography revealed marked left ventricular systolic dysfunction with reduced ejection fraction. He presented with several symptoms, including fatigue and decreased exercise ability, shortness of breath and peripheral oedema. Examination demonstrated cardiomegaly, a raised jugular venous pressure and crackles in the lungs. An ECG showed that he was in sinus rhythm.

a. Of the signs and symptoms stated, what is the main direct consequence of a reduced cardiac output?

b. Digoxin, a β-blocker and dobutamine were all considered as initial treatment for DY and were rejected. Would any of these treatments be appropriate?

c. What are the choices of diuretic open to you in treating DY?

d. Potassium loss produced by diuretics may lead to hypokalaemia, which should be avoided in patients with heart failure, particularly those taking digoxin. What is an effective way of reducing urinary K^+ loss?

e. DY was then started on an ACE (angiotensin-converting enzyme) inhibitor. What are the precautionary measures that should be taken in starting this new medication and how would its effectiveness be assessed.

f. After 4 weeks of treatement with the ACE inhibitor and a diuretic, DY's symptoms of breathlessness, fatigue and exercise tolerance were much improved. However, he developed a cough while taking the ACE inhibitor, which became intolerable. What is thought to be the reason for the cough and what alternative therapy could be given to avoid this?

The answers are provided on pages 602–603.

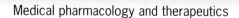

Drugs used in heart failure

Drug	Half-life	Elimination	Comments
Cardiac glycosides			
Digitoxin	8 days (3–16 days)	Metabolism + renal + bile	Once daily oral dosage, or even alternate day dosage
Digoxin	40 h (20–50 h)	Renal	Oral loading dose may be necessary
Phosphodiesterase inhibitors			
Enoximone	1.3 h	Metabolism	Intravenous dosage; half-life increased in chronic cardiac failure; metabolised to a sulfoxide which is eliminated in urine
Milrinone	0.8–0.9 h	Renal	Short-term treatment of severe failure; intravenous dosage; rapid elimination through renal tubular secretion, and low volume of distribution
Sympathomimetic inotropes			
Dobutamine	2 min	Metabolism	Given by intravenous infusion; at low doses results in vasodilation
Dopamine	7–12 min	Metabolism	Given by intravenous infusion; causes vasolidation
Dopexamine	7 min	Metabolism	Given by intravenous infusion; allow at least 15 min prior to dose incrementation; causes vasodilation

Cardiac arrhythmias

Basic electrophysiology

Myocardial cells maintain transmembrane ion gradients by movement of the ions through membrane channels. Several specific channels exist for Na^+, Ca^{2+} and K^+. These channels cycle through three states: resting, open or closed (and therefore refractory) (Ch. 1). Whether the ion channels are open or closed is determined by the membrane potential across the cell. The direction in which ions move is dependent upon both the concentration gradient of ions and also the membrane potential. The action potentials of pacemaker, Purkinje fibre and ventricular cells vary in their characteristics (Fig. 8.1) as they have different ion channels that are regulated at different membrane potentials.

The resting potential inside a cardiac cell is approximately -70 to -80 mV compared with the extracellular environment. The pacemaker cells are capable of spontaneous repetitive recycling. The intrinsic rate of firing of a pacemaker cell depends on three factors:

- the resting potential
- the threshold potential for initiating an impulse
- the rate of spontaneous depolarisation.

The upstroke in most pacemaker cells is relatively slow and results mainly from influx of Ca^{2+} into the cell (Fig. 8.1). In the sinoatrial (SA) node, the slower Ca^{2+} influx is through T-type Ca^{2+} channels, while in the atrioventricular (AV) node (and other pacemaker cells) the influx of Ca^{2+} is through L-type Ca^{2+} channels. Pacemaker cells initiate the cardiac rhythm and their action potential precedes the action potential generated in other cells. The dominant pacemaker cells (i.e. those with the fastest intrinsic rate of depolarisation) are found in the SA node. Consequently, the normal cardiac impulse arises from the SA node, and the pacemakers elsewhere in the specialised electrical conducting tissue of the heart will only be utilised if the pacemakers with a faster rate of spontaneous depolarisation slow or fail.

Action potentials in atria and ventricles can visually be divided into four phases, most clearly seen in Purkinje fibres (Fig. 8.1). Phase 0 of the action potential is initiated by a rapid influx of Na^+ through specific voltage-gated ion channels. It is triggered when sufficient Na^+ channels have been opened to allow the cell to reach the threshold potential. In the AV node, phase 0 depolarisation results from the slower influx of

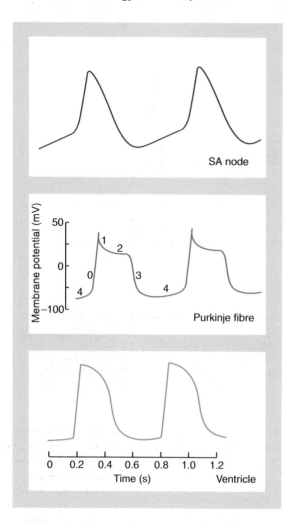

Fig. 8.1
Action potentials show patterns that vary with the region of the heart. The patterns are determined by the opening and closing of selective gates for Na$^+$, Ca^{2+} and K$^+$. The overall stability of the resting transmembrane ionic balance is maintained by active pumps such as the Na$^+$/K$^+$-ATPase pump. It is these pumps that maintain the substantial concentration gradients of 140 mmol l^{-1} Na$^+$ outside and 10–15 mmol l^{-1} Na$^+$ inside the cell and 140 mmol l^{-1} K$^+$ inside the cell and 4 mmol l^{-1} K$^+$ outside the cell. This results in an electrical gradient at rest of approximately −70 to −80 mV inside the cell relative to 0 mV outside the cell. Large ion fluxes at rest are prevented by specific pumps and closure of voltage-operated gates. The cardiac action potential is closely ordered. The sinoatrium atrioventricular node, bundle of His and ventricular action potentials are timed by the sinoatrial (SA) node in the heart when it is in sinus rhythm. The spontaneous depolarisation of the SA node determines its primary pacemaker status in the healthy heart.
Phase 0 (8.1) occurs when the membrane potential reaches a defined threshold (threshold potential) and an 'all or none' influx of Ca^{2+} and Na$^+$ through voltage-dependent channels occurs. This is transient and the gates close after a few milliseconds. Phase 0 is much slower in the SA node and depends mainly upon Ca^{2+} influx. This causes the conduction velocity in the SA node to be considerably less than that in the Purkinje fibre and the refractory period is longer in proportion to the total duration of the action potential. Phase 1 results from K$^+$ efflux and reduced Na$^+$ influx. The phase 2 plateau is primarily a result of Ca^{2+} influx over a slow time course. Phase 3 repolarisation results from inactivation of Ca^{2+} influx and increasing K$^+$ efflux.

Ca^{2+}. This results in slower conduction of the impulse than in other parts of the heart and is responsible for the conduction delay in the AV node.

At the end of phase 0, the intracellular potential briefly becomes positive, at which point a voltage-triggered 'gate' for the inward flowing Na$^+$ (pacemaker) or Ca^{2+} currents closes and prevents further inward ion flow and repetitive depolarisation. This inactivation of the channel is triggered by the same depolarising impulse that opens the channel, but the process occurs far more slowly. Recovery of the channel to the resting state, when it is closed but no longer refractory to further depolarisation, depends on repolarisation of the cell.

Repolarisation is initiated by the opening of several different types of K$^+$ channel, and begins when K$^+$ efflux exceeds Na$^+$ or Ca$^+$ influx (phase 1). In Purkinje fibres repolarisation is temporarily interrupted by a distinct period of influx of Ca^{2+} (plateau phase in Fig. 8.1), which briefly maintains depolarisation (phase 2). Finally, K$^+$ efflux increases until it is sufficient to repolarise the cell (phase 3). Most K$^+$ channels act as rectifiers (i.e. their

opening varies according to the membrane potential), giving rise to voltage dependence of membrane resistance (rectification). Repolarisation is achieved by outward rectification, when depolarisation opens K$^+$ channels.

In the resting phase, Na$^+$ and K$^+$ transmembrane concentration gradients are restored by a separate exchange pump (Na$^+$/K$^+$-ATPase) (Fig. 8.2). The resting membrane potential is maintained by high K$^+$ permeability of resting cells through inward rectifying K$^+$ channels, which close when the cell depolarises (see also Ch. 1).

During the period between phase 0 and the end of phase 2, the cell is refractory to further depolarisation (absolute refractory period), because the depolarising channels are inactivated. During phase 3, a sufficiently large stimulus can open enough Na$^+$ channels (many of which have recovered to the resting state) to overcome the K$^+$ efflux and initiate an action potential. This is the relative refractory period.

The sum of the individual electrical currents that pass from one cell to another through the heart can be recorded on the surface electrocardiogram (ECG). The

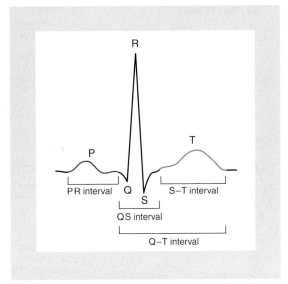

Fig. 8.3
The waveform for cardiac events seen on a surface electrocardiogram. The P wave represents the spread of depolarisation through the atria and the QRS complex is the spread through the ventricles. The T wave represents repolarisation of the ventricle. The PR interval is the time of conductance from atrium to ventricles and the QRS time is the time the ventricles are activated. The duration of the ventricle action potential is given by the QT interval.

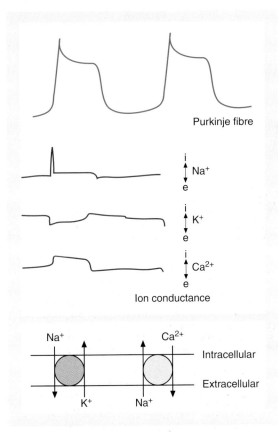

Fig. 8.2
A schematic representation of the influx and efflux of Na⁺, Ca²⁺ and K⁺ in Purkinje fibres. (a) The action potential pattern. (b) Conductance changes in relation to the action potential cycle. (c) The Na⁺/K⁺ and Na⁺/Ca⁺ ion pumps and exchangers maintaining the membrane potential. The electrogenic Na⁺/K⁺ pump also contributes to the outward current in phase 4 of the action potential. In pacemaker cells, the upstroke is dependent on Ca²⁺ rather than Na⁺ and the clear Ca²⁺ influx providing the plateau phase is absent. i, intracellular; e, extracellular

cardiac events that correspond to the ECG are shown in Figure 8.3.

Mechanisms of arrhythmogenesis

Arrhythmias are disorders of rate and rhythm of the heart, which can arise as the result of either abnormal impulse generation or abnormal impulse conduction. There are three principal mechanisms of arrhythmogenesis.

Re-entry. This is the cause of most clinically important arrhythmias. If an impulse arrives at a part of the myocardium that is refractory to the stimulus because of abnormally slow repolarisation, the impulse will be con-ducted by an alternative route that bypasses the refractory tissue (Fig. 8.4). If this impulse arrives at the 'blocked' tissue distally when it has had sufficient time to repolarise, it will then be conducted retrogradely. If there has been sufficient time for the healthy myocardium proximal to the block to repolarise, a circuit of electrical activity will be initiated (a re-entry circuit). This creates a self-perpetuating 'circus' of electrical activity that acts as a pacemaker. The re-entry circuit can be localised within a small area of myocardium that has been damaged by scarring or ischaemia, leading to heterogeneous impulse conduction. The heart can also have large re-entry circuits. Some individuals have congenital bypass pathways that conduct between the atria and ventricles. These can initiate a re-entry circuit that includes the AV node (this occurs in the Wolff–Parkinson–White syndrome).

Automaticity. Ectopic pacemakers can develop when cells in the myocardium or specialised conducting tissue develop a more rapid phase 4 depolarisation than the SA node. An ectopic pacemaker can arise in a site with natural pacemaker activity or spontaneous depolarisation can develop in cells that usually have a stable phase 4. For example, ischaemia can reduce the resting membrane potential and create the conditions in which a cell becomes a pacemaker.

Triggered activity. A cell can develop transient depolarisations during, or following, repolarisation ('after-depolarisations'), which will initiate an action

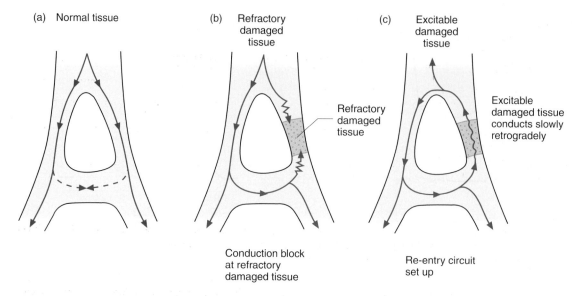

(a) Normal tissue

(b) Refractory damaged tissue

Refractory damaged tissue

Conduction block at refractory damaged tissue

(c) Excitable damaged tissue

Excitable damaged tissue conducts slowly retrogradely

Re-entry circuit set up

Fig. 8.4
Conduction in normal and damaged cardiac tissue. (a) In normal tissue, conduction is carefully ordered. When an impulse has passed, the tissue cannot be immediately reactivated because of refractoriness of the surrounding tissue. If conducted impulses meet they die out. (b) If an area of damage is present, impulses are conducted abnormally. If an impulse arrives and the damaged tissue is refractory the impulse is blocked. (c) If a distal impulse arrives when the damaged tissue is capable of being excited it will be conducted retrogradely and could set up a perpetual re-entry circuit.

potential if they reach the threshold potential. After-depolarisations are said to be 'early' if they occur during repolarisation, or 'delayed' if they occur in phase 4. Such triggered rhythms are a rare mechanism of arrhythmogenesis but may be responsible for the pro-arrhythmic activity of class I and III antiarrhythmic agents and digitalis glycosides (see below).

Classification of antiarrhythmic drugs

A widely used classification of antiarrhythmic drugs (the Vaughan Williams classification) is based on their effects on the action potential (Fig. 8.5) and explains the indications for use of each class of drug (Table 8.1). This classification has many flaws and does not take account of multiple actions possessed by some drugs, nor that the actions of drugs in diseased tissues may be different to those in healthy tissues. There are four classes.

Class I

Class I drugs slow the rate of rise of phase 0 by inhibiting fast Na^+ channels and are often called membrane stabilisers. They readily penetrate the phospholipid bilayers of the cell membrane where they concentrate in

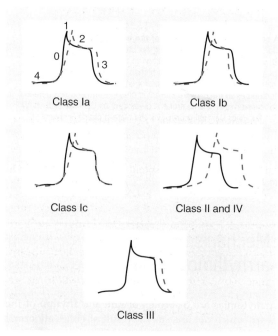

Class Ia

Class Ib

Class Ic

Class II and IV

Class III

Fig. 8.5
Effects of different classes of antiarrhythmic drug on the cardiac action potential. Class I block Na^+ channels and have variable effects on the effective refractory period. Class II decrease phase 4 slope and automaticity. Class III prolong action potential duration and delay repolarisation by acting on K^+ currents. Class IV decrease the phase 4 slope and slow conduction in the sinoatrial and atrioventricular nodes.

Table 8.1
Principal indications for antiarrhythmic drugs

Class	Examples	Supraventricular arrhythmias	Ventricular arrhythmias
Ia	Disopyramide, procainamide, quinidine	+	+
Ib	Lidocaine, mexiletine, phenytoin	−	+ (especially after myocardial infarction)
Ic	Flecainide, propafenone	+	+
II	β-Blockers, sotalol	+	+ (especially after myocardial infarction)
III	Amiodarone, sotalol, bretylium[a]	+	+
IV	Calcium channel antagonists	+	−

[a]Used only in resuscitation and life-threatening arrhythmias.

the hydrophobic core and bind to hydrophobic amino acids in the Na^+ channel. Class I drugs are subdivided according to their effects on the duration of the action potential.

- Class Ia increases the duration of the action potential. Moderate or marked Na^+ channel blockade is produced. This increases refractoriness of the cell and in addition there is blockade of the outward rectifier K^+ channel, which delays repolarisation.
- Class Ib decreases the duration of the action potential. Mild or moderate Na^+ channel blockade is produced, but there is little effect on refractoriness since there is no blockade of K^+ channels.
- Class Ic has no effect on the duration of the action potential. Marked Na^+ channel blockade is produced, and refractoriness is increased owing to some degree of outward rectifier K^+ channel blockade.

The variation in effect of the different class I subgroups results from their diverse binding characteristics to the ion channels. Class Ic drugs dissociate slowly from their binding sites in the Na^+ channel and therefore produce prolonged blockade of channels. Class Ib drugs associate rapidly with channels during depolarisation, binding preferentially to channels when they close. Therefore, they reduce the genesis of premature ectopics, particularly in depolarised tissue such as occurs in ischaemic areas. This explains their selectivity for ventricular arrhythmias in ischaemic heart disease (ischaemia mainly affects the ventricles). When the Na^+ channel returns to the resting state, class Ib drugs rapidly dissociate. Class Ia drugs have an intermediate effect between that of classes Ib and Ic.

Class II

The class II drugs are the β-adrenoceptor antagonists (β-blockers), which block the actions of catecholamines on the heart. They reduce the rate of spontaneous depolarisation of SA and AV nodal tissue and reduce conduction through the AV node. They also reduce spontaneous

depolarisation in phase 4 of some ectopic foci by indirect blockade of Ca^{2+} channels.

Class III

Class III drugs prolong the duration of the action potential, thus increasing the absolute refractory period. Amiodarone and sotalol act by inhibiting the K^+ channels involved in repolarisation (see Table 5.1, p. 88).

Class IV

The class IV drugs are Ca^{2+} channel antagonists (Ca^{2+} antagonists). Some antagonists of L-type Ca^{2+} channels stabilise phase 4 of the action potential in the SA and particularly the AV nodes. The initiation of the pacemaker depolarisation in the SA node depends largely on T-type Ca^{2+} channels and, therefore, is less affected by these drugs. The L-type channels are responsible for depolarisation in the AV node and for maintaining the plateau phase 2 of the action potential in all myocardial cells.

Unclassified drugs

Three drugs used in the treatment of rhythm disturbances do not fit into the Vaughan Williams classification: digitalis glycosides, adenosine and atropine.

Proarrhythmic activity of antiarrhythmic drugs

All antiarrhythmic drugs have the potential to precipitate serious arrhythmias, such as incessant ventricular tachycardia. Several of them (particularly class Ia agents and sotalol) prolong the Q–T interval on the ECG (Fig. 8.3). This predisposes to a polymorphic ventricular tachycardia known as torsade de pointes, which has a characteristic twisting QRS axis on the ECG and can degenerate to ventricular fibrillation. Such induced ventricular rhythm disturbances are particularly refractory to treatment.

The mechanisms of drug-induced arrhythmogenesis are probably multiple:

- electrophysiological actions (particularly triggered automaticity in the case of torsade de pointes, and excessive blockade of Na^+ channels in incessant ventricular tachycardia)
- haemodynamic changes such as depressed myocardial contractility and hypotension
- local metabolic disturbances.

Class Ia drugs

Disopyramide

Pharmacokinetics

Oral absorption of disopyramide is almost complete, but an intravenous formulation is available for rapid onset of action. Metabolism in the liver generates a less active antiarrhythmic compound but with greater anticholinergic activity. About half the drug is eliminated unchanged in the urine. Disopyramide has an intermediate half-life.

Unwanted effects

- Gastrointestinal disturbances.
- Powerful negative inotropic effect; disopyramide should be avoided in heart failure.
- Antimuscarinic effects (see Ch. 4): especially urinary retention, dry mouth and blurred vision.

Procainamide

Pharmacokinetics

Procainamide is well absorbed from the gut but is also available for intravenous use. Most of the drug is excreted unchanged by the kidney but about 40% is acetylated in the liver. The rate of acetylation is subject to genetic polymorphism and is slow in some individuals (Ch. 2). The plasma half-life is short in fast acetylators but increased two fold in slow acetylators.

Unwanted effects

- Gastrointestinal disturbances: nausea, vomiting, anorexia, diarrhoea.
- Negative inotropic effect, producing hypotension.
- Systemic lupus erythematosus-like syndrome with fever, arthralgia, rashes, pleurisy. The syndrome is more common in slow acetylators. It usually appears after at least 2 months of treatment and is common after 6 months; long-term treatment is, therefore, usually avoided and this drug is no longer widely used in the UK.

Quinidine

Pharmacokinetics

Oral absorption of quinidine is almost complete and about 30% undergoes first-pass metabolism. Metabolism in the liver is extensive and the drug has an intermediate half-life. Modified-release formulations are frequently used to reduce the peak plasma concentration and to minimise unwanted effects. An intramuscular formulation is available (but not in the UK). Quinidine is not widely used in the UK.

Unwanted effects

- Gastrointestinal disturbances: nausea, vomiting, abdominal pain, diarrhoea.
- Cinchonism: tinnitus, visual disturbance, flushing, abdominal pain, confusion, headache.
- Negative inotropic effect, producing hypotension.

Class Ib drugs

Lidocaine (lignocaine)

Pharmacokinetics

Extensive first-pass metabolism to a potentially toxic metabolite prevents oral administration. Lidocaine is usually given initially as a loading dose by intravenous bolus injection followed by an infusion. It is extensively metabolised in the liver to compounds with low antiarrhythmic activity, and one has convulsive properties. The half-life is short.

Unwanted effects

- Nausea and vomiting.
- Central nervous system (CNS) toxicity: muscle twitching, convulsions, dizziness, drowsiness.
- Negative inotropic effect, producing hypotension.
- Bradycardia.

Mexiletine

Pharmacokinetics

Oral absorption is almost complete, but an intravenous formulation is also available for rapid onset of action. Metabolism in the liver is extensive and the half-life is long.

Unwanted effects

- Nausea and vomiting.
- CNS toxicity: drowsiness, tremor, confusion, convulsions.
- Negative inotropic effect, producing hypotension.
- Bradycardia.

Class Ic drugs

Flecainide

Pharmacokinetics

Oral absorption of flecainide is complete. An intravenous formulation is also available for rapid onset of action. Most of the drug is eliminated by metabolism; the half-life is long.

Unwanted effects

- CNS toxicity: lightheadedness, anxiety, headache, blurred vision.
- Negative inotropic effect, producing hypotension.
- May be particularly proarrhythmogenic after recent myocardial infarction, when it may increase mortality.

Propafenone

Pharmacokinetics

Oral absorption of propafenone is almost complete but dose-dependent first-pass metabolism can be extensive. Elimination is by hydroxylation, which is saturable and shows genetic polymorphism (Ch. 2). The half-life is therefore dose dependent and much longer in slow metabolisers (about 7% of the Caucasian population).

Unwanted effects

- CNS toxicity (as for flecainide).
- Negative inotropic effect, producing hypotension.
- Weak β-blocking activity can cause broncho-constriction in asthmatics.

Class II drugs

Beta-adrenoceptor antagonists (β-blockers)

The $β_1$-adrenoceptor-blocking activity is responsible for the therapeutic effects of the β-blockers. The most widely used agents are atenolol and propranolol; these are also discussed in Chapter 5. Both can be given intravenously for a rapid onset of action.

Esmolol is an ultra-short-acting cardioselective β-blocker that is used exclusively for the treatment of arrhythmias. It is most often used when arrhythmias arise during anaesthesia.

Pharmacokinetics

The half-life of esmolol is very short (about 9 min) and its action is terminated by esterase activity in erythrocytes. It is given by bolus intravenous injection.

Class III drugs

Amiodarone

Pharmacokinetics

Amiodarone is incompletely absorbed orally and has a large volume of distribution as a result of extensive tissue protein binding. Metabolism in the liver produces an active metabolite and both amiodarone and its major metabolite have very long half-lives, averaging 50–60 days. An intravenous formulation is available. Because of the long half-life, a prolonged loading dose regimen is used for both routes of administration. The effects seen early after intravenous use are believed to be caused by non-competitive β-adrenoceptor antagonist activity, while the class III effect is delayed. Some of the antiarrhythmic effects may also result from class III and class IV actions.

Unwanted effects

- Gastrointestinal disturbances, for example constipation and nausea, most often occur during the loading period.
- Corneal microdeposits are almost universal and can cause dazzling by headlights when driving at night.
- Because of its iodine content, amiodarone produces thyrotoxicosis in up to one-third of patients. Inhibition of peripheral conversion of thyroxine to triiodothyronine (Ch. 41) produces hypothyroidism in other patients.
- Photosensitive skin rashes. Full sun-screening is recommended.
- Progressive pulmonary fibrosis is a rare but serious effect of long-term treatment.
- Drug interactions: the plasma concentrations of warfarin (Ch. 11) and digoxin (Ch. 7) are increased by amiodarone, with consequent potentiation of their effects. This is caused by displacement of the drugs from tissue stores; amiodarone also inhibits the renal excretion of digoxin.

Unlike most antiarrhythmic drugs, amiodarone does not have negative inotropic effects and is safe to use in heart failure.

Bretylium

Bretylium is now used only for treatment of life-threatening ventricular arrhythmias when other agents have failed. It acts by myocardial adrenergic neuron blockade.

Pharmacokinetics

Oral absorption is poor and bretylium is only available for parenteral (usually intravenous) use. Selective

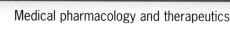

concentration occurs in the myocardium. Bretylium is excreted unchanged by the kidney and has an intermediate half-life.

Unwanted effects

- Hypotension.
- Nausea and vomiting after rapid intravenous injection.

Sotalol

Sotalol is a β-blocker (Ch. 5) with additional class III properties. As with many drugs, sotalol is a racemic mixture; both β-adrenoceptor-blocking and class III activity reside in the L-isomer, while the D-isomer only has class III activity. These additional antiarrhythmic properties also give sotalol a greater proarrhythmic potential than other β-blockers (see above). Sotalol is now reserved for treatment of significant rhythm disturbances and not for the other indications for β-blockers. Prolongation of the duration of the action potential by the class III effect tends to counteract the effect of β-blockade on myocardial contractility, which makes sotalol less negatively inotropic than most β-blockers.

Pharmacokinetics

Sotalol is almost completely absorbed from the gut and excreted unchanged in the urine. The half-life is intermediate.

Class IV drugs

Calcium channel antagonists

Verapamil and diltiazem, but not the dihydropyridine derivatives such as nifedipine, have antiarrhythmic activity. Verapamil can be given intravenously for a rapid effect, but this should be avoided in patients taking a β-blocker because of summation of myocardial depression and AV nodal conduction block. Full details of Ca^{2+} antagonists are found in Chapter 5.

Other drugs for rhythm disturbances

Several drugs used for the management of rhythm disturbances do not fit into the Vaughan Williams classification. These are considered here.

Digoxin

Digitalis glycosides (such as digoxin) are not strictly antiarrhythmic. They are, however, useful for controlling ventricular rate in atrial flutter and atrial fibrillation

through their ability to reduce conduction through the AV node. They are discussed in Chapter 7.

Adenosine

Mechanism of action and effects

Adenosine is a purine nucleotide that has potent effects on the SA node, producing sinus bradycardia. It also slows impulse conduction through the AV node but has no effect on conduction in the ventricles. Consequently, it is only useful for management of supraventricular arrhythmias, particularly those caused by AV nodal re-entry mechanisms. Its electrophysiological actions are mediated by specific adenosine receptors, particularly the A_1 subtype, which activate outward rectifier K^+ channels. This enhances the flow of K^+ out of myocardial cells and produces hyperpolarisation of the cell membrane (see Table 5.1, p. 88). This stabilises the cell membrane.

The A_2 receptor subtype is responsible for vasodilation by impairing cellular Ca^{2+} uptake. This property can be used by giving adenosine as a pharmacological stress to induce ischaemia in patients with suspected coronary artery disease who are unable to exercise. Preferential dilation of arteries to healthy tissue produces a coronary blood flow 'steal' that reduces flow in diseased arteries. Myocardial ischaemia is then assessed by radionuclide scanning or echocardiography.

Additional sites that possess adenosine A_1 receptors are the lung, placenta and T-lymphocytes, while A_2 receptors are present in the brain and placenta (see also methylxanthines, Ch. 12).

Pharmacokinetics

Adenosine is given by rapid bolus intravenous injection. The effect is terminated by uptake into erythrocytes and endothelial cells, followed by metabolism to inosine and hypoxanthine. Adenosine has a half-life of less than 10 s, and a duration of action of less than 1 min.

Unwanted effects

Unwanted effects are common, occurring in about 25% of patients; however, they are usually transient, lasting less than 1 min:

- bradycardia and AV block
- malaise, flushing, headache, chest pain or tightness, bronchospasm; adenosine should be avoided in patients with asthma
- drug interactions: dipyridamole (Ch. 11) potentiates the effects of adenosine while methylxanthines such as aminophylline (Ch. 12) inhibit its action.

Atropine

Atropine is discussed fully in Chapter 4. It is given by intravenous bolus injection and inhibits the effect of the vagus nerve on the heart. This increases the rate of firing of the SA node and increases conduction through the AV node via blockade of muscarinic M_2 receptors. The effects are mediated by activation of K^+ channels, which hyperpolarise the cell membrane. Atropine is used specifically for the treatment of sinus bradycardia and AV block. It is metabolised in the liver and has an intermediate half-life.

Drug treatment of arrhythmias

Arrhythmias can be harmless, or they can produce a variety of symptoms that vary from mild to life threatening. The probability of symptoms arising depends on several factors, the most important of which are the nature of the rhythm disturbance, the rate of an abnormal rhythm and the presence of underlying heart disease. The range of consequences of rhythm disturbances includes

● awareness of palpitation
● dizziness
● syncope
● precipitation of angina or heart failure
● sudden death.

Treatment may not be necessary for benign or self-terminating arrhythmias. Reassurance may be all that is required, but it is important to remove or treat any underlying cause. Vagotonic procedures such as the Valsalva manoeuvre or carotid sinus massage can terminate some supraventricular arrhythmias (but not atrial fibrillation)

The choice of treatment depends on the situation. With tachyarrhythmias, sinus rhythm should, if possible, be restored. Direct current (DC) cardioversion is used to achieve this in severe, life-threatening or drug-resistant arrhythmias; drug therapy is used if there is less need for immediate effect or to control the ventricular rate if the abnormal rhythm cannot be terminated. Long-term drug treatment for bradyarrhythmias is rarely used, and an implanted pacemaker may be necessary. The principle indications for antiarrhythmic drugs are given in Table 8.1.

Supraventricular tachyarrhythmias

Atrial premature beats

Atrial premature beats are very common and usually benign. However, they can be produced by digoxin toxicity, and frequent multifocal atrial ectopics can result from organic heart disease. Other than treatment of an underlying cause, specific drug therapy is rarely needed. Some patients are disturbed by a post-ectopic pause followed by a more forceful beat when sinus rhythm then recommences. A β-blocker or Ca^{2+} antagonist such as verapamil or diltiazem can be used to suppress the ectopics.

Atrial tachycardia

Atrial tachycardia is an infrequent rhythm disturbance arising from an automatic focus, and it is often accompanied by AV conduction block. It is not usually associated with significant cardiac disease but can be a manifestation of digoxin toxicity. A less common form is multifocal atrial tachycardia arising from several ectopic foci, usually in patients with severe pulmonary disease. Apart from treatment of the underlying disorder, a class Ic agent such as flecainide, a β-blocker, Ca^{2+} antagonist such as verapamil or diltiazem, or amiodarone can be used to suppress the rhythm disturbance.

Atrial flutter

The atrial rate is usually 250–350 beats min^{-1}, which is conducted to the ventricles with 2:1 or greater degrees of AV block. Flutter waves may be obvious on the ECG or appear if the ventricular rate is slowed by vagal manoeuvres or administration of adenosine. Atrial flutter usually arises from a single re-entry circuit in the right atrium. Underlying causes include cardiac surgery, cor pulmonale and congenital heart disease, but it can arise for no obvious reason. It may be paroxysmal, and it can degenerate into atrial fibrillation. Drug therapy is relatively unsuccessful for restoring sinus rhythm, and DC cardioversion (synchronised to discharge on the R wave of the ECG) or rapid 'overdrive' electrical pacing to capture the ventricle, followed by a gradual reduction in the paced rate, may be required. Class Ia, Ic and III antiarrhythmic agents can prevent recurrence in paroxysmal atrial flutter. Disopyramide should be avoided since its antimuscarinic action can increase AV conduction and speed up the ventricular response. Control of the ventricular rate in sustained atrial flutter can be achieved in a similar manner to that in chronic atrial fibrillation (see below), but treatment is often less successful. For this reason, radiofrequency ablation of the re-entrant pathway via a cardiac catheter is becoming increasingly popular. Prophylaxis against thromboembolism should be given, similar to that for atrial fibrillation.

Atrial fibrillation

Atrial fibrillation is the most common rhythm disturbance in clinical practice. It has a variety of underlying causes (Box 8.1), some of which may be treatable. In younger patients, atrial fibrillation often occurs without

---

> **Box 8.1**
>
> **Causes of atrial fibrillation**
>
> *Structural heart disease*
>   Hypertension
>   Coronary heart disease
>   Valvular heart disease (especially mitral)
>   Cardiomyopathies
>   Cardiac surgery
>   Congenital heart disease (especially atrial septal defect)
>
> *Other causes*
>   Major infections
>   Thyrotoxicosis, myxoedema
>   Alcohol intoxication
>   Systemic illness (e.g. amyloid, sarcoidosis)

any obvious underlying cause, when it is called 'lone' atrial fibrillation. The arrhythmia arises from multiple re-entry circuits in the atria, The ventricular rate will depend on AV nodal function. When this is good, atrial fibrillation is accompanied by a rapid ventricular rate. Atrial fibrillation also predisposes to atrial thrombus formation and subsequent systemic emboli, which commonly cause stroke. Management has four underlying aims.

- To identify and treat the underlying cause.
- To restore or maintain sinus rhythm (Box 8.2). It is usually desirable to attempt to restore sinus rhythm, since symptoms and exercise tolerance are usually improved and the risk of stroke is removed. Restoration of sinus rhythm is usually possible in lone atrial fibrillation or when there is a treatable underlying cause. It can occasionally be achieved with drugs, but it usually requires synchronised DC cardioversion. Pharmacological cardioversion, or maintenance of sinus rhythm after DC cardioversion, is best achieved by using class Ic drugs such as

flecainide or propafenone, or agents with class III properties such as sotalol or amiodarone. These 'antifibrillatory' drugs are also useful for prophylaxis of paroxysmal atrial fibrillation. Following successful DC cardioversion, antifibrillatory drugs can be used to prevent recurrence, which is most frequent during the first 3–6 months since this is the period of highest risk. However, long-term drug treatment is often necessary to prevent recurrent atrial fibrillation. Digoxin is ineffective for restoring or maintaining sinus rhythm in paroxysmal atrial fibrillation and should be avoided.

- To control a rapid ventricular response if sinus rhythm cannot be restored. Rate control at rest can be achieved with digoxin, but during exercise a rapid heart rate often still occurs. The addition of a β-blocker, or a rate-controlling Ca^{2+} antagonist such as verapamil or diltiazem, may then be necessary. Flecainide or amiodarone can also be used with digoxin. Sotalol has no particular value in sustained atrial fibrillation and should be avoided because of its greater pro-arrhythmic activity than other β-blockers.
- To reduce thromboembolism by long-term anticoagulation (Ch. 11). The risk of emboli is greatest in the elderly (over 75 years of age) and if there is coexisting hypertension, diabetes mellitus or recent heart failure. Poor left ventricular systolic function on echocardiography also predicts increased risk (Table 8.2). Almost all patients with atrial fibrillation, whether sustained or paroxysmal, should take either aspirin or warfarin. Warfarin is more effective than aspirin in high-risk patients but has little advantage in those at moderate or low risk of embolism. Warfarin is the anticoagulant of choice in atrial fibrillation associated with rheumatic heart disease, thyrotoxicosis and for 1 month before and 1 month after DC cardioversion.

Junctional (nodal) tachycardias

Junctional tachycardias usually arise from re-entry mechanisms, which can be within the AV node or involve an accessory AV pathway (e.g. in Wolff–Parkinson–White syndrome). Termination of an acute attack can often be achieved with vagotonic manoeuvres such as carotid sinus massage or by adenosine. Beta-blockers, diltiazem or verapamil can be used to treat acute episodes or for prophylaxis. Diltiazem, verapamil and digoxin should be avoided if there is an accessory AV pathway; selective blockade of the AV node by these drugs can predispose to rapid conduction of atrial arrhythmias through the accessory pathway. Junctional tachycardias involving an accessory pathway often respond well to flecainide, sotalol or amiodarone. Radiofrequency ablation of the re-entry circuit, via a cardiac catheter, is being employed increasingly for troublesome junctional tachycardias.

> **Box 8.2**
>
> **Factors predicting a high probability of successful restoration of sinus rhythm in patients with atrial fibrillation**
>
> Short duration of atrial fibrillation (less than 1 year)
> Younger age (<50 years)
> Absence of underlying heart disease
> Normal left ventricular function
> Little or no enlargement of the left atrium
> Withdrawal or treatment of a precipitating factor, e.g. thyrotoxicosis, alcohol

Table 8.2
Risk of stroke in 'non-rheumatic' atrial fibrillation

Patient group	Stroke risk without prophylaxis (% per year)	Anticoagulant of choice
High risk		
Previous ischaemic stroke or transient ischaemic attack	12	Warfarin
Age >75 years + one other risk factor[a]	8	Warfarin
Age 65–74 years + two or more other risk factors	8	Warfarin
Moderate risk		
Age <65 years + other risk factors	4	Aspirin
Age 65–74 years + one other risk factor	4	Aspirin
Low risk		
Age <65 years with no other risk factors	1	Aspirin

[a]Coexisting hypertension, diabetes mellitus, recent heart failure, poor left ventricular function on echocardiography (see text).

Ventricular tachyarrhythmias

Ventricular ectopic beats

Ventricular ectopic beats can occur in healthy individuals or in association with a variety of cardiac disorders such as ischaemic heart disease and heart failure. Frequent ventricular ectopic beats after myocardial infarction predict a less good long-term outcome for the patient; however, suppressing such ectopics with class I agents increases mortality, and should be avoided. Beta-blockers are useful in this situation and can improve prognosis (Ch. 5). In other situations, symptomatic ventricular ectopic beats can be suppressed by a class I drug such as mexiletine, flecainide or disopyramide.

Ventricular tachycardia

Ventricular tachycardia is often associated with serious underlying heart disease, such as ischaemic heart disease or heart failure, and is more common following myocardial infarction. It can be either sustained or non-sustained. Sustained ventricular tachycardia can be associated with a minimal or absent cardiac output ('pulseless' ventricular tachycardia), when it is treated as ventricular fibrillation (see below). Polymorphic or incessant ventricular tachycardias can occur as a complication of antiarrhythmic drug therapy (see above) and with other drugs that prolong the Q–T interval on the ECG, such as some antihistamines. For sustained ventricular tachycardias, drug options include class Ib agents such as lidocaine, or amiodarone. Sustained ventricular tachycardia is often associated with a poor long-term outlook in ischaemic heart disease, and coronary revascularisation or an automatic implantable cardiac defibrillator may be beneficial. During and after the acute phase of myocardial infarction, a β-blocker is the treatment of choice for non-sustained ventricular tachycardias.

Ventricular fibrillation

Ventricular fibrillation is a potentially lethal arrhythmia that constitutes one form of 'cardiac arrest'. An algorithm for the management of cardiac arrest is regularly updated by the European Resuscitation Working Party, and is shown in Figure 8.6. The important principles of resuscitation are maintenance of adequate cardiac output by external chest compression, and oxygenation by artificial inflation of the lungs while attempting to restore sinus rhythm. Ventricular fibrillation is the commonest arrhythmia in acute cardiac arrest and all patients should be assumed to have this, and treated with immediate DC cardioversion, if a good ECG monitor read-out is not available. Epinephrine (adrenaline) (Ch. 4) is given to vasoconstrict the peripheries and thus maintain pressure in the central arteries perfusing the heart and brain. For recurrent ventricular fibrillation, suppression is best achieved by long-term use of anti-arrhythmic drugs such as sotalol or amiodarone (often combinedvwith a β-blocker) or by an automatic implantable cardioverter–defibrillator.

Bradycardias

Sinus bradycardia

Treatment with atropine may be necessary if sinus bradycardia is causing symptoms (e.g. after myocardial infarction). Hypotension precipitated by drugs such as streptokinase (Ch. 11) or the first dose of an angiotensin-converting enzyme (ACE) inhibitor (Ch. 6)

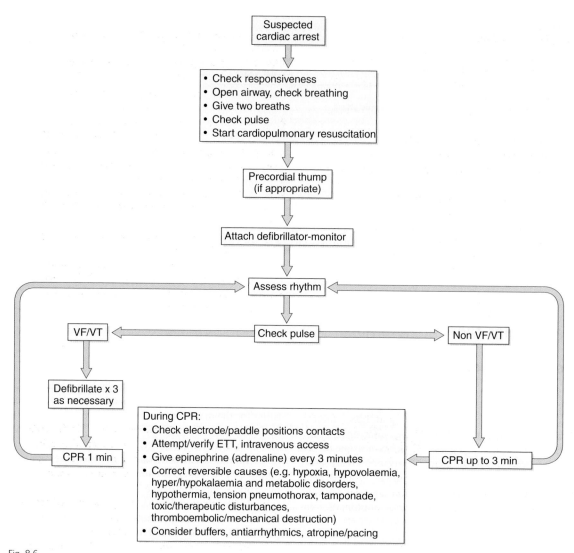

Fig. 8.6

An algorithm for the management of cardiac arrest. CPR, cardio pulmonary resuscitation; ETT, endotracheal tube; VF, ventricular fibrillation, VT, ventricular tachyarrhythmia.

is often associated with vagally mediated bradycardia, which will respond to atropine.

Atrioventricular block ('heart block')

If AV block arises suddenly, then loss of consciousness (Stokes–Adams attack) or death can occur. An AV block can be congenital or accompany a variety of heart diseases. If it occurs after myocardial infarction, it is usually temporary if the infarct is inferior but is often permanent after anterior infarction. First-degree heart block (prolongation of the PR interval on the ECG) rarely requires treatment, but higher degrees of block (with non-conducted P waves) should be treated. If the onset is acute, atropine should be given intravenously to increase AV conduction, but external or temporary transvenous electrical cardiac pacing is usually required. The β-adrenoceptor agonist isoprenaline (Ch. 4) can be given by intravenous infusion if there is likely to be delay in pacing. However, this usually produces excessive numbers of ectopic beats and rarely improves nodal conduction. If the AV block is permanent, the implantation of a permanent electrical cardiac pacemaker is usually necessary.

FURTHER READING

Advanced Life Support Working Group of the European Resuscitation Council (1998) The 1998 European Resuscitation Council guidelines for adult advanced life support. *Br Med J* 319, 1893–1899

Campbell RWF (1998) Atrial flutter. *Eur Heart J* 19(suppl E), E37–E40

Grant AO (1998) Mechanisms of atrial fibrillation and action of drugs used in its management. *Am J Cardiol* 82, 43N–49N

Hancox JC, Patel KCR, Jones JV (2000) Antiarrhythmics – from cell to clinic: past, present, and future. *Heart* 84, 14–24

Hauer RNW, Loh P (1998) 'Para' AV nodal reentry tachycardias. *Eur Heart J* 19(suppl E), E2–E9

Howard PA (1999) Guidelines for stoke prevention in patients with atrial fibrillation. *Drugs* 58, 997–1009

Katz AM (1998) Selectivity and toxicity of antiarrhythmic drugs: molecular interactions with ion channels. *Am J Med* 104, 179–195

Lip GYH, Watson RDS, Singh SP (1966) Cardioversion of atrial fibrillation. *Br Med J* 312, 112–115

Lip GYH, Watson RDS, Singh SP (1995) Drugs for atrial fibrillation. *Br Med J* 311, 1631–1634

Nademanee K, Kosar EM (1998) Long-term antithrombotic treatment for atrial fibrillation. *Am J Cardiol* 82, 27N–42N

Obel OA, Camm AJ (1998) Accessory pathway reciprocating tachycardia. *Eur Heart J* 29(suppl E), E13–E24

Reiffel JA, Estes NAM, Waldo AL et al. (1994) A consensus report on antiarrhythmic drug use. *Clin Cardiol* 17, 103–116

Reiffel JA, Reiter MJ, Blitzer M (1998) Antiarrhythmic drugs and devices for the management of ventricular tachyarrhythmias in ischaemic heart disease. *Am J Cardiol* 82, 311–401

Reiter MJ, Reiffel JA (1998) Importance of beta blockade in the therapy of serious ventricular arrhythmias. *Am J Cardiol* 82, 9I–19I

Roden DM (1994) Risks and benefits of antiarrhythmic therapy. *N Engl J Med* 331, 785–790

Sopher SOM, Camm AJ (1996) Atrial fibrillation: maintenance of sinus rhythm versus rate control. *Am J Cardiol* 77, 24A–37A

Steinbeck G, Hoffman E (1998) 'True' atrial tachycardia. *Eur Heart J* 19(suppl E), E10–E12.

Self-assessment

1. In the following questions, the first statement, in italics, is true. Is the accompanying statement also true?

   a. *Pacemaker cells in the sinoatrial node initiate cardiac rhythm discharge at a higher frequency than those in other parts of the heart.* Spontaneous or pacemaker depolarisation occurring during diastole results from the fluxes of several anions.
   b. *The influx of Na^+ during phase 0 lasts only for milliseconds and the Na^+ gates for influx are closed during the plateau phase 2. Thus muscle cells are refractory to further action potentials during this period (refractory period).* The plateau phase (phase 2) results solely from the release of Ca^{2+} from the sarcoplasmic reticulum.
   c. *Reducing the rate of rise in the slope of phase 4 will slow the normal pacemaker rate.* Beta-adrenergic stimulation, hypokalaemia and vagal stimulation reduce the slope of phase 4 depolarisation and, therefore, reduce pacemaker rate.
   d. *The sinoatrial node and the atrioventricular node have pacemaker activity.* Non-pacemaker cells always remain quiescent if not excited by an impulse arising from other regions in the heart.
   e. *Antiarrhythmic drugs reduce the automaticity of ectopic pacemakers more than that of the sinoatrial node pacemaker.* The effect of the class I antiarrhythmic drugs is to block Na^+ channels, which prolongs the refractory period of the target cell.
   f. *Sympathetic atrioventricular stimulation increases pacemaker depolarisation rate and conduction through the atrioventricular node.* Beta-adrenergic-blocking drugs are useful in stress-induced tachycardias.
   g. *Verapamil has little benefit in ventricular arrhythmias.* Verapamil will affect both the plateau phase 2 and phase 4 of the action potential cycle.
   h. *Adenosine is currently the drug of choice for prompt conversion of paroxysmal supraventricular tachycardia to sinus rhythm.* Adenosine is effective in the treatment of ventricular arrhythmias.

2. Case history question

Mr GH, aged 48 years, consulted his GP complaining of palpitations and was found to have an irregular pulse with a ventricular rate of 120 beats min^{-1}. He was suffering from shortness of breath and faintness lasting about 6 h. The symptoms had started shortly after a drinking binge 36 h previously. Examination, blood tests (including thyroid function tests), electrocardiograph (ECG) and chest radiograph revealed no coexisting heart disease, diabetes or hypertension. The ECG confirmed atrial fibrillation.

a. What are the options available for treating this patient?

Before any treatment could be instituted, the patient spontaneously reverted to sinus rhythm. Mr GH was well for a year but then returned to his GP with a 3-day history of palpitations, breathlessness, chest pain and dizziness. Examination and an ECG revealed atrial fibrillation. He was referred to a cardiologist and echocardiography showed no evidence of structural cardiac disease. Electrical DC cardioversion was carried out and the patient reverted to sinus rhythm.

Over the next 5 years, episodes of atrial fibrillation occurred with increasing frequency and eventually sinus rhythm could not be restored with a variety of antiarrhythmic drugs or by DC conversion.

b. What prophylactic treatment should be considered at the time of DC cardioversion? What drug treatments may be useful after DC cardioversion?

The answers are provided on pages 604–605.

Drugs used in the treatment of arrhythmias

Drug	Half-life (h)	Elimination	Comments[a]
Class I drugs			
Disopyramide	4–10	Renal (60%) metabolism (30%)	SVT, VF, VT; given orally, slow intravenous injection (over at least 5 min) or intravenous infusion; oral bioavailability is 90%; main metabolite is less antiarrhythmic but more anticholinergic
Flecainide	14	Renal (25%) metabolism (75%)	AFI, N; given orally, or by slow intravenous injection (over 10–30 min) or intravenous infusion; oral bioavailability is >90%; should be initiated in hospital
Lidocaine (lignocaine)	2	Metabolism	VA (especially post-MI); given by intravenous injection or intravenous infusion; metabolites retain some activity.
Mexiletine	13	Metabolism (+ some renal)	VA (especially post-MI); given orally or by intravenous injection or intravenous infusion; inactive metabolites
Moracizine (moricizine)	3	Metabolism	VA (named patient basis); given orally; bioavailability is about 30–40% owing to first-pass metabolism; induces its own metabolism by cytochrome P450 (autoinduction)
Procainamide	3	Renal (+ some metabolism)	AT, VA; given orally, by slow intravenous injection or by intravenous infusion; metabolised by N-acetylation; N-acetylmetabolite is as active as the parent drug and has a longer half-life (6–9 h)
Propafenone	4	Metabolism	SVT, N, VA; some β-blockade; given orally; low oral bioavailability (10%), which is increased at higher doses and by food; metabolised by oxidation by CYP2D6 + CYP3A4: longer half-life (17 h) in poor metabolisers of CYP2D6 substrates (e.g. debrisoquine)
Quinidine	7	Metabolism + renal	SVT, VA; specialist use; given orally; good oral bioavailability (70–80%); metabolised by oxidation; potent inhibitor of CYP2D6
Tocainide	10–40	Metabolism + renal	VT; given orally; 100% oral bioavailability; eliminated equally by renal excretion and hepatic metabolism
Class II drugs: β-blockers			Beta-blockers are used in a wide variety of indications. The list below is divided into those licensed for use in heart arrhythmias in the UK, and for completeness all other β-blockers irrespective of their value in arrhythmias
Antiarrhythmic β-blockers			Apart from esmolol, these drugs are also commonly used for angina, hypertension and other indications for β-blockers
Acebutolol	7	Metabolism + renal	AF, SVT, VT; β1-selective; 10% β1-selective PAA; given orally; oral bioavailability is 50–70%; active acetylated metabolite; drug-induced lupus reported
Atenolol	7	Renal	AF, SVT, VT; β1-selective; given orally, by injection or intravenous infusion; eliminated by glomerular filtration
Esmolol	0.15	Metabolism	SVT; β1-selective; given by intravenous infusion; rapidly hydrolysed in erythrocytes
Metoprolol	3–10	Metabolism	SVT, VT; β1-selective (< atenolol); given orally, or by injection or intravenous infusion; bioavailability is about 50%; wide variability in metabolism by CYP2D6
Nadolol	17–24	Renal + bile	SVT, VT; β-non-selective; given orally but poor absorption (30%)
Oxprenolol	2	Metabolism	SVT, VT; β-non-selective; 18% β-non-selective PAA; given orally; bioavailability is 20–80% owing to first-pass metabolism; hydroxy metabolite also active
Propranolol	4	Metabolism	AF, SVT, VT; β-non-selective; given orally or by injection; oral bioavailability is 10–50% owing to first-pass metabolism; oxidised by P450 and conjugated with glucuronic acid (17%)
Sotalol			See under Class III drugs; uses restricted to life-threatening arrhythmias

continued

Drugs used in the treatment of arrhythmias *(continued)*

Drug	Half-life (h)	Elimination	Comments[a]
Beta-blockers not normally used as antiarrhythmics			Oral dosage unless otherwise indicated (typical uses shown)
Betaxolol	13–24	Metabolism (+ some renal)	Glaucoma, hypertension; β_1-selective; high oral bioavailability (80–90%); oxidised in liver and metabolites eliminated in urine
Bisoprolol	11	Renal + metabolism	Angina, hypertension; β_1-selective (> atenolol); oral bioavailability is 90%; eliminated equally by glomerular filtration and secretion, and by metabolism in the liver
Carvedilol	6	Metabolism	Angina, hypertension; β-non-selective; vasodilator owing to α_1-blockade; oral bioavailability is 20–30% owing to first-pass metabolism; metabolites eliminated in bile and urine
Celiprolol	5	Renal (+ some biliary)	Hypertension; β_1-selective; vasodilator because of β_2-PAA; polar compound that has a bioavailability of 30–70% because of poor absorption
Labetalol	3	Metabolism	Hypertension; β_1-selective; vasodilator through α-blockade; α:β selectivity is 1:2 orally and 1:7 intravenously; given orally, or by intravenous injection or intravenous infusion; oral bioavailability is variable (10–90%) owing to first-pass metabolism; metabolised by glucuronidation
Nebivolol	10	Metabolism	Hypertension; new β_1-selective drug; metabolised by oxidation (possibly CYP2D6)
Pindolol	4	Metabolism + renal	Angina, hypertension; β-non-selective; vasodilator because of 35% β-non-selective PAA; high oral bioavailability (>90%); approximately equal elimination in urine and by metabolism
Timolol	2–5	Metabolism + some renal	Angina, hypertension, post-MI; β-non-selective; oral bioavailability is 30–50%; eliminated by metabolism and renal excretion (20%)
Class III drugs			
Amiodarone	50–60 days	Metabolism	All arrhythmias; given orally or by intravenous infusion; oral bioavailability is 20–100%; active metabolite, which also has a long half-life (50 days); accumulation
Bretylium	9	Renal	VA (resistant); given by slow intravenous injection, intramuscular injection, or intravenous infusion; clearance correlates with creatinine clearance
Sotalol	7–18	Renal	Also class II β-blocker; VT (life threatening); β-non-selective; class III antiarrhythmic activity; greater proarrhythmic risk than other β-blockers; given orally or by intravenous injection; bioavailability is >90%; eliminated largely by glomerular filtration
Class IV drugs			
Diltiazem	2–5	Metabolism	SVT; less cardioactive than verapamil; given orally; bioavailability is about 50% owing to first-pass metabolism; metabolites retain activity
Verapamil	2–7	Metabolism	SVT; main drug in this group; given orally or by intravenous injection; low oral bioavailability (about 20%); (S)-isomer is more active form; metabolised by CYP3A4 or CYP1A2
Other drugs			
Adenosine	2 seconds	Metabolism (all cells)	SVT; given intravenously; extremely rapidly cleared by metabolism
Atropine	2–5	Metabolism + renal	Bradycardia; given intravenously
Digoxin	40 (20–50)	Renal	AF; may need loading dose; oral or intravenous dosage
Phenytoin	7–60	Metabolism	VA (especially that caused by cardiac glycosides); was given by slow intravenous infusion, now obsolete for arrhythmias

The types of arrhythmias commonly treated with different drugs are AF, atrial fibrillation; AFL, atrial flutter; AT, atrial tachycardia; SVT, supraventricular tachycardia; N, nodal; VF, ventricular fibrillation; VT, ventricular tachycardia; VA, ventricular arrhythmias; PAA, partial aonist activity. Other abbreviations: MI, myocardial infarction; PAA, partial agonist activity. For other Ca^{2+} channel antagonists, see Chapter 5 compendium.

9

Cerebrovascular disease and dementia

Stroke

....

Aetiology

Strokes are a major cause of morbidity and mortality in older people. They present as a transient or permanent neurological disturbance caused by ischaemic infarction or haemorrhagic disruption of neuronal pathways in the brain. The extent and duration of the resulting functional deficit is very variable and depends on several factors. Transient cerebral ischaemic attacks (TIAs) arise from small cerebral arterial emboli which rapidly disperse. These produce short-lived neurological signs and symptoms but leave no functional deficit 24 hours later. However, there is a 30% risk of completed stroke within 5 years after a TIA. More severe cerebral ischaemia produces a cerebral infarction and the neurological disturbance persists for longer; frequently there is some permanent loss of function. Cerebral infarction can result from intracerebral arterial thrombosis or from cerebral arterial emboli. Haemorrhagic stroke commonly leaves a residual functional deficit. There are no established treatments which limit the neurological deficit in acute stroke, although there are some promising drugs in development. Most management is directed to prevention or rehabilitation after the event.

....

Prevention

There are a number of measures that can reduce the risk of stroke.

- Stopping smoking reduces the risk of stroke by up to 40% by 2–5 years after cessation.
- Hypertension is the single most powerful predictor of stroke. Results from several trials indicate that a reduction in diastolic blood pressure by 5–6 mmHg reduces the risk of stroke by about 40% (Ch. 6). For isolated systolic hypertension, a similar reduction in risk has been shown after an average 11 mmHg reduction in systolic blood pressure (with a concurrent fall of 3–4 mmHg in diastolic blood pressure).

- Aspirin at low dosage, given to patients who are in sinus rhythm following a transient ischaemic attack or a first ischaemic stroke, reduces the risk of a further non-fatal stroke by about 25% through its antiplatelet action (Ch. 11). Combining aspirin with dipyridamole (Ch. 11) is more effective than low-dose aspirin given alone, but the combination is usually reserved for recurrence of stroke during treatment with low-dose aspirin alone. Aspirin has not been shown to prevent a first stroke when taken by healthy individuals who are in sinus rhythm. By contrast, in patients with atrial fibrillation, aspirin can reduce the risk of a first event by almost one-third although it is less effective than warfarin (Ch. 8).
- Anticoagulation with warfarin reduces the risk of stroke in patients with atrial fibrillation by about two-thirds. If other risk factors for cerebral embolic disease coexist with atrial fibrillation, and after a first small stroke in patients with atrial fibrillation, warfarin is superior to aspirin for stroke prevention (see Ch. 11). Following myocardial infarction, if there is an intracardiac clot associated with an akinetic area of the left ventricular wall, warfarin reduces the risk of stroke. In patients with recurrent TIA while taking aspirin, warfarin may actually increase morbidity and mortality.
- Thrombolytic therapy with recombinant tissue plasminogen activator (rtPA) or streptokinase (Ch. 11) is still being evaluated for ischaemic stroke. There is evidence for reduced disability if treatment is started within 3 h of the onset of symptoms, but there is an associated risk of intracranial haemorrhage.
- Carotid endarterectomy reduces the risk of stroke in selected patients with arteriosclerotic disease of the carotid arteries. Greatest benefit is derived if there have already been transient focal neurological symptoms in the territory served by the diseased carotid artery. In this group of patients, if the stenosis is 70% or more of the vessel diameter, then endarterectomy reduces the risk of recurrent stroke from about 25% to 10% over the subsequent 2 years (despite a perioperative risk of stroke or death of 3–5%). The benefit is less clear in asymptomatic carotid artery disease, since the annual risk of an ischaemic stroke is low.
- Reduction of a raised plasma cholesterol with a statin (Ch. 48) produces a very modest reduction in the risk of a first stroke in patients with coronary artery disease. The effect of cholesterol reduction in secondary prevention of stroke is still under study. The main rationale for cholesterol reduction remains prevention of ischaemic heart disease, which often co-exists with cerebrovascular disease.

Subarachnoid haemorrhage

Subarachnoid haemorrhage occurs following rupture of a Charcot–Bouchard aneurysm on a cerebral artery. These aneurysms are usually found in hypertensive patients. Sudden onset of headache is the most common presenting feature, but focal neurological signs or progressive confusion and impaired consciousness can occur. The neurological disturbance is a result of cerebral ischaemia produced by vasospasm, thrombosis or metabolic disturbance following the haemorrhage. Cerebral ischaemia can occur acutely or be delayed; it leads to increased flow of calcium into the cell and further ischaemic neuronal damage.

Management

The management of subarachnoid haemorrhage is mainly surgical, with ligation of the aneurysm that produced the bleeding. Ischaemic cerebral damage can be reduced by using nimodipine in the first few days after the event.

Nimodipine

Nimodipine is a dihydropyridine Ca^{2+} channel antagonist (for mechanism of action see Ch. 5). It is a vasodilator with some selectivity for cerebral arteries that reduces the risk of vasospasm following subarachnoid haemorrhage. However, it probably produces most of its benefits by protection of ischaemic neurons from Ca^{2+} overload. There is a theoretical risk that vasodilation may actually facilitate bleeding.

Pharmacokinetics

Nimodipine is well absorbed from the gut and undergoes extensive first-pass metabolism in the liver and gut wall. It has a short effective half-life and is metabolised in the liver. It is usually given intravenously immediately after the event, followed by oral dosing for a total of 5–10 days.

Unwanted effects

These are caused by arterial dilation:

- hypotension, which can have a detrimental effect on cerebral perfusion
- headaches, flushing.

New therapies

Trials are continuing with drugs that inhibit glutamate release or inhibit glutamate receptors. The hypothesis is that these agents will inhibit glutamate-induced excitotoxicity that may be important in ischaemia. However, initial studies have been disappointing.

Drugs are also being studied that inhibit lipid peroxidation, nitric oxide synthesis or enhance the effects of the inhibitory neurotransmitter gamma-aminobutyric acid (GABA).

Dementia

Dementia usually begins with forgetfulness and is characterised by disorientation in unfamiliar surroundings, variable mood, restlessness and poor sleep. Deterioration in social behaviour with self-neglect often follows and may be accompanied by personality change with loss of inhibition. Most dementia results from Alzheimer's disease or from cerebrovascular disease (multi-infarct dementia), but other causes may be identified (Box 9.1).

Alzheimer's disease

Alzheimer's disease is the commonest cause of dementia, accounting for about 70% of cases, and affecting 2–3% of people over the age of 65 years. There is a marked loss of cholinergic neurons and acetylcholine neurotransmitter synthesis in the cerebral cortex; about half the normal synthesis has been lost by the time of diagnosis. Muscarinic receptor density appears normal but the number of nicotinic receptors is reduced. Depletion of other neurotransmitters is a late and inconsistent finding.

The cause is unknown, but there is a genetic predisposition, with persons carrying the apolipoprotein E allele 4 (apoE4) being at higher risk. Amyloid is deposited in the brain as senile plaques, which also contain typical neurofibrillary tangles.

The onset of symptoms is gradual with progressive deterioration, unlike vascular dementia.

Treatment

Several drugs are being developed for the treatment of Alzheimer's disease. Most act by increasing cholinergic transmission in the brain via inhibition of cholinesterases. They produce modest improvement in cognitive function and memory in up to 40% of sufferers and may be more effective in patients who do not carry apoE4. Efficacy should be assessed after 3 months, and treatment stopped in non-responders. The decline in mental function is delayed by about 3–6 months but not arrested, and rapid progression resumes when the drugs are stopped. They do not improve other functional measures which affect the quality of life.

- Donepezil was the first drug to become available in the UK. It is more selective for acetylcholinesterase than plasma pseudocholinesterase, and it appears to produce behavioural improvement as well as cognitive benefit. It is metabolised in the liver and has a long half-life. The major unwanted effects are diarrhoea, nausea, vomiting and insomnia.
- Galanthamine is an anticholinesterase that produces modest amelioration of cognitive impairment, especially if given early in the course of the disease.
- Rivastigmine is a reversible non-competitive inhibitor of acetylcholinesterase. It is inactivated at the site of action.

New treatment strategies are being developed that are directed either at enhancing the various neurotrophic proteins which protect neuronal systems or at altering the production of amyloid protein or Tau protein found in neurofibrillary tangles. In future, such strategies may offer a more fundamental approach to retarding the progress of Alzheimer's disease. Early studies suggest that treatment with anti-inflammatory non-steroidal drugs, indometacin and aspirin retard the progression of Alzheimer's disease, but paracetamol, an agent that has no anti-inflammatory action, did not affect progression of the disease.

Vascular dementia

Cerebrovascular disease is a particularly common cause of dementia in patients over the age of 85 years, and overall is the second most frequent cause of dementia. The deterioration in mental function is produced by multiple cerebral infarcts (multi-infarct dementia), particularly if they affect the white matter. The risk of dementia is increased nine-fold in patients with stroke. In some patients, dementia may be produced by specific strategically located infarcts, especially in the angular gyrus of the inferior parietal lobule. In contrast to Alzheimer's disease, the initial presentation is usually sudden, and cognitive decline has a stepwise course arising from recurrent cerebrovascular events.

Box 9.1

Causes of dementia

Treatable causes of dementia	Irreversible and partially treatable causes of dementia
Hypothyroidism	Vascular dementia
Neurosyphilis	Alzheimer's disease
Vitamin B₁ deficiency	Lewy body-type dementia
Normal pressure hydrocephalus	Parkinson's disease dementia
Frontal lobe tumours	Progressive supranuclear
Cerebral vasculitis	palsy
Cerebral hypoperfusion	Multisystem atrophy

Treatment

- Prophylaxis against cerebral emboli with aspirin or warfarin (see prevention of stroke above).
- Control of hypertension (Ch. 6).
- Immunosuppressive drugs (Ch. 39) in the rare cases caused by cerebral vasculitis.

- Other approaches, including the use of nootropic drugs such as oxiracetam, are under investigation. Nootropic drugs enhance learning and memory, perhaps by potentiating Ca^{2+} and Na^+ influx into neurons and by increasing the effect of the excitatory amino acid glutamate.

FURTHER READING

Stroke

Barnett HJM, Eliasziw M, Meldrum HE (1999) Prevention of ischaemic stroke. *Br Med J* 318, 1539–1543

Bronner LL, Kanter DS, Manson JE (1995) Primary prevention of stroke. *N Engl J Med* 333, 1392–1398

Diener H-C (1998) Antiplatelet drugs in secondary prevention of stroke. *Int J Clin Pract* 52, 91–97

Fotherby MD, Panayiotou B (1999) Antihypertensive therapy in the prevention of stroke. *Drugs* 58, 663–674

Gubitz G, Sandercock P (2000) Acute ischaemic stroke. *Br Med J* 320, 692–696

Howard PA (1999) Guidelines for stroke prevention in patients with atrial fibrillation. *Drugs* 58, 997–1009

Lyden PD (1999) Thrombolysis for acute stroke. *Prog Cardiovasc Dis* 42, 175–183

The International Stroke Trial Collaborative Group (1997) The International Stroke Trial (IST): a randomised trial of aspirin, subcutaneous heparin, both, or neither among 19435 patients with acute ischaemic stroke. *Lancet* 349, 1569–1581

Subarachnoid haemorrhage

Pickard JD, Murray GD, Illingworth R et al. (1989) Effect of oral nimodipine on cerebral infarction and outcome after subarachnoid haemorrhage: British Aneurysm Nimodipine Trial (BRANT). *Br Med J* 298, 636–642

Dementia

Amar K, Wilcock G (1996) Vascular dementia. *Br Med J* 312, 227–231

Forette F, Seux M-L, Staessen JA et al. (1998) Prevention of dementia in a randomised double-blind placebo-controlled Systolic Hypertension in Europe (Syst-Eur) trial. *Lancet* 352, 1347–1351

Masters CL, Beyreuther K (1998) Alzheimer's disease. *Br Med J* 316, 446–448

Mayeaux R, Sano M (1999) Treatment of Alzheimer's disease. *N Engl J Med* 341, 1670–1679.

Qizilbash N, Whitehead A, Higgins J et al. (1998) Cholinesterase inhibition for Alzheimer disease. *JAMA* 280, 1777–1782

Self-assessment

1. In the following questions, the first statement, in italics, is correct. Is the accompanying statement true?

   a. *Aspirin has not been shown to prevent a first stroke when given to patients in sinus rhythm.* Aspirin cannot prevent a first event in patients with chronic atrial fibrillation.

   b. *Approximately 85% of all strokes have a diverse ischaemic aetiology and the remaining 15% have a haemorrhagic basis.* If thrombolysis with tissue type plasminogen activator (t-PA) is given in acute stroke, antiplatelet and anticoagulant therapies should not be given concurrently.

   c. *Drugs under development for stroke include glutamate receptor antagonists that lower the neurotoxicity of the neuroexcitatory transmitter glutamate.* Cerebral ischaemia depolarises neurons and causes the release of large amounts of glutamate.

   d. *Cerebral emboli arising from the heart can be caused by atrial fibrillation, infected or damaged prosthetic valves or arise following damage to parts of the myocardium.*

Anticoagulation with warfarin or antiplatelet therapy with aspirin are equally effective for secondary prevention of recurrent transient ischaemic attacks in the presence of sinus rhythm.

2. Case history question

A 70-year-old man has a blood pressure that is currently 190/110 mmHg despite intensive treatment. He was admitted to hospital 6 h after the acute onset of unilateral weakness and sensory loss. At the time of admission to hospital most of the neurological signs had resolved. He had no headache or vomiting and remains conscious. Following clinical examination and a CT brain scan this episode was diagnosed as a transient ischaemic attack (TIA).

   a. Should this patient be given thrombolysis?
   b. What other therapies should be instituted immediately?
   c. What secondary prevention strategy should be employed?

The answers are provided on page 605.

Cerebrovascular disease and dementia (all drugs given orally)

Drug	Half-life (h)	Elimination	Comment
Donepezil	70	Metabolism + renal	Oral bioavailability is 100%; metabolised by CYP2D6, CYP3A6 and glucuronidation; given once daily at night
Galanthamine	5–7	Renal + metabolism	Complete oral bioavailability; limited data on metabolism and excretion
Nimodipine	8–9	Metabolism	Of benefit in delayed ischaemic deficit; given orally or by intravenous infusion; oral bioavailability is 10–20%; metabolised by hepatic cytochrome P450 there is a shorter distribution half-life which determines the frequency of dosage
Rivastigmine	1	Metabolism	Oral bioavailability is 40%; metabolised by acetylcholine esterase; duration of effect is 10 h
Tacrine	2–4	Metabolism	Bioavailability is 5–30% owing to extensive but variable first-pass metabolism; eliminated by CYP1A2, induction of which by cigarette smoking reduces blood levels threefold

10 Peripheral vascular disease

Atheromatous peripheral vascular disease

The risk factors for the development of atheroma in peripheral arteries (principally the aorta and lower limb arteries) are similar to those for coronary artery and cerebrovascular disease. The strongest associations are with smoking and a raised systolic blood pressure and to a lesser extent with diabetes mellitus and a raised plasma low density lipoprotein (LDL) cholesterol. Coexisting ischaemic heart and cerebrovascular disease are, not surprisingly, common in patients with peripheral vascular disease and are responsible for most of their excess mortality. Only about 50% of patients with peripheral vascular disease are alive at 10 years after diagnosis.

Intermittent claudication

Intermittent claudication is a symptom produced by atheroma of the lower limb arteries; the reduced blood flow leads to exercise-induced hypoxia of skeletal muscle. Pain is precipitated by walking, especially up a slope, and relieved by rest. Depending on the site of vascular occlusion, pain can be experienced in the calf, thigh or buttock. Peripheral pulses may be absent if vessels are occluded or bruits heard over partially occluded arteries. In three-quarters of patients the symptoms stabilise within a few months of presentation; the remainder have steady progression that can lead to severe ischaemia with pain at rest and distal gangrene (see below).

Management

Non-pharmacological treatment

- Stopping smoking slows the progression of peripheral atherosclerosis and may improve walking distance by improving blood oxygen carriage.
- Regular exercise, up to the point of claudication, can improve walking distance.

Pharmacological treatment

- Low-dose aspirin will inhibit platelet aggregation and reduce cardiac and cerebrovascular events (Chs. 11 and 29).
- Intensive management of hypertension reduces progression of atheroma, but the choice of drug is important. Non-selective β-blockers can exacerbate intermittent claudication by reducing cardiac output and impairing vasodilation of arteries supplying skeletal muscle (Ch. 5). Cardioselective β-blockers do not usually cause deterioration of walking distance if used alone but often do so if used in combination with a vasodilator such as a Ca^{2+} channel antagonist (Ch. 5) or angiotensin converting enzyme inhibitor (Ch. 6). Ischaemic tissues are usually maximally vasodilated during exercise owing to the effects of accumulated local metabolites. Vasodilators can divert blood from diseased areas to healthy tissues by preferentially vasodilating normal arteries (vascular steal). This is more likely to exacerbate intermittent claudication if cardiac output is also reduced.
- Lowering a raised serum cholesterol can stabilise or regress atherosclerotic plaques but whether this improves limb survival or reduces the need for subsequent surgery is not known. A greater benefit from cholesterol lowering may be reduced morbidity and mortality from coexistent ischaemic heart disease (Ch. 5).
- Pentoxifylline (oxpentifylline) is a xanthine-related 'haemorrheological' drug that improves leucocyte deformability and stickiness, lowers plasma fibrinogen and decreases platelet aggregability. These actions should improve blood flow through diseased arteries. However, any improvement in walking distance is usually too small to be clinically useful. Pentoxifylline (oxpentifylline) should not be used routinely, but a trial of treatment may be justified for those who remain restricted by the disease after 6–12 months of conservative treatment. Withdrawal is advised after 3–6 months of treatment to see if spontaneous improvement has occurred.
- Naftidrofuryl oxalate is a drug that promotes the production of high-energy phosphates in ischaemic tissue by activating the enzyme succinic dehydrogenase. It also has 5-hydroxytryptamine $5HT_2$ receptor-blocking activity, which leads to vasodilation and reduced platelet aggregation. These actions should improve blood flow and tissue nutrition; however, its limitations are similar to those for pentoxifylline (oxpentifylline).

Surgical treatment

Surgical treatment is usually considered if the patient's quality of life is impaired by claudication or if tissue integrity is at risk. The two options are percutaneous transluminal angioplasty, often with insertion of a stent, particularly for stenoses above the inguinal ligament, or open bypass surgery.

Critical limb ischaemia

Acute limb ischaemia in patients with peripheral vascular disease is usually caused by thrombosis superimposed on a pre-existing atheromatous plaque. A less common cause is an arterial embolus from an intracardiac thrombus, usually caused by atrial fibrillation or following a myocardial infarction. Emboli can occlude previously healthy vessels.

Management

Unless treatment is rapid, the limb may be lost through gangrene or the patient can be left with chronic limb ischaemia.

Pharmacological treatment

Intra-arterial thrombolysis (Ch. 11) is the treatment of choice. Streptokinase is most widely used. Although tissue plasminogen activator (t-PA) produces more rapid clot lysis, there is no evidence that limb salvage is any better than with streptokinase. The thrombolytic agent is usually infused for 1–3 days, but in about 25% of acute vascular occlusions lysis is not achieved.

Surgical treatment

Surgical embolectomy using a balloon-tipped catheter can be combined with a bypass operation if residual perfusion is still poor. Amputation may be required if these procedures are not feasible or successful.

Raynaud's phenomenon

Raynaud's phenomenon is a profound and exaggerated vasoconstrictor response of blood vessels in the extemities on exposure to cold or during emotional upset. This leads to episodes of ischaemia, most commonly affecting the fingers (occasionally also occurs in the toes, ear lobes or the tongue), which can be provoked by even small degrees of temperature change. About two-thirds of cases occur in women (typically presenting under the age of 40 years) in whom the overall prevalence is about 15%. Common symptoms include discomfort, loss of function and pain if the condition is severe. Digital ulceration can also occur.

The majority of cases of Raynaud's phenomenon are idiopathic (primary Raynaud's phenomenon) when the cause of the excessive vascular reactivity is unknown. Vascular function in other tissues can be abnormal in primary Raynaud's phenomenon: for example in the cerebral vessels (giving an association with migraine), the coronary circulation (producing variant angina), or more rarely in the pulmonary circulation (leading to pulmonary hypertension). In about 10% of patients, Raynaud's phenomenon is secondary to another disorder. This is most commonly scleroderma, but there are many other associations (Table 10.1). Structural damage to arteries is common in secondary Raynaud's phenomenon. Consequently, digital ulceration is much more common than in primary Raynaud's phenomenon.

Other disorders of the peripheral circulation should be considered in the differential diagnosis of Raynaud's phenomenon.

- Acrocyanosis usually affects the hands and produces persistently cold, bluish fingers which are often sweaty or oedematous. The management of this condition is similar to that of Raynaud's phenomenon.
- Chilblains is an inflammatory disorder with erythematous lesions on the hands or feet that are precipitated by damp or cold. The lesions are often painful or itchy. Treatments used for Raynaud's phenomenon may help, with the addition of topical anti-inflammatory agents.
- Erythromelalgia is a painful, burning condition of the hands and feet that, unlike Raynaud's phenomenon, is usually provoked by heat. It sometimes responds to treatment with a β-blocker (Ch. 5).

· ·

Management

Many patients with Raynaud's phenomenon are only mildly inconvenienced by their symptoms and respond to simple measures. Drug treatment is usually reserved for those suffering from more intense vasospasm, with pain, impairment of function or trophic changes. Responses to individual treatments are unpredictable and less satisfactory in secondary Raynaud's phenomenon because of the structural changes to the vessel wall.

Non-pharmacological treatment

- Often minimising changes in ambient temperature with insulating clothing is enough to reduce the numbers of attacks although electrically heated gloves or socks may be useful for more severely affected patients.
- Smoking should be strongly discouraged. Nicotine promotes vasospasm and may also reduce the threshold for other provoking factors.
- Aggravating factors should be withdrawn or corrected whenever possible (see Table 10.1).

Table 10.1
Conditions associated with Raynaud's phenomenon

Connective tissue disorders
  Systemic sclerosis
  Systemic lupus erythematosus
  Rheumatoid arthritis
  Dermatomyositis and polymyositis
Obstructive arterial disorders
  Carpal tunnel syndrome
  Thoracic outlet syndrome
  Atherosclerosis
  Thromboangiitis obliterans
Drugs and chemicals
  Ergotamine
  Beta-blockers
  Bleomycin, vinblastine, cisplatin
  Oral contraceptives
  Vinyl chloride
Occupational
  Vibrating tools
  Cold environment
Blood disorders
  Polycythaemia
  Cold agglutinin disease
  Monoclonal gammopathies
  Thrombocytosis

Beta-blockers in particular produce peripheral circulatory problems sufficient to necessitate stopping treatment in about 3–5% of hypertensive patients.

Pharmacological treatment
Arterial vasodilators

- Calcium antagonists (Ch. 5). Nifedipine is the drug of first choice for Raynaud's phenomenon. It reduces the frequency, duration and intensity of vasospastic episodes. Several other dihydropyridines are probably equally effective. Diltiazem is less effective and verapamil ineffective in this condition.
- 5-HT receptor antagonists. Naftidrofuryl is a vasodilator that selectively blocks the $5HT_2$ receptor subtype (see above) and may produce a modest reduction in the severity of attacks.
- Alpha-blockers (Ch. 6). Moxisylyte (thymoxamine) may be effective and does not lower blood pressure, unlike other α-blockers.

Drugs acting primarily on blood components

- Prostaglandins. Intravenous infusion of epoprostenol (prostacyclin, Ch. 11) produces immediate and short-lived vasodilation, but long-term improvement in symptoms and healing of ulcers over a period of 10–16 weeks after a single prolonged infusion. These effects are believed to be caused by actions on the flow properties of blood, i.e. reduced platelet aggregation, increased red cell deformability and reduced neutrophil adhesiveness.

- Pentoxifylline (oxpentifylline) (see above) may reduce the frequency of attacks of Raynaud's phenomenon.

- Inositol nicotinate produces a gradual onset of clinical response and only modest improvement. Its action may result more from fibrinolysis (reducing plasma vicosity) and reduction in platelet aggregation than from vasodilation.

FURTHER READING

Golledge J (1997) Lower-limb arterial disease. *Lancet* 350, 1459–1465

Belch JJF, Ho M (1996) Pharmacotherapy of Raynaud's phenomenon. *Drugs* 52, 682–695.

Tierney S, Fennessy F, Bouchier Hayes D (2000) Secondary prevention of peripheral vascular disease. *Br Med J* 320, 1262–1265

Self-assessment

1. In the following questions the first statement, in italics, is correct. Is the accompanying statement also true?

   a. *There is an additive effect of diabetes mellitus, hypertension and smoking as risk factors for peripheral vascular disease.* Patients with intermittent claudication do not have an increased risk of developing coronary disease.

   b. *'Statins' are indicated in patients with symptomatic atherosclerotic-peripheral vascular disease.* Simvastatin increases the expression of hepatic low density lipoprotein (LDL) receptors.

   c. *Drugs such as ergotamine, used in migraine treatment, are associated with Raynaud's syndrome.* Verapamil is the calcium channel blocker of choice in treatment of Raynaud's phenomenon.

2. Case history question

   Mr TH aged 67 years is an insulin-dependent diabetic who smokes 20 cigarettes a day. His plasma cholesterol level is raised at 7 mmol l^{-1} and his blood pressure is 160/110 mmHg. After walking 50 m he develops pain in his left calf muscle, which is relieved by rest. He occasionally but rarely has rest pain at night. On examination, both popliteal and posterior tibial pulses were absent and femoropopliteal obstruction was diagnosed.

   Comment on the use of the following drugs to treat this patient:

   a. Propranolol
   b. Atenolol
   c. Nifedipine
   d. A statin
   e. Low-dose aspirin
   f. What other therapy could be of benefit?
   g. Should the use of an electric blanket be discouraged?

   The answers are provided on pages 605–606.

Drugs for peripheral vascular disease

Drug	Half-life (h)	Elimination	Comment
Aspirin	15–20 min	Metabolism (hydrolysis)	Half-life of active salicylic acid metabolite is 3–20 h
Pentoxifylline (oxpentifylline)	1	Metabolism	Metabolised in liver and blood; clearance 3.6 l min^{-1} (that is, it greatly exceeds liver blood flow); active after oral dosage
Naftidrofuryl oxalate	3–4	Metabolism	Good oral bioavailability
Nifedipine	2–6	Metabolism	Metabolised by CYP3A4
Moxisylyte (thymoxamine)	1 (DAM)	Metabolism	Deacetylated in plasma to active metabolite (DAM)

11

Haemostasis

Platelets and platelet aggregation

When the integrity of vascular endothelium is breached, subendothelial proteins are exposed to the blood. Subendothelial glycoproteins such as von Willebrand factor, collagen and fibronectin interact with glycoprotein (GP) Ib/IX and GP Ia/IIb receptors on the surface of non-activated platelets. This results in platelets adhering to the subendothelial surface as a monolayer over the breached endothelial surface. Subsequent exposure of platelet surface receptors to specific agonists then triggers platelet aggregation. The process of platelet aggregation also involves platelet activation with release of substances from platelet vesicles that initiate or enhance the coagulation cascade. This leads to the deposition of fibrin thrombus and inhibition of fibrinolysis. In some circumstances, aggregates of platelets combined with fibrin thrombi can embolise and occlude more distal parts of the circulation. Platelets have a lifespan of 7–10 days in the circulation (Fig. 11.1).

Platelet aggregation is dependent on surface expression of the GPIIb/IIIa complex, one of a family of proteins known as integrins. At least 50 000 of these receptors are found on each platelet. The activated GPIIb/IIIa receptors bind to fibrinogen, which cross-links between platelets and produces platelet aggregation. Substances such as adenosine diphosphate (ADP), adrenaline, thrombin and collagen can trigger platelet aggregation by increasing platelet intracellular calcium concentration. This promotes phosphorylation of myosin light chains in the platelet and produces a change in platelet shape which exposes fibrinogen binding sites on the GPIIb/IIIa receptors. The conformational change in the platelet enhances exocytosis of platelet storage granules. The increase in platelet calcium also activates phospholipase A_2 which increases intracellular arachidonic acid, the precursor of thromboxane A_2. Thromboxane A_2 further enhances expression of the GPIIb/IIIa surface receptors (Fig. 11.1).

Thromboxane A_2, in addition to promoting platelet aggregation, also enhances secretion from platelet granules. These granules contain several active substances, such as platelet factor 4, β-thromboglobulin, ADP and 5-hydroxytryptamine 5HT, which have the following effects:

155

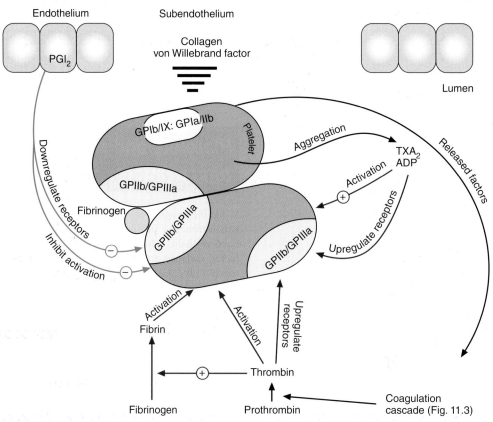

Fig. 11.1
Platelets and platelet aggregation. Subendothelial macromolecules such as collagen interact with glycoprotein receptors (GPIb/IX and GPIa/IIb) on platelets causing activation of platelets and upregulation of GPIIb/GPIIIa receptors, which are cross-linked by fibrinogen during aggregation. Synthesis of the proaggregatory thromboxane A_2 (TXA_2) and release of adenosine diphosphate (ADP) and 5-hydroxytryptamine occurs. TXA_2 and thrombin cause further platelet activation and release of proaggregatory platelet contents. This leads to further upregulation of GPIIb/GPIIIa receptors. Prostacyclin (PGI_2) from endothelial cells inhibits activation and upregulation of GPIIb/GPIIIa receptors. Thrombin is generated by the action of factor Xa on prothrombin (see Fig. 11.3).

- They impede prostacyclin production by vascular endothelium. Prostacyclin is a vasodilator and a potent inhibitor of platelet aggregation.
- They neutralise heparin produced by the same cells. This enhances activity of the coagulation cascade.
- They induce further platelet aggregation.

Both direct and thromboxane A_2-mediated expression of platelet GPIIb/GPIIIa surface receptors can be inhibited by increasing the concentration of cyclic adenosine monophosphate (cAMP) in the platelet. This is the mechanism by which prostacyclin (prostaglandin I_2), which is released from vascular endothelium, inhibits platelet aggregation. Polyunsaturated fatty acids in fish oils are precursors for thromboxane A_3 which causes less platelet aggregation than thromboxane A_2; they also increase production of prostacyclin by vascular endothelium. A high intake of fish oils therefore creates a less pro-aggregatory state.

Antiplatelet agents

Aspirin

Mechanism of action on platelets
Inhibition of platelet cyclo-oxygenase by aspirin decreases platelet thromboxane A_2 synthesis. This reduces platelet aggregation, but does not eliminate it since other pathways for platelet activation still function (Fig. 11.2). The antiplatelet action of aspirin occurs at very low doses, which have no analgesic or anti-inflammatory action. Full details of the pharmacology of aspirin are found in Chapter 29.

Dipyridamole

Mechanisms of action
Dipyridamole inhibits the enzyme phosphodiesterase and this increases intracellular concentrations of cAMP.

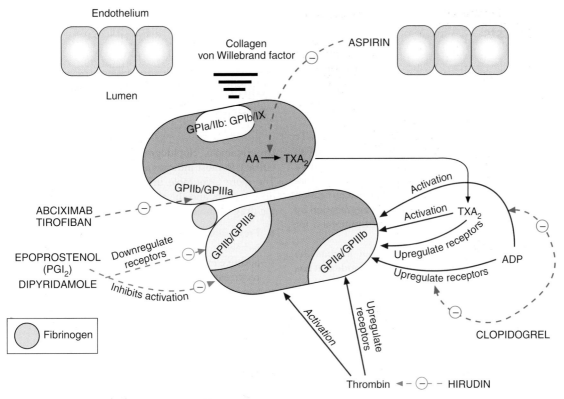

Fig. 11.2

Sites of action of major drugs used in haemostasis. Drugs act directly or indirectly to inhibit activation of platelets or to block or reduce upregulation of the glycoprotein GP IIb/IIIa receptors, which are necessary for aggregation of platelets. Abciximab is an antibody and tirofiban is a non-peptide inhibitor of these glycoprotein receptors. Epoprostenol and dipyridamole inhibit activation of platelets and downregulate the glycoprotein receptors. Clopidogrel prevents ADP-induced upregulation of the receptors and platelet aggregation. Hirudin prevents the effects of thrombin. Aspirin inhibits the generation of thromboxane A_2, which causes activation of platelets and upregulation of glycoprotein receptors. Abbreviations as in Figure 11.1.

In the platelet, this reduces activation and expression of cell surface GPIIb/IIIa receptors (Fig. 11.2).

Dipyridamole also blocks the cellular uptake of adenosine that is released by tissues when they become hypoxic. In the heart, the excess adenosine acts on specific receptors in the small resistance coronary arteries to produce vasodilation. Since these vessels are already maximally dilated in ischaemic tissue, the drug has no useful anti-anginal action. Indeed, dipyridamole can divert blood away from ischaemic tissue by dilating vascular beds in non-ischaemic myocardium (vascular steal). This effect forms the basis of a pharmacological stress test to assess the presence and extent of myocardial ischaemia (see below).

Pharmacokinetics

Dipyridamole is incompletely absorbed from the gut and is metabolised in the liver. It has an intermediate half-life.

Unwanted effects

The only unwanted effect is headache.

Clopidogrel

Mechanisms of action

Clopidogrel inhibits platelet aggregation by irreversibly binding to the purinergic P_2 receptors for ADP on the platelet surface. This reduces the mobilisation of Ca^{2+} from intracellular platelet stores, and reduces expression of GPIIb/IIIa receptors.

Pharmacokinetics

Clopidogrel is a prodrug. It is well absorbed from the gut, and activated by metabolism in the liver. It has an intermediate half-life and undergoes further metabolism to inactive derivatives in the liver.

Unwanted effects

Unwanted effects include:

- bleeding, although the risk is low
- gastrointestinal upset
- rashes.

Glycoprotein IIb/IIIa receptor antagonists

Examples: abciximab, tirofiban

Mechanism of action

Abciximab is a murine monoclonal antibody with the Fc fragment removed to prevent immunogenicity. The Fab fragment is then joined to a human Fc region to form a chimaeric molecule. Since it inhibits the receptors that form the final common pathway for platelet aggregation (Fig. 11.2) abciximab can reduce platelet aggregation by more than 90%, but the optimal level of inhibition for clinical effect is unknown.

Tirofiban is a non-peptide agent that inhibits the GPIIb/IIIa receptor and eptifibatide is a peptide that has the same effect.

Pharmacokinetics

Abciximab must be given intravenously, usually as an initial bolus followed by continuous infusion. Platelet inhibition occurs rapidly with a bolus injection and largely recovers by 48 hours after the infusion is stopped. However, small amounts of the antibody are still detected on platelets after 1 week or more.

Tirofiban also requires continuous infusion, has a short half-life and is eliminated by the kidney.

Unwanted effects

- Bleeding: especially in the elderly and those of low body weight. The risk is reduced if the dose is adjusted for the weight of the patient.
- Thrombocytopenia: occurs with abciximab, by an unknown mechanism.

Epoprostenol

Mechanism of action

Epoprostenol (prostaglandin I_2) increases platelet cAMP, which at low concentrations inhibits platelet aggregation and at higher concentrations reduces adhesion. Epoprostenol also vasodilates peripheral arteries.

Pharmacokinetics

Epoprostenol is given by intravenous infusion. Unlike most prostaglandins it is not inactivated in the lung but is rapidly metabolised by hydrolysis in peripheral tissues. The half-life is about 2 min.

Unwanted effects

These can be reduced by starting with a low dose.

- facial flushing
- headache
- nausea
- hypotension

Clinical uses of antiplatelet agents

Dipyridamole, clopidogrel and aspirin show similar efficacy in most indications for oral antiplatelet agents. The more favourable unwanted effect profile of low-dose aspirin, and the simpler dosage regimen, make it the drug of choice for the majority of patients.

- Prevention of embolic stroke and transient ischaemic attacks (aspirin; dipyridamole has an additive effect which is particularly useful for recurrent stroke) (Ch. 9).
- Secondary prevention after myocardial infarction (aspirin; clopidogrel) (Ch. 5).
- Prevention of myocardial infarction in patients with stable angina or peripheral vascular disease (aspirin; clopidogrel) (Chs. 5 and 10). The evidence for the use of aspirin for primary prevention of myocardial infarction in healthy individuals, who do not have evidence of established ischaemic artery disease, is inconclusive. However, it is recommended for people at high risk of developing ischaemic heart disease, particularly those with hypertension or diabetes.
- Treatment of unstable angina to reduce the risk of myocardial infarction or death (Ch. 5) (aspirin with the anticoagulant heparin). GPIIb/IIIa inhibitors further reduce events in high risk patients when added to aspirin and heparin, especially those with a positive plasma troponin I or T concentration.
- As an anticoagulant in extracorporeal circulations, for example cardiopulmonary bypass, and renal haemodialysis (epoprostenol).
- Symptom relief in Raynaud's phenomenon (epoprostenol) (Ch. 10).
- Abciximab (and probably other GPIIb/IIIa inhibitors in the future) is used to reduce ischaemic complications following percutaneous transluminal angioplasty with stent insertion. These complications are produced by sudden vessel closure and include myocardial infarction, the need for emergency revascularisation and death.
- Dipyridamole is used as a pharmacological stress for the coronary circulation, in order to detect myocardial ischaemia in patients who are unable to exercise. This does not rely on its antiplatelet effect. In this situation, the heart is usually imaged at rest and after stress for radio-isotope uptake (e.g. using technetium-labelled meta-iodobenzoyl isonitrile or thallium which accumulate in aerobically

metabolising myocardium) or by echocardiography to examine left ventricular wall motion.

Blood coagulation

The coagulation cascade (Fig. 11.3) involves a series of enzyme-mediated reactions which leads to generation of thrombin. Each activated clotting factor is inactivated extremely rapidly so that the coagulation process remains localised at the site of the initiating event. Once sufficient thrombin has been produced to overcome the effect of circulating antithrombin, the soluble protein fibrinogen is converted to a fibrin gel.

There are two pathways for activation of the cascade, the extrinsic and intrinsic pathways, that amplify the coagulation response and work together to produce the thrombus. The extrinsic system is triggered by the release of thromboplastin from damaged tissue and is activated rapidly within minutes of endothelial disruption. The intrinsic system is triggered by contact of blood with a negatively charged surface such as subendothelial collagen and its activation is delayed by more than 10 min after tissue disruption. Both processes are substantially slower than platelet aggregation and vasoconstriction, which initiate haemostasis.

Anticoagulant agents

Anticoagulation can be achieved with either parenteral or oral drug therapy. A comparison of some of the properties of heparin and warfarin are shown in Table 11.1.

Heparin

Mechanism of action and effects

Heparin is a highly sulfated acidic mucopolysaccharide (glycosaminoglycan) that has a variable molecular weight of 3000–30 000 Da. It forms a complex with the circulating protein antithrombin and induces a conformation change to activate it. The activated heparin–antithrombin complex interacts with and neutralises activated clotting factors (Fig. 11.3). Heparin can also bind directly to thrombin, inactivating it. This complex can then form a tertiary complex with antithrombin. Heparin is available unfractionated, or as low-molecular-weight heparin (LMWH; molecular weight less than 7000). There are several major effects of heparin on haemostasis.

- Inhibition of the activated coagulation factors Xa, thrombin and to a lesser extent other clotting factors. The higher molecular weight heparin–antithrombin complexes have greater

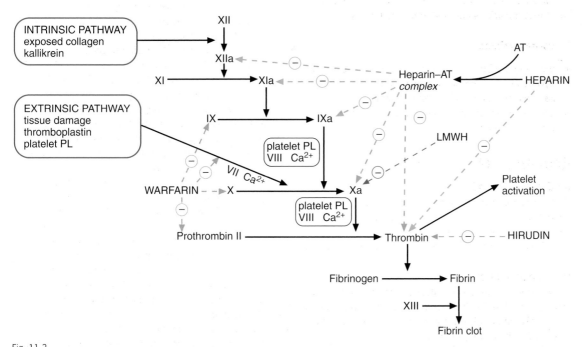

Fig. 11.3
The coagulation cascade and action of anticoagulants. The complex cascade of clotting factor synthesis is initiated extrinsically by tissue damage. Activation of the clotting factors after damage requires platelet factors and Ca^{2+} The provision of platelet products is further enhanced by the formation of thrombin, which then activates further platelets as well as causing fibrin formation. Heparin acts at various sites in the cascade by activating the anticlotting factor antithrombin (AT) and inhibiting the activating protease clotting factors shown. Low-molecular-weight heparin (LMWH) acts on factor Xa. Hirudin inhibits thrombin (IIa) formation. Warfarin inhibits the synthesis of the vitamin K-dependent clotting factors VII, IX, X and II (prothrombin). Roman numerals indicate the individual clotting factors; PL, platelet phospholipid.

Table 11.1
Comparison of heparin and warfarin

	Heparin	Warfarin
Route	Intravenous or subcutaneous	Oral
Onset	Immediate	1–3 days
Duration of action on cessation of treatment	3–6 h	3–5 days
Antagonist	Protamine	Vitamin K_I
Monitoring test	Activated partial thromboplastin time	Prothrombin time
Site of action	Activated clotting factors in plasma	Clotting factor synthesis in liver
Fate in the body	Partially degraded in liver; does not cross placenta	Inactivated in liver; crosses placenta
Individual variability in response	Little	Great: owing to genetic differences in kinetics and sensitivity and the effects of other drugs

affinity for thrombin as the heparin binds to both thrombin and antithrombin. LMWH, following its complex with antithrombin, mainly inactivates factor Xa and is four times more active in this respect than unfractionated heparin. The complex has less affinity for thrombin.

- Release of tissue factor pathway inhibitor (TFPI) from the vascular wall may also contribute to the antithrombotic effects of heparin by actions on factor Xa, vascular endothelium and platelets.
- Inhibition of platelet aggregation (unfractionated heparin only).
- Activation of lipoprotein lipase, which in addition to promoting lipolysis also reduces platelet adhesiveness.

Substances related to heparin called heparinoids are also available. These contain heparan sulfate alone or combined with dermatan sulfate and chondroitin sulfates. They have no advantages compared with heparin.

Pharmacokinetics

Heparins are inactive orally and are given intravenously or by subcutaneous injection. They have a rapid onset of action. Heparins do not cross the placenta or enter breast milk. Since the two principal forms of heparin have different structures, they also have different pharmacokinetic properties.

Unfractionated heparin. This is extracted from porcine intestinal mucosa or bovine lung, and consists of a mean of 45 polysaccharide units. Its kinetics are dose dependent: the half-life is very short (about 30 min) at low doses, increasing some fivefold at higher doses. Most is metabolised in endothelial cells after binding to surface receptors. Some is metabolised in the liver, with a small amount excreted unchanged by the kidney. It is given by repeated intravenous bolus injections or by continuous intravenous infusion for full anticoagulant effect. Low-dose subcutaneous injections are used for prophylaxis against thrombosis,

although bioavailability by this route is only about 30%.

Low-molecular-weight heparin. LMWHs have a mean of 15 polysaccharide units. They have at least twice the duration of anticoagulant action and a more predictable anticoagulant effect compared with unfractionated heparin, because they have a low affinity for endothelial cell heparin receptors and plasma protein-binding sites. They have two routes of elimination: a rapid saturable liver uptake and slower renal excretion. They are almost completely absorbed after subcutaneous administration and only need to be given once or twice daily by subcutaneous injection for full anticoagulation. The various types of LMWH form complexes with antithrombin that differ in their affinity for factor Xa, but all have a lower affinity for thrombin than the complexes formed by unfractionated heparin (see above).

Control of heparin therapy

The therapeutic index for heparin is low. The degree of anticoagulation with unfractionated heparin is usually monitored with the activated partial thromboplastin time (APTT, a global test of the intrinsic coagulation pathway) which should be prolonged by 1.5–2.0 times the control value for full anticoagulation. Monitoring is not required when low-dose subcutaneous unfractionated heparin is used (see below). The LMWHs can be monitored by factor Xa inhibition, but this is not carried out routinely, since their effect is much more predictable than that of unfractionated heparin.

Unwanted effects

Haemorrhage. The risk is greater in the elderly, especially if there is a history of heavy alcohol intake. Excessive bleeding can be reversed by infusion of fresh frozen plasma or clotting factor concentrate. The effect of unfractionated heparin can be rapidly reversed by the basic substance protamine sulphate which binds strongly to the acidic heparin components. Protamine binds poorly to LMWH and is relatively ineffective for reversing its action. Protamine is given intravenously.

Osteoporosis. This is a rare complication which can occur when heparin is given for several weeks. The risk is less with LMWH.

Thrombocytopenia. Rarely heparin induces platelet aggregation, possibly by inducing platelet antibodies, which can produce arterial thrombosis. LMWH does not affect platelet aggregation and its lower binding to endothelium also reduces interference with platelet–vessel wall interaction.

Oral anticoagulants

Example: warfarin

Mechanism of action

These drugs are antagonists of vitamin K and act by inhibiting the hepatic reductase enzyme that converts vitamin K to its active (hydroquinone) form. As a result, the hepatic synthesis of vitamin-K dependent clotting factors (II (prothrombin), VII, IX and X) is impaired (Fig. 11.3). There is a delay in the onset of the anticoagulant effect due to the presence of preformed circulating clotting factors.

Pharmacokinetics

Warfarin is the most widely used oral anticoagulant. It is almost completely absorbed from the gut and is highly protein bound to albumin in plasma. It is eliminated by cytochrome P450-mediated hepatic metabolism and has a very long half-life. The plasma concentration of warfarin does not correlate directly with the activity of the drug, which is determined by the balance between the rates of synthesis and degradation of clotting factors. The maximum effect of an individual dose is reflected in the blood coagulation time some 24–36 h later. On stopping treatment, the duration of anticoagulant action is determined largely by the time required to synthesise new clotting factors. Warfarin crosses the placenta and can adversely affect the fetus.

Control of oral anticoagulant therapy

Factor VII is the clotting factor that is most sensitive to vitamin K deficiency, and therefore a test of the extrinsic coagulation pathway – the prothrombin time – is used as a measure of effectiveness. The degree of prolongation of prothrombin time is standardised by comparison with a control plasma from a single source, and referred to as the INR (international normalised ratio). Therapeutic INR ranges differ according to the condition being treated:

- 2–2.5 for prophylaxis of deep vein thrombosis
- 2–3 for thromboprophylaxis in hip surgery and fractured femur operations, for treatment of deep vein thrombosis and pulmonary embolism, for treatment of transient ischaemic attacks and prevention of thromboembolism in atrial fibrillation.
- 3–4.5 for prevention of recurrent deep vein thrombosis and for preventing thrombosis on mechanical prosthetic heart valves.

Unwanted effects

Warfarin is an important example of a drug that has a narrow therapeutic index.

Haemorrhage. The most effective antidote to warfarin is phytomenadione (vitamin K_1), which is given intravenously and controls bleeding within 6 h. After giving a large dose of phytomenadione, it can be difficult to restore therapeutic anticoagulation with warfarin for up to 3 weeks. If this is undesirable, an immediate co-agulant effect can be achieved by intravenous infusion of fresh frozen plasma or clotting factor concentrate.

Teratogenicity. Warfarin should be avoided in the first trimester of pregnancy, except when essential, and it should not be used in the last trimester as it increases the risk of intracranial haemorrhage during delivery.

Drug interactions. These are particularly important. The anticoagulant effect of warfarin can be increased by broad-spectrum antibiotics which suppress the production of vitamin K by gut bacteria. Some non-steroidal anti-inflammatory drugs (Ch. 29) displace warfarin from its binding site on plasma proteins; this increases the plasma concentration of free (and therefore active) drug and briefly increases its effects. Amiodarone (Ch. 8) and the histamine H_2 receptor antagonist cimetidine (Ch. 33) inhibit the cytochrome P450-mediated metabolism of warfarin and enhance its effects. Drugs that induce hepatic microsomal drug-metabolising enzymes, for example phenytoin, phenobarbital (Ch. 23) and alcohol (Ch. 54), reduce the effect of warfarin by increasing its elimination.

Alopecia and allergic reactions. These conditions rarely occur.

Clinical uses of anticoagulants

Venous thromboembolism

Pulmonary embolism remains a major cause of morbidity and death and has been estimated to be responsible for 10% of all deaths in hospital. Most serious pulmonary emboli arise from lower limb deep vein thrombosis, particularly if this extends to the larger veins above the calf. Following a deep vein thrombosis, chronic post-phlebitic syndrome can develop with pain, swelling and ulceration of the affected leg.

Predisposing factors to venous thromboembolism include use of the oral contraceptive pill in some women

Table 11.2
Risk of thromboembolism in hospital patients

Risk	Procedure
Low	Minor surgery, no other risk factor
	Major surgery, age <40 years, no other risk factors
	Minor trauma or illness
Moderate	Major surgery; age ≥40 years or other risk factor
	Heart failure, recent myocardial infarction, malignancy, inflammatory bowel disease
	Major trauma or burns
	Minor surgery, trauma or illness in patient with previous deep vein thrombosis or pulmonary embolism
High	Fracture or major orthopaedic surgery of pelvis, hips or lower limb
	Major pelvic or abdominal surgery for cancer
	Major surgery, trauma or illness in patient with previous deep vein thrombosis or pulmonary embolism
	Lower limb paralysis
	Major lower limb amputation

(see Ch. 45), prolonged immobility and a variety of coexisting medical conditions such as cancer. Many episodes of deep vein thrombosis occur in hospital, particularly in patients over 40 years of age following major illness, trauma or surgery. However, within this group, and in younger patients, several additional factors predict the level of risk (Table 11.2).

Prevention of deep vein thrombosis

In hospitalised patients, the methods used to prevent deep vein thrombosis vary according to the degree of risk.

Mechanical methods. These are used for patients at moderate risk and include graduated elastic compression stockings and intermittent pneumatic compression devices to improve venous flow and limit stasis in venous valve pockets. They can also be used to supplement pharmacological prophylaxis in high risk patients.

Low-dose subcutaneous heparin. This is the treatment of choice in high risk and in many moderate risk patients. It reduces both initiation and extension of fibrin-rich thrombi at doses which have little effect on measurements of blood coagulation. Therefore, laboratory monitoring is unnecessary. Low-dose heparin reduces deep venous thrombosis and fatal pulmonary emboli by about two-thirds with minimal risk of serious bleeding, although minor bleeding is increased. For patients at highest risk, particularly during orthopaedic surgery, LMWHs are more effective than unfractionated heparin. Prophylaxis should be started before surgery.

Low-dose aspirin and warfarin. Although a meta-analysis of several studies suggests that low-dose aspirin (see below) reduces deep venous thrombosis, it is less effective than heparin. Warfarin may be more effective than heparin for prophylaxis in patients at highest risk.

Treatment of established venous thrombosis

The goals of treatment for deep vein thrombi are to prevent pulmonary emboli and to restore patency of the occluded vessel with preservation of the function of venous valves.

Full anticoagulation. This is the treatment of choice for deep vein thrombosis and for most pulmonary emboli; it substantially reduces mortality. Heparin is given initially for its rapid onset of effect. Unfractionated heparin by intravenous infusion is most widely used (in preference to intermittent bolus injection, which carries a higher risk of serious bleeding). It is important to monitor the extent of anticoagulation using the APTT (see above). LMWH given subcutaneously is a convenient and effective alternative to intravenous unfractionated heparin. Heparin is usually given for 3–5 days, with concurrent initiation of treatment with warfarin. Once warfarin has produced adequate anticoagulation (i.e. the INR is within the therapeutic range; see above) heparin can be stopped. The optimal duration of anticoagulant therapy is not well defined, but suggested periods are shown in Table 11.3.

Surgical venous thrombectomy. This may be required for massive iliofemoral thrombosis if it threatens

Table 11.3
Suggested duration of anticoagulant therapy for venous thromboembolism

Risk of recurrence	Patient type	Duration
Low	Temporary risk factors for thromboembolism	4–6 weeks
Intermediate	Continuing medical risk factors for thromboembolism	6 months
High	Recurrent thromboembolism, inherited thrombophilic tendency	Indefinite

the viability of the limb. Pulmonary embolectomy is occasionally carried out for large pulmonary emboli.

Thrombolytic treatment with streptokinase. This treatment (see below) has no advantage over warfarin in uncomplicated deep venous thrombosis but is sometimes used to disintegrate massive pulmonary emboli.

Other treatments. If patients continue to have pulmonary emboli despite adequate anticoagulation, or if anticoagulation is contraindicated, inferior vena caval plication, or insertion of a 'filter' device to trap emboli in the inferior vena cava can be considered.

Arterial thromboembolism

Warfarin is used long term in patients with prosthetic heart valves to avoid thrombosis on the valve and peripheral embolisation. Atrial fibrillation (Ch. 8) and mural thrombus in the left ventricle following a myocardial infarction also predispose patients to arterial embolism and are indications for anticoagulation.

The fibrinolytic system

Fibrinolysis is the physiological mechanism for dissolving the fibrin meshwork in a thrombus. The process is initiated by activation of plasminogen, a circulating α_2-globulin (Fig. 11.4). Tissue plasminogen activator (t-PA), released from damaged vessels, cleaves plasminogen to the active enzyme plasmin. Plasmin splits both fibrinogen and fibrin into degradation products; if this occurs at the site of a thrombus, it produces lysis of the clot matrix. The action of plasmin is regulated by circulating antiplasmins which can be useful to inhibit lysis, for example of a useful thrombus that is sealing a breach in a vessel wall.

Fibrinolytic or thrombolytic agents

Examples: streptokinase, recombinant t-PA (rt-PA), urokinase, anistreplase

Mechanisms of action

All thrombolytic drugs activate plasminogen and enhance fibrinolysis. Recombinant t-PA is a genetically engineered copy of the naturally occurring substance. A number of structurally related compounds have also

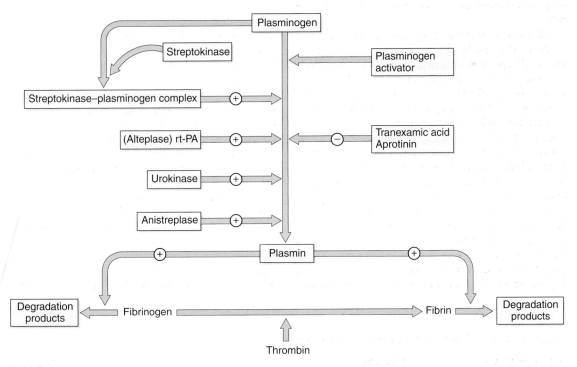

Fig. 11.4
The fibrinolytic system. The fibrinolytic system is linked intimately with the coagulation cascade and platelet function. When a clot is formed via the prothrombotic system, activation of plasminogen to the fibrinolytically active plasmin is initiated by several plasminogen activators, thus lysing the clot. The drugs promoting this act as plasminogen activators (rt-PA, urokinase) or bind to plasminogen (streptokinase, anistreplase) promoting plasmin activity. The antifibrinolytic drugs tranexamic acid and aprotinin inhibit plasminogen activation.

been produced. Urokinase is also a naturally occurring human plasminogen activator, which is derived from urine or from kidney cell culture. By contrast, streptokinase is obtained from haemolytic streptococci. Unlike rt-PA and urokinase, streptokinase is inactive until it forms a complex with circulating plasminogen; the resultant streptokinase–plasminogen activator complex substitutes for tissue plasminogen activator in the fibrinolytic cascade causing plasmin activity. Anistreplase is a preformed streptokinase–plasminogen activator complex with a blocking anisoyl chemical group at the active site. The anisoyl moiety is cleaved by enzymes liberated locally at the site of a thrombus (Fig. 11.4).

The effectiveness of any thrombolytic agent depends on the age of the thrombus and the surface area of thrombus exposed to it.

Pharmacokinetics

All thrombolytic agents are given intravenously or intra-arterially. The streptokinase–plasminogen activator complex is degraded enzymatically in the circulation. Some streptokinase is cleared from the plasma before it forms an active complex, by combining with circulating neutralising antibody formed during previous streptococcal infections. After the use of streptokinase, or following a recent streptococcal infection, neutralising antibodies can persist in high titre for several years and substantially reduce the effectiveness of subsequent therapy with streptokinase.

Urokinase and rt-PA are metabolised in the liver.

Both streptokinase and anistreplase have a slower onset of action than urokinase or rt-PA owing to slow combination with plasminogen (streptokinase) and slow activation at the clot surface (anistreplase). Consequently, the re-perfusion of occluded vessels is slower with these drugs. However, re-occlusion is less common because of their longer duration of action.

The half-lives of both streptokinase and anistreplase are longer than those of urokinase or rt-PA. Anistreplase produces prolonged thrombolysis after a single intravenous bolus injection. Streptokinase is usually given as a short (1 h) infusion for the treatment of coronary artery occlusion, although longer infusions are usual for peripheral arterial occlusions or pulmonary embolism. Infusions of rt-PA and urokinase are given over longer periods, usually for between 3 and 24 h depending on the condition being treated. Because of its short duration of action, when rt-PA has been used to lyse coronary artery thrombus, subsequent anticoagulation with heparin for 48 h is necessary to reduce the re-occlusion rate.

Unwanted effects

There are three main unwanted effects.

- Haemorrhage: this is usually minor but can occasionally be serious, for example intracerebral haemorrhage, which occurs in about 1% of patients (and is slightly more frequent with rt-PA). Bleeding can be stopped by antifibrinolytic drugs (see below) or by transfusion of fresh frozen plasma.
- Hypotension: this is dose-related and more common with streptokinase and anistreplase. It may be caused by enzymatic release of the vasodilator bradykinin from its circulating precursor. If the infusion of the thrombolytic is stopped for a brief period, the blood pressure usually recovers rapidly and treatment can be continued.
- Allergic reactions: these are rare but can occur with streptokinase or anistreplase, as a consequence of their bacterial origin.

Clinical uses of thrombolytic agents

Thrombolytic agents are used to treat the following:

- acute myocardial infarction (Ch. 5)
- pulmonary embolism or deep venous thrombosis, in a minority of cases (see above)
- peripheral arterial thromboembolism (Ch. 10)
- Restoration of patency of intravenous catheters occluded by clot: this is particularly useful for 'long-lines' inserted for intravenous nutrition or administration of cytotoxic drugs (urokinase is often used).

Haemostatic agents

Antifibrinolytic agents

Examples: tranexamic acid, aprotinin

Mechanisms of action

Aprotinin and tranexamic acid competitively inhibit the activation of plasminogen to plasmin by binding to the active site on plasmin that interacts with fibrin.

An additional action of aprotinin is inhibition of plasma kallikrein. This is involved in amplification of the coagulation cascade at the stage of activation of factor XII (Fig. 11.3). Aprotinin therefore interferes with coagulation as well as having an antifibrinolytic effect.

Pharmacokinetics

Tranexamic acid is a synthetic amino acid that is incompletely absorbed from the gut and can also be given intravenously. It has a short half-life and is excreted unchanged by the kidney. Aprotinin is a polypeptide that is not absorbed orally and must be given intravenously. It has an intermediate half-life and is metabolised in the kidney.

Unwanted effects

The theoretical risk of a thrombotic tendency does not appear to be a clinical problem. Unwanted effects are rarely seen. Tranexamic acid can produce gastrointestinal upset.

Desmopressin

Desmopressin briefly increases the plasma concentration of clotting factor VIII and von Willebrand factor, an adhesion protein in blood vessel walls. Factor VIII accelerates the process of fibrin formation and von Willebrand factor enhances platelet adhesion to subendothelial tissue. Desmopressin is more fully discussed in Chapter 4.

Clinical uses of haemostatic agents

Haemostatic agents have a number of clinical uses:

- to prevent bleeding after surgery, especially of the prostate or after dental extraction in haemophiliacs
- tranexamic acid is used for the treatment of menorrhagia, or bleeding caused by fibrinolytic drugs such as streptokinase
- aprotinin is mainly used prophylactically for reduction of bleeding during cardiovascular surgery with extracorporeal circulation
- tranexamic acid is used for treatment of hereditary angioedema
- desmopressin (Ch. 4) is used in patients with mild congenital bleeding disorders such as haemophilia A or von Willebrand's disease; it is given to reduce spontaneous or traumatic bleeding, or as a prophylactic before surgery.

FURTHER READING

Anticoagulants

Fareed J et al. (1998) Low-molecular-weight heparins: pharmacologic profile and product differentiation. *Am J Cardiol* 82, 3L–10L.

Nurmohamed MT, ten Cate H, ten Cate JW (1997) Low molecular weight heparin(oids)s. *Drugs* 53, 736–751.

Rieder M (2000) Acute pulmonary embolism 2: treatment. *Heart* 85, 351–360.

Verstraete M (1997) Prophylaxis of venous thromboembolism. *Br Med J* 314, 123–125.

Weinmann EE, Salzman EW (1994) Deep vein thrombosis. *N Engl J Med* 331, 1630–1641.

Weitz JI (1997) Low-molecular-weight heparins. *N Engl J Med* 337, 688–696.

Antiplatelet agents

Harrington RA (1999) Overview of clinical trials of glycoprotein IIb/IIIa inhibitors in acute coronary syndromes. *Am Heart J* 138, S276–S286.

Herbert J-M, Savi P, Maffrand J-P (1999) Biochemical and pharmacological properties of clopidogrel: a new ADP receptor antagonist. *Eur Heart J* Suppl A, A31–A40.

Hirsh J, Weitz JI (1999) New antithrombotic agents. *Lancet* 353, 1431–1436.

Schrör K (1996) Antiplatelet drugs. *Drugs* 50, 7–28.

Topol EJ, Byzova TV, Plow EF (1999) Platelet GPIIb/IIIa blockers. *Lancet* 353, 227–231.

Vorchheimer DA, Badimon JJ, Fuster VV (1999) Platelet glycoprotein IIb/IIIa receptor antagonists in cardiovascular disease. *JAMA* 281, 1407–1414.

Haemostatic drugs

Mannucci PM (1998) Haemostatic drugs. *N Engl J Med* 339, 245–253.

Self-assessment

1. In the following questions, the first statement, in italics, is true. Is the accompanying statement also true?

   a. *Anistreplase is a complex of plasminogen and streptokinase.* Thrombolytic infusions of recombinant tissue type plasminogen activator (rt-PA) for myocardial infarction are usually given for 1 h duration and streptokinase for 3–24 h.

   b. *Warfarin has a long half-life (36 h) in plasma.* Warfarin readily crosses the placenta.

   c. *The effect of clopidogrel is additive with warfarin and aspirin.* Clopidogrel has its antithrombotic action by enhancing the action of ADP on platelets.

   d. *Abciximab in conjunction with heparin and aspirin is used in high-risk patients undergoing coronary angioplasty.* Abciximab is an antibody directed against the glycoprotein IIb/IIIa receptor on platelets.

   e. *Aspirin irreversibly inhibits cyclo-oxygenase enzymes.* Aspirin inhibits platelet aggregation at doses below those needed for an anti-inflammatory effect.

   f. *Warfarin inhibits the activation of clotting factors II, VII, IX and X, which depend upon vitamin K for their synthesis.* Anticoagulant activity of warfarin is inhibited by broad-spectrum antibiotics.

   g. *Tranexamic acid is an antifibrinolytic agent used in the treatment of menorrhagia.* Tranexamic acid enhances plasminogen activation.

   h. *Low-molecular-weight heparin (LMWH) has a longer half-life than unfractionated heparin.* Once administered, the action of heparin cannot be reversed.

2. Case history question

   > A 51-year-old obese female has been treated with oestrogen replacement therapy for 18 months because of perimenopausal symptoms. She is scheduled for a hip replacement.

   a. Is anticoagulant therapy necessary in this patient?

   b. Should thromboprophylaxis be started before surgery?

   c. Should heparin or warfarin be chosen for prophylaxis and what routes of administration are necessary?

   > The hip replacement was carried out successfully and the patient was discharged after 5 days, although heparin therapy was continued for a further 5 days.

   d. Why was therapy continued for this extended period and what out-of-hospital therapeutic prophylaxis could be considered?

   The answers are provided on page 606.

Drugs used to effect haemostasis

Drug	Half-life (h)	Elimination	Comment
Antiplatelet drugs			
Aspirin	0.25–0.35	Metabolism	Half-life of active salicylic acid metabolite is 3–20 h
Clopidogrel	5–8 (inactive metabolite)	Metabolism	Prodrug requiring hepatic bioactivation by CYP1A; active metabolite not identified; half-life is based on an inactive metabolite
Dipyridamole	12	Metabolism	
Epoprostenol	2 min	Metabolism	Given by intravenous infusion; eliminated as glucuronide
Glycoprotein IIb/IIIa receptor inhibitors			
Tirofiban	2	Renal	A non-peptide inhibitor, used in combination with heparin for unstable angina; given intravenously
Abciximab	0.5		Antibody fragment to IIb/IIIa glycoprotein receptor on platelets; given intravenously, produces long-lasting blockade of receptors
Anticoagulants (heparin-like)			
Certoparin		Tissue uptake and degradation	Low-molecular-weight heparin
Dalteparin sodium	2–4[a]	Tissue uptake and degradation	Low-molecular-weight heparin
Danaparoid sodium		Tissue uptake and degradation	Useful in patients with heparin-induced thrombocytopenia
Enoxaparin	1–4[a]	Tissue uptake and degradation	Low-molecular-weight heparin
Heparin	0.4–2.5[a]	Tissue uptake and degradation	Dose-dependent half-life
Lepirudin			A recombinant hirudin; used for patients with heparin-associated thrombocytopenia type II
Tinzaparin		Tissue uptake and degradation	Low-molecular-weight heparin
Anticoagulants (oral)			
Nicoumalone	7 (*R*-enantiomer), 1 (*S*-enantiomer)	Metabolism	Enantiomers show different kinetics
Phenindione	5–6	Metabolism and renal	Urinary metabolites give a reddish colour to alkalinised urine
Warfarin	18–35 (*S*) 20–60 (*R*)	Metabolism	*S*-enantiomer more active and oxidised by CYP2C9; *R*-enantiomer is reduced
Thrombolytic agents			
Alteplase (rt-PA)	0.5	Hepatic uptake	Action may be limited by distribution, which has a half-life of only 3–11 min
Anistreplase	2	Deacylation	Prodrug; deacylation releases the active moiety over a prolonged period
Reteplase	0.4–0.5	Hepatic uptake	Cleared by liver and kidney
Streptokinase	1	Binding to plasminogen	Rapid initial decrease in concentrations when there is a high antibody titre
Urokinase	5–10 min	Hepatic uptake	
Haemostatic agents			
Aprotinin	7	Metabolism in kidney	Rapid uptake by kidney (half-life 1 h) where it is degraded into oligopeptides; slower uptake and release from other tissues
Ethamsylate			No published kinetic data found on MEDLINE
Tranexamic acid	1.4	Renal	Eliminated by glomerular filtration

[a]Value depends on the clotting factor measured to reflect drug presence and activity, rather than chemical analysis of the drug.

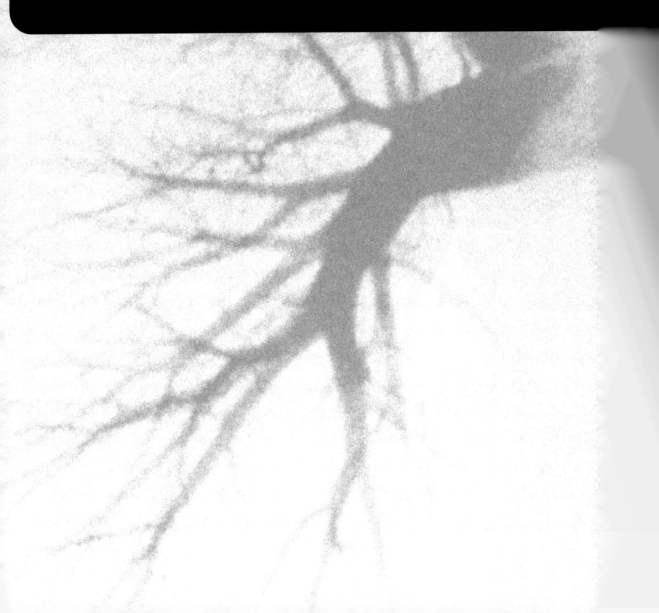

THE RESPIRATORY SYSTEM

Asthma and chronic obstructive pulmonary disease

Asthma and chronic obstructive pulmonary disease (COPD) show several similarities in their clinical features and may reflect different expressions of the same disease. It has been proposed that an inherited tendency to develop either allergy or airway hyper-responsiveness is modulated by age, gender and exposure to allergens, irritants, infection or smoking to determine the eventual outcome (Fig. 12.1).

Asthma

Reversible airways obstruction is the characteristic feature of asthma, which is often associated with an atopic disposition. Exposure to allergens, or possibly other environmental determinants, may then result in expression of the condition. The pathogenesis of asthma involves several processes (Figs. 12.2 and 12.3). Chronic inflammation of the bronchial mucosa is prominent, with infiltration of activated T-lymphocytes and eosinophils. This leads to subepithelial fibrosis and the release of several powerful chemical mediators that can damage the epithelial lining of the airway. Many of these mediators are released following activation and degranulation of mast cells in the bronchial tree, which occurs in response to a variety of immunological or irritant insults to the airway. Some of the mediators act as chemotactic agents for other inflammatory cells. They also produce mucosal oedema, which narrows the airway and stimulates smooth muscle contraction, leading to bronchoconstriction. Excessive production of mucus can cause further airway obstruction by plugging the bronchiolar lumen. Histamine, leukotrienes (LT) C_4, D_4 and E_4, prostaglandin D_2, thromboxane A_2, bradykinin, platelet-activating factor, eosinophil chemotactic factor, neutrophil chemotactic factor and nitric oxide are all thought to be involved in the genesis of asthma. These contribute in different degrees to the symptoms of bronchoconstriction, mucosal oedema, mucosal inflammation, mucus secretion and epithelial cell damage (Table 12.1)

Viral upper respiratory tract infections exacerbate the mucosal inflammatory process while exposure to allergens (such as pollen or house-dust mite faeces), irritants (such as dust or gases), or exercise can cause bronchoconstriction in sensitive airways. Attacks of

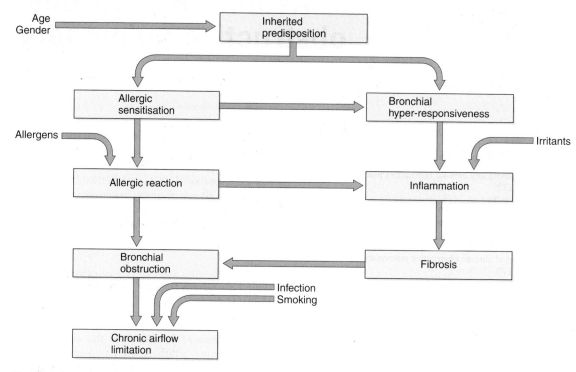

Fig. 12.1
Hypothesis for the natural history of chronic obstructive pulmonary disease.

Table 12.1
Mediators involved in the inflammatory process in asthma

	Bronchoconstriction	Mucosal oedema	Mucosal inflammation	Mucus secretion
Histamine	+	+		+
Leukotrienes C_4, D_4 and E_4	+	+		+
Prostaglandin D_2	+	+		+
Thromboxane A_2	+			+
Bradykinin	+	+	+	+
Platelet activating factor	+	+	+	+
Eosinophil chemotactic factors			+	
Neutrophil chemotactic factors			+	

asthma rapidly follow exposure to a provoking agent. Initial recovery may then be followed some 4–6 h later by a late phase bronchoconstrictor response, which can leave the bronchi hyper-reactive to various irritants for several weeks.

The most common symptoms of asthma are wheeze and breathlessness. In younger patients cough, especially at night, may be the only symptom. Treatment has two aims:

- relief of symptoms
- reduction of airway inflammation.

Chronic obstructive pulmonary disease

COPD is characterised by airflow limitation which is persistent over several months. This is usually slowly progressive and largely irreversible. Most patients with COPD are, or have been cigarette smokers. The airflow limitation results from a combination of decreased bronchial luminal diameter (produced by wall thickening, intraluminal mucus and changes in the fluid lining

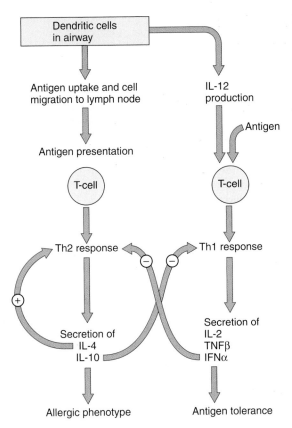

Fig. 12.2
Immune differentiation in response to antigens. In asthma, the T helper type 2 (Th2) response is consolidated in preference to the type 1 (Th1) response. Th2-generated cytokines are responsible for developing and sustaining airway inflammation in asthma. IL, interleukin; TFN, tumour necrosis factor; IFN, interferon:

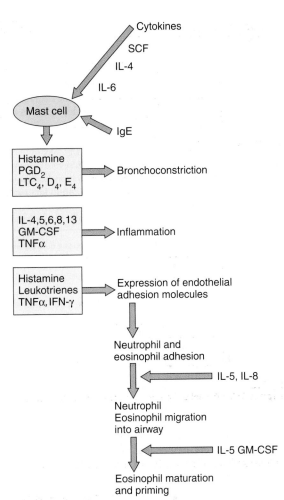

Fig. 12.3
Inflammatory mediators in asthma. Activation of mast cells results in secretion of several mediators that contribute to the pathogenesis of asthma. These mediators produce bronchoconstriction and initiate both the acute inflammatory response and attract cells responsible for maintaining chronic inflammation. IL, interleukin; SCF, stem cell factor; GM-CSF, granulocyte and macrophage colony-stimulating factor; PG, prostaglandin; TNF, tissue necrosis factor; IFN, interferon.

the small airways) and emphysema. Corresponding histological changes include an increase in goblet cells in the bronchial mucosa and an increase in muscle mass in the bronchial wall with interstitial fibrosis. Airways wall inflammation, particularly with mononuclear cells, is common especially in the early phases. Changes in small airways are most important in mild to moderate COPD.

Emphysema is largely an anatomical definition, and is characterised by enlargement of airways distal to the terminal bronchioles. This is a result of destructive changes that may involve the entire acinus (panacinar) or the central part of the acinus (centriacinar). Tissue destruction leads to a loss of lung recoil on expiration. Emphysema is probably the dominant factor in severe COPD.

There is wide variability in the rate of decline in pulmonary function in smokers. About 10–20% show an accelerated decline, which may reflect a genetic susceptibility. In the absence of smoking, or occupational exposure to some inhaled pollutants, α_1-antitrypsin deficiency is the only proven intrinsic association with COPD.

The most frequent symptoms are gradually progressive breathlessness and cough. The cough is often productive and usually worse in the morning; its severity is unrelated to the degree of airflow limitation. Repeated respiratory infections are common.

Drugs for asthma and chronic obstructive pulmonary disease

Drug delivery to the lung

For the treatment of airways disease, direct delivery of drug to the lung by aerosol spray allows the use of

Table 12.2
Comparison of aerosol and oral therapy for asthma

	Aerosol	Oral
Ideal pharmacokinetics	Slow absorption from the lung surface	Good oral absorption
	Rapid systemic clearance	Long systemic action
Dose	Low dose delivered direct to target	High systemic dose necessary to achieve an appropriate concentration in the lung
Systemic drug concentration	Low	High
Incidence of unwanted effects	Low	High
Distribution in the lung	Reduced in severe disease	Unaffected by disease
Compliance	Good with bronchodilators	Good
	Poor with anti-inflammatories	
Ease of administration	Difficult for small children and infirm patients[a]	Good
Effectiveness	Good in mild to moderate disease	Good even in severe disease

[a]May be improved by breath-activated inhalers or spacing devices. Nebulisers can be used for severe exacerbations.

smaller doses and therefore reduces the risk of unwanted effects (see Table 12.2). The size of the aerosol particle that is inhaled determines whether or not it will reach the airway. Particles larger than 5 μm will impact on the upper airway and will be swallowed. Particles smaller than 0.5 μm will not deposit in the lower respiratory tract and are exhaled. The optimal particle size for treatment is 1–3 μm. There are several methods for delivery of aerosols.

Pressurised metered dose inhaler. This is the most common delivery device. Manually activated inhalers are widely used since they are convenient and inexpensive, but they require coordination of inhalation and activation of the device. About one-third of users find this difficult. Even if coordination is optimal, about 80–95% of the aerosol is deposited in the oropharynx, then swallowed. Chlorofluorocarbon (CFC) propellant is being rapidly phased out and replaced by other propellants such as hydrofluorocarbons because of concerns over atmospheric ozone depletion. The inhaler should be shaken before use.

Large volume spacers. Plastic reservoirs of about 750 ml volume with a valve can be attached to a metered dose inhaler to remove the need to coordinate breathing. The inhaler is activated into the spacer, and the patient breathes through the mouthpiece until the aerosol has been inhaled. For young children, a small volume (350 ml) spacer is used (attached to a face mask for very young children). The spacer also allows evaporation of propellant and thus may create more droplets of the correct size to deposit in the airway. Inhalation of the contents should be completed within 10 s and when the device is washed, it should not be wiped dry since this creates an electrostatic charge which attracts particles and reduces drug delivery. Addition of a spacer makes a metered dose inhaler system less portable. To overcome this, one manufacturer has incorporated a collapsible spacer into their inhaler device.

Breath-activated devices. There are several types, delivering either an aerosol or dry powder. The aerosol type is a modified metered-dose inhaler that is activated when air is drawn through the mouthpiece provided airflow exceeds about 30 l min[-1]. Dry powder inhalers contain particles of drug of optimal size for deposition. Inspiration through the device generates turbulence which disperses the particles in the inspired air. Breath-activated devices require a high air flow and are therefore less efficient than metered-dose inhalers.

Nebulisers. These are devices that are used with a face-mask or mouthpiece to deliver drug from a reservoir solution. There are two types. Jet nebulisers use air or oxygen passing through a narrow orifice to suck drug solution from a reservoir into a feed tube with fine ligaments. The impact of the solution on these ligaments generates droplets (Venturi principle). Ultrasonic jet nebulisers use a piezoelectric crystal vibrating at high frequency. The vibrations are transmitted through a buffer to the drug solution and form a fountain of liquid in the nebulisation chamber. Ultrasonic nebulisers produce a more uniform particle size than jet nebulisers. Up to 10 times the amount of drug is required in a nebuliser to produce the same degree of bronchodilation achieved by a metered-dose inhaler. Delivery is more efficient via a mouthpiece rather than a mask.

Symptom-relieving drugs for airflow obstruction

The β₂-adrenoceptor agonists

Examples: salbutamol, salmeterol, formoterol (eformoterol)

Mechanism of action and effects

The airways are rich in β_2-adrenoceptors, which are found on bronchial smooth muscle but also on several other cell types. Effects of receptor stimulation include:

- bronchodilation via generation of intracellular cAMP
- inhibition of mediator release from mast cells
- enhanced mucociliary clearance.

Selectivity of an agonist for the β_2-adrenoceptor is desirable to minimise systemic unwanted effects from stimulation of β_1-adrenoceptors.

Pharmacokinetics

The selectivity of β_2-adrenoceptor agonists is dose-dependent. Inhalation of drug aids selectivity since it delivers small but effective doses to the airways and minimises systemic exposure. The dose–response relationship for bronchodilation is log–linear; therefore a ten-fold increase in dose is required to double the effect. A metered-dose aerosol inhaler is the most frequently used delivery mechanism, but breath-activated devices and nebuliser solutions are available.

After inhalation the onset of drug action is rapid, often within 5 min. Agents such as salbutamol have an intermediate duration of action (producing bronchodilation for up to about 6 h), far longer than the natural adrenoceptor agonists adrenaline and noradrenaline. Their chemical structure prevents neuronal uptake and reduces their affinity for catechol-O-methyl transferase, which is responsible for their metabolism (Ch. 4).

The long-acting agent salmeterol produces bronchodilation for up to 12 h by virtue of a long lipophilic side-chain on the molecule, which binds to an area adjacent to the active site of the receptor, allowing prolonged receptor activation. Formoterol (eformoterol) has a prolonged duration of action by entering the lipid bilayer of the cell membrane from which it is gradually released to stimulate the receptor. Apart from their duration of action, these drugs are no more effective than salbutamol.

The β_2-adrenoceptor agonists can also be given orally (as conventional or modified-release formulations), subcutaneously or by intravenous infusion. However, larger doses are required to deliver an adequate amount to the lungs by any of these routes and consequently the selectivity for β_2-adrenoceptors is reduced and systemic effects can be troublesome.

Unwanted effects

- Skeletal muscle tremor from β_2-adrenoceptor stimulation.
- Tachycardia and arrhythmias result from both β_1- and β_2-adrenoceptor stimulation when high doses of inhaled drug are used or after oral or parenteral administration.
- Acute metabolic responses to high-dose β_2-adrenoceptor stimulation include hypokalaemia, hyperglycaemia and hypomagnesaemia. They do not persist during long-term use.
- Salmeterol produces headache in about 10% of patients.

Concern has been expressed that regular use of high-dose inhaled β_2-adrenoceptor agonists may be linked with asthma deaths by precipitation of serious arrhythmias. A second possibility is that high doses might allow patients to tolerate initial exposure to larger doses of allergens or irritants, which then produce an enhanced late asthmatic response. However, it is more likely that the usage of high doses is really a reflection of the severity of the underlying asthma. Nevertheless, the potential link with β_2-adrenoceptor agonists and death still causes concern, and if high doses are needed, then the concurrent use of inhaled corticosteroid is strongly recommended (see below).

Methylxanthines

Examples: theophylline, aminophylline.

Mechanism of action and effects

Methylxanthines are a group of naturally occurring substances found in coffee, tea, chocolate and related foodstuffs. Theophylline, and its ester derivative aminophylline, are the only compounds in clinical use. The precise mechanisms of action of methylxanthines are not fully understood although some actions are known.

- Inhibition of the enzyme phosphodiesterase (PDE), which degrades intracellular cAMP. Theophylline appears to preferentially inhibit the PDE type IV isoenzyme, which is found in bronchial smooth muscle and several inflammatory cells, including mast cells. There is a lesser increase in intracellular cAMP in other tissues. Theophylline produces bronchodilation especially at higher plasma concentrations (10–20 mg l⁻¹). The rise in intracellular cAMP in bronchial smooth muscle leads to Ca^{2+} release from intracellular stores and its extrusion from the cell is enhanced. Influx of Ca^{2+} into the cell may also be reduced. Both effects will aid smooth muscle relaxation. In cardiac muscle, theophylline increases the force and rate of contraction (Ch. 7). This increases the cardiac output which produces a rise in glomerular filtration rate and consequent diuresis. Direct effects of methylxanthines on the renal tubule also reduce tubular Na^+ reabsorption. These actions can be useful for enhancing diuresis in heart failure.
- Other useful effects of theophylline in the chest are increased mucociliary clearance from the airway

and increased diaphragmatic contractility. The mechanisms are unknown, and these actions occur at lower plasma concentrations than those required for full bronchodilation.

- Adenosine receptor antagonism (see also adenosine; Ch. 8). This enhances smooth muscle relaxation and reduces neurotransmitter release in the central nervous system (CNS). Interference with the effects of adenosine is believed to be responsible for CNS stimulation and gastrointestinal irritation. Initial CNS effects include improved mental performance and alertness, particularly if these are impaired by tiredness or boredom.
- Theophylline has anti-inflammatory effects at concentrations well below those required for maximal bronchodilation. These include inhibition of inflammatory mediator release and a protective effect on bronchial epithelium, which reduces bronchial exudate; both actions may contribute to the ability of theophylline to block the late asthmatic reaction. Thus, improvement in symptoms of asthma can occur at low plasma theophylline concentrations even without demonstrable bronchodilation (5–10 mg l^{-1}).

Pharmacokinetics
Theophylline is absorbed erratically from the gut and is irritant to the stomach. This, and the short plasma half-life, has resulted in the widespread use of modified-release formulations. Theophylline has a narrow therapeutic index and since different formulations have dissimilar release characteristics, they are not readily interchangeable. Theophylline can also be given as a more soluble inactive ester aminophylline, which is hydrolysed rapidly after absorption from the gut to theophylline and ethylenediamine. Aminophylline can be also given by intravenous infusion. Measurement of blood theophylline concentrations is valuable as a guide to effective dosing.

Unwanted effects
Most are dose-related and can occur within the accepted therapeutic plasma concentration range.

- Gastrointestinal upset can occur including nausea, vomiting and diarrhoea.
- CNS stimulation can occur including insomnia, irritability and headache. Fits can also occur at very high plasma concentrations.
- Cardiovascular effects occur at high plasma concentrations and include hypotension from peripheral vasodilation. Unlike other peripheral vessels, cerebral arteries are constricted by methylxanthines. Cardiac stimulation produces various arrhythmias.
- Hypokalaemia can occur acutely, which also promotes cardiac arrhythmias.
- Tolerance to the beneficial effects of methylxanthines can occur.

Antimuscarinic agents

Example: ipratropium

Mechanism of action and effects
Stimulation of muscarinic receptors for acetylcholine in bronchial smooth muscle generates intracellular cGMP and leads to bronchoconstriction. Inhibition of these receptors produces bronchodilation. Direct delivery of ipratropium to the lung is mainly responsible for the lack of many of the unwanted effects characteristically associated with atropine (Ch. 4).

Pharmacokinetics
Ipratropium is a quaternary amine which is poorly absorbed from the gut and is given exclusively by inhalation from a metered-dose aerosol or a nebuliser. It has a slower onset and a longer duration of action than salbutamol, probably owing to its slow absorption from the surface of the airway.

Unwanted effects
Ipratropium causes dry mouth.

....

Anti-inflammatory drugs for airway obstruction

Corticosteroids

Examples: beclometasone dipropionate, budesonide, hydrocortisone, fluticasone, prednisolone

Mechanism of action and effects
Intracellular events involved in the action of corticosteroids are detailed in Chapter 44. The major effects in asthma probably relate to inhibition of transcription of genes coding for cytokines involved in inflammation. Powerful glucocorticoids, devoid of significant mineralocorticoid activity, are usually used. They are the most effective class of drug in the treatment of chronic asthma. Used long term, corticosteroids reduce airway responsiveness to several bronchoconstrictor mediators and block both the early and late reactions to allergen. Following a delay of 6–12 h, several anti-inflammatory actions are produced, which may be important in asthma. Immediate anti-inflammatory effects include:

- reduced inflammatory cell activation (including macrophages, T-lymphocytes, eosinophils and airway epithelial cells)

- reduced mucosal oedema and decreased local generation of inflammatory prostaglandins and leukotrienes (see also Ch. 29)
- adrenoceptor upregulation, which restores responsiveness to β_2-adrenoceptor agonists.

Long-term anti-inflammatory effects include:

- reduced T-cell cytokine production (Ch. 38) and reduced dendritic cell signalling to T-cells
- reduced eosinophil deposition in bronchial mucosa (by removing cytokine stimulation and enhancing apoptosis)
- reduced mast cell deposition in bronchial mucosa (the release of mediators from these cells is unaffected)
- reversal of the excess epithelial cell shedding and goblet cell hyperplasia found in the bronchial epithelium in asthma.

Inhaled corticosteroids are effective after a few days for the treatment of asthmatic symptoms. Reduction in airways responsiveness to allergens and irritants occurs gradually over several months. Many of the chronic structural changes in the airway in asthma are unaffected by corticosteroids.

Pharmacokinetics

Corticosteroids can be used intravenously or orally in severe asthma. However, whenever possible they are given by inhalation of an aerosol or dry powder to minimise systemic unwanted effects. Desirable properties of an inhaled corticosteroid include low absorption across mucosal surfaces (including the gut for swallowed drug) and rapid inactivation once absorbed. Beclometasone dipropionate fulfils the former condition, but once it reaches the systemic circulation it is only slowly inactivated. Budesonide (which is inactivated by extensive first-pass metabolism in the liver) and fluticasone (which is very poorly absorbed from the gut) may be preferred if high doses of inhaled drug are needed, or for the treatment of children.

Unwanted effects

The unwanted effects of oral or parenteral corticosteroids are described in (Ch. 44). Inhaled corticosteroids only have systemic actions when given in high doses. The amount of swallowed drug can be minimised by using a large volume spacer (see above); large aerosol particles, which would otherwise be deposited on the oropharyngeal mucosa, are trapped in the spacer and only the smaller particles are inhaled.

There are specific problems with inhaled corticosteroids.

- Dysphonia (hoarseness) caused by deposition on vocal cords and myopathy of laryngeal muscles, occurs in up to one-third of patients. This may be less troublesome with breath-activated delivery

since the method of inspiration leads to protection of the vocal cords by the false cords.
- Oral candidiasis can occur but can be reduced by using a spacer device or by gargling after use of the inhaler.

Cromones

Examples: sodium cromoglycate, nedocromil sodium

Mechanisms of action and effects

Mast cell stabilisation. Sodium cromoglycate was originally introduced as a mast cell stabiliser. This may be achieved by the drug enhancing phosphorylation of a protein that normally forms a substrate for the intracellular enzyme protein kinase C. This interferes with the signal transduction process in the cell and reduces release of mediators from mast cells, which probably explains the protective action of these drugs on immediate bronchoconstriction induced by allergen, exercise or cold air.

Inhibition of sensory C-fibre neurons. This is probably responsible for protection against bronchoconstriction produced by irritants such as sulfur dioxide and may occur through antagonism of the effects of the tachykinins, substance P and neurokinin B, which are involved in generation of sensory stimuli.

Prevention of 'late phase' allergy response. Cromones cause the inhibition of accumulation of eosinophils in the lungs and reduced activation of eosinophils, neutrophils and macrophages in inflamed lung tissue. These actions may be important in preventing the 'late-phase' response to allergen and the development of bronchial hyperreactivity.

Reduced IgE production. The inhibition of B-cell switching to IgE production probably also contributes to the long-term effects of these drugs.

Dosage

A single dose of either nedocromil sodium or sodium cromoglycate will prevent the early phase bronchoconstrictor response to allergen, but treatment for 1–2 months may be necessary to block the late-phase reaction. Only about one-third of patients benefit from treatment with these agents, which are generally less effective than inhaled corticosteroids but produce few unwanted effects.

Pharmacokinetics

Both sodium cromoglycate and nedocromil sodium are highly ionised and poorly absorbed across biological membranes. They are therefore retained at the site of action on bronchial mucosa after inhalation as a powder or from a metered-dose aerosol inhaler. Swallowed drug is voided in the faeces.

Unwanted effects

Cough and wheeze may be provoked transiently following inhalation.

Leukotriene synthesis inhibitors

Example: zileuton

Mechanism of action and effect

Inhibition of 5-lipoxygenase reduces the conversion of arachidonic acid to leukotrienes (see also Ch. 29), which mediate bronchoconstriction, mucosal inflammation, mucosal oedema and mucus secretion. Zileuton, therefore, has both bronchodilator and mild anti-inflammatory effects. It prevents the bronchoconstriction induced by aspirin and non-steroidal anti-inflammatory drugs (NSAIDs; see Ch. 29). Currently zileuton is not available in the UK.

Pharmacokinetics

Zileuton is well absorbed from the gut and undergoes extensive first-pass metabolism in the liver Elimination is by hepatic metabolism. It has a short half-life.

Unwanted effects

- Headache.
- Dyspepsia.

Leukotriene receptor antagonists

Example: montelukast, zafirlukast

Mechanisms of action and effect

The leukotriene receptor antagonists are given orally and inhibit the bronchoconstriction induced by LTD_4, probably by blocking a receptor for the cysteinyl leukotrienes LTD_4 and LTE_4. They prevent both the early and late bronchoconstrictor responses to allergen.

Leukotriene receptor antagonists may be most useful in mild/moderate asthma, exercise-induced asthma, and asthma provoked by NSAIDs (Ch. 29).

Unwanted effects

- Headache.
- Gastrointestinal upset.

Management of asthma

The acute attack

Mild infrequent attacks of asthma can often be controlled by occasional use of an inhaled β_2-adrenoceptor agonist. Antimuscarinic agents are most effective when asthma coexists with chronic obstructive airways disease. More severe attacks, including status asthmaticus, which is a medical emergency, require intensive treatment with bronchodilators and systemic corticosteroids. The signs of severe and life-threatening asthma are shown in Table 12.3.

Treatment of severe asthma should include

- ensuring adequate hydration
- 40–60% oxygen via a face mask
- nebulised β_2-adrenoceptor agonist such as salbutamol (preferably using oxygen)
- prednisolone orally in high dosage and/or intravenous hydrocortisone.

If there are life-threatening features, additional treatment should be given:

- nebulised ipratropium
- intravenous aminophylline or β_2-adrenoceptor agonist such as salbutamol
- consider assisted ventilation if the patient does not respond rapidly.

After a patient has recovered from a severe asthma attack, oral corticosteroids should be continued until there are no residual symptoms, especially at night, and the peak expiratory flow rate is at least 80% of the

Table 12.3
Signs of severe and life-threatening asthma

Severe	Life-threatening
Inability to complete a sentence	A silent chest
Pulse ≥110 beats min^{-1}	Bradycardia or hypotension
Peak expiratory flow rate ≤50% of predicted or previous best	Peak expiratory flow rate ≤33% of predicted or previous best
Arterial blood gas markers of severe asthma	Exhaustion, confusion or coma
Normal (5–6 kPa) or high arterial carbon dioxide ($PaCO_2$)	
Severe hypoxaemia (PaO_2 < 8 kPa)	
Low or high plasma pH	

patient's previous best. High doses of these drugs can be stopped abruptly if used for 3 weeks or less, or tapered off if they have been used for a longer period (Ch. 44).

Prophylaxis of recurrent attacks

An initial attempt should be made to identify and exclude precipitating factors, for example allergens, occupational precipitants and β-blockers (including eye drops). After initially gaining control of asthma symptoms, long-term treatment is guided by a stepwise treatment plan recommended by the British Thoracic Society.

Step 1. Inhaled short-acting β₂-adrenoceptor agonist, such as salbutamol taken as required.

Step 2. Addition of inhaled anti-inflammatory agent. For adults, a corticosteroid such as beclometasone is most often used. In children and some adults, an initial trial of cromoglycate or nedocromil can be used, substituting a corticosteroid if control is not achieved.

Step 3. Addition of high-dose inhaled corticosteroid or low-dose inhaled corticosteroid with the addition of a long-acting β₂-adrenoceptor agonist such as salmeterol or a modified-release theophylline formulation. There is increasing evidence that a long-acting β₂-adrenoceptor agonist may be the preferred option at this stage.

Step 4. High-dose inhaled corticosteroid with a short-acting β₂-adrenoceptor agonist as required plus a sequential trial of one or more of the following:

- inhaled long-acting β₂-adrenoceptor agonist
- oral modified-release theophylline formulation
- inhaled antimuscarinic agent such as ipratropium
- oral long-acting β₂-adrenoceptor agonist
- inhaled cromoglycate or nedocromil.

Step 5. Regular oral prednisolone in addition to other measures.

The role of leukotriene receptor antagonists is not yet established but probably will be at step 3 or 4, as an alternative or in addition to a long-acting β₂-adrenoceptor agonist.

Asthma resistant to treatment

For patients with resistant disease, especially those requiring oral corticosteroids, the use of immunosuppressant drugs such as ciclosporin or methotrexate (Ch. 39) has been advocated.

Management of chronic obstructive pulmonary disease

There are several important aspects of treatment for COPD, which has two goals: to prevent symptoms and to preserve lung function

Cessation of smoking. This is the most important factor. If successful, the rate of decline in lung function is slowed. Occupational exposure to inhaled pollutants should be minimised.

Antibiotics. These are used for acute exacerbation of symptoms with purulent sputum (Ch. 51).

Bronchodilator therapy. The principles are similar to those for asthma. Improvement in symptoms and functional capacity can occur without changes in lung function tests. Either a β₂-adrenoceptor agonist or an anticholinergic agent can be used, with methylxanthines as a second-line choice. Oral corticosteroid can be effective for short-term use when treating an exacerbation of symptoms. Between exacerbations, use of a long-term inhaled corticosteroid may be of value, but responsiveness should be confirmed after an initial 2–4 week treatment period. About 10% of patients will have an improvement in their forced expiratory flow rate.

Mucolytic agents. These are sometimes prescribed (Ch. 13) but there is little evidence for benefit.

Oxygen therapy. This is extremely important during acute exacerbations. Care must be taken to raise the arterial oxygen saturation (if possible to ≥90%) without increasing the arterial carbon dioxide tension. Low dose oxygen may be necessary (e.g. 24% by Venturi mask or 1–21 min⁻¹ by nasal cannulae). Long-term domiciliary oxygen treatment, usually delivered via nasal cannulae, improves symptoms and survival in COPD with respiratory failure (arterial oxygen tension 8 kPa). It should not be used unless respiratory failure persists for 3–4 weeks despite optimal drug therapy and without a clinical exacerbation. It should not be used by smokers because of the fire risk. To improve survival, oxygen must be used for at least 15 hours per day.

Ventilatory support. This may be required during exacerbations. Intubation and mechanical ventilation may be necessary, but non-invasive assisted ventilation is preferable. Nasal intermittent positive pressure ventilation (NIPPV) is being increasingly used during exacerbations for patients who fail to respond to maximal medical therapy.

FURTHER READING

Asthma

Barnes PJ (1995) Inhaled glucocorticoids for asthma. *N Engl J Med* 332, 868–875

Holgate ST (1997) The cellular and mediator basis of asthma in relation to natural history. *Lancet* 350(suppl 11), 5–9

Lipworth BJ (1997) Treatment of acute asthma. *Lancet* 350(suppl 11), 18–23

Lipworth BJ (1999) Modern drug treatment of chronic asthma. *Br Med J* 318, 380–384

Lipworth BJ (1999) Leukotriene-receptor antagonists. *Lancet* 353, 57–62

Nelson HS (1995) β-adrenergic bronchodilators. *N Engl J Med* 333, 499–506

Shrewsbury S, Pyke S, Britton M (2000) Meta-analysis of increased dose of inhaled steroid or addition of salmeterol in symptomatic asthma (MIASMA). *Br Med J* 320, 1368–1373

The British Guidelines on Asthma Management (1997) 1995 Review and position statement. *Thorax* 52 (suppl 1), S1–S20.

Chronic obstructive pulmonary disease

Bateman NT, Leach RM (1998) Acute oxygen therapy. *Br Med J* 317, 798–801

Boushey HA (1999) Glucocorticoid therapy for chronic obstructive pulmonary disease. *N Engl J Med* 340, 1990–1991

Cazzola M, Donner CF, Matera MG (1999) Long acting β₂-agonists and theophylline in stable chronic obstructive pulmonary disease. *Thorax* 54, 730–736

Celli BR (1996) Current thoughts regarding treatment of chronic obstructive pulmonary disease. *Med Clin North Am* 80, 589–609

Elliott MW (1997) Non-invasive ventilation in chronic obstructive pulmonary disease. *Br J Hosp Med* 57, 83–86

Kerrstjens HAB (1999) Stable chronic obstructive pulmonary disease. *Br Med J* 319, 495–500.

Siafakas NM, Vermeire P, Pride BN et al. (1995) Optimal assessment and management of chronic obstructive pulmonary disease (COPD). *Eur Resp J* 8, 1398–1420

Tarpy SP, Celli BR (1995) Long-term oxygen therapy. *N Engl J Med* 333, 710–714

Self-assessment

In the following questions, the first statement, in italics, is correct. Are the accompanying statements also true?

1. *In asthmatics an inherited tendency to develop allergy or airway hyper-responsiveness is exacerbated by allergens, irritants, infection and smoking.*

    a. An influx of T helper type 2 lymphocytes occurs in the late phase of response following an asthmatic attack.
    b. Leukotriene C₄ is an important bronchodilator released from eosinophils.

2. *Exercise-induced asthma appears to involve only the immediate (early) phase response.*

    a. The β₂-adrenoceptor agonists are effective in preventing exercise-induced asthma.

3. *After recovery from the bronchospasm that follows an acute attack of asthma increased hyper-reactivity and inflammation can last for weeks.*

    a. The late phase response is characterised by bronchial muscle hyper-responsiveness but a normal epithelial cell morphology.

4. *In addition to their bronchodilator action, β₂-adrenoceptor agonists enhance mucus clearance by acting on cilia.*

    a. Tolerance to β₂-adrenoceptor agonists can occur.

5. *The mechanism of the bronchodilator action of the methylxanthines is unclear but may include inhibition of* phosphodiesterases and antagonism at adenosine receptors.

    a. The plasma concentration of theophylline is increased by simultaneous administration of erythromycin and ciprofloxacin.
    b. Methylxanthines cause drowsiness.
    c. An unwanted effect of theophylline is stimulation of the heart.

6. *The muscarinic receptor antagonist ipratropium can be given in combination with β₂ adrenoceptor agonists and corticosteroids.*

    a. Ipratropium is more effective than salbutamol following challenge with an allergen.
    b. Ipratropium causes bradycardia.
    c. Ipratropium is poorly absorbed from the bronchi into the systemic circulation.

7. *Leukotriene C₄ may be important in the precipitation of asthma in subjects who are intolerant to aspirin*

    a. Montelukast inhibits the lipoxygenase enzymes that convert arachidonic acid to leukotrienes.
    b. The leukotriene antagonists (both 5-lipoxygenase enzyme inhibitors and leukotriene receptor antagonists) are only effective if given prophylactically.

8. *Glucocorticoids are ineffective in the treatment of the early-phase response in an asthmatic attack.*

    a. Glucocorticoids reduce dendritic cell signalling to T cells, T cell cytokine production and eosinophil deposition in bronchial mucosa.

The answers are provided on pages 606–607.

Drugs for use in asthma or chronic obstructive pulmonary disease

Drug	Half-life (h)	Elimination	Comment
β-Adrenoceptor agonists			
Bambuterol	8–22	Metabolism	Given orally; long-acting prodrug hydrolysed by plasma cholinesterase to terbutaline; half-life 14–18 h
Formoterol	?	?	Given by dry powder inhalation; long-acting; few data available
Fenoterol	6–7	Metabolism+renal	Given by inhalation
Reproterol	>24 h?	?	Given by inhalation; few data available
Salbutamol	4–6	Renal+metabolism	Given by inhalation, orally or intravenously; conjugated with sulfate
Salmeterol	3–5	Metabolism	Given by inhalation; long-acting; oxidised metabolite retains some activity
Terbutaline	14–18	Renal+metabolism	Given by inhalation, orally or intravenously
Tulobuterol	2–3	Metabolism+renal	Given orally
Ephedrine	6	Renal+metabolism	Given orally; direct + indirect acting sympathomimetic (obsolete)
Methylxanthines			
Aminophylline	1–13 (theophylline)	Hydrolysis	Water-soluble mixture of theophylline and ethylenediamine; given orally or by injection; very rapidly broken down to constituents
Theophylline	1–13	Metabolism +some renal	Given orally; metabolised by CYP1A2, which is induced by smoking; half-life is shorter in children (4 h) than in adults (8 h)
Antimuscarinics			
Ipratropium	2	Renal+bile +metabolism	Given by inhalation
Oxitropium	2–3	Renal+metabolism	Given by inhalation
Corticosteroids			Given by inhalation; see Chapter 44 for corticosteroids given orally or by injection
Beclomethasone dipropionate	15	Metabolism	Hydrolysed rapidly by esterases to the 17-monopropionate, which is almost 30 times more potent, or 21-monopropionate, which is inactive
Budesonide	2	Metabolism	Metabolites are inactive; oral bioavailability is about 10%
Fluticasone propionate	3	Metabolism	Oxidised by liver to acid metabolite, which is excreted in bile; any swallowed dose undergoes 100% first-pass inactivation
Leukotriene activity modulators			
Montelukast	5	Metabolism+bile	Given orally at bedtime
Zafirlukast	10	Metabolism	Given orally; not recommended for children under 12 years; believed to undergo extensive first-pass metabolism (but no intravenous formulation available for comparison)
Cromones			
Cromoglycate	1–1.5	Renal	Given by inhalation; high polarity gives slow absorption from lung; negligible absorption from gut
Nedocromil	2	Renal	See cromoglycate; oral half-life is 23 h because of absorption rate-limited kinetics

?, no data available.

Drug compendium

13

Respiratory disorders: cough, respiratory stimulants, cystic fibrosis and neonatal respiratory distress syndrome

Cough

Cough is a protective mechanism for the airway that removes mucus and foreign bodies from the upper airways. Cough is under both voluntary and involuntary control.

The cough reflex is initiated by sensory receptors located at the epithelial surface of airway mucosa. Receptors are found at and below the oropharynx and in the external auditory meatus and tympanic membrane in the ear. Afferent fibres travel in the vagus nerve to the medullary cough centre. Efferent fibres pass in somatic nerves to respiratory muscles. The cortex can also directly initiate cough, bypassing the medullary centre.

A cough is initiated by a rapid inspiration followed by closure of the glottis. Forced expiration against the closed glottis raises intrathoracic pressure, and sudden opening of the glottis expels air with secretions and debris. Flow rates can approach the speed of sound, producing vibration of upper respiratory structures and the typical sound of cough.

Cough can be a symptom of various respiratory disorders (Box 13.1). In some situations it can be considered

---

Box 13.1

Common causes of cough

Acute respiratory infection
   Upper respiratory tract infection
   Pneumonia, including aspiration
Chronic respiratory infection
   Cystic fibrosis
   Bronchiectasis
   Postnasal drip
Airway disease
   Asthma
   Chronic obstructive pulmonary disease
Parenchymal lung disease
   Interstitial fibrosis
Irritant
   Cigarette smoke
   Inhaled foreign body
Bronchopulmonary malignancy
Drug-induced
   Angiotensin-converting enzyme inhibitors
   Inhaled drugs

183

useful or productive: clearing excess secretions and inhaled foreign matter. In others it is unproductive and has no useful function. It is important to remember that asthma can present with nocturnal cough as the only symptom and chronic cough can be a sign of other underlying diseases, e.g. tuberculosis, gastro-oesophageal reflux, pertussis.

Drugs for treatment of cough

Antitussives (cough suppressants)

Cough suppressants fall into three classes.

Centrally acting drugs (opioids). These increase the threshold for stimulation of neurons in the medullary cough centre. Weak opioid analgesics (Ch. 19) are most commonly used, especially codeine and pholcodeine. They are less addictive than more powerful opioids which are reserved for terminal conditions.

Peripherally acting drugs. Local anaesthetics (Ch. 18) such as lidocaine (lignocaine) are used to reduce cough during bronchoscopy. Sprays or lozenges are also given to reduce oropharyngeal stimulation of the cough reflex. Inhalation of nebulised local anaesthetics is sometimes useful for intractable cough but can produce bronchospasm. Eating and drinking should also be avoided for an hour after their use because of impaired gag reflex and risk of aspiration. Antihistamines (Ch. 38) reduce postnasal drip from allergic rhinitis, which can stimulate cough, but probably have little direct antitussive activity.

Locally acting drugs. Demulcents line the surface of the airway above the larynx, reducing local irritation. The syrup in simple linctus acts by this mechanism.

Expectorants and mucolytics

Expectorants such as iodide, guaiacols, squill and creosotes are given to improve clearance of mucus from the airways. They appear to act by irritating the gastric mucosa; a reflex response via the vagus then stimulates bronchial secretions from goblet cells and submucous glands. There is no evidence of their clinical value.

Mucolytics such as mecysteine hydrochloride and carbocisteine can be given orally to reduce the viscosity of bronchial secretions by breaking disulfide cross-linking between molecules. The value of mucolytics is uncertain and they do not always improve lung function. They may make clearance of mucus easier, but are probably no more effective than hydration from inhaling steam or nebulised saline.

Management of cough

Cough should be treated only if it is unproductive or excessive. The most common cause of cough is a self-

limiting viral illness, for which simple linctus or a weak opioid can be used. Any cough of unknown origin that is still present after 14 days should be investigated further to identify an underlying cause. Specific treatment for left ventricular failure or asthma will eliminate the cough associated with those conditions. Mucolytics are occasionally useful in chronic bronchitis or bronchiectasis. It should be remembered that cough is an unwanted effect of angiotensin-converting enzyme (ACE) inhibitors (Ch. 6) and occurs in up to 10% of patients.

Respiratory stimulants (analeptic drugs)

Doxapram has a limited place in chronic ventilatory failure particularly in a patient with hypercapnoeic respiratory failure who is becoming drowsy. It increases respiratory drive and when combined with physiotherapy may enable a patient to cough and clear excessive secretions, thus improving ventilation. Its use has largely been superseded by ventilatory support, such as with nasal intermittent positive pressure ventilation. There is also a role in some patients with postoperative respiratory depression. Doxapram stimulates the medullary respiratory centre both by a direct action and by stimulation of the carotid body. Given by intravenous injection its action is very brief, and a continuous infusion is often used. Doxapram improves both rate and depth of ventilation but restlessness, muscle twitching and vomiting are common.

Acetazolamide (Ch. 14) stimulates the respiratory centre by creating a mild metabolic acidosis. This action may contribute to its ability to prevent acute mountain sickness by reducing periodic nocturnal apnoea and maintaining arterial oxygen saturation. Acetazolamide also reduces cerebrospinal fluid formation, which prevents the cerebral oedema that forms part of the syndrome. Use of the drug is not a substitute for gradual acclimatisation to altitude.

Cystic fibrosis

Cystic fibrosis is an autosomal recessive disorder caused by a single gene mutation on the long arm of chromosome 7. This gene encodes the cystic fibrosis transmembrane conductance regulator (CFTR), which is a Cl^- channel in epithelial cells. If the *CFTR* gene is faulty then Cl^- transport is defective in epithelial cells in many organs including the respiratory, hepatobiliary, gastrointestinal and reproductive tracts as well as the pancreas. Impaired Cl^- transport leads to reduced Na^+ and water transport. As a result, secretions become thicker causing obstruction to, and destruction of, exocrine glandular ducts.

The most common clinical problems are pancreatic exocrine insufficiency and lung disease (bronchiectasis and chronic obstructive pulmonary disease), which affect about 90% of patients. About 20% develop diabetes and a smaller number develop meconium ileus in infancy or obstructive biliary tract disease.

Drug treatment

Much of the treatment for cystic fibrosis is supportive, including intensive antibiotic therapy and physiotherapy for exacerbation of lung disease. One of the major problems is infection with Pseudomonad species, which can be treated with intravenous or nebulised aminoglycoside antibiotics (Ch. 51). There is some evidence that corticosteroids (Ch. 44), either oral or inhaled, may reduce the rate of decline in lung function.

Pancreatic enzyme supplements (pancreatin). Pancreatin is inactivated by gastric acid. Supplements must, therefore, be taken with food, concurrently with gastric acid suppression therapy (e.g. with cimetidine; Ch. 33) or as enteric-coated formulations. Most pancreatins are of porcine origin. Dosage is adjusted according to the size, number and consistency of stools. Unwanted effects include irritation of the mouth and perianal skin, nausea and vomiting and abdominal discomfort. Some higher strength formulations should be avoided in children under 15 years of age with cystic fibrosis, since they have been associated with the formation of large bowel strictures.

Ursodeoxycholic acid. This synthetic bile acid may prevent progressive liver disease by improving bile acid flow and increasing the bicarbonate content of bile.

Dornase alpha (recombinant human deoxyribonuclease I) (rhDNase I). This enzyme is capable of digesting extracellular DNA. DNA released from dying polymorphonuclear neutrophils in the airways contributes to the increased sputum viscosity. Inhaled rhDNase I reduces sputum viscoelasticity, improves lung function and results in fewer exacerbations of respiratory infection. Unwanted effects include transient laryngitis and hoarseness. Currently, use of rhDNase I is often confined to patients with reduced lung function and chronic sputum production who require regular courses of intravenous antibiotics for recurrent chest infections. Improved lung function should be measurable after 2 weeks in responders.

Neonatal respiratory distress syndrome

Pulmonary surfactant is responsible for reducing surface tension in the lung and alveoli, resisting lung collapse at resting lung pressures. Surfactant largely comprises phospholipids, with a saturated phosphatidylcholine, dipalmitoyl phosphatidylcholine, as the main surface-active component.

Surfactant is produced by alveolar cells and normally is present in adequate amounts at full-term delivery. However, preterm infants may produce too little surfactant, leading to neonatal respiratory distress syndrome.

Mortality is high in neonatal respiratory distress syndrome, but it can be reduced by administration of surfactant. There are two natural agents: beractant (bovine lung extract) and poractant (porcine lung extract). Two synthetic compounds, colfoscerib palmitate and pumactant, are also available. The natural agents have a more rapid onset of action, probably because of the presence of two associated surfactant proteins B and C. All agents are given via an endotracheal tube into the lung.

Overall, the use of a surfactant reduces the risk of neonatal death by 40% in respiratory distress syndrome, whether the treatment is given prophylactically or as a rescue treatment. The natural agents appear to be slightly more effective than the synthetic compounds. Surfactant is given via an endotracheal tube as soon as possible after delivery.

In women at risk of preterm delivery, corticosteroids such as dexamethasone will increase the production of surfactant in the fetal lung, which may prevent respiratory distress syndrome.

FURTHER READING

Cough

David CL (1997) Breathlessness, cough and other respiratory problems. *Br Med J* 315, 931–934

Cystic fibrosis

Bilton D, Mahadeva R (1997) New treatments in adult cystic fibrosis. *J Roy Soc Med* suppl 31, 2–5

Ramsey BW (1996) Management of pulmonary disease in patients with cystic fibrosis. *N Engl J Med* 445, 179–188

Rosenstein BS, Zeitlin PL (1998) Cystic fibrosis. *Lancet* 351, 277–282

Sanchez I, Guiraldes E (1995) Drug management of noninfective complications of cystic fibrosis. *Drugs* 50, 626–635

Neonatal respiratory distress syndrome

Halliday HL (1996) Natural v. synthetic surfactants in neonatal respiratory distress syndrome. *Drugs* 51, 226–237

Self-assessment

In the following questions, the first statement, in italics, is correct. Are the accompanying statements also true?

1. *Postviral cough may last for 3–6 weeks. Treatments should include increased humidity of inspired air and cough suppressants. Other drugs are of little value.*

   a. Many compound cough preparations sold over the counter contain sedating antihistamines.

   b. Dextromethorphan is a synthetic opioid but has no analgesic action.

2. *There is little evidence that any preparation can specifically facilitate expectoration; they may serve a useful placebo function.*

   a. Pulmonary surfactant increases surface tension in the alveoli.

   b. Doxapram should not be used in postoperative respiratory failure.

   c. The mucolytic mecysteine acts by inhibiting the production of mucus.

The answers are provided on page 607.

Respiratory disorders

Drug	Half-life (h)	Elimination	Comment
Cough suppressants			
Codeine	3–4	Metabolism	Undergoes *O*-dealkylation to morphine, *N*-dealkylation and glucuronic acid conjugation; metabolites are excreted in urine
Dextromethorphan	3	Metabolism (+ renal)	Opioid cough suppressant; metabolised by *O*-dealkylation followed by *N*-dealkylation and/or glucuronidation
Methadone	6–8	Metabolism + renal	Used in palliative care for the distressing cough of terminal lung cancer (used less than other opioids); eliminated by renal excretion and demethylation with excretion contributing more than metabolism for a single dose but metabolism being more important on repeated dosage
Morphine	1–5	Metabolism (+ renal)	Used in palliative care for the distressing cough of terminal lung cancer; eliminated by formation of the 3-glucuronide (which is inactive) and the 6-glucuronide (which is active – the only pharmacologically active glucuronide); about 5–10% is excreted unchanged
Pholcodine	37	Metabolism	Slowly metabolised (probably oxidation but few data are available)
Mucolytics			
Carbocisteine	–	Metabolism (+ renal)	Eliminated unchanged in urine and as *S*-oxidation and *N*-acetylation products
Dornase alfa	–	–	Recombinant human DNAase preparation used for cystic fibrosis; given by inhalation of a nebulised solution; measurable concentrations have not been found in the blood after inhalation administration; activity in sputum is measurable for at least 6 h
Mecysteine (methyl cysteine)	–	Metabolism (+ renal)	Few kinetic data available
Pulmonary surfactants			Used for respiratory distress in preterm infants
Beractant	–	–	Given by endotracheal tube; activity occurs at the alveolar surface without systemic absorption; respiratory distress syndrome may enhance permeability and uptake; (not surprisingly) radiolabelled disposition studies following clinical use have not been performed; the apparent half-life of the natural surfactant (phosphatidylglycerol) is about 30 h
Colfosceril palmitate	–	–	See beractant
Poractant alfa	–	–	See beractant
Pumactant	–	–	See beractant
Respiratory stimulants			Given only under expert supervision
Doxapram	2–4	Metabolism (+ some renal)	Given by continuous intravenous infusion; metabolised by oxidation in the liver; the keto-metabolite is less active than the parent drug but is eliminated more slowly

THE RENAL SYSTEM

14

Diuretics

Functions of the kidney

The kidney has several important functions:

- regulation of plasma electrolyte concentrations
- regulation of acid–base balance
- elimination of waste products
- conservation of essential nutrients.

Maintenance of salt and water balance

Diuretics alter the body's electrolyte and fluid balance by increasing electrolyte (essentially salt) and water elimination. This can be useful in the management of a wide range of conditions producing oedema (e.g. heart failure, cirrhosis of the liver and nephrotic syndrome) and for the treatment of hypertension. An understanding of the mechanisms of electrolyte and fluid handling by the kidney is essential for optimal usage and an appreciation of the unwanted effects of diuretics. An understanding of the reasons for combining different classes of diuretic depends on knowledge of their actions at different, complementary sites in the renal tubule.

A healthy adult will filter several hundreds of litres of plasma at the glomerulus each day. Since the urine output is only 1–2 litres in 24 h it is clear that the majority of filtered fluid and solutes is absorbed back from the tubule into the blood. Different regions of the tubule and collecting duct vary in their capacity to reabsorb solutes (Fig. 14.1).

The proximal tubule. In the proximal tubule about 60–70% of the filtered Na^+ is reabsorbed together with equivalent amounts of water. Therefore, on leaving the proximal tubule, the tubular fluid still has the same osmolarity as plasma. The proximal tubule also has many transport mechanisms for the secretion of organic acids and bases and ammonia into the tubular lumen and the reabsorption of glucose and amino acids from the lumen. Reabsorption of ions from the proximal tubule through the renal tubular cells is both passive and active (Fig. 14.1). The activity of Na^+/K^+-ATPase pump on the basolateral surface of the tubular cell drives Na^+ and glucose reabsorption and also helps to establish the electrochemical gradient for passive ion absorption. Bicarbonate is also reabsorbed from the proximal tubule by a mechanism dependent on the enzyme carbonic anhydrase (Fig. 14.1; site 2).

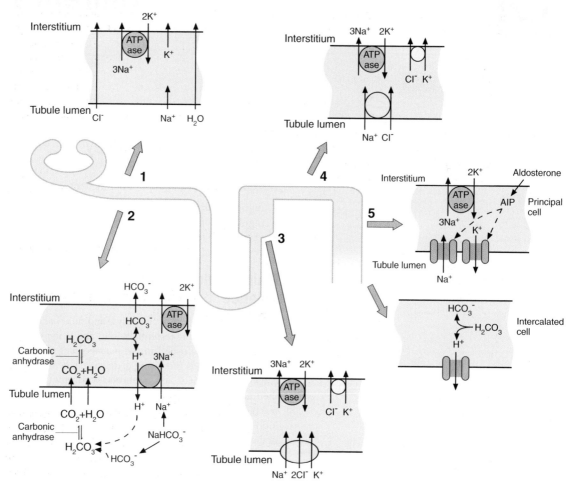

Fig. 14.1

Transport mechanisms for solutes in the kidney. In all segments of the renal tubule there is active transport of Na⁺ out of and K⁺ into the cell across the basolateral membrane using Na⁺/K⁺-ATPase. This sets up electrochemical gradients for the transport of other ions. In the proximal tubule (sites 1 and 2), considerable amounts of Na⁺ and glucose are taken up from the lumen along with water. Hydrogen ions are excreted in exchange for Na⁺ uptake and this, in part, depends upon the activity of carbonic anhydrase. In the ascending limb of the loop of Henle (site 3) the luminal membrane has a cotransport mechanism for Na⁺/Cl⁻/K⁺ but is impermeable to water. In the proximal part of the distal tubule (cortical diluting segment; site 4) Na⁺ and Cl⁻ are co-absorbed but not water. In the distal part of the distal tubule and collecting duct (site 5) Na⁺ is reabsorbed from the lumen in exchange for K⁺ through selective channels. The channels transporting these ions are dependent upon aldosterone. Water is reabsorbed in the collecting duct under the influence of antidiuretic hormone (vasopressin) acting through receptors in the basolateral membrane.

The loop of Henle. The descending limb of the loop of Henle is permeable to water but not to Na⁺. Water passes from the tubule into the interstitium of the renal medulla where the fluid is hypertonic (see below). The thick ascending limb of the loop of Henle is impermeable to water but has an active cotransporter mechanism in the luminal membrane for Na⁺, Cl⁻ and K⁺ (Fig. 14.1; site 3). The gradient for this cotransportation is maintained by activity of the Na⁺/K⁺-ATPase pump in the basolateral membrane. There is also paracellular diffusion of Ca²⁺ and Mg²⁺ from the tubular lumen into the medullary interstitium and then into blood, driven by the potential difference across the tubular cells. The active cotransporter mechanism in the ascending limb of the loop of Henle can reabsorb up to 30% of the Na⁺

filtered at the glomerulus. The reabsorption of Na⁺ and K⁺ but not water in the ascending limb establishes the hypertonicity of the medullary interstitium. This, in turn, is responsible for the osmotic gradient across the collecting ducts that permits formation of hypertonic urine.

The distal tubule. The filtrate leaving the loop of Henle is hypotonic and passes to the proximal part of the distal tubule (also known as the cortical diluting segment of the distal tubule). This part of the renal tubule is impermeable to water but has a luminal cotransporter for the reabsorption of Na⁺ and Cl⁻. The driving force for this is movement of ions, again generated by the Na⁺/K⁺-ATPase pump in the basolateral membrane. About 5% of the filtered Na⁺ load is reabsorbed at this site; however, the rich blood supply to this region allows rapid diffusion of the ions into the plasma and prevents the interstitium from becoming hypertonic. The reabsorption of Ca^{2+} is also regulated at this site under the influence of parathyroid hormone and calcitriol.

The collecting duct. The tubular fluid, which has become more hypotonic in the proximal distal tubule, is then delivered to the distal part of the distal tubule and then to the collecting duct. There are two cell types in this region. In the principal cell, Na^+ is reabsorbed in exchange for K^+. This exchange is dependent upon aldosterone-induced proteins (AIPs) that activate and increase the numbers of Na^+ and K^+ channels. The action of aldosterone is, therefore, to enhance Na^+ reabsorption and increase K^+ excretion. The driving force for the Na^+ reabsorption is again dependent upon the Na^+/K^+-ATPase, the activity of which is also increased by aldosterone. The second cell type, intercalated cells, secrete H^+ into the lumen in exchange for Na^+. Overall, only about 3–5% of filtered Na^+ is reabsorbed at the distal part of the distal tubule.

The principal cell is also the site of action of antidiuretic hormone (ADH; Ch. 43). This hormone is secreted by the posterior pituitary gland and binds to receptors in the basolateral membrane, where it increases the permeability of the cell to water. ADH increases water absorption leading to concentration of urine as it passes through the collecting duct in the hypertonic medullary region.

Maintenance of potassium homeostasis

Relatively small reductions in extracellular K^+ concentration can affect cardiac muscle, skeletal muscle and brain function. The primary site in the kidney that controls excretion of K^+ is the exchange for Na^+ in the distal part of the distal renal tubule and the collecting duct. The uptake of luminal Na^+ through aldosterone-sensitive channels creates the electrochemical gradient which results in K^+ excretion from the cell into the tubular lumen.

Diuretic drugs

Osmotic diuretics

Example: mannitol

Mechanism of action

Osmotic diuretics are filtered at the glomerulus and exert osmotic activity within the renal tubule that limits passive tubular water reabsorption. Water reabsorption throughout the renal tubule is normally driven by the osmotic gradient across the tubular cells that is created by active transport of Na^+ across the basolateral membrane. Water loss produced by an osmotic diuretic is accompanied by a variable natriuresis, a consequence of ion flow down the concentration gradient created between diluted Na^+ in tubular fluid and the higher concentration in the tubular cells. Expansion of plasma and extracellular fluid volume limits the clinical uses of osmotic diuretics.

Pharmacokinetics

Mannitol is given by intravenous infusion and has a short duration of action. It is excreted unchanged at the glomerulus.

Unwanted effects

Expansion of plasma volume resulting from the use of these drugs can precipitate heart failure.

Proximal tubular diuretics: carbonic anhydrase inhibitors

Example: acetazolamide

Mechanism of action

Acetazolamide interferes with the small proportion of Na^+ reabsorbed in the proximal tubule in exchange for H^+ (Fig. 14.2), a process dependent on the enzyme carbonic anhydrase. The final result is increased HCO_3^-, Na^+ and K^+ secretion, causing alkaline urine. A mild metabolic acidosis is produced in the blood by retention of H^+. However, the fall in plasma HCO_3^- concentration stimulates the enzyme reaction and overcomes the effect of the drug. This rapidly leads to tolerance to its diuretic action. Acetazolamide is now reserved for treatment of conditions which do not rely on its diuretic action (see below).

Pharmacokinetics

Acetazolamide is well absorbed from the gut and is eliminated unchanged by the kidney. Its duration of action is short.

Unwanted effects

- Nausea and vomiting, anorexia.
- Parasthesiae, dizziness, fatigue.
- Hypokalaemia (see loop diuretics).
- Drowsiness.

Loop diuretics

Examples: furosemide (frusemide), bumetanide

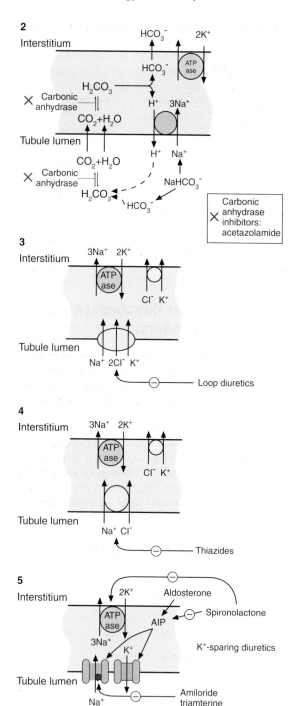

Fig. 14.2
Sites of action of diuretics. For location of these sites see
Fig. 14.1. Acetazolamide inhibits carbonic anhydrase and is a weak
self-limiting diuretic, now largely used for other situations such as
glaucoma. Osmotic diuretics increase osmotic pressure through the
tubule reducing electrolyte reabsorption across the luminal membrane.
Loop diuretics can inhibit the cotransporter for $Na^+/Cl^-/K^+$ and inhibit
up to 30% of filtered Na^+ reabsorption. Thiazide diuretics and
K^+-sparing diuretics inhibit the reuptake of a maximum of about 5%
of filtered Na^+. AIP, aldosterone-induced protein.

Mechanism of action and effects

Loop diuretics act after they are excreted into the kidney
tubule by the organic acid transporter in the proximal
tubule. At the luminal border of the thick ascending
limb of the loop of Henle, loop diuretics compete with
Cl^- for binding to the $Na^+/K^+/Cl^-$ cotransporter
complex. Inhibition of the tubular Cl^- binding site
reduces Na^+ reabsorption by diminishing the electrochemical gradient across the cell. Loop diuretics do not
affect the active transport of Na^+ at the basolateral
border of the tubular cell. Loop diuretics are powerful,
'high ceiling' diuretics, which can inhibit reabsorption
of up to 30% of the Na^+ that appears in the glomerular
filtrate. The dose–response curve is steep, and they
remain effective even in advanced renal failure.

When injected intravenously, furosemide (frusemide)
releases prostaglandins in peripheral veins causing venodilation. Pooling of blood in these capacitance vessels
reduces central blood volume, which can be useful in the
treatment of acute left ventricular failure (Ch. 7). Loop
diuretics also produce arterial vasodilation (see thiazide
diuretics) but, because of their short duration of action,
they are not widely used to treat hypertension.

Pharmacokinetics

Furosemide (frusemide) is moderately well but erratically absorbed orally and is partially metabolised by
glucuronide conjugation, principally in the kidney.
Bumetanide is more completely absorbed and partially
metabolised in the liver. In plasma, these drugs are
highly protein bound and little is filtered at the
glomerulus. Unmetabolised drug is secreted into the
proximal tubular lumen via the anion transport mechanism. The consequent rate of Na^+ excretion is directly
related to the rate of urinary excretion of the diuretic.
Natriuresis and diuresis begin about 30 min after an
oral dose and last 4–6 h. A more rapid effect can be
achieved by intravenous injection, with an onset of
diuresis within minutes, lasting about 2–3 h.

Unwanted effects

Hypokalaemia. Urinary K^+ loss is increased because
of the higher urine flow rate. In addition, delivery of
excess Na^+ to the lumen of the distal tubule stimulates
renin release, causing hyperaldosteronism. Aldosterone
enhances Na^+ reabsorption in the distal tubule at the
expense of increased K^+ excretion. Obligatory urinary Cl^-
loss with the cations creates a mild metabolic alkalosis in
the plasma. To counteract the alkalosis, H^+ are shifted out
of cells in exchange for intracellular accumulation of K^+,
which exacerbates the hypokalaemia. Magnesium depletion may accompany the hypokalaemia and make its
correction more difficult. Consequences and treatment of
hypokalaemia are discussed below.

Salt and water depletion. This can cause hypotension. Sometimes salt loss exceeds water loss, leading to
dilutional hyponatraemia.

Incontinence. This is caused by rapid increase in urine volume. In older males with prostatic hypertrophy, retention of urine can occur.

Hyperuricaemia. This is partly a result of competition between uric acid and the diuretic for proximal tubular secretion and also a result of reduced glomerular filtration of uric acid following contraction of plasma volume. Gout can occur, but is less common than with thiazide diuretics.

Increased urinary Ca²⁺ excretion. This is caused by inhibition of tubular reabsorption.

Ototoxicity. Deafness may result from cochlear damage, especially in the presence of renal failure or when very large doses are used. Vertigo may result from vestibular damage. Both are more common with furosemide (frusemide) and are usually reversible.

Thiazide and thiazide-like diuretics

Examples: bendroflumethiazide (bendrofluazide), hydrochlorothiazide, chlortalidone, metolazone

Mechanisms of action and effects

The thiazides (or more correctly benzothiadiazines) are structurally related to sulfonamides. They act at the luminal surface of the cortical diluting segment of the distal convoluted tubule to inhibit Na⁺ and Cl⁻ cotransport. Although structurally different, the thiazide-like drugs chlortalidone and metolazone share this site of action. Thiazides have a lower efficacy than loop diuretics, achieving a maximum natriuresis of about 5% of the filtered Na⁺ load. The onset of diuresis is slow, and they also have a longer duration of action than loop diuretics although this varies among the drugs; for example bendroflumethiazide (bendrofluazide) produces a natriuresis over 6–12 h and chlortalidone over 48–72 h. Most thiazide diuretics are less effective in renal failure (especially when the creatinine clearance or glomerular filtration rate is below 20 ml min⁻¹). Metolazone differs from other thiazide diuretics, probably owing to an additional effect on the proximal tubule. Its natriuretic efficacy is greater than other thiazides and it also works in advanced renal failure.

Arterial vasodilation occurs during long-term use of thiazides, which produces a useful hypotensive effect (Ch. 6). This vascular action is maximal at lower dosages than are required for diuresis.

Pharmacokinetics

The thiazides and related drugs are fairly well absorbed from the gut and extensively metabolised in the liver. They are highly protein bound and little is filtered at the glomerulus. Thiazides act from the renal tubular lumen after secretion of the parent drug via the proximal tubule anion transport mechanism (see also loop diuretics).

Unwanted effects

- Hypokalaemia (see loop diuretics): the greatest reduction in plasma K⁺ occurs within 2 weeks of starting treatment.
- Salt and water depletion. The combination of a thiazide with amiloride (see below) is particularly associated with hyponatraemia. This is usually a dilutional phenomenon caused by Na⁺ loss in excess of water loss but without true Na⁺ depletion.
- Nocturia and urinary frequency are caused by prolonged diuresis.
- Hyperuricaemia (see loop diuretics). Gout occurs infrequently and is less common in women.
- Decreased urinary Ca²⁺ excretion. This is in contrast to loop diuretics. The mechanism is not well understood.
- Glucose intolerance. A dose-related, progressive increase in plasma glucose can occur over many months during treatment with thiazides. This is in part caused by prolonged hypokalaemia, with the consequent low intracellular K⁺ concentration inhibiting insulin synthesis. The glucose intolerance usually reverses over several months if treatment is stopped.
- Hyperlipidaemia. Thiazide diuretics produce a dose-related increase in low density lipoprotein cholesterol and triglycerides. The long-term effects are small but may increase atherogenic risk (Ch. 48).
- Impotence. This is reported by up to 10% of middle-aged hypertensive males treated with high doses of thiazides.

Potassium-sparing diuretics

Examples: spironolactone, amiloride, triamterene

Mechanism of action and effects

These drugs act at the aldosterone-sensitive site in the late distal convoluted tubule and cortical collecting duct. The maximum natriuresis will be small (less than 5% of filtered Na⁺). Aldosterone increases the number and activity of Na⁺ channels via the synthesis of aldosterone-induced proteins (AIPs). Spironolactone and its active metabolite canrenone prevent this by competing with aldosterone for cytoplasmic receptors that, when bound to aldosterone, migrate to the nucleus and attach to DNA and induce AIP synthesis. Receptors occupied by spironolactone do not attach to DNA. Amiloride and triamterene block the Na⁺ channel at the luminal surface of the renal tubule.

With all these drugs, Na$^+$ and water loss is accompanied by preservation of plasma K$^+$, because of reduced Na$^+$/K$^+$ exchange.

When used together with thiazide or loop diuretics, K$^+$-sparing diuretics reduce or eliminate the excess urinary K$^+$ loss and produce an additional natriuresis that is greatest with spironolactone.

Pharmacokinetics

Spironolactone is metabolised in the wall of the gut and the liver to canrenone, which is probably responsible for most of the diuretic effect. Triamterene is also extensively metabolised but tubular secretion of the parent compound is responsible for the diuretic action. Amiloride is excreted unchanged. All three drugs are given orally, but potassium canrenoate (a salt of canrenone) is available for intravenous use.

The onset of action of amiloride and triamterene is rapid but that of spironolactone is slow, over several days.

Unwanted effects

- Hyperkalaemia. This is more common in the presence of pre-existing renal disease, in the elderly and during combination treatment with angiotensin-converting enzyme (ACE) inhibitors (Ch. 6). Magnesium retention also occurs, in contrast to the situation with the thiazides and loop diuretics.
- Hyponatraemia. This is more common with thiazide–amiloride combinations.
- Oestrogenic effects. Spironolactone has oestrogenic effects (as a result of its steroid structure) causing gynaecomastia and impotence in males. Menstrual irregularities can occur in women.
- Carcinogenesis. Spironolactone is carcinogenic in rats. It is, therefore, no longer licenced for use in hypertension, when treatment may be required for long periods.

Management of diuretic-induced hypokalaemia

A modest reduction in plasma K$^+$ concentration is common during treatment with loop or thiazide diuretics. Marked hypokalaemia (below 3.0 mmol l^{-1}) predisposes patients to cardiac rhythm disturbances, particularly in the presence of acute myocardial ischaemia, during treatment with digitalis glycosides (Ch. 7) or with antiarrhythmic agents that prolong the Q–T interval on the electrocardiogram (Ch. 8). It may also precipitate encephalopathy in patients with liver failure. The risk of hypokalaemia is greatest with:

- thiazide rather than loop diuretics, because of their longer duration of action
- low oral intake of K$^+$
- high dosages of diuretic

- co-existent high aldosterone production, for example in hepatic cirrhosis and nephrotic syndrome.

Both treatment and prevention of diuretic-induced hypokalaemia can be achieved by using either KCl supplements or a K$^+$-sparing diuretic. Potassium supplements are less effective unless used in large quantities, which often cause gastric irritation. Modified-release tablets, effervescent formulations and intravenous solutions are available. Supplements of greater than 30 mmol K$^+$ daily are usually needed but many oral formulations of K$^+$ contain no more than 8 mmol in each tablet or sachet. Intravenous K$^+$ supplements are rarely needed unless there is severe K$^+$ depletion. Rapid intravenous injection can produce potentially lethal hyperkalaemia (provoking serious cardiac arrhythmias). A maximum infusion rate of 10 mmol h^{-1} is recommended, with hourly monitoring of the plasma K$^+$ concentration if such a high infusion rate is necessary.

Potassium-sparing diuretics are more effective for preventing hypokalaemia. They are widely used together with thiazide or loop diuretics, often as fixed-dose combination tablets. Combination tablets are convenient, but they lack the facility for flexible dosage adjustments. It is unnecessary to prescribe a K$^+$-sparing diuretic for most patients who are taking a thiazide or loop diuretic. A pragmatic approach would be to reserve their use for patients at high risk from hypokalaemia or those who develop significant hypokalaemia during regular diuretic treatment.

Major uses of diuretics

Diuretics can be used to control a number of conditions.

Oedema in heart failure (Ch. 7), nephrotic syndrome and hepatic cirrhosis. Mild oedema can sometimes be controlled by a thiazide diuretic. More marked oedema usually requires the use of a loop diuretic. Modest doses of a loop diuretic provides near maximal diuresis if renal function is normal, but large doses are sometimes necessary if there is renal failure (because of a reduction in the number of functioning nephrons). The extent of diuresis is dependent on the rate of delivery of the drug to the renal tubule. Once the optimal rate is exceeded, no further diuresis or natriuresis is achieved. If fluid retention is resistant to appropriate doses of an oral loop diuretic, various strategies can be tried.

- Divided oral doses of a loop diuretic can be used to give more consistent drug delivery to the kidney.
- Oral bumetanide can be used rather than furosemide (frusemide) because of its more consistent oral absorption.
- A loop diuretic can be given by intravenous infusion if absorption of the diuretic may be impaired (e.g. with gut congestion in congestive

heart failure). Higher drug doses are more safely and effectively given by slow intravenous infusion.

- The addition of a thiazide diuretic or metolazone to a loop diuretic. Sequential inhibition of tubular Na$^+$ reabsorption can produce a dramatic diuresis and natriuresis. Hypovolaemia, hyponatraema and hypokalaemia can be troublesome with such combinations.
- If there is marked secondary hyperaldosteronism (e.g. in ascites because of cirrhosis of the liver), spironolactone can be particularly useful.

Hypertension. (Ch. 6). Low doses of a thiazide diuretic are usually used. A loop diuretic is sometimes useful for resistant hypertension.

Acute renal failure. A loop or an osmotic diuretic may prevent incipient acute renal failure from becoming established. The mechanism of action in this situation is unknown.

Hypercalciuria with renal stone formation. Thiazides can be used to reduce urinary Ca^{2+} excretion.

Glaucoma. Acetazolamide can be used to reduce intraocular pressure (Ch. 50). Tolerance does not occur to this effect, unlike the diuretic action.

Mountain sickness. Acetazolamide can be used for preventing mountain sickness by stimulating respiration (Ch. 12).

Raised intracranial pressure. An osmotic diuretic is occasionally useful, for example after neurosurgery to reduce intracerebral oedema.

FURTHER READING

Bleich M et al (1997) Mechanism of action of diuretics. *Kidney Int* 51, S11–S15

Dormans TPJ, Gerlag PGG, Russel FGM, Smits P (1998) Combination diuretic therapy in severe congestive heart failure. *Drugs* 55, 165–172

Krämer BK, Schweda F, Riegger GAJ (1999) Diuretic treatment and diuretic resistance in heart failure. *Am J Med* 106, 90–96

Self-assessment

In the following questions, the first statement, in italics, is correct. Are the accompanying statements also true?

1. *A fall in plasma K+ concentration can affect cardiac muscle and brain function.* The main renal site of K+ ion loss in the urine is in the proximal tubule.

2. *Electrogenic gradients are set up in many segments of the tubule by the Na+/K+-ATPase pump on the basolateral membrane.* The thick ascending limb of the loop of Henle is impermeable to water.

3. *Osmotic diuretics are poorly reabsorbed from the renal tubule.* Osmotic diuretics exert their activity on the proximal tubule, descending limb of the loop of Henle and the collecting ducts.

4. *Osmotic diuretics cause expansion of extracellular fluid volume.* Osmotic diuretics should not be given in heart failure.

5. *The carbonic anhydrase inhibitor, acetazolamide, is used to inhibit the formation of aqueous humour in glaucoma.* Tolerance to the diuretic effect of acetazolamide develops.

6. *20–30% of filtered Na+ is reabsorbed in the thick ascending limb of the loop of Henle.* Loop diuretics increase the hypertonicity of the interstitium in the medullary region.

7. *In addition to its diuretic properties furosemide (frusemide) has a venodilator action possibly as a result of the release of prostaglandins.*
   a. Loop diuretics are useful in the treatment of acute pulmonary oedema in chronic heart failure.
   b. Loop diuretics and thiazide diuretics should not be administered together.
   c. loop diuretics do not produce hypokalaemia.

   d. There is no upper limit to the diuretic or natriuretic activity of a loop diuretic.
   e. Loop diuretics can produce ototoxicity.

8. *Unlike loop diuretics, which are short acting, some thiazide diuretics such as chlortalidone can produce a diuresis over 48–72 h period.*
   a. Thiazide diuretics act by inhibiting the Na+ and Cl- cotransport in the basolateral membrane.
   b. Like the loop diuretics, the thiazides increase urinary Ca2+ excretion.
   c. The diuretic effect of metolazone is greater than other thiazide diuretics.
   d. Thiazide diuretics can produce glucose intolerance.

9. *Spironolactone and amiloride inhibit K+ loss by reducing the uptake of Na+ which exchange for K+ in the late distal convoluted tubule and the cortical collecting duct.*
   a. Spironolactone and amiloride act by identical mechanisms to reduce K+ loss.
   b. Potassium-sparing diuretics can interact unfavourably with angiotensin-converting enzyme (ACE) inhibitors.

10. *Thiazide or loop diuretics are given together with K+ sparing diuretics.*
    a. The combination of amiloride and hydrochlorothiazide produces no greater natriuresis than hydrochlorothiazide given alone.
    b. Spironolactone is metabolised to the inactive metabolite canrenone.

11. *Non-steroidal anti-inflammatory drugs (NSAIDs) reduce the diuretic response to thiazide and loop diuretics.* Prostaglandins synthesised within the kidney increase renal blood flow and cause natriuresis.

The answers are provided on pages 607–608.

Diuretic drugs

Drug	Half-life (h)	Elimination	Comment
Osmotic diuretics			
Mannitol	2–36	Renal	Elimination delayed in cardiac failure; half-life is 2 h in healthy subjects but very prolonged in cardiac or renal failure
Carbonic anhydrase inhibitors			
Acetazolamide	6–9	Renal	Use with caution in elderly patients with impaired renal function
Loop diuretics			
Furosemide (frusemide)	1	Renal + metabolism	Incomplete absorption from gut; limited metabolism (15%) by glucuronidation
Bumetanide	1–1.5	Renal + metabolism + bile	About 50% is conjugated with glucuronic acid and excreted in urine and bile
Torasemide	2–4	Metabolism + renal	Good oral absorption; about 25% cleared by kidney and remainder by metabolism; half-life unchanged in renal failure
Thiazide diuretics			Weak acids, therefore renal clearance affected by urine pH
Bendroflumethazide (bendrofluazide)	3–9	Metabolism and renal	30% excreted in urine unchanged; metabolites not characterised; complete absorption from gut
Chlorothiazide	15–27	Renal	Incomplete absorption from gut
Chlortalidone	50–90	Renal	Incomplete oral absorption; long half-life because of its large volume of distribution and high plasma protein binding which reduces glomerular filtration
Cyclopenthiazide	–	Renal	Limited kinetic data available
Hydrochlorothiazide	8–12	Renal	Incomplete absorption from gut
Indapamide	10–22	Metabolism + renal	Renal only 5% of dose: extensive hepatic metabolism
Mefruside	3–16	Metabolism	Oxidised in liver to active metabolites
Metolazone	4–5	Renal + metabolism + bile	Renal is main route of elimination (80%)
Polythiazide	25	Metabolism(?) + renal	Good absorption from gut; renal elimination accounts for about 25% of dose and remainder is not known.
Xipamide	5	Renal + metabolism	About 50% is excreted unchanged in the urine and 35% as a glucuronide conjugate
Potassium-sparing diuretics			
Amiloride	6–9	Renal + faecal	About 50% not absorbed from the gut
Canrenoate potassium	10–35	Metabolism	Eliminated in urine as an ester glucuronide
Spironolactone	1	Metabolism	Variable absorption from gut; metabolised to active metabolite (canrenone)
Triamterene	2	Metabolism	Variable absorption owing to first-pass metabolism; metabolised by oxidation to a hydroxy metabolite which retains activity

Disorders of micturition

The urinary bladder is a smooth muscle organ composed chiefly of the detrusor muscle, which relaxes to allow bladder filling. A smaller muscle, the trigone, is found between the ureteric orifices and bladder neck. The external urethral sphincter constricts to prevent bladder emptying; it is formed from striated muscle which in the male is below the prostate gland. Stimulation of β-adrenoceptors via the sympathetic nervous system relaxes the bladder to accommodate urine, aided by inhibition of parasympathetic supply innervating the detrusor.

Micturition is initiated by contraction of the detrusor in response to parasympathetic (muscarinic) stimulation. This is coordinated with inhibition of adrenoceptor activity, which relaxes the external sphincter and bladder neck, and bladder emptying is augmented by contraction of the diaphragm and abdominal muscles. Coordination of these activities is a function of the hind-brain.

Disorders of micturition

Disorders of micturition can arise from a disturbance of bladder function or from abnormalities affecting bladder outflow.

Detrusor instability

Detrusor instability produces uncontrolled bladder contractions and urge incontinence. Most cases are idiopathic but upper motor neuron lesions, such as those produced by stroke or multiple sclerosis can be the cause. Drugs that decrease bladder activity are sometimes helpful to treat detrusor instability.

- Oxybutinin, flavoxate, tolterodine and propiverine have antimuscarinic and possibly also local anaesthetic actions. Antimuscarinic unwanted effects can be troublesome, particularly with oxybutinin. Propantheline, another antimuscarinic agent, is now rarely used since the clinical response is poor.
- Tricyclic antidepressants can also be used, for example, imipramine and amitriptyline (Ch. 22). Although antimuscarinic effects are important for the action of these drugs, an additional membrane stabilising action on bladder smooth muscle may contribute.

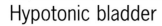

Hypotonic bladder

Hypotonic bladder is often a result of lower motor neuron lesions or can arise from bladder distension owing to chronic urinary retention. The condition leads to incomplete bladder emptying. Treatment depends on the cause.

- Chronic urinary retention is often caused by bladder outlet obstruction and should be managed by bladder catheterisation and correction of the underlying cause.
- Neurogenic problems can be helped by treatment with a muscarinic agonist (Ch. 4). This can be either an anticholinesterase, for example distigmine, or a direct-acting agonist, for example bethanechol. These drugs increase the force of detrusor contraction and should not be used in the presence of urinary outflow obstruction.

Urethral sphincter incompetence

Urethral sphincter incompetence produces stress incontinence in women or sphincter weakness incontinence in men. The most common cause in women is loss of collagenous support in the pelvic floor or perineum; other causes are pelvic trauma and prostatectomy in males. Drug treatment is not appropriate except for oestrogen replacement in postmenopausal women, either topically or as hormone replacement therapy (HRT; Ch. 45).

Benign prostatic hypertrophy

Benign prostatic hypertrophy (BPH) produces symptoms in more than 25% of men above the age of 60 years. The spectrum of symptoms is often called prostatism (Box 15.1). The severity of these symptoms can be quantified using a scoring system, which can help to guide management. If this is untreated, spontaneous improvement occurs, or symptoms remain stable, in up to half of all patients.

Medical management

The aim of drug treatment is either to reduce prostatic size or to relax smooth muscle that restricts urine outflow. There is no evidence that medical treatment avoids the need for surgery in the long term. There are two current choices:

- 5α-reductase inhibitors
- α₁-adrenoceptor blockers.

5α-Reductase inhibitors

> Example: finasteride (for more details see Ch. 46)

Inhibition of the enzyme 5α-reductase does not affect testosterone levels but reduces the level of dihydrotestosterone (DHT). DHT is involved in prostate growth, and inhibition of its production leads to a reduction in prostate volume by up to 30%. The drug often takes 2–6 months to improve symptoms, but improvements are usually maintained. Benefits may be more marked with larger volume prostates.

Unwanted effects occur in up to 5% of patients, and include:

- reduced libido
- erectile impotence
- reduction in the plasma concentration of prostate specific antigen, which must be accounted for when screening for prostatic cancer.

Alpha-1-adrenoceptor blockers (α-blockers)

> Examples: prazosin, doxazosin, alfluzosin, tamsulosin

Selective α₁-blockers block adrenoceptors in prostatic smooth muscle, and in the bladder neck, without affecting the detrusor and result in relaxation, improving urine outflow and symptoms of BPH (Box 15.1). Alfluzosin and tamsulosin are claimed to be more selective for the α₁ₐ-adrenoceptor subtype in the urinary tract and may produce fewer vasodilatory unwanted effects than the other agents. However, the extent of this selectivity and the consequent clinical advantages are equivocal. Symptomatic improvement usually occurs within 1 month, in contrast to therapy with 5α-reductase inhibitors. Symptoms improve in about two-

---

Box 15.1

Symptoms of benign prostatic hypertrophy

Obstructive	Irritative
Hesitancy	Urgency
Poor stream	Frequency
Straining to pass urine	Nocturia
Prolonged micturition	Urge incontinence
Feeling of incomplete bladder emptying	
Urinary retention	

thirds of patients. Full details of selective α_1-adreno-ceptor blockers are found in Chapter 6.

Surgical treatment

Surgical treatment is usually required for severe symptoms or complications of benign prostatic hypertrophy (Box 15.2). Options include trans-urethral resection of the prostate or open prostatectomy. Symptoms are improved in 70–90% of patients. Newer minimally invasive operations are being explored since the risk of complications, such as impotence or retrograde ejaculation, from current procedures is high.

FURTHER READING

Scientific Committee of the First International Consultation on Incontinence (2000) Assessment and treatment of urinary incontinence. *Lancet* 355, 2153–2158.

Thakar R, Stanton S (2000) Management of urinary incontinence in women. *Br Med J* 321, 1326–1331

> **Box 15.1**
>
> **Indications for surgery in patients with benign prostatic hypertrophy (BPH)**
>
> Acute retention of urine
> Chronic retention of urine
> Recurrent urinary tract infection
> Bladder stones
> Renal insufficiency owing to BPH
> Large bladder diverticula
> Severe symptoms

Self-assessment

1. In this question, the first statement, in italics, is correct. Are the accompanying statements also true?

   Urinary bladder function is controlled by parasympathetic and sympathetic innervation of the detrusor and sphincter muscles.

   a. Atropine causes urinary frequency and urge incontinence.
   b. The tricyclic antidepressant amitriptyline is effective in the management of the unstable bladder.
   c. The anticholinesterase distigmine can be safety given if there is urinary outflow obstruction.

2. Case history question

   A 65-year-old man has had developing urinary problems over a 5-year period. He has difficulty passing urine and is getting up three times in the night to pass urine. A rectal examination by his GP indicates an enlarged prostate. Ultrasound, flow tests and prostate specific antigen measurements suggest benign prostatic hypertrophy (BPH).

   a. What pharmacological approaches to the treatment of BPH could be considered?
   b. What are the unwanted effects of these treatments?
   c. What are the possible outcomes of not treating this patient?

   The answers are provided on page 608.

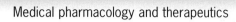

Drug compendium

Drug	Half-life (h)	Elimination	Comment
Drugs for urinary retention			
α_1-Blockers (all given orally for benign prostatic hypertrophy)			
Alfuzosin	4	Metabolism (+ some renal)	Oral bioavailability is about 70%; pathways of metabolism have not been defined; relatively selective for α_1-adrenoceptors in the genitourinary tract
Doxazosin	11(?)	Metabolism (+ some renal)	Oral bioavailability is 65%; longer half-lives (22 h) found after treatment to steady state (probably owing to minor slowly equilibrating compartment not detected after a single dose); eliminated largely by oxidative metabolism
Indoramin	5 (2–10)	Metabolism	Undergoes extensive hepatic first-pass metabolism; oral bioavailability is about 10–20% (but 70% in patients with hepatic cirrhosis); much higher blood levels (fivefold) in the elderly
Prazosin	2–3	Metabolism (+ some renal)	Oral bioavailability is about 60%; metabolised in the liver by dealkylation and conjugation
Tamsulosin	15	Metabolism (+ some renal)	Normally taken with food (to reduce side-effects) but this reduces bioavailability to about 60%
Terazosin	12	Metabolism + urine	Oral bioavailability is 90%; mainly eliminated via the faeces as parent drug and metabolites
Parasympathomimetics			
Bethanechol	?	?	Given orally; poorly absorbed from the gut; there are no adequate kinetic data available (based on quaternary nitrogen it is likely to be poorly absorbed and excreted largely unchanged)
Carbachol	?	?	Given orally or as subcutaneous injection; no data on fate in humans
Distigmine	70	Renal + hydrolysis	Given orally; very poor oral bioavailability (5%) especially if taken with food; hydrolysed by plasma esterases
Drugs for urinary frequency and incontinence			All drugs taken orally
Flavoxate	?	Metabolism + renal	Metabolised to a carboxylic acid derivative; few other kinetic data are available (high oral bioavailability in rats)
Oxybutynin	1–3	Metabolism	Very low oral bioavailability (6%) owing to extensive first-pass metabolism; cholinergic antagonism in vivo may result from metabolites formed in the liver, since the desethyl metabolite is as active as the parent compound
Propantheline	1–2 (i.v.)	Metabolism + renal	Oral bioavailability is about 5–10% (based on urinary excretion data); metabolites are inactive
Propiverine	4	Metabolism	Oral bioavailability is about 50%; metabolised mainly by *N*-oxidation
Tolterodine	2 (EM) 10 (PM)	Metabolism	High oral bioavailability (about 75%); metabolised by CYP2D6 to an active metabolite responsible for part of the therapeutic effect; subjects with low CYP2D6 activity (poor metabolisers; PM) metabolise the drug by CYP3A4; PMs have higher levels of parent drug and lower levels of the metabolite, but as both compounds are active they show similar responses as extensive metabolisers (EM); the drug shows dose-dependent kinetics in the therapeutic range

Erectile dysfunction

Physiology of erection

Penile erection results from interaction between the central nervous system and autonomic receptors in the smooth muscle of the penis; both psychological and tactile stimuli are important. Relaxation of arterial and trabecular smooth muscle in the penis increases the influx of blood into the sinusoidal spaces of the corpus cavernosum (Fig. 16.1). Compression of the veins by the trabecular smooth muscle reduces venous outflow, thus maintaining the erection. Neuronal innervation of parasympathetic and nonadrenergic-noncholinergic origin are important for erection while sympathetic stimulation inhibits erection. Nitric oxide, prostaglandins

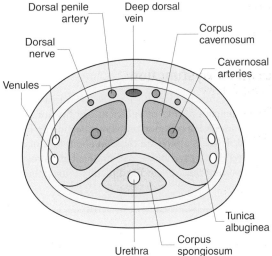

Fig. 16.1

Cross-section of the penis showing structures essential for erection. The penis contains three cylinders of erectile tissue: two corpora cavernosa and the corpus spongiosum. The corpus spongiosum contains the urethra. The cylinders of erectile tissue are divided into spaces known as lacunae, which are lined by vascular epithelium. The walls of these spaces are made up of thick bundles of smooth muscle cells within a framework of fibroblasts, collagen and elastin. The erectile tissues are supplied with blood from the two cavernosal arteries, which branch, and helicine arteries drain into the lacunar spaces. Blood is drained from the lacunae through venules that pass between the erectile tissue and the walls of the cylinders (tunica albuginea). The venules join together to form larger veins that drain into the deep dorsal vein, cavernosal and crural veins. Arterial and sinusoid dilation is important for erection, while swelling is limited by the inelastic tunica albuginea. The rising pressure during erection limits the venous outflow, thus maintaining the erection.

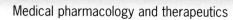

Table 16.1
Drugs that commonly cause male sexual dysfunction

	Ejaculatory dysfunction	Erectile dysfunction	Loss of libido
Antihypertensives			
β-Blockers		+	
α-Blockers	+		
Methyldopa	+	+	+
Psychotropic drugs			
Phenothiazines	+	+	+
Benzodiazepines	+	+	+
Tricyclic antidepressants		+	+
Selective serotonin (5HT) reuptake inhibitors (SSRIs)		+	+
Other			
Spironolactone			+
Digoxin		+	
Cimetidine/ranitidine		+	+
Metoclopramide		+	+
Carbamazepine		+	+
Recreational drugs			
Alcohol	+	+	
Marijuana		+	
Cocaine		+	+
Amphetamines	+	+	+
Anabolic steroids		+	+

and vasoactive intestinal peptide (VIP) may all play a role in maintaining blood flow.

Erectile dysfunction

Erectile dysfunction is defined as the consistent inability to sustain an erection of sufficient rigidity for sexual intercourse. It is a common problem, affecting up to 10% of men. There is a physical cause in about 80% of cases (Box 16.1) but a psychological component often coexists. An important cause of erectile difficulty is drug therapy, particularly antihypertensive or psychotropic drugs (Table 16.1).

Management of erectile dysfunction

A number of strategies can be used in the management of erectile dysfunction. Initially these should be an assessment and treatment of any underlying psychological or physical disease. Treatment options include

- Mechanical aids such as the vacuum erection device.
- Penile implants.
- Hypogonadism is an uncommon cause of impotence and will respond to testosterone replacement therapy.
- Hyperprolactinaemia impairs erection. It is most commonly caused by drug therapy, (e.g. with phenothiazines) and can be improved by oral bromocriptine.
- Topical glyceryl trinitrate (Ch. 5) is effective in some patients.
- Intracavernous injection of vasodilators. These are most effective if arterial flow is normal, such as with neurogenic and psychogenic impotence. Bleeding tendencies preclude this form of treatment, as does poor manual dexterity or morbid obesity.

Box 16.1

Common causes of erectile dysfunction

Diabetes
Vascular disease
Surgery
Drugs especially antihypertensives, antipsychotic drugs, antidepressants
Substance abuse, e.g. nicotine, alcohol, recreational drugs
Hormonal imbalance
Neurological disease, e.g. multiple sclerosis, Alzheimer's disease, epilepsy
Spinal cord injury
Psychological (20% as a primary cause, more commonly secondary to physical problems)

The injection is made into the side of the penis. There is a small risk of prolonged erection or priapism.

Vasodilators

Several vasolidators can be useful for the management of impotence.

Combinations of drugs can be used for synergistic actions at lower doses to reduce unwanted effects, when they are effective in about 65% of patients.

Papaverine. This is an opioid (see Ch. 19) that has additional properties. It inhibits phosphodiesterase and increases intracellular cAMP, which reduces α_1-adreno-ceptor mediated vasoconstriction. The success rate in impotence is about 50%. Fibrosis within the penis can result from the acidity of the solution.

Alprostadil. This is a synthetic prostaglandin E_1 analogue. Local pain after injection is the most common adverse effect and is reported by one third of users. The pain can be reduced by the addition of a local anaesthetic such as procaine (Ch. 18). Rapid local metabolism of alprostadil minimises systemic unwanted effects. High doses of alprostadil can be given intra-urethrally using a plastic applicator.

Phentolamine and moxisylyte (thymoxamine). These are α-adrenoceptor blockers (Ch. 6), which are relatively ineffective when used alone because they do not reduce venous outflow. However, they are better tolerated than either papaverine or alprostadil. The drugs are effective in about 65% of patients.

Sildenafil. This is an orally active selective phospho-diesterase type V inhibitor that reduces the breakdown of cGMP. Nitric oxide (which vasodilates by generation of cGMP) is involved in cavernosal smooth muscle relaxation. About 60% of men have improved erections sufficient to permit intercourse when the drug is taken orally 30–60 min before. It is well absorbed orally and is eliminated by hepatic metabolism; it has a short half-life. Some systemic unwanted effects can result from the use of sildenafil.

- Reduced blood pressure, dizziness and flushing can occur. It should not be used by patients taking nitrates (see Ch. 5) because of a synergistic effect on vascular nitric oxide, or those with recent stroke or myocardial infarction. In these situations hypotension could be dangerous.
- Phosphodiesterase type V is found in tissues other than the penis and this may explain effects on the eye, and some other vascular beds, causing nasal congestion, visual disturbance and increased intraocular pressure.

ADDITIONAL READING

Goldstein I, Lue TF, Padma-Nathan H et al. (1998) Oral sildenafil in the treatment of erectile dysfunction. *N Engl J Med* 338, 1397–1404

Lue TF (2000) Erectile dysfunction. *N Engl J Med* 342, 1802–1813

Morgentaler A (1999) Male impotence. *Lancet* 354, 1713–1718

Self-assessment

Are the following statements true or false?

1. Sildenafil should not be taken by men already taking nitrates.

2. Sildenafil can cause an increase in blood pressure if taken with nitrates.

3. Phosphodiesterase type V is only found in the vasculature in the penis.

4. Increased parasympathetic outflow to the penis causes a failure of erection.

5. Erections caused by injected drugs such as papaverine or alprostadil are not easy to control.

6. Impotence caused by hypogonadism can be treated with oestrogen.

7. Diabetes can cause impotence.

The answers are provided on page 608.

Drugs used in erectile dysfunction

Drug	Half-life	Elimination	Comments
Alprostadil	30 s	Metabolism	Given by intracavernosal injection or urethral application; prostaglandin E_2 analogue; care if partner is pregnant; can cause priapism; can be given with papaverine (see below)
Papaverine	2 h	Metabolism	Given by intracavernosal injection; eliminated by oxidation in the liver
Phentolamine	1.5 h	Metabolism + renal	Given by intracavernosal injection; eliminated in urine largely as oxidised metabolite plus some unchanged drug
Sildenafil	2 h	Metabolism	Given orally; oral bioavailability is about 40%; eliminated by oxidation catalysed by CYP3A4 and CYP2C9; incomplete oral bioavailability is due to first-pass metabolism; metabolites are eliminated mainly in the faeces (80%)

THE NERVOUS SYSTEM

General anaesthetics

General anaesthesia is the loss of awareness of general sensory inputs to the central nervous system (CNS) and includes varying degrees of analgesia, amnesia and loss of consciousness. It may also be accompanied by muscle relaxation and loss of homeostatic control of respiration and cardiovascular function. An adequate level of general anaesthesia is essential for major surgical procedures. General anaesthesia was introduced into clinical practice in the nineteenth century with the use of volatile liquids such as diethyl ether and chloroform. Major drawbacks with such compounds include the time taken to cause loss of consciousness, unpleasant taste and irritant properties. Cardiac and hepatic toxicity also limited the usefulness of chloroform. Modern general anaesthetic agents allow the rapid and smooth induction of surgical anaesthesia with a short recovery phase.

Anaesthesia was originally induced and maintained solely by inhalation of a volatile agent. If this method is used, several stages of general anaesthesia are passed through during induction and recovery. These are shown in Table 17.1. Some of these stages are undesirable. An ideal anaesthetic agent would have all the properties shown in Box 17.1 but since no single anaesthetic possesses all of these properties it is now usual practice to use a combination of agents. To minimise the initial excitement phase, anaesthesia is usually rapidly induced in adults with a non-volatile agent given as an intravenous bolus dose and is subsequently maintained by an inhalation anaesthetic. In children, anaesthesia is often both induced and maintained with an inhalational

---

Box 17.1

Properties of an ideal inhalational anaesthetic

Inherently stable
Non-flammable and non-explosive when mixed with air, oxygen or nitrous oxide
Potent, allowing the use of a high inspired oxygen concentration
Low blood solubility, allowing rapid induction (with minimal excitation stage); rapid emergence from anaesthesia, with no hangover; and rapid adjustment of the depth of anaesthesia
Non-irritant to the airway
Non-toxic
Lack of sensitisation of the heart to catecholamines

Table 17.1
The stages of anaesthesia

Stage	Description	Effects produced
I	Analgesia	Analgesia without amnesia or loss of touch sensation; consciousness retained
II	Excitation	Excitation and delirium with struggling: respiration rapid and irregular; frequent eye movements with increased pupil diameter; amnesia
III	Surgical anaesthesia	Loss of consciousness; subdivided into four levels or planes of increasing depth; *plane I* shows a decrease in eye movements and some pupillary constriction; *plane II* shows loss of corneal reflex; *planes III and IV* show increasing loss of pharyngeal reflex, and a progressive decrease in thoracic breathing and general muscle tone
IV	Medullary depression	Loss of spontaneous respiration and progressive depression of cardiovascular reflexes: should be considered as an overdose requiring respiratory and circulatory support

agent. For some short surgical procedures in adults, total intravenous anaesthesia is now used.

Anaesthesia for surgical procedures usually involves the use of several drugs in addition to the anaesthetic agent(s). The patient will normally be given a premedication which may include an opioid analgesic (Ch. 19), an antimuscarinic agent (Ch. 4) and a benzodiazepine (Ch. 20) or neuroleptic (Ch. 21). These are used to dry secretions, reduce anxiety, to produce amnesia and for postoperative pain relief. In addition, an anti-emetic such as metoclopramide (Ch. 32) may be given. A neuromuscular junction blocking drug (Ch. 27) is given before or after tracheal intubation for procedures that require muscle relaxation.

Mechanism of action

General anaesthesia can be produced by compounds of widely differing chemical structure from simple gases such as nitrous oxide to organic liquids such as isoflurane (Fig. 17.1). Despite this diversity of chemical structures, all general anaesthetics interfere with the propagation of nerve impulses by a non-specific mechanism involving the cell membrane. General anaesthetics are characterised by a number of properties.

1. Anaesthetic potency of different agents is proportional to their lipid solubility.
2. Anaesthesia is produced when the concentration of the compound in the cell membrane is about 0.05 mol l^{-1}, irrespective of the agent.
3. Anaesthesia appears to be reversed if the body is subjected to a high atmospheric pressure (50 atmospheres; although data on this are conflicting).
4. The potency ranking of different agents is consistent across organisms of widely different phylogenetic origins (e.g. protozoa to humans).
5. Different stereoisomers (where these occur) show the same potency.

Anaesthetic potency is measured as the minimum alveolar concentration (MAC) of an agent necessary to

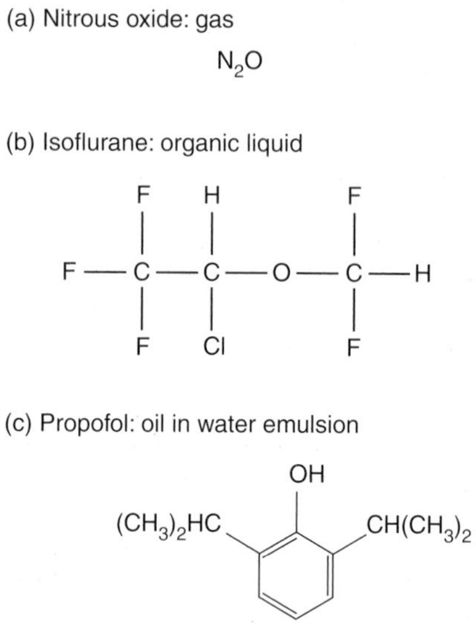

(a) Nitrous oxide: gas

$$N_2O$$

(b) Isoflurane: organic liquid

(c) Propofol: oil in water emulsion

Fig. 17.1
Examples of general anaesthetics of different chemical natures.

immobilise 50% of subjects exposed to a noxious stimulus (which in humans is a surgical skin incision). Therefore, MAC is the equivalent of the ED$_{50}$ (the 50% effective dose) for other drugs (Ch. 1). The MAC for inhaled anaesthetics correlates closely with their lipid solubility or oil:gas partition coefficient (see Table 17.2).

The ability of diverse chemical structures to produce general anaesthesia might indicate that non-specific mechanisms are responsible for anaesthesia. General anaesthetics act at cell membranes, and the characteristic (1 above) led to the hypothesis that incorporation into lipids altered the cell membrane, perhaps resulting in increased membrane fluidity and neural volume expansion that are known to accompany anaesthesia.

With many anaesthetics, hyperbaric pressure (3 above) reverses anaesthesia and at the same time reverses membrane fluidity and volume expansion. However, in some studies these effects are not unequivocally causal. Other more recent theories propose effects upon protein domains including receptors for gamma-aminobutyric acid (GABA) and other neurotransmitters,

Table 17.2
Inhalation anaesthetics[a]

Compound	Blood:gas partition coefficient	Oil:gas partition coefficient	Induction time (min)[b]	MAC (%)[c]	Metabolism (%)[d]
Nitrous oxide	0.5	1.4	2–3	>100[f]	0
Isoflurane	1.4	91	–	1.12	0.2
Enflurane	1.9	96	–	1.7	2.10
Halothane	2.3	224	4–5	0.8	15
Sevoflurane	0.6	53	–	2.1	approx 5
Diethyl ether[e]	12.1	65	10–20	2	5–10

[a]Most cause cardiac and respiratory depression and muscle relaxation. They have varying effects on cerebral blood flow.
[b]Inhalation time necessary if used as the sole anaesthetic; correlates with blood:gas coefficient.
[c]Minimum alveolar concentration necessary for surgical anaesthesia (equivalent to potency); correlates inversely with oil:gas coefficient.
[d]Percentage eliminated as urinary metabolites; most of the remainder is eliminated in the expired air; influenced by volatility and blood:gas coefficient.
[e]No longer available for clinical use.
[f]Theoretical value.

alteration of ion channel function and changing membrane excitability.

The different stages of anaesthesia (Table 17.1) probably arise from the size of different neurons and their accessibility to the anaesthetic agent. A rapid action on small neurons in the dorsal horn of the spinal cord (nociceptive impulses; Ch. 19) and inhibitory cells in the brain (cf. effects of alcohol; Ch. 54) explain the early analgesic and excitation phases. By contrast, neurons of the medullary centres are relatively insensitive and are affected last.

General anaesthetics can be grouped according to their route of administration, which is either intravenous or inhalational.

Drugs used in anaesthesia

Intravenous anaesthetics

Examples: propofol, thiopental, ketamine, etomidate

Intravenous anaesthetics are generally given for rapid induction of anaesthesia and supplemented by inhalation anaesthetics. Propofol and ketamine can, however, be given continuously for short operations. Some properties of commonly used intravenous anaesthetics are shown in Table 17.3.

Pharmacokinetics

Thiobarbiturates, such as thiopental, have a very rapid onset of action (about 10 s) owing to their high lipid solubility and ease of passage across the blood–brain barrier. The delay in onset of action is largely a consequence of the circulation time between the site of injection in the arm and the brain. The duration of action after a bolus dose is very short (about 2–5 min) owing to redistribution from rapidly equilibrating tissues (including the brain) into more slowly equilibrating tissues such as muscle (Fig. 17.2; see also Ch. 2). With thiopental, total intravenous anaesthesia is not

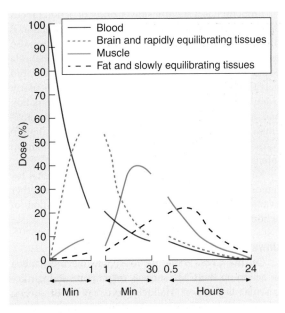

Fig. 17.2
The amounts of thiopental in blood, brain (and other rapidly equilibrating tissues), muscle and adipose tissue (and other slowly equilibrating tissues) after an i.v. infusion over 10 seconds. NB: the time axis is not linear: the continued uptake into muscle between 1 and 30 min lowers the concentration in the blood and in all rapidly equilibrating tissues (including the brain); the terminal elimination slopes are parallel for all tissues; metabolism removes about 15% of the body load per hour.

Table 17.3
Some properties of common intravenous anaesthetics

Drug	Type	Speed of induction	Recovery	Hangover effect	Analgesia	Comment
Thiopental	Barbiturate	Rapid	Slow owing to redistribution	Yes	No	Widely used; sloughing of tissue if extravascularisation occurs from the blood vessel or the site of injection; cannot be given by long-term continuous infusion; can cause bradycardia
Propofol	Phenol	Rapid	Rapid. Liver metabolism	Low	No	Does not accumulate during infusion; continuous infusion can be used in intensive care; occasional bradycardia
Etomidate	Imidazole	Rapid	Fairly rapid. Liver metabolism	Low	No	Not infused continuously; cardiac depressant; enhances GABA activity; repeated doses suppress adrenocortical function
Ketamine	Cyclohexanone	Slower	Slower	No	Yes	Hallucinations on recovery; cardiac stimulant raises blood pressure; can be given continuously; analgesia that outlasts anaesthesia; bronchodilator

practicable since the blood and slowly equilibrating tissues would reach equilibrium during anaesthesia; the cessation of anaesthetic action would then depend on the elimination half-life (12 h for thiopental) not the distribution half-life (about 3 min). Therefore after induction of anaesthesia with thiopental, an inhaled agent is used for maintenance of anaesthesia.

Propofol has a slightly slower onset of action (about 30 s) compared with thiopental; its duration of action is limited by redistribution after a bolus dose. It can also be given as an infusion for total intravenous anaesthesia when its duration of action is determined by rapid hepatic clearance (half-life 1 h). Propofol is particularly useful for day surgery because of its rapid elimination and absence of hangover effects. It also has an antiemetic action. Propofol can also be used for sedation in conscious patients requiring controlled ventilation in an intensive care unit.

Ketamine has some advantages over thiopental for minor procedures. It produces analgesia unlike all other available intravenous anaesthetics. The duration of action after bolus injection is about 15 min.

Unwanted effects

On the CNS. Some are related to the mechanism of action on the CNS, such as respiratory and cardiovascular depression. Hallucinations can occur during recovery from ketamine.

On the heart. All intravenous anaesthetics (except ketamine) have a negative inotropic effect on the heart. Such effects are particularly likely if there is pre-existing circulatory failure in which case the distribution rate is reduced. This may lead to prolonged high plasma concentrations of the drug. Ketamine produces cardiac stimulation and tachycardia.

Pain. Some intravenous anaesthetics, such as propofol, are lipid soluble and therefore are given in a complex vehicle. Intravenous injection of propofol may be associated with pain and possibly thrombophlebitis. Thiobarbiturates and ketamine are produced in aqueous solution.

Intravenous opioids

Examples: fentanyl, remifentanil

Intravenous opioids are given for intra-operative analgesia and not as primary induction agents. They can reduce the tachycardia and hypertension produced by the sympathetic nervous system during endotracheal intubation and surgical stimulation. The ability of opioids to stabilise the circulation makes them particularly useful during anaesthesia in patients with ischaemic heart disease.

Pharmacokinetics

Fentanyl has a long duration of action so that prolonged ventilatory support is necessary after surgery. Details of the metabolism of opioids are given in Chapter 19. Remifentanil is an opioid ester that has a very short half-life of about 6 min owing to metabolism by plasma esterases. After an initial bolus dose of remifentanil, continuous intravenous infusion is necessary to maintain its effects.

Unwanted effects

Muscle rigidity. This can be controlled during surgery with muscle relaxants, but after recovery myoclonus and rigidity can persist, requiring assisted ventilation.

Profound respiratory depression. This means that assisted ventilation is usually necessary during surgery.

Inhalational anaesthetics

Examples: isoflurane, halothane, nitrous oxide, sevoflurane

Inhaled anaesthetics are given with oxygen to avoid hypoxia during anaesthesia. The concentration of anaesthetic used in the inhaled gas (potency) and the duration of inhalation necessary to give sufficient concentration of drug within the membranes of the CNS to produce general anaesthesia depend on the relationships shown in Fig. 17.3 and Table 17.2. There are four factors that are important.

1. The rate of absorption across the alveolar membranes. This depends on both the concentration of drug in the inspired air and the rate of drug delivery, that is the rate and depth of inspiration. Lung conditions such as emphysema, which result in poor alveolar ventilation, will slow the induction of anaesthesia; premedication with drugs that depress respiratory rate (e.g. opioid analgesics) can increase the duration of induction.
2. The rate at which the concentration of drug in the blood reaches equilibrium with that in the inspired air. An important factor in this context is the solubility of the anaesthetic in blood and rapidly equilibrating tissues which include the brain. A high solubility in blood will be associated with a slow attainment of equilibrium. Anaesthesia could be achieved more rapidly if the concentration inhaled during induction is higher than the maintenance concentration, since this would be equivalent to a loading dose (see Ch. 2).
3. The cardiac output, which will determine circulation time and drug delivery to the brain.
4. The relative concentrations of the drug in the brain and blood at equilibrium, which depends on the partition coefficient. The rate of entry of drug into the brain is not limiting because for lipid-soluble drugs, which are relatively insoluble in blood, the brain is part of the rapidly equilibrating central compartment. The rate-limiting step is the rate of delivery via the inhaled gas compared with the total amount in the body at equilibrium. The time to onset of anaesthesia, and maintenance concentrations for a range of anaesthetic compounds, are given in Table 17.2. This table also contains data on partition coefficients.

The blood:gas partition coefficient. This indicates the relative solubility of the drug in blood (or water) and air. A high solubility in water, and therefore all rapidly equilibrating body tissues, means that a greater amount of the agent will need to be administered before the partial pressure of the agent in the blood equilibrates with that in the inspired air. Diethyl ether, although no longer available, has been included in Table 17.2 since this illustrates well the relationship between a high blood:air partition coefficient and a long induction period. (Note: the data in Table 17.2 conform to the basic pharmacokinetic principle that compounds with a large apparent volume of distribution take longer to reach steady state during a constant rate of drug input.)

The oil:gas partition coefficient. This reflects the ratio between the concentration in the lipid membranes of brain cells and the inhaled concentration. Since all anaesthetic agents must achieve approximately the same concentration in the membrane lipids of CNS neurons for effective anaesthesia, the higher the partition coefficient then the lower will be the inhaled concentration of gas required to maintain anaesthesia. This is well illustrated by the data in Table 17.2. Nitrous oxide is of such low potency that surgical anaesthesia could only be achieved with an inspired concentration of drug that would not allow an adequate inspired oxygen concentration. However, nitrous oxide has the advantage of producing analgesia (unlike the other inhalational anaesthetics) and is often used in combination with other anaesthetics, thus reducing the required dose of the other agent. Nitrous oxide can be used as the sole inhalational agent when combined with an intravenous opioid and a neuromuscular junction blocking agent (Ch. 27). Sevoflurane is widely used for children since it has a pleasant odour, an advantage when using it for induction. Recovery is rapid as it is eliminated more quickly than halothane or isoflurane.

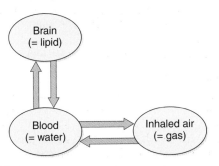

Fig. 17.3
Equilibration of inhaled general anaesthetics between air, blood and brain. The concentration in ratio between blood and air at equilibrium is estimated from in vivo studies of the blood:gas partition coefficient (Table 17.2). The concentrations in brain and blood at equilibrium reflect the different affinities of the two media for general anaesthetics. The brain:blood ratio is 1–3:1 for all commonly used anaesthetics. The concentration in the inspired air required to give the necessary concentration in brain membranes (minimum alveolar concentration; MAC) is an indication of the potency of the compound.

Pharmacokinetics

The major route of elimination of inhaled anaesthetics is via the airways. Factors that influence the duration of the induction phase, such as ventilation rate and the blood:gas partition coefficient, will also affect the time taken to eliminate the anaesthetic and thus the recovery phase. The recovery time may also depend on the duration of inhalation, which can affect the extent to which the drug enters slowly equilibrating tissues. Elimination from these tissues can maintain the plasma concentration of the drug and delay recovery. During recovery, the depth of anaesthesia reverses through the stages discussed above to consciousness; a rapid recovery which minimises stage II is beneficial. Comparing the data in Table 17.2, it is hardly surprising that diethyl ether is no longer used.

General anaesthetics are also partly eliminated by metabolism, the extent of which depends on the time that the agent is retained in the body and available to the metabolising enzymes. Thus exhalation and metabolism can be regarded as alternative pathways of elimination, the use of which is determined largely by the volatility of the agent and its blood:gas partition coefficient (see Table 17.2).

Unwanted effects

A number of unwanted effects are common to most clinically useful inhaled anaesthetics; however each agent also shows a unique profile of additional unwanted effects.

Cardiovascular system. Most agents are negatively inotropic and depress myocardial contractility by interfering with transmembrane calcium flux. This decreases cardiac output and blood pressure and is a particular problem with halothane. Halothane also sensitises the heart to catecholamines, which can lead to arrhythmias. Nitrous oxide has less depressant effect on the heart and circulation and its use in combination with other agents may permit reduction in their dosage and, therefore, their depressant effect on the heart. Inhaled anaesthetics often increase cerebral blood flow, which can exacerbate an elevated intracranial pressure.

Respiratory system. All agents depress the response of the respiratory centre in the medulla to carbon dioxide and hypoxia. They also decrease tidal volume and increase respiratory rate. Some agents, e.g. isoflurane, are irritant and can cause coughing and laryngospasm during inhalation.

Liver. Most agents decrease liver blood flow. Mild hepatic dysfunction because of specific hepatic toxicity is common after treatment with halothane. However, about 1 in 30 000 patients develop severe hepatic necrosis following the use of halothane especially after repeat exposure. This is because of interaction of reactive metabolites with cellular proteins, which initiates an autoimmune reaction. Obese patients, and those who become hypoxic during anaesthesia, appear to be at greatest risk of this complication. This toxic effect has resulted in the decreased use of halothane in adults, although the problem has not been reported in children.

Kidney. Both renal blood flow and renal vascular resistance decrease, resulting in a reduced glomerular filtration rate.

Uterus. There is relaxation of the uterus, which may increase risk of haemorrhage if used in labour. Nitrous oxide has little effect on uterine muscle compared with the other agents.

Skeletal muscle. Most agents produce some muscle relaxation which enhances the activity of neuromuscular blocking drugs (Ch. 27). With sevoflurane, this may be sufficient to enable tracheal intubation without the use of a neuromuscular blocker.

Chemoreceptor trigger zone. Inhalational anaesthetics trigger postoperative nausea and vomiting. This may be most pronounced with nitrous oxide.

FURTHER READING

Dodds C (1999) General anaesthesia: Practical recommendations and recent advances. *Drugs* 58, 453–467

Fox AJ, Rowbottam DJ (1999) Anaesthesia. *Br Med J* 319, 557–560

Wiklund RA, Rosenbaum SH (1997) Anaesthesiology Parts I and II. *N Engl J Med* 337, 1132–41, 1215–1219

Self-assessment

In questions 1–6, the initial statement, in italic, is true. Are the accompanying statements also true?

1. *The minimum alveolar concentration of an inhalation anaesthetic required to produce surgical anaesthesia correlates with the oil:gas partition coefficient of drug.*

   a. Inhalation anaesthetics have their effect by interacting with specific receptors in neurons.
   b. Inhalation anaesthetics are all gases.
   c. Most inhalation anaesthetics are sulphated compounds.

2. *Properties of an ideal inhalation anaesthetic are that it is stable, non-flammable, potent, low lipid solubility, non-irritant, non-toxic and does not sensitise the heart to catecholamines.*

   a. Halothane closely approaches the properties of an ideal inhalation anaesthetic.
   b. The risk of hangover effects with inhalation anaesthetics increases if the operation is long.
   c. Nitrous oxide, when administered alone, reaches the minimum alveolar concentration necessary for surgical anaesthesia if its concentration in inspired air is 50%.
   d. Nitrous oxide is frequently given with oxygen and a fluorinated anaesthetic agent to produce effective surgical anaesthesia.

3. *Isoflurane is now the most widely used volatile anaesthetic.*
   Isoflurane is metabolised by the same pathway as halothane.

4. *The short duration of action of thiopental is due to its redistribution into richly perfused tissues such as muscles.*

   a. The elimination half-life of thiopental is similar to the distribution half-life.
   b. Propofol cannot be given as a continuous infusion for intravenous anaesthesia.
   c. Accidental injection of thiopental into an artery can have serious consequences.
   d. Ketamine is sedative but is without analgesic action.

5. *Fentanyl is a lipid-soluble opioid analgesic*
   Fentanyl should not be administered concurrently with inhalation anaesthetics.

6. *Because of the rapid activity of modern anaesthetics, the individual well-defined stages of anaesthesia are not clearly seen.*

   a. When administering an inhalational anaesthetic, the excitement stage of anaesthesia is prolonged if an intravenous anaesthetic is not given beforehand.
   b. Most inhalational anaesthetics have a depressant effect on the cardiovascular system.
   c. Inhalational anaesthetics reduce the sensitivity of the respiratory centre to carbon dioxide and hypoxia.
   d. Sevoflurane has the advantage of a fast onset of action and eliminaton.

7. Case history question

   A 40-year-old lady is scheduled for a laparotomy because of an abdominal swelling. She has not had a previous operation and is otherwise healthy with normal cardiovascular and respiratory function. The patient was premedicated with pethidine (meperidine) and atropine.

   a. Why is atropine used less as preanaesthetic medication nowadays?
   b. Do the muscarinic antagonists atropine and hyoscine have the same properties?

   The patient was intubated after the administration of thiopental, fentanyl and suxamethonium (succinylcholine).

   c. Why has the routine use of suxamethonium to facilitate endotracheal intubation been reduced.

   Following intubation, pancuronium and fentanyl were given and she was ventilated with nitrous oxide, enflurane and oxygen. An ovarian cyst was removed and the operation took 40 min.

   d. Is pancuronium a suitable choice of muscle relaxant? What alternatives are available?

   After the operation, the patient did not breathe spontaneously despite the administration of neostigmine and glycopyrrolate.

   e. What are the possible reasons for the apnoea and how could they be treated?
   f. Would mivacurium (a short duration muscle relaxant) have been a preferable muscle relaxant to use in this patient?
   g. What is the reason for administering glycopyrrolate with neostigmine at the end of the operation?

   The answers are provided on pages 608–610.

General anaesthetics

Drug	Half-life (h)	Elimination	Comment
Intravenous anaesthetics			
Etomidate	2–11	Metabolism	Hydrolysed in liver but not blood and oxidised to inactive products
Ketamine	2–4	Metabolism	Hepatic metabolism to numerous oxidation products
Methohexital	1–2	Metabolism	Hepatic metabolism terminates drug action; clearance limited by liver blood flow
Propofol	0.5–1	Metabolism	Duration of action partly determined by redistribution; rapid glucuronidation in the liver and other tissues contributes to recovery
Thiopental	4–12	Metabolism	Duration of action determined by redistribution; slow oxidation to an inactive product
Intravenous opioids			
Alfentanil	0.7–2	Metabolism	Oxidised in liver by CYP3A4, and conjugation with glucuronic acid
Fentanyl	2–14	Metabolism	Rapid initial uptake by lungs, followed by redistribution and elimination; very variable kinetics; metabolised in the liver
Remifentanil	0.1	Metabolism	Very rapid clearance by blood and tissue esterases (clearance, 3 l min^{-1}); given as an infusion; metabolite inactive
Inhalation anaesthetics			
Desflurane		Exhalation	< 0.1% metabolised by CYP2E1; brain:blood ratio 1.3:1; rapid recovery (minutes) but present in exhaled air for days
Enflurane		Exhalation + metabolism	About 8% metabolised by CYP2E1; brain:blood ratio 1.4:1; rapid recovery; multiple phases in elimination curves with half-lives ranging from 2 min to 34 h owing to uptake and release from tissues
Halothane		Exhalation + metabolism	About 20% metabolised; oxidation by CYP2E1 produces trifluoroacyl chloride, which may be linked to hepatotoxicity; brain:blood ratio 2.9:1; half-lives similar to enflurane
Isoflurane		Exhalation	<0.2% metabolism by CYP2E1; brain:blood ratio 2.6:1; multiple half-lives reported, <1 min to 40 h, requires a five-compartmental mathematical model; rapid recovery during redistribution phases
Sevoflurane		Exhalation + metabolism	About 5% metabolism by CYP2E1; complex elimination kinetics; recovery slower than with desflurane
Nitrous oxide		Exhalation	Rapid recovery owing to low potency and low tissue affinities; brain:blood ratio 1.0:1; may reduce cerebrovascular effects of halothane when used in combination

18

Local anaesthetics

Local anaesthetics are drugs that reversibly block the transmission of pain stimuli locally at their site of administration.

Examples: lidocaine (lignocaine), cocaine, bupivacaine, benzocaine, ropivacaine, tetracaine (amethocaine) prilocaine

Mechanism of action

Local anaesthetics block the nerve transmission of pain by reducing the ion fluxes that are responsible for depolarisation of excitable cells, particularly the very rapid influx of Na^+ as well as the slower efflux of K^+. Because local anaesthetics act by such a ubiquitous mechanism, they inhibit both afferent and efferent pathways as well as neuroeffector systems such as the neuromuscular junction. The effect is most rapid and intense on small diameter and/or myelinated fibres such as pain afferents and these fibres also show the greatest duration of effect. This gradation of sensitivity is probably related to the ease of entry of the compound into the neuron based on its surface area/volume relationship. Therefore, pain pathways are considerably more sensitive to blockade by local anaesthetics than the larger fibres involved in touch or pressure (Table 18.1). Local anaesthesia is produced by a variety of different mechanisms inhibiting nerve transmission.

Non-specific membrane effects. Local anaesthesia can be produced by a wide range of compounds including acidic, basic and neutral molecules. Many drugs used for their action at specific receptors, for example atropine and propranolol, also have potent local anaesthetic activity. The structural requirements for local anaesthetic activity appear to involve a minimum of a lipid-soluble centre and an ester or amide bond (Fig. 18.1).

Specific intraneuronal receptor activity. The principal site of action of local anaesthetics is the inner sites on the Na^+ channel and the drug must be in a lipid-soluble form to penetrate the nerve and reach its site of action. As most local anaesthetics are weak bases, the drug is in its least ionised and most lipid-soluble form at high pH. However, it is the ionised form of the drug that binds to

Table 18.1
Nerve fibres and their responsiveness to local anaesthetics

Fibre type	Site	Myelination	Diameter (μm)	Sensitivity to anaesthesia[a]
A				
Alpha	Motor	+	12–20	+
Beta	Touch, pressure	+	5–12	+
Gamma	Muscle spindle	+	3–6	++
Delta	Pain, temperature	+	2–5	+++
B	Preganglionic			
	Autonomic	(+)	1–3	+++
C	Dorsal horn	–	0.4–1.2	+++
	Postganglionic	–	0.3–1.3	+++

[a]Increasing number of + indicate increasing sensitivity to local anaesthesia.

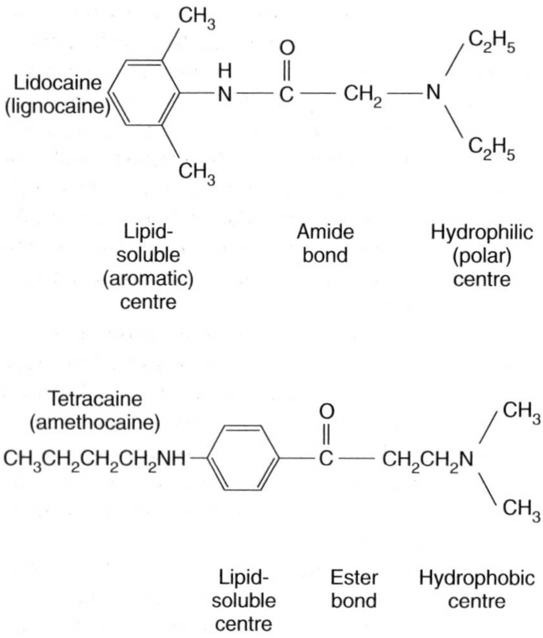

Lidocaine (lignocaine)

Lipid-soluble (aromatic) centre   Amide bond   Hydrophilic (polar) centre

Tetracaine (amethocaine)

Lipid-soluble centre   Ester bond   Hydrophobic centre

Fig. 18.1
General structure of local anaesthetics. Differences in structure alter the speed of onset, duration of action and the metabolism of the drugs (see the drug compendium table).

the Na^+ channel. The general form of most local anaesthetics is shown in Figure 18.1. Variation to the structures of the aromatic and polar centres alters the onset and duration of action and penetrability. Their effectiveness is dependent on the frequency of firing of the neuron. The open Na^+ channel has a much higher affinity for local anaesthetics and is blocked more readily than the resting channel. These observations have given rise to the concept that the ionised (protonated) form of the local anaesthetic binds to an intracellular 'receptor' which is accessible when the channel is open (Fig. 18.2). Once the local anaesthetic has bound to the channel, the influx of Na^+ is blocked but the channel remains inactivated. It only slowly reverts to the resting state with consequent loss of local anaesthetic binding. This mechanism of action results in faster onset of local anaesthesia in rapidly firing neurons.

Pharmacokinetics

The duration of action of local anaesthetics is dependent on their rate of removal from the site of administration rather than their systemic elimination by metabolism. Therefore, the duration of action as well as potency of local anaesthetics is proportional to their lipid solubility: the larger, lipid-soluble drugs such as bupivacaine have a longer duration of action than smaller molecules such as lidocaine.

The duration of action is also affected by the extent of vasodilation locally at the site of administration. Cocaine (which has restricted medical use) blocks noradrenaline reuptake (uptake 1; Ch. 4) by noradrenergic neurons, produces vasoconstriction and has a longer duration of action than would be expected given its polarity.

The duration of action of any local anaesthetic can be extended considerably by co-administration of a vasoconstrictor such as an α_1-adrenoceptor agonist, for example epinephrine (adrenaline). There are numerous local anaesthetic preparations available as combinations of a local anaesthetic and a vasoconstrictor.

Once the local anaesthetic has diffused away from the site of administration it enters the general circulation and undergoes elimination from the body. Because local anaesthetics are lipid-soluble molecules they are eliminated by metabolism, mainly in the liver, which frequently involves the hydrolysis of the central amide bond. The half-life within the circulation is generally short (between 1 and 3 h).

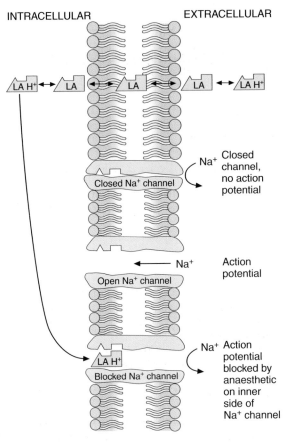

INTRACELLULAR   EXTRACELLULAR

Na⁺ Closed channel, no action potential

Closed Na⁺ channel

Na⁺ Action potential

Open Na⁺ channel

Na⁺ Action potential blocked by anaesthetic on inner side of Na⁺ channel

Blocked Na⁺ channel

Fig. 18.2
Site and mechanism of action of local anaesthetics. Weakly basic local anaesthetics exist as an equilibrium between ionised (LAH⁺) and unionised (LA) forms. The ionised form binds to the intracellular receptor and the unionised form is lipid soluble and crosses the axonal membrane. Local anaesthesia may also result from incorporation of the compound into a ring of lipid around the Na⁺ channel, which becomes rigid and cannot open.

Unwanted effects

Local effects. These occur at the site of administration and include irritation and inflammation. Local hypoxia can occur if they are co-administered with a vasoconstrictor, therefore this should be avoided in the extremities of digits. Tissue damage/necrosis can follow inappropriate administration (e.g. accidental intra-arterial administration or spinal administration of an epidural dose).

Systemic effects. These are related to the local anaesthetic action. High systemic doses can affect other excitable membranes such as the heart (see antiarrhythmic action of lidocaine; Ch. 8). Excessive amounts can cause cardiovascular collapse owing to systemic vasodilation and a negative inotropic effect. Cardiotoxicity with serious arrhythmias is a particular problem with bupivicaine and is caused by its avid tissue binding in the heart. This problem has been reduced by the intro-

duction of ropivacaine, the less cardiotoxic (*S*)-isomer of bupivacaine. The cardiotoxic actions of bupivacaine reside in its *R*(+) isomer. Ropivacaine also has vasoconstrictor activity. In the central nervous system (CNS) local anaesthetics can produce sedation and loss of consciousness. Metabolites of lidocaine can cause generalised excitation and convulsions. Because of its pronounced CNS effects (see Ch. 54), cocaine has restricted use as a local anaesthetic. For more details of individual local anaesthetics see the drug compendium table.

Techniques of administration

The extent of local anaesthesia depends largely on the technique of administration.

Surface administration. High concentrations (up to 10%) of drug in an oily vehicle can slowly penetrate the skin to give a small localised area of anaesthesia. The same effect can be produced more efficiently by infiltration anaesthesia. Benzocaine is a relatively non-polar local anaesthetic that produces useful anaesthesia of mucous membranes such as the throat and is included in some throat pastilles. Cocaine is restricted to ophthalmological procedures (where it combines anaesthesia with mydriasis as a result of the inhibition of reuptake of noradrenaline by sympathetic nerve terminals) and for nasal surgery (to produce vasoconstriction and reduce mucosal bleeding).

Infiltration anaesthesia. A local injection of an aqueous solution of a water-soluble salt of the base (such as the hydrochloride), sometimes used with a vasoconstrictor, produces a local field of anaesthesia.

Nerve trunk block anaesthesia. Injection of an aqueous solution similar to that described above around a nerve trunk to produce a field of anaesthesia distal to the site of injection.

Epidural anaesthesia. Injection or slow infusion of an aqueous solution adjacent to the spinal column but outside the dura mater produces anaesthesia both above and below the site of injection. The extent of anaesthesia depends on the volume of anaesthetic administered. This technique is used extensively in obstetrics. The concentration of drug used is the same as that for spinal anaesthesia but the volume and, therefore, the dose is greater.

Spinal anaesthesia. This involves injection of an aqueous solution into the lumbar subarachnoid space, usually between the third and fourth lumbar vertebrae. The spread of anaesthetic within the subarachnoid space depends on the density of the solution (a solution in 10% glucose is more dense than cerebrospinal fluid) and the posture of the patient during the first 10–15 min while the solution flows up or down the subarachnoid space. Sympathetic fibres are particularly sensitive to local anaesthetics and this can result in cardiovascular complications, particularly hypotension.

FURTHER READING

Foster RH, Markham A (2000) Levobupivacaine: a review of its pharmacology and use as a local anaesthetic. *Drugs* 59, 551–579

French RJ, Zamponi GW, Sierralta IE (1998) Molecular and kinetic determinants of local anaesthetic action on sodium channels. *Toxicol Lett* 100/101, 247–254

McClellan KJ, Spencer CM (1998) Levobupivacaine. *Drugs* 56, 355–362

Wiklund RA, Rosenbaum SH (1997) Anaesthesiology Part II. *N Engl J Med* 337, 1215–1219

Self-assessment

In the following questions, the first statement, in italics, is true. Are the accompanying statements true or false?

1. *Local anaesthetics exhibit use dependence. The block is more rapid and complete when the nerve is actively firing. This is because local anaesthetics bind more readily to open Na⁺ channels.*

   a. Local anaesthetics have no systemic unwanted effects.

   b. The main mechanism by which the effect of local anaesthesia wears off is through liver metabolism of the anaesthetic.

   c. Local anaesthetics block smaller myelinated axons more effectively than large myelinated axons.

   d. The α_1-adrenoceptor blocker prazosin is added to local anaesthetics to extend their duration of activity.

2. *Local anaesthetics must be lipid soluble to penetrate the axon and reach the innerside of the Na⁺ channel before blocking it.*

   a. Ropivacaine is a long-acting local anaesthetic.

   b. $S(+)$-bupivacaine (levobupivacaine; ropivacaine) exhibits greater cardiotoxicity than its enantiomer $R(+)$-bupivacaine.

The answers are provided on page 610.

Self-assessment questions

Local anaesthetics[a]

Drug	Half-life (h)	Elimination	Comment
Bupivacaine	1–3	Metabolism (+ renal)	Used for local infiltration, peripheral nerve block, epidural block and sympathetic block; slow onset of action (30 min); metabolised mainly by N-dealkylation and hydroxylation; less than 10% is excreted in urine (see ropivacaine)
Ropivacaine	2	Metabolism	Used for epidural, major nerve block and field block; metabolised by hepatic CYP1A2 and CYP3A4 isoenzymes; ropivacaine is the (S)-isomer form of bupivacaine (racemic) and has less cardiotoxicity
Lidocaine (lignocaine)	1.5	Metabolism	Used for local infiltration, intravenous regional anaesthesia and nerve blocks and dental anaesthesia; also used topically; metabolised by dealkylation, catalysed by CYP3A4, followed by hydrolysis
Prilocaine	1–2	Metabolism	Used for local infiltration anaesthesia, intravenous anaesthesia, nerve blocks and dental anaesthesia; may cause methaemoglobinaemia (especially in infants); metabolised mainly by amide hydrolysis in the liver
Procaine	Not relevant	Metabolism	Seldom used now; local infiltration anaesthesia; very rapid ester hydrolysis at site of injection; any which escaped into the blood would be rapidly hydrolysed by plasma esterases with a half-life of less than 1 min
Tetracaine (amethocaine)	Not relevant	Metabolism	Mostly used topically; poorly absorbed; hydrolysed by plasma pseudocholinesterase
Articaine	1	Metabolism	Used in dentistry; concentrations in tooth alveolus are 100 times those in circulation; half-life data are from patients treated to produce regional anaesthesia; hydrolysed to inactive articainic acid by serum esterases
Mepivacaine	2–3		Used in dentistry; metabolised in liver by N-dealkylation and hydroxylation
Benzocaine	Not relevant	Metabolism	Used in throat lozenges; minimal absorption; metabolised in liver

[a]All are given by injection apart from benzocaine.

19 Opioid analgesics and the management of pain

Pain and pain perception

Pain is a complex phenomenon that involves both the generation of specific neuronal activity and the response of the patient to that activity. Stimuli that produce tissue damage initiate activity in the nervous system, which is called nociception. Similar neuronal activity can also be generated by damage to, or functional change in, the neural pathways (neuropathic mechanisms). Pain is the subjective sensation that results from the perception of these impulses. The response of the individual to the painful stimulus will be influenced by psychological factors; this will determine whether or not the pain produces or contributes to suffering or distress (Fig. 19.1).

Nociceptive pain can arise from somatic or visceral structures. Somatic pain is typically aching, stabbing, throbbing or pressure-like. Visceral pain is gnawing or cramp-like if it arises from a hollow viscus, or similar to somatic pain when arising from other structures. Sharp pain stimuli are transmitted to the central nervous system (CNS) by fast fibres in the neospinothalamic pathway; chronic visceral pain is transmitted by slow fibres in the paleospinothalamic pathway (Fig. 19.2).

Non-steroidal anti-inflammatory drugs (NSAIDs) (Ch. 29) and opioids are the major classes of pain-relieving (analgesic) drug. They act at different levels in the pain-transmitting pathways to influence the production and recognition of pain as indicated in Figure 19.3. Neuropathic pain responds poorly to both classes of analgesic.

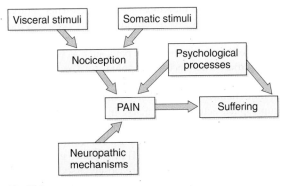

Fig. 19.1
The origin of pain and suffering.

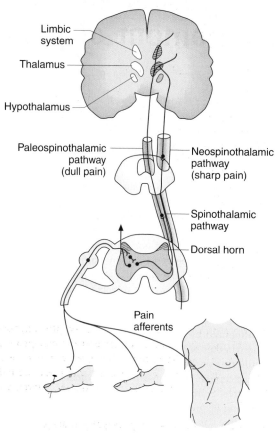

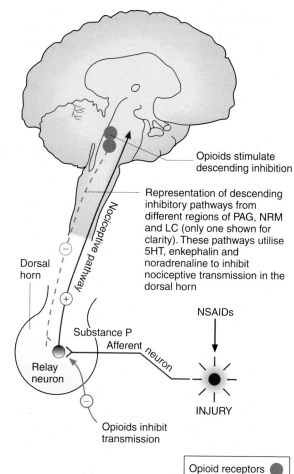

Fig. 19.2
Pathways of pain perception. Shaded areas are rich in opioid receptors Opiod receptors are also found in medullary areas and the spinal cord. This shows in simplified form the pathways activated following stimulation of peripheral nociceptive nerve terminals. Many mediators are involved during afferent stimulation of the nociceptive pathway. Mediator release (bradykinin, 5-hydroxytryptamine, prostaglandins) stimulates the nerve terminals of pain fibres. Onward afferent transmission of ascending nerve impulses at the synapses in the dorsal horn involves neuropeptides such as substance P. Hyperexcitability of pain fibres can also be promoted by other mediators. The ascending pathways innervate areas of the midbrain and thalamus.

Fig. 19.3
Transmitters and receptors for pain perception. The nociceptive pathways use a variety of transmitter substances and promoters of transmission in neurones, substance P, other neuropeptides and nitric oxide all appear to be involved. The afferent pathways are subject to inhibitory control. Opioids act at opioid receptor-rich sites in the periaqueductal grey matter (PAG), the raphe magnus nucleus (NMR) and other spinal sites to stimulate descending inhibitory fibres that inhibit nociceptive transmission in the dorsal horn. Descending pathways from the locus ceruleus (LC) that are noradrenergic are also involved. Opioids also act directly in the dorsal horn to inhibit transmission. The inhibitory pathways associated with 5-hydroxytryptamine (5HT) and noradrenergic neurons may also explain the analgesic properties of antidepressants and anticonvulsants in certain types of pain. NSAIDs, non-steroidal anti-inflammatory drugs.

Non-steroidal anti-inflammatory drugs. These act mainly by blocking the generation of the original nociceptive impulses and are most effective against peripheral pain of musculoskeletal origins. They inhibit the production of prostaglandins thereby reducing the sensitivity of nerve endings to agents released by damaged tissue which initiate pain, such as bradykinin.

Opioids. These act in the spinal cord, especially in the dorsal horn pathways associated with the paleo-spinothalamic pathway, and also have important supraspinal actions particularly in the periaqueductal grey matter, the nucleus reticularis paragigantocellularis and raphe magnus nucleus. The contribution of peripheral actions is smaller. They produce their effects via specific receptors which are closely associated with the neuronal pathways that transmit pain from the periphery to the CNS.

Opioid analgesics

Examples: morphine, diamorphine (heroin), buprenorphine, pethidine, codeine, pentazocine, fentanyl

Opioid is a term used for both naturally occurring and synthetic molecules that produce their effects by combining with opioid receptors. Use of the term opiate analgesics (specifically drugs derived from the juice of the opium poppy, *Papaver somniferum*) or narcotic analgesics (which literally means a 'stupor-inducing pain killer') is no longer preferred.

Mechanism of action

The brain produces several neuropeptides known as endorphins ('endogenous morphine'), which act as neurotransmitters via specific opioid receptors. Among the endorphins are the pentapeptide enkephalins: these contain the amino acid sequence Tyr-Gly-Gly-Phe linked to either leucine or methionine and are called leu- and met-enkephalin. Endorphins are formed from larger precursor peptides. It is possible that the most important peptide neurotransmitter in this family is β-endorphin, a peptide consisting of 31 amino acid residues with met-enkephalin at its carboxyl end; this is extremely potent. It is uncertain whether met-enkephalin is a breakdown product of β-endorphin that retains partial activity or is a major neurotransmitter in its own right. Recent studies support the latter possibility.

There is a distinctive regional distribution of enkephalins in the CNS with high concentrations in the limbic system and spinal cord, a distribution similar to that for opioid receptors. These regions also contain high concentrations of a neutral endopeptidase (enkephalinase), which rapidly hydrolyses the pentapeptides into fragments (i.e. analogous to acetylcholine and acetylcholinesterase; Ch. 4). Opioid receptors are found on the presynaptic membrane of neurons in the main pain pathways of the CNS; they have also been identified in the peripheral nervous system.

Morphine and related analgesics produce their effects by acting at specific opioid receptors in the CNS. Three major classes of opioid receptor have been identified, which mediate distinct effects (Box 19.1). Each of these receptors has subtypes (μ_1 and μ_2; κ_1, κ_2 and κ_3; δ_1 and δ_2) that have different distributions; for example μ_1, κ_3 and δ_2 are mainly supraspinal while μ_2, κ_1 and δ_1 are mainly found in the spinal cord. Opioid receptors are coupled to inhibitory G-proteins; stimulation reduces the intracellular generation of cAMP by adenylate cyclase. The G-proteins are also directly coupled to K^+ channels. When these channels are opened by an opioid, neurons in the pain pathways become hyperpolarised. Consequent inhibition of voltage-gated Ca^{2+} channels in the presynaptic neurons reduces neurotransmitter release. In the periaqueductal grey matter, supraspinal analgesia is achieved by enhanced descending neuronal activity. At the spinal level analgesia probably results from inhibition of the release of substance P from dorsal afferent neurons.

The various endogenous opioid peptides show preferential receptor-binding affinities, for example

> **Box 19.1**
>
> **Effects of opioid receptors**
>
> Mu (μ)
>   Analgesia (supraspinal μ_1, spinal μ_2)
>   Respiratory (μ_2)
>   Euphoria
>   Miosis
>   Physical dependence
>   Sedation
> Kappa (κ)
>   Analgesia (spinal)
>   Sedation
>   Miosis
>   Dysphoria
> Delta (δ)
>   Analgesia (spinal)
>   Respiratory depression

β-endorphin binds mainly to μ- and δ-receptors, dynorphin binds mainly to κ-receptors and the enkephalins binds mainly to δ-receptors. Therapeutic agents also show receptor selectivity. While many are pure opioid receptor agonists, others have a different pharmacological profile.

- Pure agonists: these act principally at the μ-receptors and include morphine, diamorphine, pethidine (meperidine), codeine and dextropropoxyphene. The drugs also have variable agonist activity at δ- and κ-receptors.
- Mixed agonist–antagonist: pentazocine has partial agonist effects at the κ-receptor and is a weak μ-antagonist.
- Partial agonist: buprenorphine is a partial agonist at the μ-receptor and has antagonist activity at K opioid receptors.
- Opioids with additional properties; for example meptazinol is a μ_1-receptor agonist with muscarinic receptor agonist activity, while tramadol is a μ-receptor agonist that also inhibits neuronal noradrenaline and 5-hydroxytryptamine (5HT) re-uptake. Enhanced amine-mediated neurotransmission may potentiate descending inhibitory pain pathways.

Clinical uses and side-effects

Analgesia. The paleospinothalamic pathway and limbic system are rich in opioid receptors, therefore, the analgesia produced by morphine is most effective for chronic visceral pain. In addition to its antinociceptive effect, morphine alters the patient's perception of the pain making it less unpleasant. Opioids have no anti-inflammatory effect and morphine can even release the inflammatory mediator histamine locally at the site of an injection. Analgesia produced by morphine is often associated with an elevated sense of well being (euphoria, mediated by μ-receptors) whereas opioid administration to a pain-free subject can produce the opposite effect (dysphoria, mediated by κ-receptors). Pure μ-receptor agonists are the most powerful opioid analgesics. However, some pure μ-receptor agonists are only useful for moderate pain either because the affinity of the drug for the receptor is low (e.g. dextropropoxyphene) or because unwanted effects prevent the use of high doses (e.g. codeine). The ceiling effect of partial agonists is lower. If a person receiving high doses of a potent pure μ-receptor antagonist is given a μ-receptor partial agonist (e.g. buprenorphine) or a μ-receptor partial antagonist (e.g. pentazocine) then some of the pure agonist molecules will be displaced from receptor

sites by the less effective molecules, and the level of analgesia may be reduced (Table 19.1). In dependent patients, withdrawal symptoms can be produced (see below).

Respiratory depression. The sensitivity of the respiratory centre to stimulation by carbon dioxide is reduced by morphine, which decreases respiratory drive. Respiratory paralysis is a common cause of death in opioid overdose. Occasionally, the effect on respiratory rate can be of clinical benefit, for example, when intravenous morphine relieves the dyspnoea associated with acute pulmonary oedema by lowering central respiratory drive and reducing the associated stress and anxiety. Meptazinol and tramadol are claimed to cause less respiratory depression because of their selectivity for μ-receptors. Meptazinol is being used for obstetric analgesia because of this.

Suppression of the cough centre. Opioids possess a useful antitussive action although the mechanism is

Table 19.1
Opiate analgesics

Compound	Analgesic potency	Tolerance and dependence	Clinical uses and comment
Morphine	+++	+++	See text
Diamorphine (heroin)	++++	++++	Clinical uses restricted because of high abuse potential; given orally or by infusion for the pain of terminal cancer; given for acute severe pain, e.g. myocardial infarction
Buprenorphine	++++	++	Used as an alternative to morphine for analgesia, but nausea may limit its tolerability; a partial agonist at μ opioid receptors
Codeine	+	+	See text; also used when the non-analgesic effects such as antitussive or antidiarrhoeal actions are needed; produces little respiratory depression
Pethidine	++	+	Not useful for antitussive or antidiarrhoeal effects
Pentazocine	+++	++ (but not cross-tolerance to morphine)	See text; will provoke a withdrawal syndrome in a morphine-dependent subject because of weak antagonist or partial agonist action on μ-receptors
Methadone	+++	++	Major use is for withdrawal from morphine/heroin dependence
Dextropropoxyphene	(+)	+	Widely used for mild analgesia (usually in combination with paracetamol as coproxamol despite its low therapeutic index; reports of fatalities with overdose, especially when taken with alcohol)
Fentanyl	++	+	Increasingly used by transdermal patch for intractable pain; intravenous adjunct in anaesthesia
Tramadol	+	+	Obstetric analgesia; less potential for respiratory depression; WHO classified step II agent. It is also a monoamine reuptake blocker
Meptazinol	+	–	Behaves as a mixed agonist/antagonist and lacks withdrawal and dependence symptoms

Increasing + signs indicate increasing effect.

unclear. Compounds such as codeine and dextro-methorphan are highly effective for cough suppression despite having relatively weak analgesic effects (Ch. 13).

Sleep. Opioids are not hypnotics, but often the relief of pain is associated with relaxation so that sleep is an indirect consequence of opioid administration.

CNS excitation

Vomiting. Opioids stimulate the chemoreceptor trigger zone (Ch. 32). Emesis is more common in ambulatory patients, but tolerance can occur.

Miosis. Stimulation of the third nerve nucleus results in pupillary constriction. Pinpoint pupils, together with coma and slow respiration, are signs of opioid overdose (Ch. 53).

Peripheral effects

Gastrointestinal tract. There is a general increase in resting tone of the gut wall and sphincters, but a decrease in propulsive activity. Thus opioid administration is associated with constipation and opioids are useful in the treatment of diarrhoea (Ch. 35). An increase in biliary pressure caused by spasm at the sphincter of Oddi can exacerbate biliary colic (especially at low doses). Pethidine has less activity in the gastrointestinal tract than equi-analgesic doses of morphine. The effects of morphine on the gut are largely a result of hyperpolarisation of cells in the myenteric plexus, but there is some additional central action.

Cardiovascular and respiratory systems. Opioids have limited effects on the circulation and lungs; hypotension and bronchoconstriction can occur with morphine, possibly because of histamine release.

Other systems. Opioids have minor effects on other systems, for example there is an increase in tone of the bladder wall and sphincter, which can lead to urinary retention. Changes in the release of some pituitary hormones may be mediated via interference with the actions of opioid peptide hormones.

Tolerance and dependence

Tolerance and dependence are inter-related phenomena probably resulting from changes in the functioning of opioid receptors during continuous opioid administration. In response to the inhibitory effects of morphine on intracellular cAMP generation, there is increased synthesis of stimulatory G-proteins and adenylate cyclase in an attempt to restore homeostasis. As a consequence of these adaptive changes, more drug is necessary to produce the same effect (tolerance) and withdrawal of the drug produces adverse physiological effects until the compensatory changes are reset (dependence).

Tolerance is associated with increased firing of neurons in the noradrenergic pathways of the locus ceruleus which is rich in inhibitory opioid receptors. Dependence may be in part caused by effects on opioid neurons radiating from this region to the ventral tegmental area. The dopaminergic pathway projecting from the ventral tegmental area to the nucleus accumbens is believed to be involved in the euphoria of opioid administration.

Tolerance occurs rapidly during chronic opioid administration, despite constant plasma drug concentrations. Tolerance develops to analgesia, euphoria, respiratory depression and emesis but much less to the constipatory effects or miosis. A high degree of cross-tolerance is shown by many opioids; consequently, individuals who develop tolerance to one opioid will usually be tolerant to another. However, not all opioids show cross-tolerance. The non-uniform nature of tolerance and cross-tolerance may be a result of the multiplicity of opioid receptors.

Dependence manifests itself as a withdrawal syndrome, which can be precipitated when patients who are taking long-term opioid therapy (or individuals who are abusing the drug) have their intake stopped or are given an opioid antagonist or partial agonist. The withdrawal effects during the first 12 h, such as nervousness, sweating and craving, are largely psychological since they can be alleviated by the administration of a placebo. Following this period the effects of physiological dependence manifest themselves, for example dilated pupils, anorexia, weakness, depression, insomnia, gastrointestinal and skeletal muscle cramps, increased respiratory rate, pyrexia, piloerection with goose-pimples and diarrhoea. The time course for the development and loss of these symptoms varies among the opioids. In the case of morphine, the maximum withdrawal effects occur quickly (about 1–2 days) and subside rapidly (about 5–10 days) but the intensity of the symptoms may be intolerable. In contrast, withdrawal from methadone is a slow process because of its very long half-life, but the effects are far less intense (peak effect at almost 1 week and symptoms persist for about 3 weeks). Therefore, morphine- or heroin-dependent subjects are often transferred from their drug of abuse to methadone prior to withdrawal. Methadone also produces less euphoria than morphine or heroin. After a period of chronic treatment with methadone, the methadone dosage is gradually reduced and the person undergoes a more tolerable withdrawal.

Pharmacokinetics of individual agents

The pharmacokinetic properties of individual opioid analgesics are summarised in the drug compendium table. Opioids can be given by intravenous or intramuscular injection, by subcutaneous infusion, or orally. Morphine can also be given as a suppository, while buprenorphine is formulated for buccal absorption. Other opioids such as fentanyl or tramadol can be delivered transdermally for prolonged analgesia. Some opioids (e.g. morphine) show a low and variable absorption from the gut so that they are usually given by injection for treatment of acute pain, for example postoperative pain. Oral treatment with larger doses of an opioid such as morphine is mainly used to establish adequate control of severe chronic pain. Because of the short half-life of morphine, a modified-release formulation is often used to prolong the duration of action when it is given for long-term pain control. Fentanyl has a short half-life, but its effects persist for several hours after removing the transdermal patch owing to build up of a subcutaneous drug reservoir. Short acting opioids such as fentanyl are also used as analgesic supplements in anaesthesia. This use is considered in Chapter 17.

Unwanted effects

The unwanted effects of opioids are caused by their actions on those opioid receptors that are not the primary site for therapeutic benefit. For example, respiratory depression and constipation are unwanted effects when an opioid is used as an analgesic. Tolerance and dependence can also be regarded as unwanted problems associated with chronic use. However, concerns about tolerance and dependence should not inhibit the administration of adequate analgesia for patients with severe chronic pain, for example the pain experienced by terminally ill patients with cancer.

··

Pain management

Appropriate management of pain depends on its origin and severity. Minor pain can be effectively treated with a peripherally acting analgesic such as paracetamol or aspirin (Ch. 29). If there is an inflammatory component, for example soft tissue injuries, then a drug with combined anti-inflammatory and analgesic properties from the NSAID class (Ch. 29) will be particularly useful. More severe pain may require centrally acting drugs, for example an opioid either alone or in combination with a peripherally acting compound.

Acute pain

Acute pain usually has an obvious cause and is accompanied by anxiety. For rapid pain relief in a self-limiting condition, for example migraine, a readily absorbed, short-acting drug will be appropriate. For more protracted conditions, for example sprains, a long-acting drug may be helpful to improve compliance by reducing the frequency of administration. More severe acute pain can be treated with paracetamol and a weak opioid such as codeine, often in combined formulation such as co-proxamol (paracetamol and dextropropoxyphene) or co-codamol (paracetamol and codeine). Very severe acute pain, for example with myocardial infarction, will require a strong opioid such as morphine. This should be given parenterally for rapid effect. Intramuscular injection should be avoided if possible, since severe pain is often accompanied by sympathetic nervous system stimulation, which produces peripheral vasoconstriction and delays drug absorption.

Chronic pain

Chronic pain (usually defined as pain lasting for 6 months or more) can be a result of chronic nociceptive stimulation or can have a neuropathic origin. Drug therapy is not the only solution for chronic pain. Depending on the cause, non-pharmacological or local treatments are often appropriate. Examples include:

- surgery for neoplastic, structural or ischaemic disorders
- physical methods such as acupuncture, transcutaneous electrical nerve stimulation (which activates spinal inhibitory neurons by counter-irritation), local anaesthetic nerve block
- behavioural modification, for example biofeedback, relaxation techniques, hypnosis.

The principles of drug control of chronic pain are common to many clinical disorders. The concept of the World Health Organization's 'analgesic ladder' is useful for choosing drug therapy appropriate to the level of pain experienced by the patients (Box 19.2).

Step 1 drugs. Paracetamol (Ch. 29) is a simple analgesic, suitable for mild pain. However, if there is local inflammation, an NSAID (Ch. 29) may be more appropriate. Examples of pain that respond better to an NSAID are soft tissues injury, tissue compression, visceral pain caused by pleural or peritoneal irritation and bone pain caused by metastatic deposits (see case notes). Bone metastases cause local secretion of prostaglandins and NSAIDs can be particularly effective. Individual responses to an NSAID vary; about 60% of patients can respond to an alternative drug even if the first was ineffective.

Step 2 drugs. Opioids suitable for mild to moderate pain include codeine, dihydrocodeine and dextropropoxyphene. These are often used in combination with paracetamol, although the dose of opioid in these combinations is sometimes too low to produce additional analgesia. Tramadol has been advocated at this stage, but claims that it has a lesser effect on respiration

---

Box 19.2

The 'analgesic ladder'

Step 1: simple analgesics, e.g. paracetamol, NSAIDs
Step 2: opioid suitable for moderate pain ± simple analgesics
Step 3: opioid suitable for severe pain ± simple analgesics

Adjuvant analgesics may be required at any step (see text).

or gastrointestinal motility have not been shown to be clinically important.

Step 3 drugs. The drug of choice for severe pain is morphine. It is usually effective orally, using a rapid onset formulation for initial pain control. Doctors are often unwilling to give adequate doses of strong opioid because of concern about addiction. In severe chronic pain, especially with terminal illness, this is not a major concern. If the pain remains severe with a low initial dosage of morphine, the dosage should be increased by 50–100% every 24 h; once the pain is moderate in intensity, increments of 25–50% daily are usually sufficient to achieve control without excessive unwanted effects. A modified-release formulation of morphine can be substituted once a stable dosage has been determined, although a rapid-acting formulation may still be required to treat breakthrough pain. Oral administration may not be possible if the patient is vomiting or has dysphagia or intestinal obstruction. In these circumstances, rectal administration or subcutaneous infusion using a syringe driver can be used. For subcutaneous delivery, diamorphine is preferred since it is more soluble than morphine and can be given in a much smaller volume. Diamorphine can also be given by epidural or intrathecal injection for intractable pain. Transdermal delivery of the opioid fentanyl from an adhesive patch is an alternative to modified-release oral morphine.

Adjuvant analgesics. These are a heterogeneous group of drugs that can be used to enhance the effect of a conventional analgesic. Examples include tricyclic antidepressants or antiepileptic drugs for neuropathic pain (see below). Corticosteroids can be helpful for relieving nerve compression, by reducing local inflammation and reducing neuronal excitability. Neuralgic and neuropathic pain responds poorly to conventional analgesia. Examples include trigeminal neuralgia, postherpetic neuralgia and phantom limb pain after an amputation. In addition to spontaneous pain, the area involved may be painful to touch (dysaesthesia), show exaggerated response to normal stimulus (hyperaesthesia) or a painful response to trivial stimuli (allodynia). Tricyclic antidepressants (Ch. 22) can be effective for neuropathic pain and probably inhibit the spinal neurons in the pain pathways by increasing synaptic noradrenaline and 5HT concentrations in the inhibitory pathways (Fig. 19.3). Selective serotonin reuptake inhibitor (SSRI) antidepressants are ineffective for neuropathic pain. Anticonvulsant drugs such as phenytoin, carbamazepine or sodium valproate reduce the lancinating component of neuropathic pain by stabilising neuronal membranes (Ch. 23).

FURTHER READING

Ashburn MA, Staats PS (1999) Management of chronic pain. *Lancet* 353, 1865–1869

Besson JM (1999) The neurobiology of pain. *Lancet* 353, 1610–1615

Carr DB, Goudas LC (1999) Acute pain. *Lancet* 353, 2051–2058

Cherny NI (1996) Opioid analgesics. *Drugs* 51, 713–737

Kost RG, Graus SE (1996) Postherpetic neuralgia – pathogenesis, treatment and prevention. *N Engl J Med* 335, 32–42

Levy MH (1996) Pharmacologic treatment of cancer pain. *N Engl J Med* 335, 11124–11132

McQuay H (1999) Opioids in pain management. *Lancet* 353, 2229–2232

Portenoy RK, Lesage P (1999) Management of cancer pain. *Lancet* 353, 1695–1700

Thürlimann B, de Stoutz ND (1996) Causes and treatment of bone pain of malignant origin. *Drugs* 51, 383–398

Ward J, Hall W, Mattick RP (1999) Role of maintenance treatment in opioid dependence. *Lancet* 353, 221–226

Woolf CJ, Mannion RJ (1999) Neuropathic pain: aetiology, symptoms, mechanisms and management. *Lancet* 353, 1959–1964

Self-assessment

In questions 1–4, the initial statement, in italics, is true. Are the accompanying statements also true?

1. *Opioids are analgesic by acting at the level of the dorsal horn to inhibit transmission in the ascending nociceptive pathway. They also act at the level of the periaqueductal grey matter to stimulate descending inhibitory pathways that further inhibit dorsal horn synaptic transmission.*

   a. Opioids can cause euphoria or dysphoria.
   b. Tolerance develops uniformly to all of the biological effects of the opioids.
   c. Methadone is rapid in onset and has a short half-life.

2. *Concerns about dependence potential should not inhibit the administration of adequate doses of opioids to patients with severe chronic pain.*

   a. Meptazinol is a pure μ-receptor stimulant.
   b. Naloxone is a short-acting opioid agonist.

3. *Opioids are not very effective in treatment neuropathic pain.*

   a. Drugs that inhibit the reuptake of noradrenaline can be effective analgesics in some cases of neuropathic pain.
   b. Anticonvulsants are ineffective in treatment of neuropathic pain.

4. *Pentazocine and buprenophine are partial agonists at opioid receptors and have less abuse liability than morphine.* Pentazocine can precipitate withdrawal symptoms in morphine addicts.

5. Case history questions
   Pain control in terminal cancer. These case notes have been modified from original material written by Martin Church and Richard Hillier at the University of Southampton and gratefully reproduced with their permission. The casenote highlights the pharmacology of analgesic usage and concomitant drugs.

   A 60-year-old man was admitted to a hospice. He had previously had a left nephrectomy because of renal cell carcinoma and now had intense metastatic bone pain in his ankles, right iliac crest and left upper arm. He also has periods of dyspnoea. Prior to admission his medication was the compound analgesic co-proxamol and diclofenac (150 mg) at night. He was also taking cimetidine (400 mg) twice daily. His pain was not well controlled on admission. After a week of assessment and optimisation of drug therapy, his treatment comprised the following drugs:

morphine, slow release (MST)	260 mg	twice daily
morphine, oral solution	50 mg	when required
diclofenac, slow release	150 mg	at night
dexamethasone	2 mg	three times daily
metoclopramide (anti-emetic)	10 mg	three times daily
cimetidine	400 mg	twice daily
docusate sodium (laxative)	100 mg	three times daily
temazepam	20 mg	at night.

   Morphine is the optimum drug of choice for pain control in the vast majority of patients with cancer.

   a. How does morphine exert its pharmacological action as an analgesic?
   b. Why is morphine oral solution (which is an immediate release form) also made available in addition to the slow-release formulation?
   c. Is the addictive potential of morphine likely to present a problem in this patient?
   d. What alternative opioids as an immediate replacement for morphine might you consider?
   e. How does diclofenac control inflammation and inflammatory pain?
   f. Why is diclofenac useful in this patient?
   g. What was the rationale for the use of dexamethasone in this patient?
   h. Metoclopramide is an anti-emetic. Why do you think that this patient is likely to suffer from nausea and possibly vomiting?
   i. How does metoclopramide act to alleviate nausea?
   j. What other drugs could be used to alleviate nausea?
   k. Why may gastric or duodenal ulceration be a problem in this patient?
   l. How may cimetidine reduce the problem of gastric or duodenal ulceration?
   m. Why is constipation likely to be a problem in this patient and what form is it likely to take?
   n. What is the mechanism of action of docusate sodium?
   o. What alternative laxative agents or docusate sodium may be used?
   p. Why is temazepam given?

The answers are provided on pages 610–611.

Opioid analgesics

Drug	Half-life (h)	Elimination	Comments
Alfentanil	0.6–1.2	Metabolism	Used at surgery; given by intravenous injection
Buprenorphine	4–6	Metabolism	Bioavailability sublingual > oral; action only partly reversed by naloxone
Codeine	3–4	Metabolism (+ renal)	Demethylated to morphine (5–15%)
Dextromoramide	6–22	Metabolism	Rapid and complete absorption orally
Dextropropoxyphene	8–24	Metabolism	Undergoes 60% first-pass metabolism
Diamorphine	2–5 min	Hydrolysis	Acetylated prodrug which is hydrolysed to morphine
Dihydrocodeine	3–5	Metabolism	Undergoes extensive first-pass metabolism; role of metabolites in activity is unknown
Diphenoxylate	2–3	Metabolism	Low oral bioavailability owing to incomplete dissolution in gut
Dipipanone	No data available	No data available	Clinical effects suggest good oral absorption
Fentanyl	1–6	Metabolism (+ renal)	Usually given by injection, transdermally or buccally
Meptazinol	2–6	Metabolism (+ renal)	Extensive and rapid absorption
Methadone	6–8	Metabolism + renal	Good oral bioavailability
Morphine	1–5	Metabolism	Oral bioavailability is low (10–50%)
Nalbuphine	2–4 (intravenous), 3–8 (oral)	Metabolism + renal	Extensive first-pass metabolism (bioavailability, 10–20%)
Naloxone	1–1.5	Metabolism	Opioid antagonist: given by injection
Oxycodone	5–6	Metabolism (+ renal)	Oral and rectal bioavailability is about 50–90%
Pentazocine	2	Metabolism (+ renal)	Oral bioavailability (11–32%)
Pethidine (meperidine)	3–8	Metabolism + renal	Oral bioavailability about 50%
Phenazocine	no data available	No data available	
Remifentanil	0.1	Metabolism	Very rapid hydrolysis in blood and tissues (not redistribution)
Tramadol	5–6	Metabolism (+ renal)	Oral bioavailability about 60–70%

20

Anxiolytics, sedatives and hypnotics

There is considerable overlap in the pharmacology of drugs that have anxiolytic and hypnotic properties. Compounds with sedative properties (moderating excitement and calming) at low doses often have hypnotic (sleep-inducing) effects at higher doses. In addition, sedative drugs may have anxiolytic properties when used at doses that are too small to produce sedation. However, compounds such as buspirone have been developed, which act in a different way, and have anxiolytic properties but do not sedate.

Biological basis of anxiety disorders

The clinical manifestations of anxiety are both psychological and physical. Anxiety is only pathological when it is inappropriate to the degree of stress to which the individual is exposed. A variety of anxiety disorders are recognised (Box 20.1). Of these, mixed anxiety and depressive disorder is the most common, followed by generalised anxiety disorder.

The symptoms vary among the disorders, but usually include apprehension, worry, fear and nervousness. Increased sympathetic nervous system activity frequently accompanies these feelings, causing sweating, tachycardia and epigastric discomfort. Sleep is often disturbed, with difficulty getting to sleep being a common feature.

Dysfunction of neurotransmission in the limbic region of the brain underlies the genesis of anxiety. The

---

Box 20.1

Simplified classification of anxiety disorders

Phobic anxiety disorder
Other anxiety disorder (including panic disorder and mixed anxiety and depressive disorder)
Obsessive compulsive disorder
Reaction to severe stress (including post-traumatic stress disorder)
Conversion disorders
Somatoform disorders
Other neurotic disorders (including neurasthenia)

hippocampus and amygdala are a central part of the system which receives input from the locus ceruleus and dorsal raphe, and in turn projects to the subcortical and cortical nuclei. This system is involved in the integration of internal and external sensory perception.

Excessive serotonergic, and to a lesser extent noradrenergic, excitatory neurotransmission in the limbic system has been implicated in some forms of anxiety, but peptide neurotransmitters may also be important. Deficient inhibition of limbic neurotransmission by gamma-aminobutyric acid (GABA) receptors may also be important. Endogenous modulators of GABA receptors have recently been identified and a defect in their synthesis or the excessive production of an inverse agonist at GABA receptors may promote anxiety states. The understanding in anxiety of the role of neurotransmitters and their many receptors is unclear. Drugs acting to stimulate 5HT receptors but also to inhibit 5HT reuptake (Ch. 22) and to stimulate GABA receptors and block adrenergic β-receptors can be effective.

Drug therapy for anxiety

Drugs used to treat anxiety are called anxiolytics.

Benzodiazepines

Examples: diazepam, temazepam.

Mechanism of action and effects

Benzodiazepines act at three specific binding sites (ω_{1-3} subtypes of the benzodiazepine receptor), which are closely linked to the $GABA_A$ receptor (Ch. 4). When a benzodiazepine binds to its receptor, it induces a conformational change that enhances the action of the inhibitory neurotransmitter GABA. When GABA binds to its receptor, the influx of Cl^- into the cell increases, leading to membrane hyperpolarisation and decreased cell excitability. Benzodiazepines act only in the presence of GABA to enhance GABA-mediated opening of the ion channel; they have no direct action on the channel (Fig. 20.1). The consequent increased inhibitory neurotransmission produces the following potentially useful effects:

- sedation because of reduced sensory input to the reticular activating system
- sleep induction at high concentrations of drug
- anxiolysis as a consequence of actions on the limbic system and hypothalamus
- anticonvulsant activity (Ch. 23).

Pharmacokinetics

Most benzodiazepines are well absorbed from the gut. Many, including diazepam, are subsequently metabolised in the liver to active compounds that contribute to a prolonged duration of action through relatively slow elimination from the body. Metabolism of some benzodiazepines, for example temazepam, produces inactive derivatives. The pharmacokinetics of individual benzodiazepines determine their major clinical uses.

Hypnotic benzodiazepines are rapidly absorbed and their lipid solubility ensures ready penetration into the brain. This produces a fast onset of sedation, then sleep. A brief duration of action is desirable to avoid hangover sedation in the morning; this can be achieved if the drug is inactivated in the liver (e.g. temazepam). Repeated dosing, particularly with long-acting compounds such as diazepam, increases the risk of accumulation with a prolonged sedative effect (see compendium).

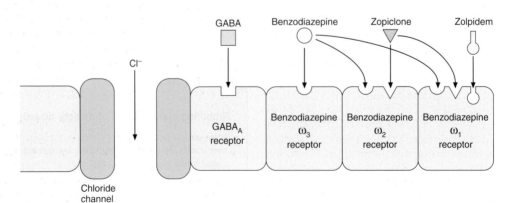

Fig. 20.1
Subtypes of benzodiazepine receptors (ω_{1-3}) modulate the activity of the gamma-aminobutyric acid (GABA) type A receptor, which facilitates the opening of Cl^- channels. Compounds such as zolpidem are thought to act selectively on the ω_1 subtype of the benzodiazepine receptor and this may explain why it lacks anticonvulsant and muscle relaxant activity. Barbiturates have similar effects on the Cl^- channel but act by modulating the channel rather than the benzodiazepine receptor.

The anxiolytic properties of benzodiazepines are best exploited by using a compound with a long duration of action. Smaller doses can then be used to minimise sedation, and the rebound in anxiety symptoms that can occur between doses of a short-acting drug is avoided. A long- acting drug can also be useful for the treatment of epilepsy (Ch. 23).

Diazepam and some other benzodiazepines can also be given by intravenous injection for rapid onset of effect. This can be useful for treatment of epilepsy (Ch. 23) or for rapid sedation pre-operatively or before procedures such as endoscopy. Diazepam is available in solution for rectal administration.

Unwanted effects

Benzodiazepines have several unwanted effects:

- drowsiness, which may cause problems with driving or operating machinery
- confusional states especially in the elderly
- impaired memory
- Incoordination or ataxia
- potentiation of the sedative effects by other CNS depressant drugs, for example alcohol
- tolerance and dependence.

Flumazenil is an antagonist of benzodiazepines and can be used in acute overdosage.

Tolerance. Tolerance to the therapeutic effects of benzodiazepines is common. Hypnotic effects are lost quite early but the rebound insomnia on withdrawal can perpetuate benzodiazepine use.

Dependence. Dependence with physical and psychological withdrawal symptoms during long-term treatment. The risk is highest in patients with personality disorders, or a previous history of dependence on alcohol or drugs, and more likely to occur if high doses of benzodiazepine are used. Restricting their use to a maximum of 4 weeks will minimise the risk of dependence. With long-acting drugs, withdrawal symptoms may be delayed by up to 3 weeks. Anxiety is the most frequent symptom and can take up to a month to resolve. Insomnia, depression or abnormalities of perception such as altered sensitivity to noise, light or touch also occur. More severe reactions include toxic psychosis or convulsions. Gradual withdrawal of a benzodiazepine over 4 to 8 weeks is desirable after long-term use although complete withdrawal may take up to a year. Lorazepam is a potent benzodiazepine with a relatively short action that proves particularly difficult to stop because of the intensity of withdrawal symptoms, which occur a few hours after withdrawal. Substitution by the longer-acting drug diazepam may be helpful before withdrawal is attempted. There are no proven treatments for reducing symptoms associated with withdrawal, but β-blockers (Ch. 5) and sedative tricyclic antidepressants such as amitriptyline (Ch. 22) have been used.

Azapirones

Example: buspirone.

Mechanism of action and effects

Buspirone has no effect on GABA receptors. It is a full agonist at presynaptic 5-hydroxytryptamine (5HT) type 1A ($5HT_{1A}$) receptors, a partial agonist (Ch. 1) at postsynaptic 5HT receptors and also a presynaptic α_2-adrenoceptor agonist. The actions at presynaptic receptors produce negative feedback to inhibit neurotransmitter release. Initial exacerbation of anxiety may occur, possibly caused by postsynaptic 5HT receptor stimulation. The onset of action of buspirone is slow over several days. It has no sedative action and it does not relieve benzodiazepine withdrawal symptoms.

Pharmacokinetics

Buspirone is well absorbed from the gut and undergoes extensive first-pass metabolism in the liver. The half-life is short.

Unwanted effects

Buspirone has few unwanted effects:

- gastrointestinal upset
- dizziness and headache.

Neither tolerance nor dependence has been reported.

Management of anxiety

Symptoms of anxiety, if mild, may respond to counselling and psychotherapy such as relaxation training. If they are more severe or persistent, benzodiazepines are the most effective drugs, with a rapid onset of action over a few minutes. Problems with dependence should limit their use to a maximum of 4 weeks, and the dose should be gradually reduced after the first 2 weeks. A minority of patients may require long-term treatment. Buspirone is equally effective but the slow onset of action (1–2 weeks) makes it less versatile for managing short-term anxiety. Somatic symptoms of anxiety (e.g. tremor, palpitations) are often helped by a β-blocker (Ch. 5).

Anxiety frequently coexists with depression and antidepressants (Ch. 22) provide a useful alternative in this situation. Tricyclic antidepressants and selective serotonin reuptake inhibitors (SSRIs) appear to be equally effective. However, antidepressants can initially exacerbate anxiety and a benzodiazepine may be necessary for the first week to prevent this. The optimal duration of antidepressant treatment in this situation is uncertain, but similar treatment periods as for depression (Ch. 22) are usually recommended.

Phobic disorders usually need a different approach. Behavioural techniques are often most effective in the long term. Social phobia in particular responds to monoamine oxidase inhibitors (MAOIs) better than to most other agents (Ch. 22). Moclobemide is the treatment of choice, but phenelzine is also used.

Panic disorder is usually treated with tricyclic antidepressants or SSRIs; MAOIs are used for those who do not respond.

Insomnia

Defining insomnia is complicated by the considerable variability in the normal pattern of sleep. It is considered to be present if there is 'inability to initiate or maintain sleep'. There are three major categories of insomnia (Table 20.1).

The reticular formation in the midbrain, medulla and pons is responsible for maintaining wakefulness. This is dependent on sensory input via collateral connections from the main sensory pathways. Neurotransmitter systems involved in the regulation of sleep include noradrenergic pathways from the locus ceruleus and cholinergic ascending tracts, which are involved in cortical arousal. By contrast, GABA neurotransmission inhibits these neurons, and release of serotonin from the rostral raphe nucleus also induces sleep.

Sleep patterns

The two main types of sleep pattern are non-rapid eye movement sleep (non-REM) and rapid eye-movement sleep (REM). These sleep patterns occur in cycles (Fig. 20.2), with non-REM sleep varying between light sleep (stages 1 and 2) and slow wave sleep (stages 3 and 4). Two thirds of sleep is usually spent in stages 2–4, characterised by continuous or intermittent delta waves (slow waves) on the electroencephalogram. These deeper stages of sleep are the recuperative phase, while most dreaming occurs during the REM sleep periods.

Table 20.1
Types of insomia

Type of insomnia	Duration	Likely causes
Transient	2–3 days	Acute situational or environmental stress (e.g. jet lag, shift work)
Short term	<3 weeks	Ongoing personal stress
Long term	>3 weeks	Psychiatric illness, behavioural reasons, medical reasons

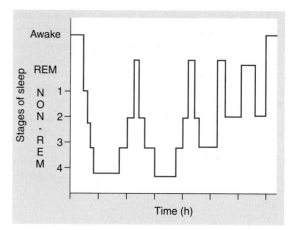

Fig. 20.2
Typical sleep pattern in a young adult. REM, rapid eye-movement sleep.

Increasing age is associated with more nocturnal awakening and longer periods of REM sleep.

Drug therapy for insomnia

Drugs used to treat insomnia are called hypnotics.

Benzodiazepines

Benzodiazepines are both anxiolytics and hypnotics depending on the dose. See above for details.

Cyclopyrrolones

Example: zopiclone

Mechanism of action and effects
Zopiclone interacts with the $GABA_A$ receptor on postsynaptic neuronal membranes. It appears to be more selective than benzodiazepines for the ω_1- and ω_2-subtypes of benzodiazepine receptor. Like the benzodiazepines, zopiclone increases Cl^- influx into the cell, which inhibits neurotransmission and produces a marked hypnotic effect. Although it possesses anxiolytic and anticonvulsant activity its short duration of action makes it unsuitable for these indications.

Pharmacokinetics
The rapid absorption and short half-life of zopiclone make it ideally suited to its role as a hypnotic. Metabolism in the liver is responsible for elimination.

Unwanted effects
Unwanted effects include:

- bitter metallic taste
- gastrointestinal disturbance
- drowsiness (that may persist to the next day), headache and fatigue
- depression, confusion.

There is only anecdotal evidence for tolerance, but dependence with withdrawal symptoms has been reported.

Imidazopyridines

Example: zolpidem

Mechanism of action
Zolpidem binds preferentially to benzodiazepine ω_1-receptors and modulates the $GABA_A$–Cl^- channel complex.

Pharmacokinetics
Zolpidem is rapidly absorbed from the gut. It is metabolised by the liver and has a short half-life.

Unwanted effects
Unwanted effects include:

- gastrointestinal disturbance
- headache, confusion
- daytime drowsiness
- brief psychotic episodes, depression

Dependence with a withdrawal syndrome can occur.

Clomethiazole

Mechanism of action, effects and clinical uses
Clomethiazole is structurally similar to thiamine (vitamin B_1). It probably enhances GABA receptor activity by interaction with a site similar to that of the barbiturates (Fig. 20.1 and Ch. 23). Clomethiazole has sedative, hypnotic and anticonvulsant properties but is rarely used as a hypnotic. Clinical uses are limited, but it is sometimes used in the management of alcohol withdrawal (Ch. 54), status epilepticus (Ch. 23) and control of agitation in the elderly.

Pharmacokinetics
Clomethiazole is readily absorbed from the gut but undergoes extensive first-pass metabolism in the liver. The half-life is short. It can also be given in smaller doses by continuous intravenous infusion, which avoids first-pass metabolism.

Unwanted effects
Unwanted effects include:

- nasal and conjunctival irritation early in use

- hangover effects
- respiratory depression in overdose, especially if taken with alcohol.

Dependence is common, which restricts the drug's usefulness. To reduce the incidence of dependence, treatment should not be given for more than 9 days.

Chloral derivatives

Examples: chloral hydrate, cloral betaine, triclofos

Mechanism of action and effects
The alcohol metabolite trichloroethanol is mainly responsible for the hypnotic effects of chloral derivatives. It may act in part by potentiating GABA-ergic inhibitory neurotransmission by binding to the GABA receptor. Chloral derivatives have a narrow therapeutic index and therefore are not ideal hypnotic drugs. Their use is not recommended.

Pharmacokinetics
Chloral is a prodrug that is well absorbed from the gut, then rapidly metabolised to trichloroethanol by alcohol dehydrogenase. The drug competes with ethanol for metabolism.

Unwanted effects

- Unpleasant taste and gastric irritation (less common with triclofos).
- Ataxia and nightmares.
- Hangover effects.
- Tolerance and dependence are frequent, as with benzodiazepines.
- Respiratory and myocardial depression can occur in overdose.

Management of insomnia

Drugs play only a small part in the treatment of insomnia. Explanation of the normal variations in sleep patterns and avoidance of diuretics or of drinks containing caffeine or alcohol in the hours before retiring can help. Eliminating excessive noise or heat in the bedroom, encouraging regular exercise in the day and minimising daytime napping may also be useful. Hypnotic drugs are reserved for when abnormal sleep markedly disrupts the patient's life. The ideal hypnotic will induce good quality prolonged sleep without disturbance of the normal sleep pattern. It should have a rapid onset of action, with no 'hangover' sedation in the morning and not produce tolerance or dependence. Few drugs have this ideal profile. Benzodiazepines reduce sleep latency (the time between settling down and falling asleep) and prolong sleep duration. However, they disturb the structure of sleep with loss of REM sleep. Progressive shortening of the deeper stages of sleep is also seen with more time spent in stage 2 sleep. Of the other hypnotic drugs, zopiclone may produce less disturbance of sleep 'architecture', having little effect on the amount of REM sleep and increasing the duration of slow-wave sleep.

Hypnotic drugs should only be used for short periods and intermittently if possible; tolerance to hypnotics frequently occurs after 2 weeks. If benzodiazepines are used continuously for 4 to 6 weeks rebound insomnia is common when the drug is stopped, caused by mild dependence. However, benzodiazepines are widely used since they are safe in overdose. Short-acting benzodiazepines may produce wakefulness early in the morning but longer-acting drugs carry the risk of hangover effects the following day. Zopiclone and zolpidem are probably equally as effective as a benzodiazepine but also carry a risk of dependence. Of the other hypnotics, chloral derivatives and clomethiazole should usually be avoided. Compounds with sedative actions as a part of their therapeutic profile can be useful to aid sleep, for example, a sedative antihistamine such as promazine (Ch. 38) for children suffering from somnambulism (sleep walking) or night terrors. Antidepressants (Ch. 22) should be considered if there is an underlying depressive illness, for example sedative tricyclic antidepressant such as amitriptyline. If less-sedative antidepressants are used, short-term concurrent use of a benzodiazepine may be necessary while awaiting the onset of the antidepressant effect.

FURTHER READING

Aranda M, Hanson CW (2000) Anesthetics, sedatives and paralytics. Understanding their use in the intensive care unit. *Surg Clin North Am* 80, 933–947

Doble A (1999) New insights into the mechanism of action of hypnotics. *J Psychopharmacol* 13, S11–S20

Gale C, Oakley-Browne M (2000) Anxiety disorder. *BMJ* 321, 1204–1211

Hale AS (1997) Anxiety. *Br Med J* 314, 1886–1889

Kupfer DJ, Reynolds CF (1997) Management of insomnia. *N Engl J Med* 336, 341–345

Lader M (1994) Treatment of anxiety. *Br Med J* 309, 321–324

Lader MH (1999) Limitations on the use of benzodiazepines in anxiety and insomnia: are they justified? *Eur Neuropsychopharmacol* 9(suppl 6), S399–S405

Lerch C, Park GR (1999) Sedation and analgesia. *Br Med Bull* 55, 76–95

Longo LP, Johnson B (2000) Addiction: Part l. Benzodiazepines – side effects, abuse risk and alternatives. *Am Fam Physician* 61, 2121–2128

Maczaj M (1993) Pharmacological treatment of insomnia. *Drugs* 45, 44–55

Moller HJ (1999) Effectiveness and safety of benzodiazepines. *J Clin Psychopharmacol* 19, 2S–11S

Monti JM, Monti M (1995) Pharmacological treatment of chronic insomnia. *CNS Drugs* 4, 182–194

Scott MK, Demeter DA, Nortey SO, Dubinsky B, Shank RP, Reitz AB (1999) New directions in anxiolytic drug research. *Prog Med Chem* 36, 169–200

Tancer ME, Uhde TW (1995) Social phobia: a review of pharmacological treatment. *CNS Drugs* 3, 267–278

Young C, Knudsen N, Hilton A, Reves JG (2000) Sedation in the intensive care unit. *Crit Care Med* 28, 853–866

Self-assessment

In questions 1–3, the first statement, in italics, is true. Are the accompanying statements true?

1. *Benzodiazepines with a medium to long duration of action are useful for treating anxiety states.*

   a. Long-term use of benzodiazepines is desirable in anxiety states.
   b. Potentiation of central nervous system (CNS) effects occurs with concurrent alcohol administration.

2. *Central nervous system (CNS) depressant effects of benzodiazepines can be reversed with the antagonist flumazenil*

   a. Lower doses of benzodiazepines should be used in the elderly.
   b. Buspirone is more sedative than temazepam.

3. *Benzodiazepines used to treat anxiety should be administered for as short a time as possible in the lowest dose possible*
   Benzodiazepines have no effect on sleep patterns as measured by duration of rapid eye movement (REM) sleep.

4. Case history question

> Mrs FL is a 46-year-old mother of three who has found it very hard to cope following the sudden death of her husband 5 weeks previously. She has returned to work from bereavement leave but does not sleep properly, experiences occasional panic attacks when driving to work and feels that she is at risk of losing her job because tiredness and anxiety about her financial difficulties prevent her concentrating on her work.

   a. What drug might you prescribe to help Mrs FL's insomnia? What factors may determine your choice of this drug?
   b. How does your chosen drug work to reduce insomnia and anxiety? What potential unwanted effects and drug interactions should you warn her about?
   c. She returns 2 weeks later, saying that she regularly wakes at 4 a.m. and cannot get back to sleep. Consider the 'pros' and 'cons' of changing her to a longer-acting drug. What non-benzodiazepine drug may be useful in this situation?
   d. What are the problems associated with long-term use of benzodiazepines? What other options should be considered to help to manage Mrs FL's problems in the long term?

The answers are provided on pages 611–612.

Drug compendium

Anxiolytics, sedatives and hypnotics

Drug	Half-life (h)	Elimination	Comments (all given orally unless otherwise stated)
Anxiolytics			
Alprazolam	6–16	Metabolism + renal	Almost complete oral bioavailability; eliminated largely by oxidation followed by conjugation with glucuronic acid; about 20% excreted unchanged
Bromazepam	23	Metabolism	Good bioavailability (but reduced when taken with food); eliminated by hepatic oxidation
Buspirone	2–11	Metabolism	Rapid absorption but extensive first-pass metabolism; metabolised by oxidative dealkylation and hydroxylation
Chlordiazepoxide	15	Metabolism	Complete oral bioavailability; slowly eliminated by hepatic metabolism; a number of the metabolites retain activity and contribute significantly to the effect
Clorazepate	10	Metabolism	Complete oral bioavailability; metabolised by oxidation to hydroxy metabolites which are conjugated with glucuronic acid and sulfate
Diazepam	20–100	Metabolism	May be given orally, rectally or by intramuscular or slow intravenous injection; complete oral bioavailability; metabolised to N-desmethyl metabolite which has a longer half-life (30–200 h) and to temazepam; N-desmethyldiazepam is oxidised to oxazepam
Lorazepam	4–25	Metabolism	May be given orally or by intramuscular or slow intravenous dosage; high bioavailability, eliminated mainly as the glucuronicacid conjugate
Meprobamate	8	Metabolism	Very few published data available
Oxazepam	4–25	Metabolism	High bioavailability; eliminated mainly as the glucuronic acid conjugate
Sedatives and hypnotics			
Clomethiazole	4–6	Metabolism	Used only in the elderly (with little hangover); may be given orally (or by intravenous infusion for acute alcohol withdrawal); rapid absorption but extensive (40–95%) first-pass metabolism; metabolised by dechlorination and oxidation
Chloral hydrate	0.1, 8–12 (trichloroethanol), 67 (trichloroacetic acid)	Metabolism	Limited current use; not recommended; extensive first-pass metabolism; rapidly reduced to trichloroethanol (TCE) and oxidised to trichloroacetic acid; the hypnotic effect is believed to be caused by trichloroethanol
Flunitrazepam	23	Metabolism	Good oral bioavailability; a large number of metabolites, some of which retain pharmacological activity
Loprazolam	7	Metabolism (+ biliary)	Good oral absorption; metabolised by formation of a more polar N-oxide; metabolite and parent drug are eliminated in bile
Lormetazepam	8–10	Metabolism	Unlike many benzodiazepines it is not extensively oxidised but is eliminated as the glucuronic acid conjugate of the parent drug; limited oxidation (about 10%) to the glucuronide of lorazepam (the N-demethyl analogue)
Nitrazepam	20–48	Metabolism	Rapid absorption but variable bioavailability (50–90%); metabolism is mainly by nitro-reduction, followed by N-acetylation of the resultant amino group; only the parent drug is active
Promethazine	7–14	Metabolism	Hypnotic antihistamine that has a prolonged effect; incomplete oral bioavailability (about 20%); metabolised by S-oxidation and N-dealkylation in the liver; the S-oxide (which is the main metabolite) is inactive
Temazepam	5–12	Metabolism	High oral bioavailability; oxidised by N-demethylation to oxazepam and by conjugation with glucuronic acid; most activity is probably due to the parent compound
Triclofos (triclos)	–	Metabolism	Similar to chloral hydrate (see above); few published data available; phosphate ester of trichloroethanol which is hydrolysed in vivo; causes fewer gastrointestinal effects than chloral hydrate
Zolpidem	2–4	Metabolism	Good oral bioavailability (about 70%); metabolised largely by CYP3A4 to inactive metabolites
Zopiclone	4–6	Metabolism (+ some renal)	Rapid absorption and a high bioavailability (about 80%); metabolised by N-dealkylation, N-oxidation and decarboxylation; metabolites (+ about 5% of parent drug) are eliminated in the urine

The major psychotic disorders: schizophrenia and mania

Psychotic disorders

The term psychosis indicates that the patient has lost contact with reality. This is usually experienced as hallucination, delusion or a disruption in thought processes. The two most profound functional psychotic conditions are schizophrenia and mania. These disorders probably form extremes of a continuum that embraces the so-called schizo-affective disorders (Box 21.1). Organic disease caused by metabolic disturbance, toxic substances or psychoactive drugs can also cause psychosis.

Schizophrenia

Schizophrenia is more common in males and usually presents relatively early in life. The onset is usually gradual but can be abrupt. Once established, it can have a relapsing or persistent course. Clinical features are often categorised as positive or negative (Table 21.1), although none are pathognomonic of the disorder. The positive features are disordered versions of thinking, perception, formation of ideas or sense of self. They include hallucinations (false sensory perceptions) and delusions (false beliefs held with absolute certainty and unexplained by the patient's socioeconomic background). The negative features are often the most debilitating in the long term.

Biological basis of schizophrenia
The dopaminergic systems in the central nervous system (CNS) arise from the midbrain (Fig. 21.1).

Box 21.1

Classification of major psychotic disorders

Schizophrenia
Persistent delusional disorders (includes paranoid
    psychosis, paraphrenia)
Acute and transient psychotic disorders
Schizo-affective disorders
Manic episode
Bipolar affective disorder

Table 21.1
Clinical features of schizophrenia

Features	Characteristics
Positive features	
Hallucinations	Third person auditory hallucinations (voices talking about patient as 'he' or 'she')
	Second person commands
	Olfactory, tactile or visual hallucinations
Delusions	Thought withdrawal (thoughts being taken from your mind)
	Thought insertion (alien thoughts inserted in your mind)
	Thought broadcast (thoughts are known to others)
	Actions are caused or controlled from outside
	Bodily sensations are imposed from outside
	Delusional perception (a sudden, fully formed delusion, in the wake of a normal perception)
Negative features	Loss of interest in others, initiative or sense of enjoyment
	Blunted emotions
	Limited speech

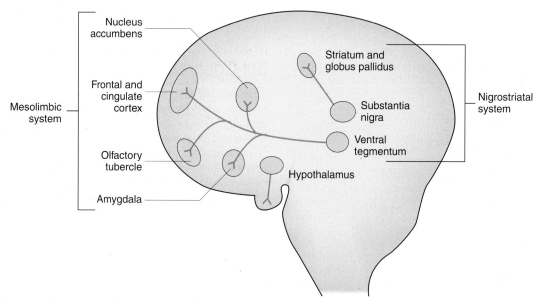

Fig. 21.1
Major dopaminergic pathways in the central nervous system.

Dopaminergic neurons from the substantia nigra ascend to the striatum via the nigrostriatal pathways (Ch. 24) and modulate motor function. Neurons from the ventral tegmental area connect via the mesolimbic projections to the limbic region and via the mesocortical projections to the prefrontal cortex. The limbic region and prefrontal cortex are involved in cognition, emotional memory and the initiation of behaviour. The positive symptoms of schizophrenia are believed to result from dopaminergic overactivity in the mesolimbic system of the dominant hemisphere, although direct evidence for this hypothesis is still patchy. Amphetamines can release dopamine and result in schizophrenia-like episodes. There is a positive correlation between the potency of antipsychotic drugs and their ability to bind and inhibit dopamine D_2 receptors.

Several receptors for the neurotransmitter dopamine are found in the brain. CNS dopamine receptors belong to two families, D_1 and D_2. The D_2 subtype is prominent in the nigrostriatal and mesolimbic systems, while the frontal cortex has few D_2 receptors. Additional D_2 receptor subtypes have been discovered (known as D_3 and D_4) that form part of the D_2 receptor family. Of these, the D_4 receptor is found in both the mesolimbic system and the frontal cortex, although there is a low density of these receptors in the nigrostriatal pathways. It has been suggested that D_4 receptors may be involved in the pathogenesis of schizophrenia, although this is still unclear.

Abnormalities of other neurotransmitter systems, neuropeptides and modulatory substances may also be important in schizophrenia. Reduced noradrenergic activity has been demonstrated, and excitatory amino acids such as glutamate or aspartate may also be involved. 5-Hydroxytryptamine (5HT) inhibits dopaminergic neurons both in the midbrain and in the forebrain. In the forebrain, excessive serotonergic activity may be important in determining negative symptoms.

Our knowledge of the biology of schizophrenia is becoming increasingly complex, and it may represent several disease processes. However, there is increasing evidence that it is a disorder with a genetic basis, expressed in response to environmental influences.

Mania

Mania is a disorder of elevated mood that can occur alone or be interspersed with episodes of depression (bipolar affective disorder or manic-depressive illness); unipolar mania is uncommon. Mild mania is termed hypomania. In some patients the fluctuations of mood are less marked, and the disorder is termed cyclothymia.

Mania can occur gradually or suddenly and varies in severity from mild elation, increased drive and sociability, to grandiose ideas, marked overactivity, overspending and socially embarrassing behaviour. Onset is usually early in adult life and it has a stronger genetic component than any other major psychiatric disorder.

Biological basis of mania

The biological basis for mania is less well understood than that of depression. Increased CNS monoamine neurotransmitter activity may be important, leading to complex changes in neuronal function caused by altered levels of intracellular second messengers such as inositol trisphosphate or cAMP.

Antipsychotic drugs

Classification

Antipsychotic drugs (also known as neuroleptics or major tranquillisers) belong to various chemical classes that vary in their sedative, antimuscarinic and extrapyramidal effects (Table 21.2).

The phenothiazines. These have a tricyclic structure and a side-chain. Structural differences give variations in profiles of biological activities. According to the nature of the side-chain they are subdivided into:

- aliphatic, e.g. chlorpromazine
- piperidine, e.g. thioridazine
- piperazine, e.g. fluphenazine.

The thioxanthenes. These also have a tricyclic structure but a different side-chain, e.g. flupentixol.

The butylpiperidines. These have a different core structure and are subdivided into:

- butyrophenones, e.g. haloperidol
- diphenylbutylpiperidines, e.g. pimozide.

The substituted benzamides. The most commonly used is sulpiride.

Table 21.2
Consequences of receptor antagonist activity among antipsychotic drugs

	Example	Sedative	Anticholinergic	Extrapyramidal	Hypotension
Phenothiazines					
Aliphatic	Chlorpromazine	+++	++	++	+++
Piperidine	Thioridazine	++	+++	+	++
Piperazine	Fluphenazine	++	+	+++	+
Thioxanthenes	Flupentixol	+	+	+++	+
Butylpiperidines					
Butyrophenones	Haloperidol	+	+	+++	++
Diphenylbutylpiperidines	Pimozide	+	+	+++	+
Other agents					
Substituted benzamides	Sulpiride	+	+	0	0
Dibenzodiazepines	Clozapine	++	+	0	+
Benzisoxazoles	Risperidone	+	+	+	+

+++, high risk; ++, moderate risk; +, low risk; 0, minimal risk.

The atypical antipsychotics. These include the:

- dibenzodiazepines, e.g. clozapine, olanzapine
- benzisoxazoles, e.g. risperidone.

The first three groups are most widely used. The antipsychotic drugs differ mainly in the degree of associated or unwanted effects (Table 21.2).

Mechanism of action and effects

The antipsychotic action involves blockade of CNS dopamine receptors in mesolimbic pathways. Blockade of the D_2 family of receptors is common to all effective neuroleptics.

For most 'classical' antipsychotic drugs, efficacy is directly related to their ability to bind to the D_2 receptor: about 70% or higher occupancy is required for clinical benefit. However, 80% or more D_2 receptor blockade in the striatum will produce extrapyramidal unwanted effects (see below). Newer 'atypical' antipsychotic drugs (e.g. clozapine) show more selective affinity for D_4 receptors than D_2 receptors. This property could explain their effectiveness in some patients who do not respond to classical antipsychotics, and their relative lack of extrapyramidal unwanted effects. Clozapine acts on dopamine receptors mainly in the ventral tegmental area and less on those in the substantia nigra which are associated with movement disorders (Ch. 24). However, other atypical antipsychotics, for example risperidone, also block $5HT_2$ receptors, which may explain their greater efficiency in controlling the negative symptoms of schizophrenia.

The lack of brain region selectivity of most antipsychotics means that they act on many different dopamine receptors including those in the hypothalamus, basal ganglia (Ch. 24) and the chemoreceptor trigger zone (CTZ) in the brainstem (Ch. 32). These actions are responsible for many of the unwanted effects of the drugs; effects at the CTZ give their anti-emetic activity.

Many antipsychotic drugs are also antagonists at several other receptors including α_1-adrenoceptors and histamine H_1 receptors. In this respect they resemble tricyclic antidepressants. These actions do not influence their efficacy in psychotic illness but can produce unwanted effects, the severity of which varies considerably among the individual drugs.

There are a number of clinically useful effects produced by antipsychotic drugs.

- A depressant action on conditioned responses and emotional responsiveness. In psychoses this is particularly helpful for management of thought disorders, abnormalities of perception and delusional beliefs.
- A sedative action, which is useful for treatment of restlessness and confusion. Sensory input into the reticular activating system is reduced by blockade of collateral fibres from the lemniscal pathways, but spontaneous activity is preserved. Arousal stimuli therefore produce less response. Risperidone does not produce sedation.
- An anti-emetic effect through dopamine receptor blockade at the CTZ, which is useful to treat vomiting such as that associated with drugs (e.g. cytotoxics, opioid analgesics) and uraemia. Some of the drugs are also effective in motion sickness through muscarinic receptor blockade (Ch. 32).
- Antihistaminic activity produced by histamine H_1 receptor blockade can be used for treatment of allergic reactions (Ch. 38).

Pharmacokinetics

Antipsychotics are rapidly absorbed from the gut but undergo extensive first-pass metabolism involving up to 90% of the parent drug. The plasma concentration of active drug (including metabolites) can vary some tenfold among individuals. However, the relationship between plasma drug concentration and clinical response is not close. The half-lives of the antipsychotics vary widely; for example, that of droperidol is short while that of pimozide is long. Many antipsychotics can be given by intramuscular injection for more rapid onset of action in disturbed patients. Since compliance with treatment is often poor in psychotic disorders, depot formulations of many antipsychotics have been developed. They are given by intramuscular injection in an oily base which slowly releases the drug for between 1 and 12 weeks. When given as a depot preparation or by intramuscular injection, the doses used are smaller than those for oral treatment, because of lack of first-pass metabolism in the liver.

Unwanted effects

The profile of unwanted effects varies widely among the different groups of drug (Table 21.2).

- Extrapyramidal effects such as akathisia (restlessness), acute dystonias (tongue protrusion, torticollis, oculogyric crisis) or parkinsonism arise from D_2 receptor blockade in the nigrostriatal pathways. Extrapyramidal effects occur in more than half of patients receiving treatment but are usually reversible if the drug is stopped. Their management is discussed in Chapter 24. With prolonged use, tardive dyskinesias or dystonias can develop. These consist of choreo-athetoid and repetitive orofacial movements, which arise after months or years of continued treatment and often do not resolve when the drug is withdrawn. Their aetiology is uncertain: upregulation of D_2 receptors may contribute but damage to inhibitory GABA-ergic neurons or dysfunction in other neurotransmitter pathways probably participate. Atypical antipsychotics have a lower risk of extrapyramidal effects.

- Drowsiness and cognitive impairment can occur as a result of dopamine receptor blockade. Risperidone, by contrast, causes insomnia and agitation.
- Galactorrhoea, amenorrhoea, infertility and impotence can result from dopamine receptor blockade in hypothalamic pathways, which causes hyperprolactinaemia and reduced gonadotrophin secretion.
- Antimuscarinic effects (Ch. 4). In addition to peripheral antimuscarinic actions, CNS muscarinic receptor blockade predisposes to acute confusional states.
- Alpha$_1$-adrenoceptor blockade produces postural hypotension, nasal stuffiness and impaired ejaculation.
- Hypothermia as a consequence of depressed hypothalamic function. Altered 5HT neuronal activity may be responsible.
- There is an increased risk of epileptic seizures.
- Hypersensitivity reactions include cholestatic jaundice, photosensitivity and skin discoloration (especially with chlorpromazine).
- Agranulocytosis is a particular problem with clozapine (1–2% risk) and regular blood tests are mandatory during treatment with this drug.
- Sudden withdrawal after long-term use can produce a prolonged syndrome of insomnia, sweating and dyskinesias.
- Neuroleptic malignant syndrome is a rare genetically determined disorder in which antipsychotic drugs produce high fever, muscle rigidity, autonomic instability with hypertension and sweating, and altered consciousness. Immediate withdrawal of the antipsychotic and treatment with dantrolene or a dopamine agonist (Ch. 24) may be life saving.
- Cognitive impairment. This is less marked with atypical antipsychotics.

Management of psychotic disorders

Management of schizophrenia

Acute psychotic symptoms such as hallucinations and delusions can be controlled relatively rapidly with an antipsychotic drug such as haloperidol or chlorpromazine. The initial sedative actions of these drugs can be particularly helpful. However, reduction in thought disturbance, withdrawal and apathy are delayed. Therefore, the full clinical benefit is gradual over several weeks, despite rapid dopamine receptor blockade. This suggests that the major effects of these drugs involve modification of complex intracellular events, initiated by receptor blockade.

Treatment for schizophrenia is not curative, and long-term maintenance therapy is usually required to prevent relapse. The duration of this treatment is determined by the number of acute episodes, and is usually at least 2–5 years. Intermittent treatment introduced only for early relapses is associated with a higher overall relapse rate (50%, compared with 25% taking prophylactic therapy). Depot injections given every 1–4 weeks can be used to improve compliance with maintenance treatment, which is often poor in schizophrenia. Continuous antipsychotic treatment provides relief of symptoms for more than 70% of patients. Various psychological treatments to improve social skills are important as an adjunct to drug treatment and should be provided along with social support.

Some patients prove resistant to classical antipsychotics particularly if negative symptoms predominate. For these patients, increasing use is made of the atypical antipsychotics. These are also increasingly used for newly diagnosed patients, because of their better unwanted effect profile. Risperidone was initially believed to be useful for patients with predominantly negative symptoms, although the evidence for this is very limited. Clozapine was the first drug shown to be effective in drug-resistant schizophrenia, and is more effective than the classical antipsychotics. The risk of agranulocytosis has limited the use of this drug. There is less secure evidence for efficacy of newer atypical drugs in resistant patients.

Management of mania

When symptoms of mania are mild they can usually be controlled by lithium alone (Ch. 22), or in combination with a benzodiazepine (Ch. 20). If symptoms are more severe, an antipsychotic drug may be necessary in combination with lithium. As an alternative to lithium, the anticonvulsants carbamazepine or sodium valproate (Ch. 23) are effective, but in the acute phase supplementary treatment with benzodiazepines is still necessary. Anticonvulsants can also be used in combination with lithium.

Lithium is the treatment of choice for prophylaxis of mania and can also be particularly helpful for bipolar illness, since it prevents the depressive episodes as well. Patients who relapse with manic episodes despite lithium are often treated with additional antipsychotic drug therapy.

As for schizophrenia, psychological treatments are an essential adjunct to drug therapy in patients with mania.

FURTHER READING

Daly I (1997) Mania. *Lancet* i, 1157–1160

Geddes J, Freemantle N, Harrison P, Bebbington P (2000) Atypical antipsychotics in the treatment of schizophrenia: systematic overview and meta-regression analysis. *Br Med J* 321, 1371–1376

Kane, JM (1996) Schizophrenia. *N Engl J Med* 334, 34–41

McGrath J, Emmerson WB (1999) Treatment of schizophrenia. *Br Med J* 319, 1045–1048

Reynolds GP (1996) The importance of dopamine D_4 receptors in the actions and development of antipsychotic agents. *Drugs* 51, 7–11

Shale H, Tanner C (1996) Pharmacological options for the management of dyskinesias. *Drugs* 52, 849–860

Turner T (1997) Schizophrenia. *Br Med J* 315, 108–111

Self-assessment

The following statements, in italics, are true. Are the accompanying statements also true?

1. *Some antipsychotic drugs such as clozapine have relatively few effects on the extrapyramidal system and have low affinity for the dopamine receptors in the substantia nigra.*

   a. The phenothiazine fluphenazine has greater antimuscarinic activity than chlorpromazine.
   b. Clozapine causes agranulocytosis.
   c. Chlorpromazine given as decanoates in a depot preparation has to be injected weekly.

2. *The beneficial effects of antipsychotics take several weeks for full effect to be seen.*

   a. The 'positive' symptoms of schizophrenia (e.g. delusions) are more readily controlled than negative (withdrawal) symptoms.
   b. There is a close correlation between plasma levels of chlorpromazine and its antipsychotic effect.

3. *Antipsychotics are effective in treating only about 70% of schizophrenics.*
   Clozapine and thioridazine cause relatively few extrapyramidal symptoms.

4. Case history question

   > A 25-year-old man (Mr PS) with schizophrenia has been treated with high-dose oral chlorpromazine for 2 years. His main symptoms of auditory hallucinations and delusional thoughts ('*The people in the flat above are broadcasting my thoughts on their radio*') have been improved, but he remains socially withdrawn and apathetic and has described a number of new problems including feeling very tired, faintness on standing up, dry mouth, sexual problems, blurred and darkened vision, occasional difficulty with fine control of movement (writing/typing) and weight gain.

   a. Which neural pathways are thought to be dysfunctional in schizophrenia and what is the evidence for this? How does chlorpromazine exert its antipsychotic action?
   b. Which adverse effect(s) reported by Mr PS are likely to be caused by chlorpromazine acting at dopamine receptors? Why are movement disorders caused by chlorpromazine relatively mild compared with those associated with some other antipsychotic drugs?
   c. Which unwanted effects reported by Mr PS are likely to be caused by blockade of histamine receptors, muscarinic receptors and adrenoceptors?
   d. Mr PS has had two severe relapses requiring hospitalisation within the last 18 months and is vague on whether he always takes his medication as directed. How might you improve compliance with treatment?
   e. Consider alternative antipsychotic drugs that might help Mr PS. What special care is required with the drug(s) you suggest?

   The answers are provided are pages 612–613.

Antipsychotic drugs

Drug compendium

Drug	Half-life (h)	Elimination	Comments
Amisulpride[a]	12	Metabolism (?)	Oral dosage; D_2/D_3 antagonistic with presynaptic and limbic system selectivity; data on metabolic fate have not been published
Benperidol	7	Metabolism	Oral dosage; metabolites are inactive; incomplete oral bioavailability (about 40%)
Chlorpromazine	8–35	Metabolism	Oral, suppository and injection formulations available; incomplete oral bioavailability (10–33%); numerous pathways of metabolism with some metabolites detectable months after cessation of treatment
Clozapine[a]	12 (6–33)	Metabolism	Oral dosage; high affinity for D_1 and D_4 receptors; high bioavailability; metabolised by hepatic oxidation (CYP1A2 and CYP3A4)
Droperidol	2–3	Metabolism	Given orally or by injection (i.m. or i.v.); good oral bioavailability (about 75%); metabolised in liver
Flupentixol	35	Metabolism	Given orally (as hydrochloride) or by depot injection (as the decanoate ester prodrug); oral bioavailability is about 40%; the half-life for release from the depot injection is about 17 days; parent drug undergoes enterohepatic circulation following biliary excretion as a glucuronide
Fluphenazine (and decanoate)	16	Metabolism	Given orally (as hydrochloride) or by depot injection (as the decanoate ester prodrug); oral bioavailability is about 50%; the half-life for release from the depot injection is about 26 days; metabolites of fluphenazine retain activity and may be responsible for about 50% of the total activity
Haloperidol (and decanoate)	20 (9–67)	Metabolism	Given orally and by injection, or by depot injection (as the decanoate prodrug); oral bioavailability is about 60%; the half-life for release from the depot injection is about 21 days; reduced to an active metabolite in liver and extrahepatic tissues; undergoes enterohepatic circulation
Levomepromazine (methotrimeprazine)	15–30	Metabolism	Given orally or by injection (i.m. or i.v.); oral bioavailability is about 50%; numerous metabolites
Loxapine	4	Metabolism	Given orally; bioavailability is about 30%; extensive metabolism
Olanzapine	30 (21–54)	Metabolism	Given orally; antagonist at D_1, D_2, D_4 and $5HT_2$ receptors; oral bioavailability is 60%; metabolised by CYP1A2 and CYP2D6 to inactive products
Oxypertine	Not available	Metabolism	Given orally; early drug and few published data available
Pericyazine	Not available	Metabolism(?)	Given orally; early drug and few published data available
Perphenazine	9	Metabolism	Given orally; low oral bioavailability (30–40%); extensive hepatic metabolism
Pimozide	55	Metabolism	Given orally; oral bioavailability is about 60–80%; metabolised to inactive products by CYP3A4
Pipotiazide palmitate	15–16 days	Metabolism	Depot injection formulation; long half-life results from slow release from depot injection; the active drug (pipotiazide) has a circulating half-life of a few hours only
Prochlorperazine	6–7	Metabolism	Given orally, rectally or by deep i.m. injection; variable absorption of oral doses
Promazine	Not available	Metabolism	Given orally or by i.m. injection; it is a low-potency analogue of chlorpromazine
Quetiapine[a]	6	Metabolism	Given orally; antagonist at $5HT_2$ and D_2 receptors; metabolised by hepatic CYP3A4
Risperidone[a]	2–4 (EM), 17–22 (PM)	Metabolism (+ renal in PM)	Given orally; oral bioavailability is about 70%; antagonist at $5HT_2$ and D_2 receptors; metabolised by hepatic CYP2D6 with extensive metabolisers (EM) eliminating the drug 5–10 times more rapidly than poor metabolisers (PM), who excrete about 30% unchanged in urine
Sertindole[a]	60–90	Metabolism	Given orally; selective antagonist at $5HT_2$ receptors; metabolised by CYP2D6 and CYP3A4
Sulpiride	6–8	Urine + metabolism	Given orally; incomplete oral bioavailability (about 30–40%) owing to poor absorption; water-soluble compound eliminated largely unchanged in urine and faeces
Thioridazine	10	Metabolism	Given orally; oral bioavailability is about 60%; metabolised in liver to a number of S-oxidised products of which the simple sulfoxide (SO) and sulfone (SO_2) analogues retain activity

continued

Antipsychotic drugs (*continued*)

Drug	Half-life (h)	Elimination	Comments
Trifluoperazine	14 (7–18)	Metabolism	Given orally; oral bioavailability has not been defined (because of the absence of intravenous reference data); numerous metabolites formed
Zotepine[a]	12–24	Metabolism	Given orally; low oral bioavailability (7–13%); antagonist at $5HT_2$ and D_2 receptors; numerous metabolites formed
Zuclopenthixol (and acetate and decanoate)	20 (13–23)	Metabolism	Given orally or as deep intramuscular depot injection (acetate and decanoate); oral bioavailability (of zuclopenthixol dihydrochloride) is about 60%; the half-lives of the depot forms (acetate and decanoate) are about 19 days; zuclopenthixol is converted into numerous inactive metabolites

i.m., intramuscular; i.v., intravenous.
[a]Atypical antipsychotic.

22

Depression

Clinical depression is characterised by diverse psychological symptoms such as low mood, loss of interest and enjoyment of activities and reduced energy. It is often accompanied by a sense of guilt and worthlessness as well as physical symptoms including sleep disturbance, reduced appetite and loss of libido. If severe, there may be marked suicidal tendencies and psychotic symptoms (hallucinations and delusions). Many patients present with physical rather than psychological symptoms. The existence of mixed anxiety–depression disorder is now also well accepted.

Biological basis of depression

The cause of depression is unknown but current views centre around the monoamine receptor sensitivity hypothesis. Abnormalities in neurotransmission and receptor numbers and responsiveness to monoamines such as noradrenaline and 5-hydroxytryptamine (5HT, serotonin) in the limbic system are believed to underlie depressive disorders. There is particular evidence that reduced serotonergic neurotransmission is involved in depression. Simplistically it is hypothesised that in depression the following occur:

- low levels of monoamine transmitters
- upregulation of postsynaptic monoamine receptors
- upregulation of the presynaptic and somatodendritic autoreceptors that control monoamine release.

Correction of these abnormalities forms the basis of the actions of antidepressant drugs (Fig. 22.1).

There is a plethora of 5HT receptor subtypes in the limbic system situated presynaptically in the terminal end of the neuron ($5HT_{1D}$) and in the cell body (somatodendritic $5HT_{1A}$) and also postsynaptically ($5HT_{1A}$, $5HT_2$ (several subtypes), $5HT_3$, $5HT_4$ and others) (Fig. 22.1). Stimulation of the presynaptic cell body $5HT_{1A}$ receptor reduces 5HT release at the terminal; thus it is an autoreceptor exerting inhibitory control. Although unequivocal evidence for a primary role of these receptors in the genesis of depression is lacking, $5HT_2$ receptors in the frontal cortex of patients who committed suicide are significantly increased.

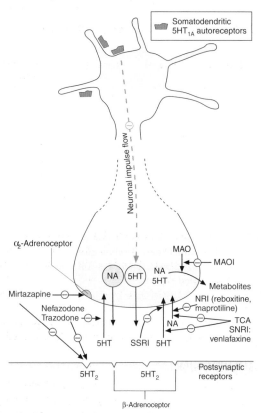

Fig. 22.1

The effect of drugs used in the treatment of depression. Some of the bewildering array of adrenergic and 5-hydroxytryptamine (5HT, serotonin), receptor subtypes are omitted for clarity. In the normal neuron, stimulation of the somatodendritic $5HT_{1A}$ autoreceptors inhibits the neuronal impulse flow in the axon and reduces 5HT release. It is hypothesised that there is a reduction in amine neurotransmission in depression resulting in upregulation of postsynaptic *and* somatodendritic receptors. Using 5HT as an example, it is considered that the depletion of 5HT results in an upregulation of postsynaptic $5HT_2$ receptors and presynaptic (somatodendritic) $5HT_{1A}$ receptors. There is now a range of antidepressants having a variety of different actions on serotonin and noradrenaline neurotransmission. It is not clear whether the different types of antidepressants have advantages in terms of their antidepressant activity. The major difference from the 'classical' TCAs is the lower incidence of sedation, antimuscarinic and antihistaminergic activities. The figure shows the sites of action of antidepressants and examples. Similar actions may occur at somatodendritic sites. TCA, 'classical' antidepressants; SSRI, selective serotonin reuptake inhibitors; SNRI, serotonin *and* noradrenaline reuptake inhibitors; NRI, (selective) noradrenaline reuptake inhibitor. Other drugs act by significantly blocking pre- and postsynaptic receptors. NA, noradrenaline; MAO, monoamine oxidase.

Reduced neurotransmission in pathways dependent on excitatory amino acids (particularly *N*-methyl-D-aspartate, NMDA) has also attracted interest in the investigation of depressive illness, while the ability of increased plasma cortisol (or corticotrophin-releasing factor) to depress serotonergic transmission in the brain may also be implicated. Additional pathogenic factors may include excessive immunological activity with production of interleukins (IL) 2 and 6 and prostaglandin E_2 (PGE_2) by central nervous system (CNS) monocytes (which differentiate into microglial cells in the brain).

These mediators may depress central monoaminergic neurotransmission.

Antidepressant drug action

Enhancement of monoamine levels

The primary action of several classes of drug used in the treatment of depression is to increase central monoaminergic transmission. However, although they rapidly increase synaptic concentrations of monoamines, clinical improvement is delayed. The delayed response is the same regardless of whether the drug increases noradrenaline or serotonin concentrations. This paradox may be explained by the observation that it requires considerable time for adaptive changes, such as downregulation of receptors, to occur in response to altered monoamine levels. The time course of downregulation of receptors more closely parallels the time course of clinical improvement.

In addition to the effects on 5HT receptors, antidepressants also enhance binding of the excitatory amino acids glycine and glutamate to the NMDA receptor complex. These changes only occur after 1–2 weeks of treatment. Effects on other pathways of neurotransmission are also possible. Upregulation of CNS glucocorticoid receptors, reduced release of IL-2 and IL-6 from CNS macrophages and decreased CNS production of PGE_2 also occur during antidepressant use.

Therefore, the therapeutic effects of drug therapy in depression may result from modulation of several central pathways of neurotransmission. See later for mechanisms of action of individual drugs.

Blockade of monoamine receptors

Several antidepressant drugs act by inhibiting noradrenaline or 5HT receptor subtypes postsynaptically, thus 'normalising' the upregulation of receptors that occurs in depression.

Inhibition of monoamine oxidase

Some antidepressants elevate monoamine levels by inhibiting their breakdown by monoamine oxidase.

Antidepressant drugs

Tricyclic antidepressant drugs and related compounds

Examples: tricyclic compounds: amitriptyline, imipramine, protriptyline, lofepramine
non-tricyclic compounds: maprotiline

Table 22.1
Comparative properties of some commonly used antidepressants that inhibit 5-hydroxytryptamine (5HT, serotonin) and noradrenaline reuptake

	Active metabolites	Uptake inhibition	Anticholinergic	Sedative	Stimulant	Epileptogenic	Toxicity in overdose
Amitriptyline	Yes	5HT > NA	+++	+++	0	++	+++
Imipramine	Yes	5HT > NA	+++	++	0	++	+++
Nortriptyline	No	NA > 5HT	++	0	+	+	++
Lofepramine	Yes	NA >> 5HT	+	+	0	0	+
Venlafaxine	Yes	NA = 5HT	0	+	0	0	+
Reboxetine	No	NA	0	0	0	0	+
Fluoxetine	No	5HT	0	0	0	0	+

+++, high risk; ++, moderate risk; +, low risk; 0, minimal risk.

Mechanism of action

The first-generation compounds in this class have a triple carbon ring structure (tricyclic antidepressants; TCAs). Many of the newer drugs are structurally unrelated to tricyclic compounds despite having a similar mechanism of action. These include bicyclic, tetracyclic and non-cyclic structures.

Most TCAs and related drugs inhibit the reuptake of monoamine neurotransmitters into the presynaptic neuron by competitive inhibition of the ATPase in the membrane pump (Fig. 22.1). Some drugs show little monoamine selectivity while other compounds are highly selective for noradrenaline (Table 22.1). However the specificity has not been shown to influence the efficacy of the drug.

A major contribution to the unwanted effects of these drugs is their ability to block other postsynaptic receptors to varying degrees (e.g. muscarinic and histamine H_1 receptors and α_1-adrenoceptors). This probably does not influence their antidepressant action.

Drugs such as mirtazapine do not block reuptake of monoamines but instead increase monoamine neurotransmission by blocking autoreceptors. Presynaptic α_2-adrenoceptors and 5-HT_{1A} receptors in the cell body are inhibited, thus reducing negative feedback control on monoamine release (Ch. 4).

Pharmacokinetics

All TCAs and related drugs are well absorbed from the gut and highly protein bound in plasma. Those with a tertiary amine structure, for example imipramine and amitriptyline, undergo extensive first-pass metabolism by demethylation in the liver. Active secondary amines such as desipramine and nortriptyline are formed and are partially responsible for the long duration of action of the parent drugs. Half-lives vary from long (for example the active metabolite of imipramine) to up to 4 days (for example protriptyline).

Unwanted effects are dose related but there is no clear dose relationship for therapeutic effects. This may reflect the considerable interindividual variability in the first-pass metabolism of most TCAs, and the difficulty in quantifying the contribution of both parent drug and active metabolites to the clinical response. Plasma concentrations of the parent drug show up to a 40-fold variation among individuals. Because of these differences, dose titration is usually necessary to optimise the therapeutic response; this should be gradual to minimise unwanted effects. However, the need for routine use of maximally tolerated doses is not universally accepted.

Unwanted effects

The incidence and nature of unwanted effects vary widely among the different drugs. In general, tertiary amine TCAs have greater α_1-adrenoceptor, histamine H_1 and cholinergic receptor blocking activity. TCAs tend to be cardiotoxic, especially in overdose. These differences are outlined in Table 22.1, which compares the profile for selected compounds.

- Sedation. Some compounds are highly sedative, for example amitriptyline, and others less so, for example imipramine. Sedation is a result of histamine H_1 receptor blockade (Ch. 38). It can be useful to help restore sleep patterns in depressed patients (using a larger dose at night) but can be troublesome or dangerous during the day. Protriptyline has mild stimulant effects: doses should be given early in the day to avoid sleep disturbance.
- Antimuscarinic effects (see Ch. 4). These are common with older drugs, especially causing dry mouth. Tolerance can occur and gradual increases in dose may reduce these problems.
- Excessive sweating and tremor. The mechanisms behind these effects are uncertain.
- Postural hypotension produced by peripheral α_1-adrenoceptor blockade (Ch. 4).
- Epileptogenic effects. Fits can be provoked even when there is no previous clinical history.
- Cardiotoxicity in overdosage. Most tricyclic drugs depress myocardial contractility or produce tachycardia and severe arrhythmias when taken in overdose. Anticholinergic effects and excessive noradrenergic stimulation both contribute to the

genesis of arrhythmias. Lofepramine appears to be the safest drug in this group after overdose.

- Weight gain. Appetite stimulation is common with tricyclic drugs.
- Sudden withdrawal syndrome. During long-term treatment, doses should be progressively reduced to avoid agitation, headache, malaise and gastrointestinal upset which accompany sudden withdrawal of treatment in some patients. This may be a result of excessive cholinergic activity following prolonged muscarinic receptor blockade.
- Hyponatraemia leading to drowsiness, confusion and convulsions. This is possibly because of inappropriate antidiuretic hormone (ADH) secretion.

Drug interactions

Several important drug interactions are recognised. TCAs potentiate the central depressant activity of many drugs, including alcohol. A dangerous interaction can result from giving a monoamine oxidase (MAO) inhibitor (MAOI; see below) and a TCA together. Potentiation arises from the prolonged action of excess serotonin released from the neuron and leads to hyperpyrexia, convulsions and coma. The long duration of MAO inhibition means that the interaction can occur up to 2 weeks after stopping an MAO inhibitor.

When TCAs are taken with drugs that prolong the Q–T interval on the electrocardiogram, and are therefore potentially arrhythmogenic (Ch. 8), the risk of serious arrhythmias is increased. Such drugs include sotalol, class I antiarrhythmics and antihistamines such as astemizole and terfenadine (Ch. 38).

Selective serotonin reuptake inhibitors and related antidepressants

Examples: fluoxetine, paroxetine, sertraline, citalopram, fluvoxamine

Mechanism of action

Unlike the tricyclic antidepressants, the selective serotonin reuptake inhibitors (SSRIs) reduce the neuronal reuptake of serotonin but have no effect on noradrenaline reuptake (Fig. 22.1). Their efficacy is similar to that of the TCAs but they have a more favourable profile of unwanted effects because of low affinity for muscarinic, histaminergic and adrenergic receptors. The hypothetical mechanism of action of SSRIs is as follows:

1. Initial increase in 5-HT concentration in the somatodendritic area and downregulation of cell body $5\text{-}HT_{1A}$ receptors.
2. As a consequence of reduced inhibitory autoreceptor activity ($5\text{-}HT_{1A}$), there is increased 5-HT release at the axon terminal. The prolonged

increase in synaptic 5-HT concentration results in downregulation of postsynaptic $5\text{-}HT_2$ receptors.

Pharmacokinetics

SSRIs are well absorbed from the gut and metabolised in the liver. Fluoxetine has a very long half-life of 2 days and that of its active metabolite norfluoxetine is 7 days. The long duration of action of fluoxetine can be a disadvantage if a MAOI is subsequently used (see below). Paroxetine has a long half-life, and citalopram a very long half-life of 1–3 days. Compared with tricyclic antidepressants, therapeutic doses of SSRIs are less likely to cause side-effects.

Unwanted effects

In contrast to the tricyclic antidepressants, SSRIs have few antimuscarinic effects, cause little sedation or weight gain and are not cardiotoxic in overdose. However, they may cause:

- nausea (can be frequent), abdominal pain or diarrhoea (less frequent)
- insomnia, anxiety and agitation
- anorexia with weight loss.

Drug interactions

The most serious interaction is with MAOIs (see tricyclic antidepressants above). An interval of 5 weeks is recommended after stopping fluoxetine before an MAOI is prescribed. Some SSRIs (especially fluoxetine) inhibit hepatic cytochrome P450 CYP2D6. When they are coprescribed with carbamazepine or phenytoin (Ch. 23) the plasma concentration of the anti-epileptic drug is increased.

Serotonin and noradrenaline reuptake inhibitors

Example: venlafaxine

Mechanism of action

Serotonin and noradrenaline reuptake inhibitors (SNRIs) have properties that place them between the tricyclic and SSRI antidepressants. Like the TCAs, they inhibit neuronal reuptake of both noradrenaline and 5HT, but they share with SSRIs a low affinity for muscarinic, histaminergic and adrenergic receptors. Their unwanted effect profile is therefore closer to that of the SSRIs than TCAs.

There is some evidence that clinical improvement with venlafaxine may begin earlier than with other antidepressant drugs.

Pharmacokinetics

Venlafaxine is rapidly absorbed from the gut and undergoes limited first-pass metabolism. The active metabolites have long half-lives. Elimination is by hepatic metabolism.

Unwanted effects

Unwanted effects are:

- somnolence
- dry mouth, nausea, constipation
- dizziness, confusion.

Selective noradrenaline reuptake inhibitors

Examples: reboxetine, maprotiline

Mechanism of action

Reboxetine and maprotiline selectively inhibit noradrenaline reuptake. Selective inhibition of noradrenaline reuptake is believed to enhance serotonergic transmission, possibly by augmenting postsynaptic $5HT_{1A}$ neurotransmission. Selective noradrenaline reuptake inhibitors (NRIs) do not affect 5HT reuptake. Reboxetine, in common with the SSRIs, has no activity at histamine H_1, muscarinic and adrenergic receptors. It has fewer cardiovascular unwanted effects than TCAs. Maprotiline also has a similar mechanism of action to reboxitine but does, however, have antimuscarinic effects and other unwanted effects similar to TCAs.

Pharmacokinetics

Reboxetine is rapidly absorbed orally with a long half-life. It is metabolised in the liver by P450 enzymes. Maprotiline is slowly but completely absorbed orally and has a long half-life. It is metabolised in the liver to an active metabolite. Neither drug inhibits MAO.

Unwanted effects

Unwanted effects are:

- insomnia
- antimuscarinic effects with maprotiline
- rashes, common with maprotiline
- sedation with maprotiline.

Specific serotonin and adrenergic receptor blocker

Example: mirtazapine

Mechanism of action

Mirtazapine is a tetracyclic piperazinoazepine unrelated to the tricyclic antidepressants. In addition to potent $5HT_2$ receptor-blocking activity, mirtazapine blocks presynaptic α_2-adrenoceptors (Fig. 22.1). Presynaptic α_2-adrenoceptors act as autoreceptors; stimulation inhibits noradrenaline release. Blockade with mirtazapine has 10-fold greater effect on central α_2-adrenoceptors than peripheral receptors. Mirtazapine blocks histamine H_1 receptors but has a low affinity for muscarinic receptors and dopaminergic receptors. Mirtazapine has minimal effects on monoamine reuptake.

Pharmacokinetics

Mirtazapine is fairly well absorbed orally with about 50% bioavailability. It is metabolised in the liver by cytochrome P450 enzymes and has a very long half-life of about 30 h.

Unwanted effects

Mirtazapine has the following unwanted effects:

- drowsiness and sedative, especially at lower doses; at higher doses, increased noradrenergic neurotransmission offsets some of the sedative effects of histamine H_1 receptor blockade
- increased appetite and weight gain.

Serotonin $5HT_2$ receptor blockers

Examples: nefazodone, trazodone

Mechanism of action

Nefazodone and trazodone are phenylpiperazines unrelated to tricyclics. A significant action of these drugs is to block $5HT_2$ postsynaptic receptors in addition to weak inhibition of presynaptic 5HT reuptake, which may also contribute to their antidepressant activity; they do not inhibit noradrenaline reuptake. Nefazodone also blocks postsynaptic α_1-adrenoceptors but not muscarinic or histamine H_1 receptors. Trazodone also blocks α_1-adrenoceptors and weakly blocks muscarinic and histamine H_1 receptors. The antidepressant activity may take several weeks to be noticeable.

Pharmacokinetics

Nefazodone is rapidly absorbed and undergoes extensive first-pass metabolism. It is metabolised to active metabolites, one of which, hydroxynefazodone, has the same profile of activity as nefazodone. The half-life is short. Trazodone is well absorbed orally and the half-life is intermediate. Liver metabolism is extensive.

Unwanted effects

Unwanted effects are less common with nefazodone than trazodone:

- sedation
- hypotension and reflex tachycardia as a result of α-adrenoceptor blockade
- nausea.

Classical (non-selective) monoamine oxidase inhibitors

Examples: phenelzine, tranylcypramine.

Mechanism of action

The mechanism of action of classical (non-selective) monoamine oxidase inhibitors (MAOIs) is complex. However, their primary action is to inhibit intracellular MAO, which is the enzyme responsible for degrading free monoamines. The accumulation of monoamine neurotransmitters in the presynaptic neuron leads to increased release when the nerve is stimulated (Fig. 22.1). Two MAO isoenzymes have been identified (Fig. 22.2). MAO-B is the predominant enzyme in many parts of the brain, but MAO-A is present in noradrenergic and serotonergic neurons, especially in the locus ceruleus and other cells of the brainstem, as well as being the main enzyme in peripheral tissues. MAO-A inhibition in the brain produces the therapeutic effects of these drugs, but classical inhibitors (MAOIs) are not selective for this isoenzyme. MAO-A inhibition in the gut wall and liver also has important consequences (see below). MAOIs also inhibit various drug-metabolising enzymes in the liver; this predisposes to drug interactions but does not contribute to clinical efficacy.

Pharmacokinetics

All drugs in this group are well absorbed from the gut. Structurally, they are either derivatives of hydrazine (e.g. phenelzine) or similar to amphetamine (e.g. tranylcypramine). They are irreversible enzyme inhibitors so the short half-lives of these drugs, as a result of extensive liver metabolism, has no influence on their duration of action. Withdrawal is followed only gradually by restoration of normal MAO activity over about 2 weeks as new enzyme is synthesised.

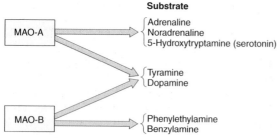

Fig. 22.2
Actions of monoamine oxidase (MAO). The relative selectivity of the substrates for MAO is shown. MAO-A is the target for drugs useful in treating depression. Non-selective inhibition of both MAO-A and MAO-B blocks the metabolism of tyramine, which is responsible for the food reaction that occurs with these drugs. Reversible inhibition of MAO (RIMA) blocks only type MAO-A. Therefore tyramine is still metabolised by type B and the food reaction is reduced.

Unwanted effects

- Compared with the TCAs, anticholinergic effects are unusual and there is no predisposition to fits.
- Postural hypotension is dose-related and, unlike the tricylic compounds, tolerance does not occur. The mechanism may involve conversion of tyramine (normally degraded by MAO) to octopamine, a false neurotransmitter which competes with noradrenaline at sympathetic nerve terminals.
- CNS stimulation with tranylcypromine leads to irritability and insomnia. These are amphetamine-like actions (Ch. 54) and doses should be given early in the day to avoid disturbing sleep. The stimulant effect of tranylcypromine makes it more hazadous than phenelzine.
- Hepatitis is a rare idiosyncratic reaction to the hydrazine derivative phenelzine.
- Acute overdose produces delayed toxic effects after some 12 h. Excessive adrenergic stimulation leads to chest pain, headache and hyperactivity, progressing to confusion and severe hypertension with eventually profound hypotension and fits.
- Food interactions can occur because MAO in the gut wall and liver usually prevents the absorption of natural amines, particularly tyramine, which is an indirect-acting sympathomimetic (Ch. 4). If food containing tyramine, for example cheese, yeast extracts (such as Bovril®, Oxo® or Marmite®), pickled herrings, chianti and caviar, or broad bean pods (which contain L-dopa), is eaten, the increased release of noradrenaline produces vasoconstriction and severe hypertension. The first indication of this is a throbbing headache. A warning card should be supplied to patients.
- A number of drug interactions can occur. Indirect-acting sympathomimetics (Ch. 4) in cold remedies (e.g. ephedrine, phenylpropanolamine) will be potentiated. Levodopa given for treatment of Parkinson's disease (Ch. 24) will also be more active. The combination of MAOIs with TCAs (see above) can be dangerous. Other important interactions are because of impaired hepatic metabolism of drugs, especially opioid analgesics.

Reversible inhibitors of monoamine oxidase A

Example: moclobemide.

Mechanism of action and effects

Moclobemide is a selective reversible inhibitor of MAO-A (RIMA). This isoenzyme is the target for the antidepressant action of classical MAOIs. If tyramine is absorbed from the gut, MAO-B is able to degrade it and the food reaction seen with classical MAOIs is very unlikely to occur. Also since the action of moclobemide on MAO-A is reversible, high concentrations of tyramine will displace the drug from the enzyme, further facilitating tyramine degradation. If moclobemide is taken after meals, then inhibition of MAO-A in the gut during absorption of tyramine will be minimised, providing further protection. Enzyme inhibition by moclobemide lasts less than 24 h after a single dose.

Pharmacokinetics

Oral absorption is good but there is substantial first-pass metabolism, partially to an active metabolite. Extensive hepatic metabolism gives a short half-life.

Unwanted effects

Unwanted effects are:

- CNS stimulation can produce sleep disturbance or agitation
- nausea
- dizziness, headache.

Drug interactions

Inhibition of cytochrome P450 activity in the liver by cimetidine (Ch. 33) substantially reduces the metabolism of moclobemide and smaller starting doses are recommended in this situation.

Lithium

Mechanism of action

The mechanism of action of lithium is not well understood. One possible sequence of events is as follows:

1. Inhibition of G-protein function, reducing the intracellular generation of cAMP in response to some monoamine neurotransmitters such as dopamine, noradrenaline (via β-adrenoceptors) or 5HT (via $5HT_{1A}$ receptors).
2. Stimulation of other G-proteins, increasing the intracellular production of diacylglycerol in response to acetylcholine (muscarinic M_1 receptors), noradrenaline (via α_1-adrenoceptors) or 5HT (via $5HT_2$ receptors).

These actions produce changes in intracellular function, with stimulation of protein kinase C and activation of K^+ channels, leading to Ca^{2+} channel opening and intracellular Ca^{2+} accumulation. However, the role of these mechanisms in the regulation of mood remains speculative.

Pharmacokinetics

Lithium is given as a salt (e.g. carbonate, citrate), which is rapidly absorbed from the gut. To avoid high peak plasma concentrations (which are associated with unwanted effects), modified-release formulations are normally used. Lithium is widely distributed in the body but enters the brain slowly. It is selectively concentrated in bone and the thyroid gland. Excretion is by glomerular filtration with 80% reabsorbed in the proximal tubule by the same mechanism as Na^+. Unlike Na^+, lithium is not reabsorbed from more distal parts of the kidney. When the body is depleted of salt and water, for example by vomiting or diarrhoea, then enhanced reabsorption of Na^+ in the proximal tubule is accompanied by lithium reabsorption which can produce acute toxicity. Lithium has a long half-life of about 1 day and has a narrow therapeutic index. Regular monitoring of plasma concentrations (which should be measured 12 h after dosing so that the absorption and distribution phases are completed) is mandatory at least every 3 months during long-term treatment.

Unwanted effects

- Nausea and diarrhoea can occur at low plasma concentrations.
- CNS effects, including tremor, giddiness, ataxia and dysarthria, occur commonly with moderate intoxication.
- Severe intoxication produces coma, convulsions, and profound hypotension with oliguria.
- Hypothyroidism caused by interference with thyroxine synthesis during long-term treatment.
- The distal renal tubule becomes less responsive to ADH. This occasionally produces reversible nephrogenic diabetes insipidus with polyuria.

Drug interactions

Diuretics can reduce lithium excretion by producing dehydration (see above). This is most marked with thiazides (Ch. 14) because of their prolonged action.

Management of depression

Drugs form only part of the management of the depressed patient but are usually necessary for moderate, severe or protracted symptoms. However, in mild to moderate depression, cognitive therapy is as effective as drug treatment. All antidepressant drugs have a delayed onset of action and severely ill patients should be considered for electroconvulsive therapy.

The TCAs or related compounds are still considered by some psychiatrists to be the drugs of choice for initial management, although other drugs such as the SSRIs are being prescribed more frequently because of their more favourable unwanted effect profile, more predictable dosages and safety in overdosage. About 70% of depressed individuals will respond to drug therapy if the dosage is adequate, compared with about half that number taking placebo. Responders show an initial improvement in sleep pattern within a few days.

Psychomotor retardation responds more gradually over several days leading to greater involvement with everyday activities and to enjoyment of life. Improvement in the depressed mood is delayed, beginning up to 2 or more weeks after treatment with adequate dosages. The response of most symptoms tends to be erratic with good and bad days.

Persuading patients to comply with treatment with TCAs may initially be difficult since antimuscarinic unwanted effects can be troublesome before any benefit is perceived. Starting with a small dose with gradual dose titration is desirable. Older TCAs have serious cardiotoxic effects when taken in overdose and should usually be avoided when treating patients who are at high risk of attempting suicide. The newer drugs, for example SSRIs, are no more effective and do not work any faster than TCAs, but they are better tolerated and safer when treating patients with a high risk of suicide.

One of the most frequent reasons for treatment failure is the use of dosages that are too small for too short a time. Treatment with adequate dosages of an antidepressant should be given for 6 weeks before the patient is considered to be a non-responder. If there is no response after this time, and the patient is believed to be compliant with treatment, then either the dose should be increased further if unwanted effects permit or an alternative drug can be substituted. Up to 15% of patients will respond to a different drug after failure of the initial treatment. If a good response occurs the dosage can usually be reduced but maintenance treatment should be continued for at least 6 months after the first episode of depression to minimise the risk of relapse. A longer period of treatment (up to 2 years) is often recommended for elderly patients. About half of all depressed patients only have a single episode. For recurrent depressive episodes a small maintenance dose of antidepressant may be effective. In recurrent illness, relapse occurs in up to 65% of patients who stop treatment within a year, but only in 15% of those who continue.

Classical MAOIs are usually reserved for atypical depression with hypochondriacal and phobic symptoms, or when TCAs have failed. The place of the newer antidepressants such as SNRIs and RIMAs in therapy is yet to be fully established. Small doses of a phenothiazine such as flupentixol (Ch. 21) are often recommended for elderly depressed patients. Evidence for a true antidepressant effect is slight, but some symptoms undoubtedly do improve.

Treatment is most difficult in severe depression, especially if there are psychotic features, or where depression forms part of a bipolar affective disorder (Ch. 21). For such patients, a combination of a TCA with an antipsychotic drug (Ch. 21) is often used. Electroconvulsive therapy is frequently very effective for severe depression, but must be combined with prolonged antidepressant drug treatment.

Lithium is reserved for patients with severe recurrent depressive episodes and for prophylaxis of those with bipolar affective disorder. The effect of lithium can take several months to become fully established.

FURTHER READING

Edwards JG (1995) Drug choice in depression. *CNS Drugs* 4, 141–159

Edwards JG, Anderson I (1999) Systematic review and guide to selection of selective serotonin reuptake inhibitors. *Drugs* 57, 507–533

Hale AS (1997) Depression. *Br Med J* 315, 43–46

Herbert J (1997) Stress, the brain, and mental illness. *Br Med J* 315, 530–535

Kent JM (2000) SNaRIs, NaSSAs, and NaRIs: new agents for the treatment of depression. *Lancet* 355, 911–918

Leonard BF (1995) Mechanisms of action of antidepressants. *CNS Drugs* 4(suppl 1), 1–12

Möller H-J, Volz H-P (1996) Drug treatment of depression in the 1990s. *Drugs* 52, 625–638

Self-assessment

In questions 1–4, the first statement, in italics, is true. Are the accompanying statements also true?

1. *Despite the fact that the monoamine hypothesis does not adequately explain all the processes of depression, alteration of monoamine transmission remains the mainstay of successful drug treatment.*

   a. Downregulation of 5-hydroxytryptamine type 2 (5HT$_2$) receptors occurs during antidepressant treatment.
   b. Most tricyclic antidepressants (TCAs) inhibit the reuptake of noradrenaline and 5HT equally.
   c. TCAs have a less satisfactory therapeutic ratio than selective serotonin (5HT) reuptake inhibitors (SSRIs).

2. *Although there are variations in responses of individuals, inhibitors of noradrenaline or 5HT reuptake are equally effective as antidepressants.*

   a. Lofepramine is more cardiotoxic than amitriptyline.
   b. Co-administration of an SSRI and a monoamine oxidase inhibitor (MAOI) can cause cardiovascular collapse.

3. *Atypical antidepressants include compounds such as trazodone; which have a different mechanism of action to the TCAs.*

   a. Trazodone is an antidepressant that is only a weak inhibitor of monoamine reuptake.
   b. Venlafaxine has marked sedative and antimuscarinic actions.
   c. Venlafaxine requires longer than most antidepressants to produce clinical improvement.

4. *During antidepressant treatment only 30–40% of patients improve as a result of the drug*

   a. Tricyclic antidepressants potentiate the central depressant effects of alcohol.
   b. The half-life of lithium is about 30 min.
   c. Lithium is only used in patients with bipolar effective disorder.

5. Case history question

DW is a 30-year-old female financier, and a former Olympic athlete. In 1994 she was appointed manager of the Emerging Countries Fund of a large Unit Trust Company. In early 1996 the Company was taken over and DW had a new boss and was moved to assistant manager of the Fund. From 1994 to 1996 she had put on 10 kg in weight, and in January 1996 started a strict diet and worked out at a gym four times a week. In June 1996 she visited her GP with a 6 month history of increasing insomnia, lack of concentration, irritability and anxiety. She had begun to withdraw from a busy social calendar and was becoming indecisive. This was now affecting her work. For the last 4 weeks she has recurrent thoughts of suicide. She had also lost 4 kg in weight during that period. The GP diagnosed that she was depressed, arranged a psychiatric consultation for her and started her on a tricyclic antidepressant (TCA).

   a. What are the causes of depression?
   b. What are the risk factors for depression; was DW at risk prior to the diagnosis.
   c. What neurochemical and receptor changes are associated with depressive illness.
   d. Are TCAs an appropriate first choice of drug for this patient?
   e. What are the unwanted effects of TCAs?
   f. How successful is antidepressant treatment? After therapy for 3 months and some improvement, DW decided that the side-effects of the TCAs were unacceptable. What alternative antidepressant therapies could be given and what are the unwanted effects?

The answers are provided on pages 613–614.

Antidepressant drugs[a]

Drug	Half-life (h)	Elimination	Comments
Tricyclic antidepressants and related compounds			Most show high apparent volumes of distribution (10–50 l kg^{-1}), which explains the combination of high first-pass metabolism and high clearance with a long half-life
Amitriptyline	10–28	Metabolism	Bioavailability is 30–60%; oxidised by hepatic CYP3A4 mediated demethylation to nortriptyline (see below) which has a slightly longer half-life
Amoxapine	8–14	Metabolism	Bioavailability is 18–54%; metabolised to the 7-, and 8-hydroxy compounds which are eliminated as conjugates; 8-hydroxyamoxapine is active and has a longer half-life (30 h) and is present at two-fold greater concentrations than amoxapine during repeated dosage
Clomipramine	12–36	Metabolism	Given orally or by intramuscular injection or intravenous infusion; oral bioavailability is about 50%; oxidised by demethylation followed by hydroxylation and conjugation; selective and potent inhibitor of 5HT uptake
Dosulepin (dothiepin)	11–40	Metabolism	Absolute bioavailability has not been defined; oxidised by demethylation and S-oxidation
Doxepin	8–25	Metabolism	Bioavailability is about 30%; extensive demethylation in the liver; desmethyl metabolite retains some activity
Imipramine	8–20	Metabolism	Bioavailability is about 50%; metabolised by demethylation to an active metabolite (desipramine) and by hydroxylation; desipramine is metabolised by CYP2D6
Lofepramine	5	Metabolism	Absolute bioavailability not known; metabolised to desmethylimipramine, which is probably responsible for much of the activity; few data available
Maprotiline	30–60	Metabolism	Tetracyclic compound; oral bioavailability is 40–70%; extensively metabolised with metabolites eliminated in urine and bile
Mianserin	10–20	Metabolism	Tetracyclic compound; oral bioavailability is 20–30%; major metabolite is desmethyl compound (demethylation product) which has weak α_2-adrenoceptor agonist properties
Nortriptyline	18–60	Metabolism	Bioavailability is 50–60%; oxidised by CYP2D6 to a 10-hydroxy metabolite (which retains some activity) that is conjugated and excreted
Protriptyline	50–200	Metabolism	Bioavailability is 75–90%; undergoes extensive oxidation with the metabolites eliminated in urine
Trazodone	7–13	Metabolism	Tetracyclic compound; complete oral bioavailability (100%); rapidly metabolised by CYP3A4 oxidation to an active metabolite (that has higher plasma concentrations than the parent compound)
Trimipramine	7–23	Metabolism	Bioavailability is 40%; metabolised by demethylation and hydroxylation; activity of desmethyl metabolite is not known
Viloxazine	2–5	Metabolism	Bicyclic compound; good absorption (bioavailability 85%); few data available
Selective serotonin (5HT) reuptake inhibitors (SSRIs)			
Citalopram	23–75	Metabolism	Oral bioavailability is 80%; oxidised in liver by cytochrome P450 to a range of metabolites some of which retain weak activity; weak inhibitor of, but not a substrate for, CYP2D6
Fluoxetine	48–72	Metabolism	Essentially complete bioavailability; metabolised by CYP2D6; poor metabolisers have a two-fold longer half-life and excrete more of the parent compound in the urine; the major desmethyl metabolite (norfluoxetine) is as active as the parent drug and has a longer half-life (6 days); both parent drug and metabolite are potent inhibitors of CYP2D6 (which metabolises desipramine)
Fluvoxamine	7–70 (mean 15)	Metabolism	High oral bioavailability (absolute bioavailability is not known); extensively metabolised by oxidation (not by CYP2D6)

continued

Antidepressant drugs[a] *(continued)*

Drug	Half-life (h)	Elimination	Comments
Selective serotonin (5HT) reuptake inhibitors (SSRIs) *(continued)*			
Paroxetine	10–20 (EM), 30–50 (PM)	Metabolism	Good but variable absorption; eliminated by CYP2D6 catalysed oxidation; the half-life in poor metabolisers (PM) is longer than in extensive metabolisers (EM); the metabolites are inactive; during repeated dosage the steady-state plasma concentrations are similar in EM and PM subjects because CYP2D6 is saturated in both groups, and other non-saturable enzymes determine the clearance
Sertraline	26	Metabolism	Oral bioavailability is low and increased if given with food (absolute bioavailability is not known); undergoes demethylation and oxidation to largely inactive metabolites
Serotonin and noradrenaline reuptake inhibitors (SNRIs)			
Venlafaxine	5	Metabolism	High oral bioavailability (>90%); oxidised by hepatic CYP2D6 to the active *O*-desmethyl metabolite which is responsible for much of the therapeutic activity and has a longer half-life (11 h); other minor metabolites, such as *N*-desmethyl- are inactive
Classical (non-selective) monoamine oxidase inhibitors (MAOIs)			
Isocarboxazid	2–3	Metabolism	Essentially complete bioavailability; rapidly hydrolysed by esterases; duration of action is measured in days; slow onset of clinical action (weeks)
Phenelzine	1	Metabolism	Extensively absorbed; rapidly metabolised by *N*-acetylation; produces profound and prolonged inhibition of MAO with a slow onset of clinical action (weeks)
Tranylcypromine	2–3	Metabolism	Extensively absorbed; metabolised by oxidation, *N*-acetylation and *N*-glucuronidation (rare reaction); onset of action is more rapid than the other drugs in this group
Reversible inhibitors of monoamine oxidase-A (RIMAs)			
Moclobemide	1–2	Metabolism	Bioavailability is about 50%; numerous metabolites formed; metabolised by CYP2C19 (CYP2C19 metabolises mephenytoin); poor metabolisers of mephenytoin (low CYP2C19) have a half-life of moclobemide which is 4 h, compared with 2 h in extensive metabolisers of mephenytoin (high CYP2C19)
Other antidepressant drugs			
Flupentixol (flupenthixol)			Antipsychotic drug given orally for depression (Ch. 21)
Lithium	8–45	Renal	Complete oral absorption; filtered at the glomerular and reabsorbed (about 80%) in the proximal, but not distal, parts of the renal tubule
Mirtazapine	20–40	Metabolism	Principal action is inhibition of central presynaptic α_2-adrenoceptors and blocking of postsynaptic $5HT_2$ receptors; bioavailability is about 50%; metabolised by oxidation followed by glucuronidation; metabolised by CYP2D6 and CYP3A4

continued

Antidepressant drugs[a] *(continued)*

Drug	Half-life (h)	Elimination	Comments
Other antidepressant drugs (continued)			
Nefazodone	3–10	Metabolism	A structural analogue of trazodone (tetracyclic); inhibits postsynaptic $5HT_2$ receptors, and weakly inhibits presynaptic 5HT uptake with little effect on noradrenaline uptake; low bioavailability (15–20%) because of first-pass metabolism; undergoes numerous pathways of oxidative metabolism
Reboxetine	15	Metabolism (+ renal)	Selective inhibitor of noradrenaline uptake; complete oral bioavailability; oxidised by hepatic CYP3A4 plus some renal clearance (10%)
Tryptophan	2	Metabolism	Actively absorbed from the intestinal tract and transported across the blood:brain barrier (in competition with other amino acids); undergoes decarboxylation and deamination

[a] All drugs given orally unless otherwise stated; they are all lipid soluble and well absorbed but many undergo extensive first-pass metabolism, which limits their bioavailability.

23

Epilepsy

Pathological basis of epilepsy

All epilepsies are characterised by sudden and transient episodes of motor, sensory, autonomous or psychic disturbance. These are usually triggered by abnormal electrical discharges in the brain. Epileptic fits present in several different forms depending on the site of the discharge and whether the discharge remains localised, or spreads (Table 23.1). Identification of the type of seizure is useful as a guide to treatment.

The origin of epilepsy is complex. In some patients, structural damage can be identified in the brain, such as that resulting from trauma or haemorrhage, but in most patients there is probably a genetic component. In some cases it may be caused by metabolic events such as hypoglycaemia or by alcohol abuse, in which case treatment should be for the underlying cause.

Neurotransmitters and epilepsy

Coordinated activity among neurons depends on a controlled balance between excitatory and inhibitory influences on the electrical activity across the cell membrane. The pathophysiology of epilepsy probably involves a local imbalance among these factors, which leads to a focus of neuronal instability.

A reduction in the activity of membrane-bound ATPases linked to neuronal transmembrane ion pumps has been found in the brains of epileptic patients. A defect in those pumps that exchange Na^+ and K^+ or extrude Ca^{2+} from the cell will reduce the transmembrane electrical potential until the threshold potential in the cell is reached. This process could initiate the burst of firing that produces epileptiform activity. Once an electrical discharge is triggered, spontaneous repetitive firing of the focus is maintained by a feedback mechanism known as post-tetanic potentiation.

There is additional evidence that activity in the inhibitory gamma-aminobutyric acid (GABA)-ergic neurons is reduced in epilepsy. The involvement of other mediators such as adenosine or enkephalins remains speculative.

Most anti-epileptic drugs act either by blockade of neuronal Na^+ channels (thus reducing the likelihood of depolarisation) or by enhancing the inhibitory actions of GABA.

Table 23.1
Simplified classification of epileptic seizures

Seizure type	Characteristics
Partial (focal) seizures	
Simple partial seizures	Motor, somatosensory or psychic symptoms; consciousness is not impaired
Complex partial seizures	Temporal lobe, psychomotor; consciousness is impaired
Secondary generalised seizures	These begin as partial seizures
Generalised seizures	Affect whole brain with loss of consciousness
Clonic, tonic, or tonic–clonic	Initial rigid extensor spasm, respiration stops, defecation, micturition and salivation occur (tonic phase, ~ 1 min); violent synchronous jerks (clonic phase, 2–4 min),
Myoclonic	Seizures of a muscle or group of muscles
Absence	Abrupt loss of awareness of surroundings, little motor disturbance (occur in children)
Atonic	Loss of muscle tone/strength
Unclassified seizures	

Antiepileptic drugs

Sodium valproate

Mechanism of action and uses

Sodium valproate has a wide spectrum of activity and is effective for all forms of epilepsy. It produces use-dependent blockade of transmembrane Na^+ channels, thus stabilising neuronal membranes. It also facilitates the action of the inhibitory amino acid GABA, although the mechanism by which it achieves this is unknown. The full benefit of treatment may be delayed by several weeks. Sodium valproate is also used for the prophylaxis of migraine (Ch. 26) and in the management of neuropathic pain (Ch. 19).

Pharmacokinetics

Sodium valproate is well absorbed from the gut. To reduce the risks of gastric upset, conventional tablets should be taken with food or enteric-coated tablets can be given. Protein binding of sodium valproate is high in plasma, but the proportion of free (and therefore active) drug rises with increasing blood concentration of the drug. The drug concentration in plasma does not correlate well with therapeutic effect and routine monitoring of blood concentrations is only useful to assess compliance or to avoid toxicity. Sodium valproate is extensively metabolised in the liver and the half-life is long. The dose should be increased slowly to minimise unwanted effects.

Unwanted effects

Sodium valproate has a number of unwanted effects:

- gastrointestinal upset: nausea, vomiting, anorexia, abdominal pain (which can be caused by pancreatitis) and bowel disturbance
- weight gain caused by appetite stimulation
- transient hair loss
- tremor (dose related)
- thrombocytopenia
- rarely, severe hepatotoxicity, especially in children under age 3 years receiving multiple drug therapy for seizures
- teratogenicity (see below)
- inhibition of hepatic drug-metabolising enzymes
- interactions with other antiepileptic drugs (discussed below).

Carbamazepine and oxcarbazepine

Mechanism of action and uses

Carbamazepine and oxcarbazepine are used in all types of epilepsy except myoclonic epilepsy or absences, which may be exacerbated. Inhibition of repetitive neuronal firing is produced by reduction of transmembrane Na^+ influx, by use-dependent blockade of Na^+ channels. They also used in the management of neuropathic pain (Ch. 19).

Pharmacokinetics

Absorption of carbamazepine is slow and incomplete after oral administration. The major epoxide metabolite, which is produced in the liver, is also active but present in lower concentrations than the parent drug. The half-life of carbamazepine is initially very long at about 1.5 days but decreases by two-thirds over the first 2 to 3 weeks of treatment because of 'autoinduction' of its own metabolising enzymes in the liver. Seizure control may then require an increase in dose. During long-term therapy the half-life is extremely variable among individuals. The plasma or salivary concentration of carbamazepine correlates well with its clinical efficacy, but substantial fluctuations in plasma concentration between doses make interpretation of a single value difficult. A modified-release formulation is available that minimises the transient neurological adverse effects which can occur in association with the peak plasma drug concentration when using the standard formulation.

Oxcarbazepine is well absorbed orally and rapidly converted to an active metabolite 10-monohydroxy oxcarbazepine, which has an intermediate half life and is largely excreted by the kidney after conjugation in the liver.

Unwanted effects

The nature of unwanted effects with carbamazepine and oxcarbazepine are similar, but they are less frequent and severe with oxcarbazepine.

- Nausea and vomiting can occur especially early in treatment.
- Central nervous system (CNS) toxicity leads to double vision, dizziness, drowsiness. Ataxia occurs at high doses.
- Transient leucopenia is common, especially early in treatment, but severe bone marrow depression is rare.
- Hyponatraemia is caused by potentiation of the action of antidiuretic hormone, which can lead to confusion and decreased control of seizures.
- Teratogenicity is common especially with carbamazepine (see below).
- Induction of hepatic drug-metabolising enzymes with carbamazepine (Ch. 2). The most common interaction is with the oral contraceptive pill. To avoid failure of contraception, the dose of estrogen should be increased. The metabolism of warfarin and ciclosporin are also accelerated. Interactions of carbamazepine with other antiepileptic drugs are discussed below. Oxcarbazepine produces little induction of cytochrome P450 and therefore has fewer drug interactions than carbamazepine.

Phenytoin and fosphenytoin

Mechanism of action and effects

Phenytoin and its analogue fosphenytoin have a wide spectrum of activity and are effective against all forms of epilepsy except absences. Phenytoin produces use-dependent blockade of Na^+ channels, inhibiting Na^+ influx across the cell membrane and therefore reduces cell excitability. Phenytoin is also used in the management of neuropathic pain (Ch. 19) and occasionally for cardiac arrhythmias (Ch. 5).

Pharmacokinetics

Phenytoin is well but slowly absorbed from the gut. Slow intravenous injection can be used if a rapid onset of action is needed. Intramuscular injections of phenytoin should be avoided since absorption by this route is erratic and unpredictable and muscle damage can occur. By contrast, fosphenytoin is well absorbed after intramuscular injection and it can also be given intravenously. Extensive metabolism by liver microsomal enzymes is responsible for elimination of phenytoin. However, the enzyme is saturable at plasma drug con-

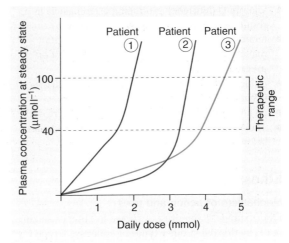

Fig. 23.1
Increasing the daily dose of phenytoin results in marked interindividual variation in plasma concentrations of phenytoin at steady state. The figure illustrates the types of relationships between dose and plasma concentration that can be seen in three patients. The non-linear relationship within the desired therapeutic range leads to difficulties in dosage adjustment.

centrations near the lower end of the therapeutic range. Once the enzyme is saturated the pharmacokinetics then change from first order (linear) kinetics to zero order (Ch. 2; Fig. 23.1). Therefore, when the plasma concentration is close to, or within, the therapeutic range a small change in dose produces a large change in plasma concentration. Once the metabolising enzymes are saturated, the elimination half-life is lengthened fourfold to almost 2 days. Plasma phenytoin concentrations are closely related to effect and their measurement is useful as a guide to dosing. Assay of salivary phenytoin concentration only measures free drug and can be useful if protein binding is altered (e.g. pregnancy, renal failure) or in children. Phenytoin is highly protein bound and can be displaced by valproate and salicylates, which therefore enhance the effect of phenytoin to an unpredictable extent.

Unwanted effects

Most unwanted effects of these drugs are dose related:

- impaired brainstem and cerebellar function producing nystagmus, double vision, vertigo, ataxia, dysarthria, drowsiness, cognitive impairment
- chronic connective tissue effects: gum hyperplasia, coarsening of facial features and hirsutism (for this reason it is usual to avoid phenytoin in young women)
- skin rashes including acne
- folate deficiency producing megaloblastic anaemia with a macrocytic blood picture (this may be because folate is used as a cofactor by enzymes that are induced by phenytoin)

- vitamin D deficiency producing osteomalacia as a result of increased vitamin D metabolism
- teratogenic effects, including facial and digital malformations; these can occur in up to 10% of pregnancies
- induction of hepatic drug-metabolising enzymes (Chapter 2)
- metabolism of warfarin and ciclosporin increased
- interactions with other anticonvulsants, discussed below.

Ethosuximide

Mechanism of action and uses

Ethosuximide is the drug of choice in absence seizures but is ineffective in other types of epilepsy. T-type Ca^{2+} channels probably contribute to the generation of thalamocortical activity in absence seizures and ethosuximide is thought to inhibit these channels.

Pharmacokinetics

Absorption of ethosuximide from the gut is almost complete. Metabolism in the liver is extensive and the half-life is very long at 2 to 3 days. Plasma and salivary drug concentrations correlate well with control of seizures and can be used to monitor treatment.

Unwanted effects

Ethosuximide can cause:

- nausea, vomiting, anorexia (less frequent if the drug is taken with food and if the dose is gradually increased)
- teratogenicity
- drowsiness and headaches.

Phenobarbital and primidone

Mechanism of action and effects

The major effect of phenobarbital and primidone is prolongation of the opening time of postsynaptic neuronal transmembrane Cl⁻ channels. This effect is independent of the presence of the inhibitory amino acid GABA, which has a similar action, but phenobarbital will also potentiate the effect of GABA (Ch. 20). The action of primidone is a result partly of its conversion to phenobarbital. These drugs have a wide spectrum of activity and are effective in most forms of epilepsy.

Pharmacokinetics

Oral absorption of phenobarbital is almost complete. Elimination is by hepatic metabolism and renal excretion, with up to 40% excreted unchanged in the urine. The half-life is very long, ranging between 2 and 6 days.

Primidone is well absorbed orally and converted in the liver to two active metabolites, phenobarbital and phenylethylmalonamide, producing rather more of the former. Enzyme induction increases the conversion to phenobarbital. Primidone has no advantage over phenobarbital and is less well tolerated.

The plasma concentrations of phenobarbital and primidone relate poorly to control of seizures; they are only useful as a guide to compliance with treatment. Control of seizures or unwanted effects should determine dosages.

Unwanted effects

Phenobarbital has a number of unwanted effects:

- CNS effects: sedation and fatigue are common in adults, hyperactivity and aggression can occur in children; poor memory and depression are also seen
- nausea and vomiting (especially after the first dose of primidone)
- tolerance to both toxic and therapeutic effects tends to occur during long-term administration
- dependence with a physical withdrawal reaction is seen after long-term treatment.
- teratogenicity (see below)
- induction of hepatic drug-metabolising enzymes (Ch. 2) leads to increased metabolism of warfarin, ciclosporin and estrogen (reducing the effectiveness of oral contraception)
- interactions with other antiepileptic drugs, considered below.

Vigabatrin

Mechanism of action and uses

Vigabatrin is only used for epilepsy that is resistant to other drug therapy but it is useful as a potential adjunct in all types of epilepsy. Vigabatrin is a structural analogue of GABA and produces irreversible inhibition of GABA transaminase (GABA-T), which inactivates GABA. The increase in CNS concentrations of GABA inhibits the spread of epileptic discharges.

Pharmacokinetics

Vigabatrin is rapidly absorbed from the gut and excreted unchanged by the kidney. The half-life is intermediate, but irreversible binding to the target enzyme results in a long duration of action which is unrelated to the plasma drug concentration. Blood concentration monitoring is therefore of no value.

Unwanted effects

Vigabatrin can cause:

- sedation and fatigue
- psychotic reactions, especially in patients with a history of psychiatric disorder
- severe peripheral visual field defects during prolonged use (monitoring is recommended)
- weight gain.

Lamotrigine

Mechanism of action and uses

Lamotrigine is believed to inhibit neuronal Na^+ currents in a use-dependent manner. It has a wide spectrum of efficacy for partial and generalised seizures.

Pharmacokinetics

Lamotrigine is well absorbed orally and extensively metabolised in the liver. The half-life is long.

Unwanted effects

Lamotrigine causes:

- nausea, vomiting
- skin rashes: some disappear despite continued treatment; occasionally severe skin reactions occur
- CNS effects: headache, dizziness, double vision and ataxia; tremor can be troublesome at high dosages.

Gabapentin

Mechanism of action and uses

The major use of gabapentin is in partial seizures. Although designed as a structural analogue of GABA, gabapentin does not mimic GABA in the brain although it may enhance its effects. Binding sites for gabapentin are present in the superficial neocortex and hippocampus, but how these produce an anticonvulsant effect is unclear.

Pharmacokinetics

Gabapentin is incompletely absorbed from the gut and excreted unchanged by the kidney. It has a short half-life.

Unwanted effects

CNS effects can occur including drowsiness, dizziness, ataxia, fatigue and diplopia.

Topiramate

Mechanism of action and uses

Topiramate is used as an add-on treatment for drug-resistant partial or generalised seizures. The mechanism of action is not fully understood. The drug blocks Na^+ channels, and also enhances the action of GABA, by binding to a modulatory site on the receptor complex distinct from that for benzodiazepines. It is possibly also an antagonist at the kainite subtype of receptor for the excitatory amino acid glutamate.

Pharmacokinetics

Topiramate is rapidly absorbed orally and undergoes limited metabolism in the liver. The main route of elimination is the kidney. The half-life is long.

Unwanted effects

Topiramate can cause:

- CNS effects including cognitive difficulty, tremor, dizziness, ataxia, and headache
- gastrointestinal upset.

Tiagabine

Mechanism of action and uses

Tiagabine is currently used as an adjunctive therapy for partial seizures. It decreases neuronal and astrocyte uptake of the inhibitory amino acid GABA. This is the mechanism that limits the activity of GABA in the brain. The increase in synaptic GABA accounts for the antiepileptic actions of tiagabine.

Pharmacokinetics

Tiagabine is well absorbed from the gut. It is metabolised in the liver by P450 CYP3A and has an intermediate half life.

Unwanted effects

Tiagabine can cause:

- dizziness
- lethargy, somnolence.

Benzodiazepines

Examples: clonazepam, diazepam, clobazam

Mechanism of action and uses

These drugs enhance the action of the inhibitory neurotransmitter GABA (Ch. 20). Clonazepam and clobazam are used orally for prophylaxis, usually as an adjunct to other drugs, whereas diazepam can be used intravenously or rectally to control individual fits.

Pharmacokinetics

These are long-acting benzodiazepines. Their pharmacokinetics are considered fully in Chapter 20.

Unwanted effects

These are discussed in Chapter 20. Partial or complete tolerance to the anti-epileptic action of benzodiazepines often occurs after about 4 to 6 months of continuous treatment.

Drug interactions among anticonvulsants

Since many antiepileptics affect drug-metabolising enzymes in the liver, interactions are frequent. They have major clinical implications for seizure control or toxicity when two or more antiepileptics are used together. Plasma drug concentration monitoring is often advisable when more than one drug is used.

Sodium valproate. Inhibition of hepatic drug metabolism often increases the plasma concentrations of phenobarbital and lamotrigine as well as those of an active metabolite of carbamazepine. Sodium valproate can displace phenytoin from plasma protein binding sites but also inhibits the metabolism of phenytoin. The net result is a reduction in total plasma phenytoin concentration but an increase in the active free component.

Carbamazepine. This hepatic enzyme inducer often lowers the plasma concentrations of carbamazepine, clonazepam, lamotrigine, tiagabine, topiramate, sodium valproate and the active metabolite of oxcarbazepine.

Phenytoin. This is also a hepatic enzyme inducer and it often lowers the plasma concentrations of carbamazepine, clonazepam, lamotrigine, tiagabine, topiramate, sodium valproate and the active metabolite of oxcarbazepine.

Phenobarbital and primidone. These hepatic enzyme inducers often lower the plasma concentration of carbamazepine, clonazepam, lamotrigine, tiagabine, phenytoin, sodium valproate and the active metabolite of oxcarbazepine.

Vigabatrin. This drug reduces plasma phenytoin concentration by an unknown mechanism.

Management of epilepsy

Treatment of individual seizures

Prolonged or repetitive seizures (status epilepticus) usually require urgent parenteral drug treatment. Particular attention must also be given to maintaining the airway and ensuring adequate oxygenation. Diazepam is the drug of choice and is given either intravenously or as a rectal solution (particularly useful for children) with close observation for signs of drug-induced respiratory depression. Intravenous phenytoin is an alternative choice and can be given if diazepam is ineffective or to prevent recurrence after initial control of the seizure is achieved. Alternative treatments that can be useful in status epilepticus are intravenous clonazepam, phenobarbital or chlomethiazole. If seizures are not controlled with these measures then full anaesthesia with assisted respiration in an intensive care unit will be necessary.

Prophylaxis for seizures

A diagnosis of epilepsy requires two or more spontaneous seizures. After a single event up to 80% of patients will have a second fit within 3 years. If a predisposing cause cannot be identified and avoided (e.g. alcohol withdrawal, photosensitive epilepsy precipitated by viewing a television from too close a distance), drug treatment will usually be recommended after a second fit unless the fits were separated by very long intervals, or were mild.

Treatment should begin with a single drug, the choice depending on the type of epilepsy and relative toxicity of the drugs (Table 23.2). If the type of epilepsy is uncertain then sodium valproate is often recommended since it has the broadest spectrum of activity. If fits are not controlled with the first choice drug, it becomes more important to accurately identify the type of seizure. A second single drug should then be tried while the first is gradually withdrawn (Table 23.2). A single drug will usually control fits in up to 90% of people with epilepsy, although this may not be achieved with the first drug chosen. Refractory epilepsy can indicate poor compliance, inappropriate drug choice or that the fits are 'pseudo seizures' rather than true epilepsy. Multiple drug treatment (e.g. with two first-line, or a first- and a second-line drug) should be reserved for patients resistant to two or three drugs used alone. Drugs like vigabatrin, gabapentin or topiramate are only used in combination with other agents.

It is not usually necessary to monitor plasma drug concentrations to determine whether the drug concentration is within the 'therapeutic range' unless seizure control is poor, or if poor compliance or drug toxicity are suspected. Many patients will achieve good seizure control at plasma drug concentrations that are below the accepted therapeutic range and an increase in dosage will not be necessary unless there are recurrent fits. Conversely, other patients who continue to have fits may need plasma drug concentrations above the standard therapeutic range to achieve control, provided there is no evidence of toxic effects. The only drug for which monitoring is of proven benefit for dosage adjustment is phenytoin. Adjustment of the dosages of carbamazepine or ethosuximide may be easier if the plasma concentration is known, but for other drugs monitoring is of value only to confirm that the drug is being taken.

Once started, treatment should usually be continued for at least 2 to 3 years after the last fit. If there is a continuing predisposing condition or the patient wishes to drive (in the UK, a driving licence is revoked until the patient has been fit-free for 1 year, or has only suffered nocturnal fits for 3 years), treatment should probably be life-long. If withdrawal is undertaken it should be gradual to minimise the risk of rebound fits.

Prophylaxis for fits is often given following neurosurgical procedures or head injury (particularly if there was a depressed skull fracture or an associated intracranial haematoma) for up to 3 months. However, the evidence that such routine use is beneficial is not secure.

Table 23.2
Drug choice in the treatment of epilepsy

Type of seizure	First-line drugs	Second-line drugs
Partial seizures	Carbamazepine, or phenytoin, or valproate[a]	Phenobarbital/primidone[b] Clonazepam/clobazam[b] Gabapentin[b] (as adjunct) Lamotrigine[b] Vigabatrin[b] (as adjunct) Topiramate[b] (as adjunct)
Generalised seizures Tonic–clonic (grand mal)	Valproate, or carbamazepine or phenytoin[a]	Phenobarbital/primidone[b] Lamotrigine[b] Vigabatrin[b] (as adjunct)
Myoclonic	Valproate[a]	Clonazepam[b] Ethosuximide[c]
Absence	Ethosuximide[c] or valproate	Clonazepam[b] Lamotrigine[b]
Atonic	Valproate[a]	Phenytoin[a] Lamotrigine[b] Clonazepam[b] Ethosuximide[c] Phenobarbital[b]

Valproate, sodium valproate.
[a]Blocks Na^+ channels.
[b]Enhances gamma-aminobutyric acid activity.
[c]Inhibits T-type Ca^{2+} channels.

Febrile convulsions occur commonly in infancy and usually do not lead to epilepsy or produce CNS damage. About 4% of children have them and they recur in about one-third. Measures to reduce pyrexia during febrile episodes are essential, for example removal of clothes and use of paracetamol (Ch. 29). Routine prophylaxis with antiepileptic drugs is not recommended, but rectal diazepam is sometimes given when a child who has previously had a febrile convulsion becomes pyrexial.

Anticonvulsants in pregnancy

No anticonvulsant has a proven safety record in pregnancy and many carry a high risk of teratogenesis if the fetus is exposed in the first trimester. Fetal abnormalities are most frequent if more than one drug is used. Neural tube defects are particularly common with carbamazepine and sodium valproate (1–2% of pregnancies) and other developmental abnormalities occur with phenytoin. Women taking antiepileptic drugs who wish to become pregnant should be counselled about the risk and offered antenatal screening during pregnancy with α-fetoprotein measurement (to detect neural tube defects) and ultrasound scanning. Folic acid supplements may reduce the risk of neural tube defects. Of all the anticonvulsant drugs, cautious optimism has been expressed for the lack of teratogenicity with lamotrigine.

It is important to advise a potential mother with epilepsy that the risks of uncontrolled fits during pregnancy, both to her and to the fetus, may be greater than the risk associated with drug therapy.

FURTHER READING

Anon (1998) Consensus Statements: medical management of epilepsy. *Neurology* 51(suppl 4), S39–S43

Beghi E, Perucca, E (1995) The management of epilepsy in the 1990s. *Drugs* 49, 680–694

Bourgeois BFD (1998) New anti-epileptic drugs. *Arch Neurol* 55, 1181–1183

Brodie MJ, Dichter MA (1996) Antiepileptic drugs. *N Engl J Med* 334, 168–175

Brodie MJ, French JA (2000) Management of epilepsy in adolescents and adults. *Lancet* 356, 323–329

Dichter MA, Brodie MJ (1996) New antiepileptic drugs. *N Engl J Med* 334, 1583–1590

Eadie MJ (1997) The single seizure. To treat or not to treat? *Drugs* 54, 651–656

Feely M (1999) Drug treatment of epilepsy. *Br Med J* 318, 106–109

Leach JP, Brodie MJ (1998) Tiagabine. *Lancet* 351, 203–207

Lowenstein DH, Alldredge BK (1998) Status epilepticus. *N Engl J Med* 338, 970–976

Neville BRG (1997) Epilepsy in childhood. *Br Med J* 315, 924–930

Nulman I, Laslo D, Koren G (1999) Treatment of epilepsy in pregnancy. *Drugs* 59, 525–533

Self-assessment

In questions 1–6, the first statement, in italics, is true. Are the accompanying statements also true?

1. *Generalised seizures involving the whole brain include tonic–clonic seizures (grand mal) and absences (petit mal).*
   Absences occur mainly in adults.

2. *Partial (or focal) seizures are localised and can involve motor, sensory or psychic symptoms without loss of consciousness.*
   In partial seizures, generalised muscle contractions do not occur.

3. *The excitatory amino acid glutamate acting on NMDA (N-methyl-D-aspartate) receptors is increased in some seizures and can lead to excitotoxic damage to cells.*
   a. Control of glutamate is an important approach to current drug therapy.
   b. Gamma-aminobutyric acid (GABA) is useful for treating epilepsy by decreasing Na⁺ influx.

4. *The two main mechanisms by which drugs act as anticonvulsants is to inhibit Na⁺ channel actions and enhance the activity of GABA.*
   The effect of phenytoin diminishes with long-term use.

5. *Phenytoin is highly protein bound.*
   a. Salicylates and sodium valproate reduce the effectiveness of phenytoin.
   b. The plasma concentration of phenytoin varies in a linear manner with the dose administered over the whole therapeutic dose range.

6. *The abrupt withdrawal of anti-epileptics should be avoided.*
   Vigabatrin is a first-line drug for the treatment of all types of epilepsy.

7. Case history 1

A 7-year-old boy is described as dreamy by his mother. He is making slow progress at school and his mother and teachers both comment that he cannot concentrate and has frequent episodes of staring vacantly for a few seconds and then carrying on as normal. Following an electroencephalogram (EEG), a synchronous discharge characteristic of petit mal or absence form of epilepsy was demonstrated.

a. Which of the following drugs would you prescribe: phenytoin, phenobarbital, sodium valproate, ethosuximide?
b. What are the major relevant unwanted effects of those drugs you should have prescribed in this child?
c. If control of absence seizures is inadequate with your chosen antiepileptic, can combination therapy be given?

8. Case history 2

A 19-year-old woman has a long-term history of epilepsy of the complex partial seizure type, which often gravitates to generalised seizures. For several years her epilepsy has been well controlled with a stable drug regimen. She is seeking advise on contraception.

a. What anti-epileptic drugs might be effective in the type of epilepsy this patient has?
b. What suitable options are available for contraception?
c. What potential problems can arise if the patient takes the oral combined contraceptive?
d. Would an injected progestogen contraceptive be worth considering?
e. If the oral combined contraceptive is the chosen method, what strategies should be adopted?
f. Would the progestogen-only pill be a suitable method of contraception?

The answers are provided on pages 614–615.

Drugs used for epilepsy

Drug	Half-life (h)	Elimination	Comments
Epilepsy			
Acetazolamide	6–9	Renal	Low efficacy; second-line drug only
Carbamazepine	30–40	Metabolism	Good oral bioavailability; epoxide metabolite has anticonvulsant actions
Clobazam	10–50	Metabolism	N-desmethyl metabolite is active and plasma concentrations are 5–10 times those of the parent drug
Clonazepam	18–45	Metabolism	Oral bioavailability about 80%; metabolites have negligible activity
Ethosuximide	50–60	Metabolism + renal	About 80% is metabolised; half-life is shorter in children (30 h)
Gabapentin	5–7	Renal	Clearance approximates to glomerular filtration rate; absorption from gut is rapid but dose dependent (possibly because of saturation of active amino acid transporter)
Lamotrigine	29	Metabolism + renal	>50% forms a N-glucuronide (unusual reaction)
Oxcarbazepine	1–2.5 (8–14 10-OH)	Renal	The keto analogue of carbamazepine; active metabolite (10-hydroxy oxcarbazepine 10-OH) has most of the antiseizure activity
Phenobarbital	50–150	Metabolism + renal	Oral bioavailability >90%
Phenytoin	7–60	Metabolism + renal	Dose-dependent elimination because of saturation of metabolism; renal elimination is 7% of dose at low doses
Primidone	4–22	Metabolism	Active metabolites (phenobarbital and phenylethyl malonamide) have longer half-lives than primidone and, therefore, accumulate thus accounting for most activity during chronic treatment
Sodium valproate	9–21	Metabolism	Oral bioavailability is >95%; some metabolites have activity but their importance is not known
Tiagabine	5–8	Metabolism	Does not induce cytochrome P450; elimination is increased by drugs which induce cytochrome P450
Topiramate	20–30	Renal + metabolism	Elimination is enhanced by cytochrome P450 inducers
Vigabatrin	7–8	Renal	Clearance correlates with glomerular filtration rate
Drugs used for status epilepticus			
Clomethiazole	4–6	Metabolism	Intravenous formulation available
Clonazepam	8–45	Metabolism	Intravenous formulation available
Diazepam	30–200	Metabolism	Active N-desmethyl metabolite; rectal and intravenous formulations available
Fosphenytoin	0.15–0.25	Hydrolysis (to phenytoin)	Given by intravenous injection as sodium salt for status epilepticus; prodrug for phenytoin
Lorazepam	8–25	Metabolism	Major metabolite is a glucuronide; intravenous formulation available
Paraldehyde	10 (neonates)	Metabolism	Given rectally using a glass syringe (it dissolves plastic!); can be given as an intravenous infusion after dilution in physiological saline (but this is no longer recommended practice)
Phenytoin sodium	see above	–	The solution for injection contains sodium hydroxide and is highly alkaline (pH 12)

Drug compendium

24

Extrapyramidal movement disorders and spasticity

The neuronal connections of the area of the brain known as the basal ganglia are intimately involved in the co-ordination of motor function in conjunction with the motor cortex, cerebellum and spinal cord. Several major neurotransmitters are involved in regulating the function of the basal ganglia (Fig. 24.1). Disordered regulation of neuronal activity following degeneration of vital neurons in these pathways is thought to be the reason for the dysfunctional motor activity. Treatment for these disorders is directed at restoring the balance among the neurotransmitters.

Parkinson's disease

Parkinson's disease is a disorder characterised by a triad of resting tremor, skeletal muscle rigidity and brady-kinesia (poverty of movement). The underlying pathology involves degeneration of the nigro-striatal pathway which produces dopamine as a neurotransmitter (Fig. 24.1). The cause for the progressive degeneration of these neurons is not known; it may be related to the production of free radicals during dopamine biosynthesis and metabolism, or to the presence of environmental toxins. More than 70% of neurons have degenerated before symptoms show. The proposed changes in some transmitter substances in the basal ganglia that may contribute to the disordered motor function are shown in Figure 24.1. Overall, these events are still poorly understood. In addition, increased cholinergic activity which affects motor control has also been demonstrated.

In some conditions which have similarities to Parkinson's disease, for example the Steele–Richardson and Shy–Drager syndromes, the γ-aminobutyric acid (GABA) neurons also degenerate which explains the poor response of these conditions to treatment with dopamine replacement therapy. Drugs can produce a parkinsonian syndrome by blockade of striatal dopamine receptors. Antipsychotic drugs (Ch. 21) most commonly produce this syndrome, which also responds poorly to dopamine replacement therapy.

Drugs for Parkinson's disease

Treatment of Parkinson's disease involves enhancing dopaminergic activity (Fig. 24.2) or inhibiting

273

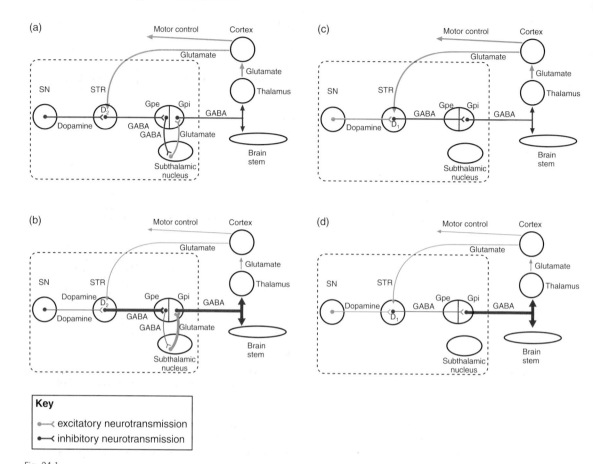

Fig. 24.1

A simplified model of events occurring in the basal ganglion that help to explain the disordered motor control in Parkinson's disease. For the purposes of clarity only selected interconnections and anatomical areas are shown. Many other complex excitatory and inhibitory interconnections exist.

The basal ganglia contains the substantia nigra (pars compacta SN), the striatum (STR), the globus pallidus externa (Gpe) and interna (Gpi) segments and the subthalamic nucleus. The green interconnections mark excitatory neurotransmitter function and the red inhibitory. The thickness of the lines in interconnecting pathways between structures shows the relative differences in function of that pathway in parkinsonism. In parkinsonism there are relative increases or decreases in the activity of different neurons. The figure shows two different pathways where the degeneration of dopaminergic neurons results in a change in neuronal firing rates between different brain regions resulting in dysfunctional motor control. (a,c) Healthy individuals, (b,d) changes in parkinsonism. (a,b) Pathways in which dopamine neurotransmission in nigrostriatal pathways utilises mainly D_2 receptors in the striatum. In parkinsonism (b), reduction in the inhibitory dopaminergic control to the striatum following degeneration of the pathways from the nigra compacta (SN) leads to increased firing rates of neurons from the subthalamic nucleus to the Gpi. This leads to greater gamma-aminobutyric acid (GABA)-mediated inhibitory control in the motor thalamus causing dysfunctional motor control. (c,d) Another nigrostriatal dopaminergic pathway utilises predominantly D_1 receptors in the striatum. The degeneration of the neurons in this pathway also leads to dysfunctional motor activity (d). Oscillatory bursts of neuronal activity from the subthalamic nucleus and Gpi are seen in parkinsonism and may contribute to the excessive thalamic and brainstem locomotor area inhibition. (For more detail see Lang and Lozano (1998) from whom this figure was adapted.)

cholinergic activity. Experimental work is also being carried out with glutamate antagonists.

Dopaminergic drugs

Levodopa

Mechanism of action

Dopamine cannot be given to replace the deficiency in the basal ganglia since it does not cross the blood–brain barrier. However, the large neutral amino acid levodopa can enter the brain, where it is taken up into dopaminergic neurons and converted to dopamine by L-aromatic amino acid decarboxylase (Ch. 4).

Pharmacokinetics

Levodopa is absorbed from the small intestine by an active transport mechanism for large neutral amino acids. A similar transport system is used to transfer levodopa across the blood–brain barrier. Decarboxylation of levodopa to dopamine occurs extensively in peripheral tissues such as the gut wall and liver. This reduces the

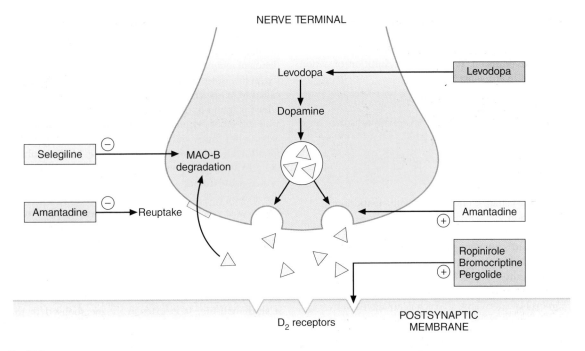

Fig. 24.2
The major effects of drugs on the dopaminergic nerve terminal. Ropinirole, bromocriptine and pergolide may act at other dopamine receptor subtypes, which is important for their therapeutic actions. coloured △, dopamine; MAO-B, monoxamine oxidase B; +, stimulation; −, inhibition.

amount of levodopa that reaches the brain (to about 1% of an oral dose) and generates substantial amounts of extracerebral dopamine which produces unwanted effects. Therefore, levodopa is usually given in combination with a peripheral dopa decarboxylase inhibitor (with carbidopa as co-careldopa or with benserazide as co-beneldopa) that does not cross the blood–brain barrier. About 80% of the peripheral metabolism of levodopa can be inhibited by this means, thus increasing the amount of levodopa that crosses the blood–brain barrier to 5–10% of the oral dose.

The half-life of levodopa is short. In the early stages of the disease, storage of dopamine in striatal neurons can ensure a stable response despite infrequent doses of levodopa. Modified-release formulations of levodopa are also available to provide a more continuous supply of drug to the neurons. Transition from conventional levodopa to a modified-release formulation requires care since the latter have a lower bioavailability which makes estimations of dosage equivalence difficult.

Unwanted effects
Unwanted effects fall broadly into two categories.

- Effects arising mainly from peripheral dopamine generation. These can be reduced by a peripheral decarboxylase inhibitor. They include nausea and vomiting, caused by stimulation of the chemoreceptor trigger zone (CTZ) of the medullary vomiting centre, which lies outside the blood–brain

barrier (Ch. 32), and postural hypotension caused by vasodilation.
- Effects arising from excessive central dopamine generation. These include dyskinetic involuntary movements, especially of the face and neck, or akathisia (restlessness). Psychological disturbance can also occur including hallucinations and confusion.

Dopamine receptor agonists

Examples: bromocriptine, pergolide, apomorphine, ropinirole

Mechanism of action
In contrast to levodopa, these drugs act as direct agonists of central dopaminergic receptors. They have a longer duration of action than levodopa. Bromocriptine and ropinirole are selective for the inhibitory dopamine D_2 receptor subtype, showing little activity at excitatory D_1 receptors (see Ch. 4), while pergolide and apomorphine are non-selective. Bromocriptine also has weak α-adrenoceptor agonist properties. Pergolide and ropinirole may also stimulate D_3 receptors.

Pharmacokinetics
Bromocriptine, pergolide and ropinirole are incompletely absorbed from the gut and undergo extensive

presystemic metabolism in the liver. The half-lives vary from short to very long (see compendium).

Apomorphine is given parenterally by injection or continuous infusion. It has a short duration of action because of liver metabolism.

Unwanted effects

Gradual dosage titration over several months may limit the following unwanted effects:

- nausea and vomiting (particularly with apomorphine)
- dyskinesias
- neuropsychiatric effects with hallucinations and confusion
- peripheral vasospasm especially in patients with Raynaud's phenomenon taking bromocriptine
- postural hypotension (especially with bromocriptine)
- retroperitoneal fibrosis (with bromocriptine)
- respiratory depression with apomorphine (a morphine derivative), which is antagonised by naloxone (Ch. 19).

Nausea and vomiting can be prevented by giving domperidone (Ch. 32), a dopamine receptor blocker, for at least 3 days before starting apomorphine. Domperidone does not cross the blood–brain barrier.

Amantadine

Mechanism of action

Amantadine was introduced originally as an antiviral drug. It is believed to act in Parkinson's disease by stimulating release of dopamine stored in nerve terminals and by reducing reuptake of released dopamine into the presynaptic neuron. Its usefulness tends to be short lived, because of the development of tolerance.

Pharmacokinetics

Amantadine is well absorbed from the gut and has a variable but long half-life. It is excreted unchanged by the kidney.

Unwanted effects

Amantadine can cause:

- ankle oedema
- postural hypotension
- insomnia or hallucinations with high doses
- livedo reticularis (skin vasoconstriction caused by local catecholamine release).

Selective monoamine oxidase B inhibitors

Example: selegiline.

Mechanism of action and effects

Selegiline inhibits the enzyme monoamine oxidase (MAO), which is responsible for the intraneuronal degradation of monoamine neurotransmitters (Ch. 4). It is selective at low doses for the isoenzyme found in the striatum, called MAO-B. This isoenzyme is distinct from MAO-A, which is found in the central nervous system (CNS), gut wall and other peripheral tissues; consequently, the interaction with drugs and foods containing tyramine that is found with conventional non-selective MAO inhibitor (MAOI) antidepressants do not occur (Ch. 22). Selegiline prolongs the duration of action of levodopa and reduces the levodopa dosage requirement by about one-third. It produces a small degree of clinical benefit when used alone. It may also reduce the production of toxic free radicals in the striatum but it remains unproven whether this will alter progression of the disease.

Pharmacokinetics

Selegiline is completely absorbed from the gut and has a short half-life. It is extensively metabolised in the liver, in part to amphetamine metabolites that have long half-lives.

Unwanted effects

Selegiline can cause:

- transient nausea, dizziness or lightheadedness (common)
- agitation, confusion, hallucinations caused by production of active amphetamine metabolites (Ch. 54).

Catechol-*O*-methyl transferase inhibitors

Example: entacapone

Mechanism of action and effects

Catechol-*O*-methyl transferase (COMT) is responsible for breakdown of between 10 and 30% of levodopa both peripherally and in the CNS (Ch. 4). In the presence of a peripheral dopamine decarboxylase inhibitor, COMT is responsible for most of the peripheral metabolism of levodopa. Inhibition of COMT in conjunction with a dopamine decarboxylase inhibitor doubles the half-life of levodopa and produces a 50% increase in the motor response to each dose of levodopa. Entacapone is given together with levodopa to improve the 'end-of-dose' motor fluctuations in response to levodopa. Levodopa doses may need to be reduced. Entacapone does not cross the blood–brain barrier.

Pharmacokinetics

Entacapone is rapidly absorbed from the gut. It is metabolised in the liver and has a short half-life.

Unwanted effects

Entacapone can cause:

- dyskinesia, hallucinations
- nausea, vomiting, diarrhoea.

Antimuscarinic drugs

Examples: trihexyphenidyl hydrochloride (benzhexol), orphenadrine, procyclidine.

Mechanism of action and effects

Drugs that block central muscarinic receptors (Ch. 4) restore the balance between cholinergic and dopaminergic activity by reducing the former. They have little effect on bradykinesia, and are less effective than levodopa for treating tremor and rigidity.

Pharmacokinetics

Oral absorption of the antimuscarinic drugs is moderate, and most of these drugs undergo extensive hepatic metabolism with intermediate to long half-lives. High lipid solubility ensures ready transfer across the blood–brain barrier.

Unwanted effects

These are predictable and a result of blockade of peripheral muscarinic receptors (Ch. 4). Reduced saliva production can be helpful in some parkinsonian patients, in whom sialorrhoea is a problem. Blockade of CNS muscarinic receptors can produce confusion in the elderly.

Management of Parkinson's disease and parkinsonian syndromes

Levodopa (with a peripheral decarboxylase inhibitor) is the mainstay of treatment for idiopathic Parkinson's disease and is particularly useful for reducing bradykinesia. Clinical response is achieved in about 70% of patients with idiopathic Parkinson's disease, whereas by contrast those with drug-induced parkinsonism respond poorly. Frequent doses may be needed, especially in advanced disease, to prevent the response 'wearing off'. Some neurologists advocate a dopamine agonist as initial therapy in younger patients or selegiline for those with mild symptoms. The evidence to support their use in preference to levodopa is controversial, although recent evidence suggests that ropinirole used as initial treatment causes significantly less

dyskinesia after 5 years compared to levodopa. Earlier dopamine receptor agonists were less effective than levodopa for preventing disability.

A further problem late in the disease is the 'on–off' phenomenon with rapid swings between severe bradykinesia and toxic dyskinesias. Fluctuating delivery of levodopa to the striatum is believed to be responsible; there are too few surviving neurons to store dopamine and smooth out the response when delivery of levodopa is not constant. Modified-release formulations of levodopa, combining levodopa with selegiline or entacapone or the addition of a dopamine receptor agonist may be helpful in some patients. Other patients find the rapid action of subcutaneous apomorphine invaluable to abort the 'off' component of the phenomenon. Antimuscarinic agents are most useful for tremor that responds inadequately to levodopa. They can also be helpful in reducing excessive salivation. Amantadine is well tolerated but effective only in mild parkinsonism, with rapid loss of clinical benefit after a few weeks. Combinations of drugs are often necessary in advanced disease but unwanted effects can be troublesome: confusion is a particular problem, especially in the elderly.

Drugs improve symptoms and quality of life in idiopathic Parkinson's disease but they do not appear to alter the underlying rate of neuronal degeneration. Nevertheless, levodopa therapy does increase life expectancy probably by reducing complications. Initial encouraging evidence that selegiline might delay the neuronal degeneration of Parkinson's disease has not been confirmed by more recent studies in previously untreated patients.

In advanced Parkinson's disease, surgical treatment is sometimes advocated. Severe tremor may respond to stereotactic thalamotomy or pallidotomy. Pallidotomy can also be helpful for severe dyskinesias.

Parkinsonism associated with antipsychotic drug therapy responds best to drug withdrawal. If this is not possible, then an antimuscarinic drug is the treatment of choice.

Dyskinesias and dystonias

Tardive dyskinesias and dystonias most frequently occur after long-term use of antipsychotic drugs because of their antagonist action at the inhibitory dopamine D_2 receptor (see Ch. 21). Dyskinesias are usually choreiform movements that affect the oral region or extremities; dystonias commonly affect the neck or trunk. These movement disorders can occur during treatment or arise when it is stopped. They are more common in the elderly, and especially women. Antimuscarinic drugs often exacerbate dyskinesias but may help dystonias. Dystonias can also be hereditary.

Choreiform movements can occur after a group A streptococcal infection in children (Sydenham's chorea). It does not usually require specific treatment. Huntington's chorea is an autosomal dominant hereditary disease that presents in adult life with progressive impairment of motor coordination and bizarre limb movements. The pathology is a loss of GABA inhibitory neurons within the neostriatum, which connect with the substantia nigra. There is a consequent reduction of inhibitory activity on dopaminergic cells in the substantia nigra and cells in the globus pallidus. Therefore, these cells generate uncoordinated discharges that produce bursts of excess motor activity. Treatment aims to reduce the excessive dopaminergic activity.

Drug treatment

Tetrabenazine

Mechanism of action
Tetrabenazine produces selective monoamine depletion from neurons in the CNS. Storage vesicles become leaky and the released contents are degraded by MAO. It is more effective for choreiform movements than the antipsychotic drugs, which block dopamine receptors.

Pharmacokinetics
Tetrabenazine has a low oral bioavailability. It is metabolised to an active derivative. The half-life is intermediate.

Unwanted effects
Unwanted effects include:

- drowsiness
- postural hypotension
- Dysphagia, which may be caused by extrapyramidal dysfunction.

Management of dyskinesias and dystonias

There are several options for management of dyskinesias and dystonias.

- Cessation of the provoking drug. Symptoms may initially be exacerbated but usually settle. Withdrawal dyskinesias usually respond to gradual drug discontinuation.
- Tetrabenazine is effective in some patients.

- Enhanced inhibitory GABA neurotransmitter activity with baclofen (see below), sodium valproate or clonazepam (Ch. 23).
- Botulinum toxin (Ch. 27), which impairs acetylcholine release from nerve endings in the neuromuscular junction, can be injected into dystonic muscles to provide temporary relief. Spread of the paralytic effect to adjacent muscles can cause problems, for example, dysphagia after injection of neck muscles for torticollis.

Spasticity

Spasticity is a state of sustained muscle tone or tension which is often associated with an increase in stretch reflexes. The increase in muscle tone can arise from continued spinal reflex activity in the absence of inhibitory input from the motor cortex, such as can result from a stroke or in multiple sclerosis. Spasticity in skeletal muscles is often associated with partial or complete loss of voluntary movement and can produce painful and deforming contractures. Drugs that block the neuromuscular junction are not used to treat spasticity since their main effect would probably be a further loss of voluntary movement.

Drugs for spasticity

The primary sites of action of drugs for spasticity are the spinal reflexes and the release of Ca^{2+} in the muscle fibre. Muscular hypotonia is a common problem in the drug therapy of spasticity.

Diazepam

Diazepam enhances spinal inhibitory pathways by facilitating GABA-mediated opening of Cl^- channels (Ch. 20). The main disadvantage is sedation as a result of inhibitory activity in higher centres at the doses necessary for a spasmolytic action.

Baclofen

Mechanism of action
Baclofen inhibits excitatory activity at mono- and polysynaptic reflexes at the spinal level. It binds stereoselectively to, and is an agonist at, $GABA_B$ receptors. This is believed to increase presynaptic inhibition of reflex pathways by reducing presynaptic Ca^{2+} influx and thus reducing excitatory neurotransmitter release. Baclofen also has an analgesic action, probably by inhibition of the release of substance P.

Pharmacokinetics

Baclofen is absorbed rapidly from the gastrointestinal tract. It has a short half-life and is eliminated largely in the urine in the unchanged form. It can be given by intrathecal injection if severe spasticity is resistant to oral therapy.

Unwanted effects

Baclofen can cause:

- sedation and drowsiness
- nausea
- various CNS effects (e.g. lightheadedness, confusion, dizziness and headache)
- hallucinations (caused by sudden withdrawal).

Dantrolene

Mechanism of action and uses

Dantrolene inhibits the release of Ca^{2+} from the sarcoplasmic reticulum of skeletal muscles. This impairs activation of the contractile apparatus and relaxes the muscles. In patients with spasticity this may improve functional capacity, but generalised muscle weakness is a potential problem. Dantrolene is also used for the treatment of malignant hyperthermia (Ch. 17) and as an adjunctive treatment in neuroleptic malignant syndrome (Ch. 21).

Pharmacokinetics

Dantrolene is well absorbed from the gut but can also be given intravenously. It is metabolised in the liver and has a variable and unpredictable half-life, which is short in some individuals and long in others.

Unwanted effects

Dantrolene can cause:

- drowsiness, dizziness, weakness and malaise (usually transient)

- hepatitis (risk is dose-related)
- diarrhoea.

Tizanidine

Mechanisms of action

Tizanidine is an α_2-adrenoceptor agonist that results in an increase in excitatory amino acids and increases presynaptic inhibition of motor neurons. Inhibition of imidazoline receptors may also be contributory (see also Ch. 6). Its actions are both spinal and supraspinal; it inhibits descending noradrenergic pathways but has only 10% of the antihypertensive activity of clonidine. Inhibition is greatest in polysynaptic rather than monosynaptic pathways.

Pharmacokinetics

Tizanidine is well absorbed but undergoes extensive first-pass metabolism. Its elimination half-life is short.

Unwanted effects

Unwanted effects include:

- dry mouth
- drowsiness and tiredness
- dizziness.

Management of spasticity

In many patients mild spasticity is useful since the increased tone provides support for a weak limb. Excessive spasticity following a stroke is most effectively prevented by adequate physiotherapy. For patients with deforming or painful spasticity drug therapy can be useful, particularly if they are not ambulant. In severe spasticity, intramuscular injection of botulinum toxin (see above) can be helpful for up to 3 months.

FURTHER READING

Parkinson's disease

Hughes AJ (1997) Drug treatment of Parkinson's disease in the 1990s. *Drugs* 53, 195–205

Lang AE, Lozano AM (1998) Parkinson's disease. Part 1 and Part 2. *N Engl J Med* 339, 1130–1143

Olanow CW, Koller WC (1998) An algorithm (decision tree) for the management of Parkinson's disease. *Neurology* 50(suppl 3), S1–S38

Rehman H-ur (2000) Diagnosis and management of tremor. *Arch Intern Med* 160, 2438–2444

Schapira AHV (1999) Parkinson's disease. *Br Med J* 318, 311–314.

Tanner CM (2000) Dopamine agonists in early therapy for Parkinson disease. *JAMA* 284, 1971–1973

Dyskinesias and dystonias

Shale H, Tanner C (1996) Pharmacological options for the management of dyskinesias. *Drugs* 52, 849–860

van Harten PN, Hoek HW, Kahn RS (1999) Acute dystonia induced by drug treatment. *Br Med J* 319, 623–626

Self-assessment

In questions 1–4, the first statement, in italics, is true. Are the accompanying statements also true?

1. *In Parkinson's disease there is abnormally reduced dopaminergic transmission which results in overexpression of GABA-ergic, glutaminergic and cholinergic transmission.*

   a. In patients showing symptoms of Parkinson's disease, approximately 25% of dopaminergic neurons have been lost.
   b. Glutamate antagonists are being investigated for use in Parkinson's disease.
   c. Levodopa has a long half-life.

2. *In patients with young-onset disease (below 40 years of age), treatment with levodopa will lead to complications such as dyskinesias and on/off fluctuations in all patients after about 5 years.*

   a. In very early Parkinson's disease, ropinirole is as effective as levodopa.
   b. Anticholinergic drugs such as benzhexol have a low incidence of unwanted effects.

3. *The motor complications associated with long-term use of levodopa may be helped by reducing the dosage and increasing the frequency of administration.*

   a. Bromocriptine is a potent agonist at dopamine (D_2) receptors.
   b. Some of the movement disorder in Parkinson's disease arises from abnormalities in non-dopaminergic innervated areas of the brain.
   c. The chemoreceptor trigger zone (CTZ) is stimulated by peripheral dopamine as the CTZ lies outside the blood–brain barrier.
   d. Monoamine oxidase inhibitor (MAOI) selegiline causes the 'cheese' reaction.
   e. Entacapone is a drug acting directly at dopamine receptors.

4. *Dantrolene is useful in spasticity as it reduces the Ca^{2+} release that contributes to contraction of skeletal muscle.*

   a. Baclofen enhances muscle spasticity.
   b. Botulinum toxin has a duration of action of up to 3 months.

5. Case history

   > Mrs FT is 75 years of age and has been suffering from progressive symptoms of Parkinson's disease for 5 years. From the outset she has been treated continuously with levodopa but problems have now developed in controlling the symptoms with this drug.

   a. What is the cause of Parkinson's disease?
   b. What symptoms is Mrs FT likely to have?
   c. Levodopa was given as co-beneldopa. What are the benefits of this formulation?
   d. What difficulties can arise in controlling symptoms with levodopa in the early stages and later stages of treatment, and what changes in therapy could be considered?
   e. What precautions need to be followed if Mrs FT was given vitamin supplements?
   f. Could a β-blocker drug be of use as part of Mrs FT's treatment?
   g. Can any treatment protect against the progressive deterioration in this patient?

6. Case history

   > Mr JJ is a married man aged 40 and has been newly diagnosed as suffering from Parkinson's disease. His symptoms are tremor, bradykinesia, hypokinesia and rigidity, which are sufficiently mild that he is still able to carry out his work and pursue his hobbies. He is a security guard and had previously fought as a relatively unsuccessful professional boxer for 10 years before retiring from the ring at the age of 35.

   Suggest possible treatment regimens for this patient, with reasons for your suggestions.

   The answers are provided on pages 615–616.

Drugs used for extrapyramidal movement disorders and spasticity

Drug	Half-life (h)	Elimination	Comments
Parkinson's disease			Given orally unless otherwise stated
Dopaminergic drugs			
Amantadine	10–15	Renal	Complete oral bioavailability: renal clearance (400 ml min^{-1}) indicates extensive tubular secretion
Apomorphine	0.5	Metabolism	Given by subcutaneous injection; not effective orally, probably as a result of presystemic metabolism; fate in humans has not been studied (D$_2$ agonist)
Benserazide	No data	Renal + biliary	Incomplete absorption; peripheral decarboxylase inhibitor used in combination with levodopa (co-beneldopa)
Bromocriptine	15	Metabolism	Low oral bioavailability (30–40%) as a result of first-pass metabolism
Cabergoline	60–90	Metabolism (+ renal)	Metabolites excreted in bile and urine (D$_2$ agonist); used as an adjunct to levodopa
Carbidopa	2–3	Renal + metabolism	Variable oral bioavailability (40–90%); peripheral decarboxylase inhibitor used in combination with levodopa (co-careldopa)
Entacapone	2–3	Metabolism	Oral bioavailability is about 30–50%; metabolised by glucuronidation
Levodopa	1.3	Metabolism	Precursor of dopamine; normally given with carbidopa or benserazide to reduce first-pass metabolism and increase duration of action
Lisuride	2–3	Metabolism	Low oral bioavailability (about 10%) with large interpatient variability because of first-pass metabolism
Pergolide	27	Metabolism	Rapid absorption but high first-pass metabolism; metabolites (unidentified) eliminated in urine and bile
Pramipexole	8–12	Renal	High oral bioavailability; selective for D$_3$ receptors; eliminated by renal tubular secretion + filtration.
Ropinirole	6	Metabolism (+ renal)	Bioavailability is about 50%; main metabolic pathway is oxidation by CYP1A2 in the liver
Selegiline	1–2	Metabolism	High bioavailability; metabolised in the liver; desmethyl metabolite is an irreversible inhibitor of monoamine oxidase type B
Antimuscarinic drugs			
Benzatropine	No data	Metabolism	Given orally or by intramuscular or intravenous injection; few data available; numerous metabolites found in rat studies
Biperiden	18	Metabolism	Bioavailability about 30% because of first-pass metabolism; very high volume of distribution (4000 l) contributes to long half-life
Orphenadrine	14–16	Metabolism (+ renal)	Bioavailability is about 70%; eliminated by P450-mediated oxidation
Procyclidine	13	Metabolism	Given orally, or by intramuscular or intravenous injection; about 75% oral bioavailability; eliminated by oxidation and conjugation
Trihexyphenidyl hydrochloride (benzhexol)	3–7	Metabolism	High bioavailability; 56% recovered as hydroxy metabolites within 3 days

Drugs used for essential tremor, chorea, tics and related disorders

Given orally unless otherwise indicated

Drug	Half-life (h)	Elimination	Comments
Chlorpromazine	8–35	Metabolism	Oral, suppository and injection formulations available; incomplete oral bioavailability (10–33%); numerous pathways of metabolism with some metabolites detectable months after cessation of treatment
Clonidine	20–25	Renal + metabolism	Approximately 60% renal and 40% hepatic metabolism
Haloperidol (and decanoate)	20 (9–67)	Metabolism	Given orally and by injection, or by depot injection (as the decanoate prodrug); oral bioavailability is about 60%; the half-life for release from the depot injection is about 21 days; reduced to active metabolite in liver and extrahepatic tissues; undergoes enterohepatic circulation

continued

Drug compendium

Drug compendium

Drugs used for extrapyramidal movement disorders and spasticity *(continued)*

Drug	Half-life (h)	Elimination	Comments
Drugs used for essential tremor, chorea, tics and related disorders *(continued)*			Given orally unless otherwise indicated
Pimozide	53	Metabolism	Given orally; oral bioavailability is about 60–80%; metabolised to inactive products by CYP3A4
Piracetam	4	Renal	Mostly eliminated by glomerular filtration; non-renal elimination (route undefined) accounts for about 30% of elimination
Primidone	4–22	Renal + metabolism	Chronic treatment induces metabolism so that elimination by the kidneys decreases from 60% to 40%
Propranolol	3–6	Metabolism	Low oral bioavailability and wide interindividual differences
Riluzole	12	Metabolism	Used only in motor neuron disease; bioavailability is 60%; oxidised by cytochrome P450
Sulpiride	6–8	Renal + metabolism	Given orally; incomplete oral bioavailability (about 30–40%) owing to poor absorption; water-soluble compound eliminated largely unchanged in urine and faeces
Tetrabenazine	7	Metabolism	Low oral bioavailability (5%); response is probably caused by a metabolite dihydrotetrabenazine which is as active as the parent drug, and has a longer half-life (12 h)
Trihexyphenidyl hydrochloride (benhexol)			See above.
Spasticity			Given orally except where indicated
Baclofen	3–4	Renal (+ metabolism)	Good oral bioavailability (95%)
Dantrolene	4–24	Metabolism	Good oral bioavailability (80%); metabolites eliminated in urine and bile
Diazepam	20–100	Metabolism	Given orally, by intramuscular injection or by intravenous injection or infusion; N-desmethyl metabolite (nordiazepam) is one of three active metabolites and it has a longer half-life
Tizanidine	3–4	Metabolism	Oral bioavailability is about 20–40% because of first-pass metabolism; metabolites are inactive
Other muscle relaxants			Orally active
Carisoprodol	6–8	Metabolism	Rapid absorption; numerous metabolites including meprobamate formed by CYP2C19 (which shows genetic polymorphism)
Methocarbamol	1–2	Metabolism	Rapid and complete absorption (more published data for race horses than for humans!)

25 Other neurological disorders: multiple sclerosis, motor neuron disease and Guillain–Barré syndrome

Multiple sclerosis

Multiple sclerosis is characterised by initial immunologically mediated inflammation of perivascular white matter in the central nervous system (CNS). The blood–brain barrier is breached by lymphocytes and macrophages which cause loss of myelin sheaths around nerves, a reduction in the numbers of oligodendrocytes that produce the myelin and the generation of demyelinated plaques which disturb normal conduction of electrical impulses in the CNS. The process of demyelination is enhanced by inflammatory cytokine production. If the damage is severe enough, myelin repair is no longer possible and scar tissue forms. The cause of multiple sclerosis is unknown, but it may result from exposure of individuals with susceptible immune systems to exogenous triggers (possibly viruses) in childhood.

Multiple sclerosis usually begins in the second and third decade of life and most often presents with relapsing and remitting symptoms and signs of multifocal CNS dysfunction. Such episodes must be disseminated in both time and place to secure the diagnosis. In most patients, the clinical course is one of stepwise or eventually progressive deterioration. The areas of the CNS most often involved are the optic nerves, spinal cord, brainstem and cerebellum. Common presentations are optic neuritis, spasticity, weakness, bladder and bowel involvement.

Drug treatment

There is no proven cure for multiple sclerosis but drugs can be used to reduce the symptoms.

- Corticosteroids (Ch. 44) are often used to treat acute relapse (e.g. intravenous methylprednisolone for 3 days or oral prednisolone for 3 weeks). They probably shorten the duration of an attack but have no effect on long-term outcome.
- Interferon-β can reduce the inflammatory response in an acute attack and reduce the frequency of relapses. Proposed mechanisms include downregulation of the production of inflammatory interferon-γ, enhanced activity of suppressor T cells and inhibition of the expression of class II major histocompatibility complex antigens. It is given by subcutaneous injection. Its place in treatment

283

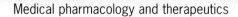

remains unclear; current recommendations reserve its use for ambulant patients who have had at least one attack of relapsing and remitting disease per year for the previous 2 years. The most frequent adverse effects are 'flu-like' symptoms, which may persist for several months, and pain or ulceration at the injection site.

- Symptomatic treatment of spasticity may be necessary, for example with baclofen (Ch. 24).

Motor neuron disease

Motor neuron disease is an uncommon, rapidly progressive disorder of motor neurons that occurs most often in middle-aged males. It leads to both upper motor neuron signs (hypertonia, impaired fine movement and hyperreflexia) and peripheral motor signs (fasciculations, muscle cramps, weakness and muscle atrophy). Neuronal death occurs but the cause is unclear. An autoimmune origin is said to be unlikely since immunosuppression is ineffective for treatment. One hypothesis proposes excessive activation of the excitatory glutamate receptors in the CNS. Overstimulation of the motor neurons may lead to Ca^{2+} overload and cell death, perhaps involving excessive free radical generation.

Drug treatment

Riluzole is the only available agent that alters the course of the disease. This crosses the blood–brain barrier and may block the release and actions of glutamate at presynaptic terminals at motor neuron cells. Glutamate, although an excitatory neurotransmitter, can under some circumstances cause excitotoxicity by excessive elevation of Ca^{2+} within cells out of control. This leads to release of reactive oxygen species, activation of proteases and nitric oxide generation leading to cell damage. An alternative possible mechanism of action of riluzole involves an interaction with adenosine receptors. Treatment does not

arrest the disease but may slow its progression to a modest extent. Adverse effects include lethargy, nausea and dizziness.

Symptomatic treatment is often necessary for pain, breathlessness or dysphagia.

Guillain–Barré syndrome

Guillain–Barré syndrome is an autoimmune disorder, probably triggered by a bacterial or viral infection. It produces rapid onset of limb weakness with loss of tendon reflexes, few sensory signs, and autonomic dysfunction. It only affects the peripheral nervous system. About 10% of patients die in the acute illness and a further 10% are left with severe long-term disability.

The pathological process involves acute lymphocytic infiltration into peripheral nerves and spinal roots, which results in demyelination. However, in about 10% of patients, the macrophages invade the nerve especially in the spinal root (and cause axonal degeneration).

Management

Several methods can be used to manage Guillain–Barré syndrome.

- Supportive treatment may be life-saving, for example, ventilatory support if breathing is affected. Haemodynamic disturbance can also result from autonomic involvement.
- Plasma exchange, when used within 2 weeks of the onset, improves the long-term outcome. Removal of autoantibodies probably underlies the benefit.
- High-dose intravenous IgG is an equally effective alternative to plasma exchange, and more readily available.
- Corticosteroids are of no benefit alone but their use with immunoglobulin therapy is being studied.

FURTHER READING

Hahn AF (1998) Guillain–Barré syndrome. *Lancet* 352, 635–641

Noseworthy JH, Lucchinetti C, Rodriguez M, Weinshenker BG (2000) Multiple sclerosis. *N Engl J Med* 343, 938–952

Orrell RW, Lane RJ, Guiloff RJ (1994) Recent developments in the treatment of motor neuron disease. *Br Med J* 309, 140–141

Rowland W (1994) Riluzole for the treatment of amyotrophic lateral sclerosis – too soon to tell? *N Engl J Med* 330, 626–627

Rudick RA, Cohen JA, Weinstock-Guttman B et al. (1997) Management of multiple sclerosis. *N Engl J Med* 337, 1604–1611

Shaw PJ (1999) Motor neuron disease. *Br Med J* 318, 1118–1121

Tselis AC, Lisak RP (1999) Multiple sclerosis. A therapeutic update. *Arch Neurol* 56, 277–280

van Oosten BW, Truyen L, Barkolf F, Polman CH (1998) Choosing drug therapy for multiple sclerosis. *Drugs* 56, 555–559

Self-assessment

Are the following statements true or false?

1. Treatment with interferon gamma is of benefit in reducing relapses in multiple sclerosis.

2. Multiple sclerosis is characterised in the early years by a steady progressive worsening of symptoms in most patients.

3. Glutamate can cause neuronal damage.

4. Riluzole is of benefit in motor neuron disease by blocking the release of γ-amino butyric acid.

5. In multiple sclerosis prednisolone appears to shorten relapses.

The answers are provided on page 616.

Drugs used in multiple sclerosis, motor neuron disease and Guillain–Barré syndrome

Drug	Half-life (h)	Elimination	Comments
Interferon beta	2–4	Metabolism	Given by subcutaneous or intramuscular injection; rapid elimination is because of tissue uptake and catabolism (especially in the liver)
Riluzole	12	Metabolism	Given orally; eliminated by hepatic CYP1A2-mediated oxidation

Migraine

Headache has many causes (Box 26.1). Of the primary causes of headache, tension is by far the most common cause accounting for about two-thirds. Migraine is the second most frequent cause. In prolonged or recurrent headache, secondary causes should be excluded by a full history and examination for associated neurological symptoms and signs.

Migraine is characteristically a unilateral throbbing headache often associated with nausea and occasionally with vomiting and with light and noise sensitivity. In the majority of patients these are the only symptoms (common migraine). In up to one-third of migraineurs the headache is preceded by an aura (classical migraine) which often consists of visual disturbances but occasionally more severe focal neurological episodes.

Pathogenesis of migraine

The pathogenesis of migraine, and other related types of headache, is as yet imperfectly understood but it is believed to involve neuronal and vascular dysfunction (Fig. 26.1). Intracranial vessels are innervated by many neuronal sources utilising a multitude of neurotransmitter substances. Vasoconstrictor sympathetic innervation involves noradrenaline (norepinephrine) but is also associated with peptidergic neuropeptide Y and purinergic adenosine triphosphate (ATP) transmission. Vasodilator parasympathetic innervation is associated

---

Box 26.1

Causes of headache

Primary headache
   Tension-type headache
   Migraine
   Idiopathic stabbing headache
   Exertional headache
   Cluster headache

Secondary headache
   Systemic infection
   Head injury
   Drug-induced headache
   Vascular disorders
   Brain tumour

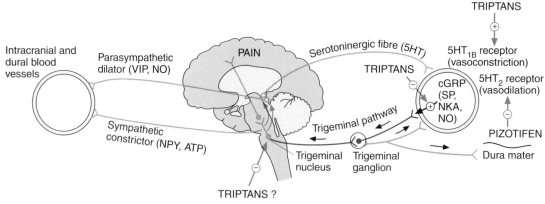

Fig. 26.1
Some factors associated with the genesis of migraine and putative sites of action of antimigraine drugs. The sequence and nature of neurogenic and vascular involvement in migraine are vigorously debated and may vary in different types of migraine-type headache. The trigeminal system (red) is activated by cGRP. This transmitter is elevated in migraine in association with the pronounced blood vessel dilatation. Antidromic stimulation (green) via the trigeminal ganglion, which has cGRP receptors, causes dilatation and inflammation of blood vessels and dura mater. Bipolar activation of the trigeminal ganglion also stimulates the trigeminal nucleus (which is rich in $5HT_{1B/D}$ receptors) and activates fibres responsible for pain, nausea and vomiting. 5HT, SP, NKA and NO also play a role in these vascular and neurological phenomena. Parasympathetic outflow may also be stimulated. Triptans ($5HT_{1B/D/F}$ agonists) are thought to relieve the symptoms of migraine activity at presynaptic receptors to inhibit cGRP release ($5HT_{1D}$ agonist) and inhibit vasodilatation ($5HT_{1B}$ agonist). Serotoninergic fibres to blood vessels can also cause vasodilatation by stimulating $5HT_2$ subtype receptors; this may explain the benefit of pizotifen, which blocks $5HT_2$ receptors. Some triptans (e.g. naratriptan) will act on trigeminal nucleus but the significance of this is not clear. cGRP, calcitonin gene-related peptide; SP, substance P; NKA, neurokinin A; NO, nitric oxide; VIP, vasoactive intestinal peptide; ATP, adenosine triphosphate; NPY, neuropeptide Y; 5HT, 5-hydroxytryptamine.

with vasoactive intestinal peptide, other neuropeptides and perhaps nitric oxide. Neuronal pathways utilising 5-hydroxytryptamine (5HT, serotonin) and causing vasodilatation or vasoconstriction have also been shown. The $5HT_{1B}$ and $5HT_2$ subtype receptors are found on cerebral blood vessels; stimulation of $5HT_{1B}$ receptors causes vasoconstriction and that of $5HT_2$ receptors results in vasodilatation. Lastly there is a complex vasodilator pathway utilising the trigeminal system (Fig. 26.1). In the early stages of migraine activation of the trigeminal ganglion (perhaps by dilation of blood vessels) results in antidromic release of calcitonin gene-related peptide (and possibly substance P, neurokinin A and nitric oxide) resulting in further dilation of blood vessels and dura mater neurogenic inflammation. In addition, stimulation of the trigeminal ganglion relays signals to the trigeminal nucleus. Nociceptive impulses from these regions pass to the thalamus and cortex and other brain regions causing pain, nausea and vomiting. This dysfunction may also activate parasympathetic and related vasodilator pathways. The trigeminal nucleus is also rich in $5HT_{1B/1D}$ receptors and trigeminal neurons can be inhibited by the action of 5HT at presynaptic $5HT_{1D}$ autoreceptors.

The aura of migraine is now believed to be caused by a cortical depolarisation wave that transiently depresses spontaneous and evoked neuronal activity (cortical spreading depression). This wave is preceded by intense but brief neuronal excitation producing cortical hyperaemia. The depressant wave is associated with vasoconstriction, which accounts for the focal neurological symptoms and signs.

Drugs for migraine

Specific drugs for the acute migraine attack

Ergotamine and dihydroergotamine

Mechanism of action

Ergotamine and dihydroergotamine probably have an antimigraine action similar to the triptans, stimulating $5HT_{1D}$ receptors (see below). Unwanted effects arise from the agonist activity of these compounds at several other receptors (including vascular $5HT_2$ receptors and dopamine D_2 receptors in the brainstem). Both drugs have similar clinical effects.

Pharmacokinetics

Oral administration of ergotamine is often accompanied by nausea. It is better tolerated when given sublingually, as a rectal suppository or by inhalation from a pressurised aerosol (dihydroergotamine). Absorption is poor and erratic whichever route is chosen. Ergotamine undergoes extensive metabolism in the liver and has a short half-life. However, tight receptor binding produces a long duration of action.

Unwanted effects

● Nausea and vomiting are caused by dopaminergic

stimulation at the chemoreceptor trigger zone (Ch. 32).

- Abdominal cramps and diarrhoea can occur.
- Severe vasoconstriction is a result of α_1 adrenoceptor stimulation that can lead to peripheral gangrene (acute ergotism). These drugs should be avoided in patients with known vascular disease (including ischaemic heart disease) or those concurrently receiving β-blockers, which reduce cardiac output (Ch. 5).
- Chronic intoxication with dependence can occur after prolonged use. Withdrawal produces nausea and headache similar to an acute migraine attack. For this reason, these drugs should not be used more than twice a month.

Triptans

Examples: sumatriptan, zolmitriptan

Mechanisms of action and effects
The mechanisms of action of the triptans are reviewed in Figure 26.1. Sumatriptan is a selective $5HT_{1D}$ agonist but also has actions at $5HT_{1B}$ and $5TH_{1F}$ receptors that may be important in its antimigraine actions. Sumatriptan does not cross the blood–brain barrier. Zolmitriptan and other 'second-generation' triptans penetrate the blood–brain barrier and may directly inhibit excitability of the trigeminal ganglion and trigeminal nucleus caudalis. Zolmitriptan is an agonist at $5HT_{1B}$ and $5HT_{1D}$ receptors on cerebral arteries, produces vasoconstriction and may block the peptide-mediated neurogenic inflammation. Triptans also relieve both the pain and the nausea associated with migraine.

Pharmacokinetics
Absorption of sumatriptan from the gut is rapid but erratic, whereas second-generation triptans such as zolmitriptan have better absorption. Effective plasma concentrations are usually reached within 30 min. Sumatriptan is also available for subcutaneous injection or administration by nasal spray. Triptans are extensively metabolised in the liver. Sumatriptan and zolmitriptan have short half-lives. Nasal or subcutaneous administration rapidly relieves symptoms in most patients within 15 min and these routes are particularly useful if the patient is vomiting.

Unwanted effects
The triptans can cause:

- pain or irritation at the injection site, or in the nose after local use
- nausea or vomiting
- tingling or sensation of warmth

- dizziness or vertigo
- chest discomfort or pressure in up to 40% of patients, which is probably not caused by myocardial ischaemia.
- angina caused by coronary artery vasoconstriction if there is pre-existing coronary artery disease; such individuals should not take a triptan.

Prophylactic drugs

Beta-adrenoceptor antagonists (β-blockers)

Examples: propranolol, atenolol

Mechanism of action in migraine
Full details of the β-adrenoceptor antagonists (β-blockers) are found in Chapter 5. In migraine, drugs with partial agonist activity that cause vasodilation (e.g. pindolol) are ineffective, suggesting that vasoconstriction may contribute to their action. Some β-blockers (e.g. propranolol) are also weak $5HT_2$ receptor antagonists.

Pizotifen

Mechanism of action
Pizotifen is an antagonist at $5HT_2$ receptors resulting in vasoconstriction and may have central actions that prevent the onset of the inflammatory response associated with established migraine attacks.

Pharmacokinetics
Oral absorption is almost complete and extensive metabolism occurs in the liver. The half-life of pizotifen is long.

Unwanted effects
Pizotifen can cause:

- appetite stimulation with weight gain (may be caused by enhanced insulin release)
- drowsiness.

Methysergide

Mechanism of action
Methysergide is similar to pizotifen, having $5HT_2$ antagonist activity and some additional partial agonist activity at $5HT_{1D}$ receptors.

Pharmacokinetics
Oral absorption is complete and liver metabolism extensive. Methysergide has an intermediate half-life.

Unwanted effects

Methysergide can cause:

- drowsiness
- retroperitoneal fibrosis with long-term use: producing ureteric compression, hydronephrosis and renal failure; it is reversible, but methysergide should only be given for a maximum of 6 months, followed by a 1-month drug-free interval.

Management of migraine

The acute attack

Withdrawal of possible triggers such as cheese, chocolate, citrus fruits or alcoholic drinks may reduce the frequency of attacks by up to 50%. The oral contraceptive pill is a potential exacerbating factor.

For relief of a mild acute attack, simple analgesia, for example with aspirin, paracetamol or a non-steroidal anti-inflammatory drug (NSAID; Ch. 29) may be sufficient. Nausea delays gastric emptying and frequently accompanies a migraine attack; absorption of the analgesic will be more rapid if an antiemetic such as metoclopramide or domperidone (Ch. 32) is given. Gastric emptying is also enhanced by metoclopramide. If vomiting is prominent, rectal or intramuscular analgesia, for example with the NSAIDs diclofenac or naproxen, may be needed. Analgesics are usually more effective when given early after the onset of pain. Opioid analgesics are not recommended since they are short-acting, produce dependence and frequent use can also promote 'analgesic headaches' (pain which appears as the effect of the drug wanes). Analgesic headaches

are also more common with compound analgesics, especially those that contain caffeine. Ergotamine can be used but the risk of vasospasm and habituation means that it should be avoided in older patients (who may have cardiovascular disease) and in those with frequent attacks. If attacks are poorly controlled by standard therapies or are severe, sumatriptan or a related drug is usually highly effective. It can relieve pain even if taken more than 4 h after the onset of an attack.

Prophylaxis

Prophylaxis is usually recommended for patients experiencing at least two attacks of migraine each month. Beta-blockers are widely held to be the best choice if there are no contraindications. Pizotifen is an alternative but weight gain limits its acceptability especially in young women. Methysergide can be given provided there are brief drug-free periods. The anti-epileptic drug sodium valproate (Ch. 23) is an effective prophylactic drug. Its major disadvantage is the risk of teratogenicity in women of child-bearing age. Clonidine (Ch. 6) is an effective prophylactic but is not recommended because of its propensity to cause depression or insomnia.

Small doses of a tricyclic antidepressant, such as amitriptyline, are sometimes recommended for the management of migraine either alone or in combination with a β-blocker. However, this may be more effective for tension-type headache, which can coexist with migraine. The efficacy of all current prophylactic treatments is limited. Although the response to an individual drug class is unpredictable, only about half of all migraineurs can expect to have a 50% reduction in the frequency of attacks

FURTHER READING

Diener H-CD, Kaube H, Limroth U (1998) A practical guide to the management and prevention of migraine. *Drugs* 56, 611–624

Ferrari MD (1998) Migraine. *Lancet* 351, 1043–1051

Groadsby PJ, Olesen, J (1996) Diagnosis and management of migraine. *Br Med J* 312, 1279–1283

Johnson KW, Phebus LA, Cohen ML (1998) Serotonin in migraine: theories, animal models and emerging therapies. *Progress Drug Res* 51, 219–244

Self-assessment

In the following questions the first statement, in italics, is true. Are the accompanying statements also true?

1. *Both antagonists at 5-hydroxytryptamine type 2 (5HT$_2$) receptors and agonists at 5HT$_{1D}$ receptors are used for the treatment of migraine.*

   a. Ergotamine is used prophylactically for migraine.
   b. Sumatriptan is not of use for acute attacks of migraine as it is slow acting.

2. *The contraceptive pill can enhance the frequency of migraine attacks in some women.*
   There is a large release of 5HT (possibly from platelets) in a migraine attack.

3. *Headache in migraine is thought to be caused by stimulation of sensory nerve endings in arteries.*

   a. Pizotifen is used prophylactically and inhibits 5HT$_2$ receptors.
   b. Ergotamine is safe to use in patients with ischaemic heart disease.
   c. Sumatriptan causes chest discomfort in 40% of patients as a result of coronary vasoconstriction.
   d. Prophylactic treatment for migraine is highly effective.

4. *A variety of drugs such as tricyclic antidepressants, β-blockers and pizotifen may be useful in prophylaxis of migraine.*
   Where migraine is associated with vomiting, metoclopramide and paracetamol given together is a useful combination.

5. *Beta-blockers are widely used in the prophylaxis of migraine.*
   Dietary or stress factors play little part in the precipitation of migraine attacks.

The answers are provided on pages 616–617.

Drugs used in migraine

Drug	Half-life (h)	Elimination	Comments
Dihydroergotamine	1–2	Metabolism	Very low oral bioavailability (1%); there is a terminal half-life of about 18 h, but this contributes minimally to elimination
Ergotamine	2	Metabolism	Very low oral bioavailability (2%)
Methysergide	10	(Renal + metabolism)?	Rapid and complete absorption; extent and routes of metabolism are poorly defined
Naratriptan	6	Metabolism/renal 50% unchanged	Inactive metabolites. Unlike sumatriptan, inhibits trigeminal nucleus
Pizotifen	26	Metabolism	Good oral bioavailability (80%)
Rizatriptan	2	Metabolism + renal	More rapid absorption than sumatriptan
Sumatriptan	2	Metabolism	Low oral bioavailability (14%), good subcutaneous bioavailability (100%)
Zolmitriptan	3	Metabolism	Oral bioavailability about 40%; one of the three main metabolites (the N-desmethyl metabolite) is a 5HT$_{1D}$ agonist

THE MUSCULOSKELETAL SYSTEM

The neuromuscular junction and neuromuscular blockade

Neuromuscular transmission

Acetylcholine (ACh) is the neurotransmitter at the nicotinic N_2 receptor of the neuromuscular junction. The processes of synthesis and release of ACh have been described briefly in Chapter 4, in relation to the general properties of neurotransmitters in the nervous system. The neuromuscular junction represents a specialised part of the sarcolemma of skeletal muscle, the motor endplate (Fig. 27.1a). In mammals, depolarisation of the

(a)

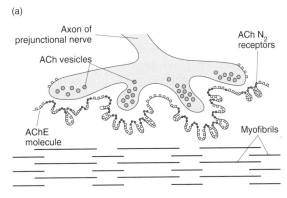

(b)

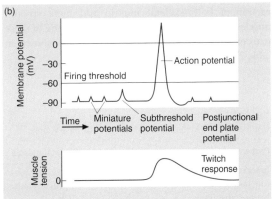

Fig. 27.1
Acetylcholine (ACh) at the neuromuscular junction. (a) Released ACh acts upon a postsynaptic nicotinic (N_2) receptor on the motor endplate opening a cation channel and an influx of Na^+ occurs, resulting in depolarisation. (b) At rest, insignificant amounts of ACh are released, and miniature endplate potentials generated are insufficient to reach the threshold potential to cause a propagated action potential. If sufficient ACh is released, an action potential is propagated causing muscle contraction. Non-depolarising muscle relaxants prevent the generation of the action potential by blocking N_2 receptors.

postsynaptic membrane at the motor endplate causes contraction of the muscle fibre in an all or none response. For stronger contractions, more motor units (the fibres innervated by one nerve) are recruited. The presynaptic nerve terminal contains 300 000 or more vesicles, each of which may contain up to 5000 molecules of ACh (known as a quantum). In response to an action potential, up to 500 vesicles are discharged over a very short period (0.5 ms). Rapid depolarisation of the motor endplate arises from binding of ACh to the nicotinic N_2 receptors. Each receptor has five subunits, two of which (the α-subunits) bind ACh. When two molecules of ACh are bound, the Na^+ channel in the centre of the receptor opens (Ch. 1), allowing an influx of Na^+. The extent of channel opening is dependent on the amount of ACh that is released and binds to nicotinic N_2 receptors; a minimum amount of depolarisation is necessary in order to reach the firing threshold at which full depolarisation is triggered (Fig. 27.1b). The action potential passes along the sarcolemma into the T tubules, where Ca^{2+} is released from the sarcoplasmic reticulum bringing about the processes of contraction. This usually requires the release of 50–200 quanta, which will activate 10–15% of motor endplate receptors. The action of ACh on nicotinic N_2 receptors is very short lived (about 0.5 ms) since the motor endplate has large amounts of acetylcholinesterase (AChE) associated with it (mouse diaphragm endplate has 12 000 AChE molecules per square micrometre). Another esterase, plasma or pseudocholinesterase, which is present in plasma and other cells, hydrolyses ACh more slowly than acetylcholinesterase but it is important pharmacologically because of its broad spectrum of activity in metabolising a number of ester drugs.

Although ACh is the neurotransmitter causing contraction of both skeletal muscle and most smooth muscles, the basic organisation and functioning of these neuroeffector systems are very different, as shown in Table 27.1.

Drugs acting at the neuromuscular junction

Acetylcholinesterase inhibitors

AChE inhibitors block the breakdown of ACh following its release in synapses and neuroeffector junctions. The mechanisms of action of different types of AChE inhibitor have been described in Chapter 4, but it should be appreciated that they are non-selective and affect the actions of ACh at nicotinic N_1, N_2 and muscarinic receptors. A major clinical use for these drugs is in the treatment of myasthenia gravis and details of this use are presented in Chapter 28.

Inhibitors of release of acetylcholine

Botulinum toxin A from the anaerobic bacillus *Clostridium botulinum* probably works by decreasing the release of ACh from vesicles. It is extremely toxic, as seen by occasional outbreaks of botulinum poisoning, but it has a clinical role, producing local muscle paralysis in patients with involuntary movements such as blepharospasm (spasm of the eyelids) or torticollis (wry-neck) (Ch. 24). It is given by injection as botulinum A toxin–haemagglutinin complex into the affected muscles, after which is can be effective for many weeks. It is used as a local injection for excessive sweating because of its action in inhibiting ACh at sweat glands and it is also being use for cosmetic reasons to remove frown lines and wrinkles.

Antagonists/blockers at the neuromuscular junction

Relaxation of skeletal muscles is an essential prerequisite for many surgical operations. To avoid the need for

Table 27.1
Comparison of skeletal and smooth muscle innervation

Property	Skeletal muscle	Smooth muscle
Innervation	Single	Multiple
Junction	Highly organised motor endplate	Simple
Neurotransmitter	ACh	ACh
Receptor subtype	Nicotinic N_2	Muscarinic (mainly M_3)
Receptor distribution	Only at motor endplate, only one motor endplate per muscle fibre	Widely on the muscle surface
Effects of stimulation	Single nerve contracts the whole muscle fibre (all or none response)	Each nerve contracts part of muscle fibre (graded response)
Overdose by inhibition of AChE	Flaccid paralysis	Spasticity

ACh, acetylcholine; AChE, acetylcholinesterase.

deep anaesthesia, this is achieved by drugs that specifically block the neuromuscular junction without affecting autonomic functioning (that is the actions of ACh on muscarinic and nicotinic N_1 receptors). Drugs that block the neuromuscular junction almost all resemble ACh to the extent that they contain a quaternary amino group, which produces strong binding to the anionic site of the nicotinic N_2 receptor.

Competitive antagonists

Examples: vecuronium, atracurium, pancuronium, mivacurium, cistracurium, rocuronium

Mechanism of action and effects

The competitive antagonists bind to the nicotinic N_2 receptor without causing depolarisation of the post-synaptic membrane and, therefore, blocking the depolarising effect of ACh. Inhibition of ACh breakdown by an AChE inhibitor (usually neostigmine, see Ch. 28) will reverse the blockade. The blockade is characterised by post-tetanic stimulation. A period of continuous nerve stimulation (tetanic stimulation) decreases neuronal ACh stores and increases ACh synthesis. If tetanic stimulation occurs during partial blockade of the N_2 receptor, the release of ACh decreases, the extent of blockade increases and the tetanic contraction fades. However, after cessation of tetanic stimulation, there is an enhanced response to a subsequent single stimulation, which is known as post-tetanic potentiation.

Pharmacokinetics

Because of their high polarity, conferred by the quaternary N atom (Fig. 27.2), these drugs are not absorbed from the gastrointestinal tract (hence the successful use of curare as an arrow tip poison in hunting) and they are given by intravenous injection. They have a low volume of distribution and do not cross the blood–brain barrier or placenta. Some are eliminated unchanged by glomerular filtration (tubocurarine, atracurium), while others are also metabolised partially in the liver and excreted in the bile (vecuronium, pancuronium). Their speed of onset of action and duration of action vary (Table 27.2).

Atracurium undergoes non-enzymatic spontaneous degradation as well as ester hydrolysis in the liver, which is an advantage in patients with hepatic or renal impairment. Mivacurium, like suxamethonium (succinylcholine; see below), is metabolised by plasma cholinesterase. The duration of effect of atracurium and mivacurium is about 20 min. This is longer than predicted from their plasma half-lives and may be a consequence of high-affinity binding sites close to the ACh receptor acting as a reservoir for the drug. With the exception of atracurium and mivacurium, the duration of action of competitive antagonists at the neuromuscular junction (from about 20 min for vecuronium up to 60 min for pancuronium) is determined by redistribution of the drug into the body tissues, which lowers the plasma concentration (see Ch. 2) and, therefore, the

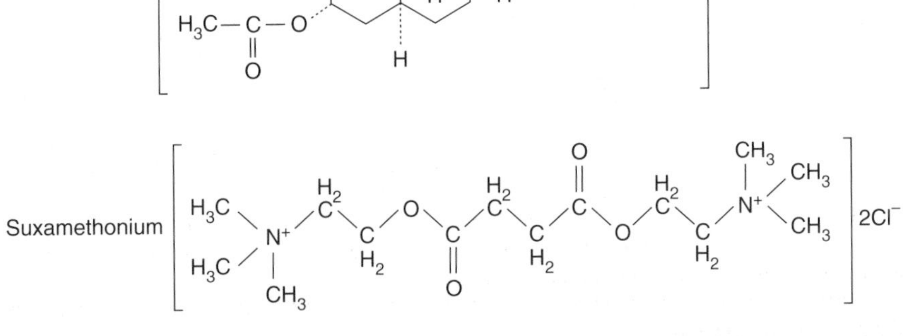

Fig. 27.2
The structures of pancuronium, a non-depolarising blocking drug, and suxamethonium, a depolarising blocker.

Table 27.2
Properties of non-depolarising skeletal muscle relaxants

Muscle relaxant	Time to onset (min)[a]	Duration (min)	Comment
Pancuronium	4–5	60	Tachycardia, hypertension
Vecuronium	5–6	20	Metabolite 3-desacetyl vecuronium is active leading to rare prolonged paralysis
Atracurium	5–6	20–25	Histamine release
Cisatracurium	5–6	20–25	Low histamine release
Rocuronium	2	20	
Mivacurium	2–3	15–20	Histamine release; metabolised by plasma cholinesterase

[a]90% reduction in muscle twitch.

concentration at the motor endplate. The drugs are removed by metabolism or degradation, which results in a duration of action of about 30 min.

Unwanted effects

- Blockade of ganglionic nicotinic N_1 receptors (tubocurarine) and cardiac muscarinic receptors (pancuronium), which leads to tachycardia.
- Tubocurarine, atracurium and mivacurium can cause the release of histamine from mast cells, producing flushing, hypotension, bronchospasm and a rash.
- Mivacurium can cause prolonged muscle paralysis in patients with pseudocholinesterase deficiency (see suxamethonium below).
- The other agents have few unwanted effects at clinically used doses.

Depolarising blockers

Example: suxamethonium (succinylcholine)

Mechanism of action and effects

Suxamethonium structurally resembles ACh and binds to the nicotinic N_2 receptors where it acts as an agonist to cause depolarisation of the motor endplate.

Suxamethonium is not hydrolysed by AChE and, therefore, causes more prolonged depolarisation of the motor endplate. This leads to a conformational change in the receptor that allows the Na^+ channel to close despite the continued presence of an agonist. As a result, the muscle repolarises and although it can respond to direct electrical stimulation, it can no longer be stimulated via the neuronal release of ACh. Indeed if the amount of Ach is enhanced (such as occurs with the use of an AChE inhibitor), it will add to a partial depolarising blockade and not reverse it. Suxamethonium produces a complex 'dual block', because after about 20 min of blockade the nature of the effect resembles that of a non-depolarising competitive antagonist. At this stage, tetanic stimulation no longer produces a sustained contraction and is accompanied by post-tetanic potentiation; in addition the blockade can now be partially reversed by an AChE inhibitor.

Pharmacokinetics

Suxamethonium contains two quaternary amino groups (Fig. 27.2), and because of its very high polarity it is not absorbed orally and must be given intravenously. It has a low volume of distribution and does not cross the blood–brain barrier or placenta. It is rapidly hydrolysed by plasma pseudocholinesterase and this results in a very short duration of action (about 5 min); therefore, an infusion is necessary to give a prolonged effect. A very prolonged paralysis occurs in about 1 in 2000–3000 individuals who have a genetically determined deficiency of plasma pseudocholinesterase. In this population, the action of suxamethonium is terminated after some 2–3 h by renal excretion.

Unwanted effects

- There is an initial depolarisation of the motor endplates prior to blockade; this results in muscle fasciculation and postoperative muscle pain.
- Prolonged apnoea occurs if there is a low circulating concentration of pseudocholinesterase through either a genetic deficiency or a decreased synthesis of the enzyme in patients with severe liver disease.
- The use of suxamethonium during anaesthesia has been linked with the development of a rare but potentially fatal disorder of muscles known as malignant hyperthermia; predisposition to this condition has an autosomal dominant inheritance, producing a defect in Ca^{2+} flux across the cell membrane.
- Stimulation of ACh receptors at autonomic ganglia (nicotinic N_1) and muscarinic receptors by high doses produces salivation and tachycardia.

- Profound bradycardia or cardiac arrest with repeated doses, especially in the presence of hyperkalaemia (which can be produced by suxamethonium, especially in the presence of tissue trauma).

Indications for neuromuscular-blocking drugs

The neuromuscular-blocking drugs are used in both surgical procedures and intensive care.

Tracheal intubation. Suxamethonium is used when there are residual gastric contents, since its rapid onset of action minimises the risk of aspiration. This is the only current major use for this drug. Because of frequent unwanted side-effects, the use of suxamethonium is declining. This change is especially driven by the advent of rapidly acting non-depolarising blocking drugs.

During surgical procedures. Neuromuscular blockade produces muscle relaxation for procedures such as abdominal incisions. It can be achieved either by single injection or by intravenous infusion for more prolonged surgery.

In intensive care. Neuromuscular blockade is used in addition to analgesia and sedation during mechanical ventilation, particularly if respiratory drive is suppressed (e.g. in adult respiratory distress syndrome), in status asthmaticus, for status epilepticus or tetanus, and in patients with elevated intracranial pressure.

FURTHER READING

Denborough M (1998) Malignant hyperthermia. *Lancet* 352, 1131–1136

Hunter JM (1995) New neuromuscular blocking drugs. *N Engl J Med* 332, 1691–1699

Miinchau A, Bhatia KP (2000) Uses of botulinum toxin injection in medicine today. *Br Med J* 320, 161–165

Wiklund RA, Rosenbaum SH (1997) Anesthesiology Part 1. *N Engl J Med* 337, 7132–7141

Self-assessment

In the following questions, the initial statement, in italics, is true. Are the accompanying statements also true?

1. *Vecuronium, unlike atracurium, has no haemodynamic effects as it does not cause histamine release.*

   a. Suxamethonium blockade is antagonised by lowered body temperature.
   b. All non-depolarising muscle relaxants cause similar amounts of histamine release.

2. *Malignant hyperthermia is a rare genetically determined disorder that causes hyperthermia and muscle spasms in response to suxamethonium, halothane and other drugs.*

   a. Dantrolene is used to treat malignant hyperthermia.
   b. A skeletal muscle fibre is innervated by one motor endplate
   c. The nicotinic receptor on skeletal muscle is identical to the nicotinic receptor in autonomic ganglia.

3. *Except for mivacurium and atracurium, the action of competitive neuromuscular junction-blocking drugs is mainly limited by redistribution of the drug*

   a. Suxamethonium is the only muscle relaxant used for tracheal intubation.
   b. Competitive neuromuscular blocking drugs such as vecuronium are relatively well absorbed orally.

4. *Botulinum toxin poisoning results from long-lasting blockade of parasympathetic and motor function.*

   a. Botulinum toxin acts postsynaptically to block acetylcholine-induced depolarisation.
   b. Botulinum toxin is administered only by discrete local injection.
   c. Botulinum toxin inhibits pathological excessive sweating as sweat glands are innervated by sympathetic cholinergic nerve fibres.

The answers are provided on page 617.

Self-assessment questions

Drugs acting at the neuromuscular junction

Drug	Half-life (h)	Elimination	Comments
Acetylcholine esterase inhibitors			
Distigmine	? (long)	Renal + hydrolysis	Given orally; very poor oral bioavailability (1–2%) especially if taken with food; hydrolysed by plasma esterases
Edrophonium	1.8	Renal + metabolism	Given intravenously over 30 s; eliminated mainly by renal excretion
Neostigmine	0.4–1.7 (i.v.)	Hydrolysis + renal	Given orally or by subcutaneous or intramuscular injection; very poor oral bioavailability (1–2%); elimination after oral dosage is probably longer than after i.v. dosage (absorption rate limited); metabolised by plasma and hepatic esterases
Pyridostigmine	0.4–1.9 (i.v.)	Renal + hydrolysis	Given orally; low and variable bioavailability (10–20%); most of the absorbed fraction is excreted in the urine unchanged; terminal half-life after oral dosage is probably longer than after i.v. dosage (absorption rate limited)
Non-depolarising blockers			All show negligible oral absorption and are given parenterally
Atracurium	0.3	Spontaneous + hydrolysis	Very rapidly breaks down within blood; unaffected by hepatic or renal failure
Cisatracurium	0.5	Spontaneous	Spontaneous degradation; therefore, low interpatient variability
Gallamine	2–2.5	Renal	Increased half-life in elderly
Mivacurium	2 min (*trans–trans*); 50–60 min (*cis–cis*)	Plasma hydrolysis	Consists of three isomers; the *cis–trans* and *trans–trans* have similar half-lives, are 10 times more potent than the *cis–cis* isomer, and are responsible for the clinical response
Pancuronium	0.5	Renal + biliary + metabolism	Hydrolysis product (3-hydroxy metabolite) retains activity
Rocuronium	1.2	Renal + metabolism	
Vecuronium	1.0	Bile + metabolism	Bile is major route of elimination (molecular weight 638 Da)
Depolarising blockers			
Suxamethonium	2–5 min	Plasma hydrolysis	Half-life shorter in infants and children

i.v., intravenous

28

Myasthenia gravis

Myasthenia gravis is a comparatively rare autoimmune disease in which there is an autoantibody to the acetylcholine nicotinic N_2 receptor system that impairs the responsiveness of the neuromuscular junction. The antibody causes increased receptor destruction; cross-links receptors, which causes increased receptor turnover; and blocks receptors by steric hindrance. This leaves a reduced number of functional nicotinic N_2 receptors on the motor endplate. In order to depolarise enough receptors to reach the firing potential in the muscle cell, a higher percentage than normal of receptors must be occupied by acetylcholine. As a result, myasthenic patients experience voluntary muscle weakness. Physiologically in a healthy neuromuscular junction, repetitive nerve impulses result in a decrement in the availability of sensitive receptors. In the myasthenic patient, the smaller receptor pool leads to a more rapid reduction in receptor availability with repetitive stimulation and increasing numbers of muscle fibres fail to fire. This produces the characteristic rapid muscle fatigue on exertion. Patients with myasthenia gravis show altered sensitivity to muscle relaxant drugs: they are more sensitive to competitive non-depolarising receptor antagonists but are resistant to depolarising blockers (Ch. 27).

The thymus gland plays a part in the genesis of the immune response in myasthenia gravis although the precise role is as yet uncertain. There are associated abnormalities of the thymus in 80% of patients with myasthenia gravis, usually lymphoreticular hyperplasia if the onset of the condition is at an early age or thymoma if the onset is over the age of 40 years.

Drug treatment of myasthenia gravis is based on prolongation of the action of acetylcholine by inhibiting its breakdown.

Acetylcholinesterase inhibitors

Examples: neostigmine, pyridostigmine, edrophonium

Mechanism of action and effects

Acetylcholinesterase (AChE) inhibitors block the breakdown of released acetylcholine (Ch. 4). They are non-selective and produce beneficial effects in myasthenia gravis through their action at nicotinic N_2 receptors (Ch. 4); unwanted effects arise from the excessive actions of acetylcholine at nicotinic N_1 and muscarinic receptors.

Pharmacokinetics and clinical uses

Neostigmine and pyridostigmine are quaternary amines that are slowly and incompletely absorbed from the gut; as a result, oral doses need to be approximately 10 times greater than parenteral doses to be effective. They have short half-lives and are eliminated by a combination of hepatic metabolism and renal excretion. They do not readily cross the blood–brain barrier. Both can be used to treat myasthenia gravis, and neostigmine is also used by intravenous injection to reverse the effect of competitive neuromuscular blockers (Ch. 27). Neostigmine has a faster onset of action and a shorter duration of action than pyridostigmine.

Edrophonium is given as an intravenous bolus to test the therapeutic response to AChE inhibitors in myasthenia gravis (see below); it has a very short duration of action (2–5 min) largely owing to tissue redistribution and is of no value in treatment.

Physostigmine is a tertiary amine isolated from the Calabar-bean and is readily absorbed from the gut. It is sufficiently lipid soluble to cross the blood–brain barrier and has a short half-life because of its rapid metabolism. It is therefore reserved for topical use in the eye but is now little used (Ch. 50).

Unwanted effects

Unwanted effects arise from the non-specific inhibition of AChE and the actions of accumulating acetylcholine on the autonomic nervous system (particularly a problem with neostigmine). They include effects on:

- the gastrointestinal tract: diarrhoea, abdominal cramps, excessive salivation
- heart: bradycardia
- eye: miosis
- airways: bronchoconstriction (see Ch. 12).

These peripheral muscarinic receptor effects can be blocked by administration of atropine or propantheline.

Excessive dosage will lead to a depolarising neuromuscular blockade by acetylcholine, and weakness through the build up of excess acetylcholine (see below).

Management of myasthenia gravis

Diagnosis

When the diagnosis of myasthenia is suspected (often because of ptosis, intermittent diplopia, facial weakness,

nasal speech or weakness of limb and trunk muscles with exertional fatigue) useful information can be rapidly obtained by pharmacological testing. An intravenous injection of the short-acting AChE inhibitor edrophonium will produce clinical improvement within 1 min, lasting about 5 min. Electromyographical tests that demonstrate abnormal fatiguability in multiple muscle fibres or abnormal contractile patterns in single fibres are confirmatory.

Treatment

Myasthenia gravis is treated with an AChE inhibitor, which reduces the normal rapid breakdown of acetylcholine and thereby enhances the activity of acetylcholine released by nerve stimulation. Pyridostigmine is commonly used since its action is more consistent than that of neostigmine, the dosing frequency is less and there are fewer muscarinic unwanted effects. An antimuscarinic agent (such as propantheline) may be necessary to block any parasympathomimetic actions of pyridostigmine, especially if large doses are given.

Excessive dosage of an AChE inhibitor can lead to prolonged stimulation of the N_2 receptors by acetylcholine, resulting in a depolarising blockade of the neuromuscular junction similar to that produced by suxamethonium (Ch. 27). Therefore, muscle weakness in myasthenia gravis can be the result of either inadequate dosage ('myasthenic crisis') or excessive dosage ('cholinergic crisis') of AChE inhibitor. The safest way to distinguish these problems is to use assisted ventilation and temporarily withdraw the AChE inhibitor.

Muscle groups do not all respond equally well to AChE treatment; ptosis and diplopia appear to be the most resistant. Patients who do not respond adequately to an AChE inhibitor are usually treated by immunosuppression with the corticosteroid prednisolone (Ch. 44) given alone or with azathioprine (Ch. 39). Corticosteroids are also used for initial immunosuppression in severely ill patients; they probably act by suppressing T-cell proliferation and reducing antibody synthesis. Azathioprine produces a clinical response over 2–4 months and its use can allow a reduction in the long-term dosage of prednisolone. Ciclosporin (Ch. 39) is used if there is a poor response to other immunosuppressive therapy. Plasma exchange to remove circulating acetylcholine receptor antibodies can produce a short-term response in severe disease. Immunosuppression is effective in most patients, but long-term treatment is usually necessary since relapse frequently occurs on withdrawal of therapy.

Thymectomy can induce remission and should always be carried out if there is a thymoma. In the absence of a thymoma, thymectomy is usually reserved for generalised disease.

FURTHER READING

Drachman DB (1994) Myasthenia gravis. *N Engl J Med* 330, 1797–1810

Evoli A, Batocchi AP, Tonali P (1996) A practical guide to the recognition and management of myasthenia gravis. *Drugs* 52, 662–670

Lindstrom JM (2000) Acetylcholine receptors and myasthenia. *Muscle Nerve* 23, 453–477

Self-assessment

In questions 1 and 2, the first statement, in italics, is true. Are the accompanying statements also true?

1. *Caution is required when administering pyridostigmine to patients with asthma.*

   a. Overdosage causing respiratory depression can be treated with atropine.
   b. In severe myasthenia gravis, the response to an anticholinesterase may be poor because of increased breakdown of the drug.

2. *Pyridostigmine produces less muscarinic receptor activity than neostigmine.*

   a. An acetylcholinesterase inhibitor should not be given with depolarising muscle relaxants such as suxamethonium (succinylcholine).
   b. A cholinergic crisis should be confirmed by administering pyridostigmine.

3. Case history question

   A 35-year-old woman with no previous illness noticed that she had ptosis and occasional diplopia. Over a period of time she became aware that on exertion she suffered from leg weakness although her coordination was normal. Following a sustained upward gaze for a minute, ptosis and diplopia could be elicited. Myasthenia gravis was suspected.

   a. What tests should be performed to verify the diagnosis?
   b. What is the pathogenesis of myasthenia gravis?
   c. Why is edrophonium injection used as a test for myasthenia gravis?

   Treatment was commenced following diagnosis.

   d. What principles should treatment follow?

   The answers are provided on pages 617–618.

Acetylcholine esterase inhibitors for the treatment of myasthenia gravis

Drug	Half-life (h)	Elimination	Comments
Distigmine	? (long)	Renal + hydrolysis	Very low oral bioavailability (1–2%) which is increased five-fold when taken on an empty stomach; given orally or by intramuscular injection; maximum effect is 9 h after the latter and the effect lasts for 24 h
Edrophonium	1.8	Renal (+ metabolism)	Given intravenously over 30 s; severe renal impairment reduces total clearance by more than 50%; not given orally
Neostigmine	0.4–1.7 (i.v.)	Renal and hydrolysis (of absorbed drug)	Very low oral bioavailability (1–2%); food delays absorption but does not affect AUC; elimination after oral dosage is probably longer than after i.v. dosage (absorption rate limited); metabolised by plasma and hepatic esterases
Pyridostigmine	0.4–1.9 (i.v.)	Renal (+ hydrolysis)	Low oral bioavailability (10–20%); food delays absorption but does not alter bioavailability; most of the absorbed fraction is excreted in the urine unchanged; terminal half-life after oral dosage is probably longer than after i.v. dosage (absorption rate limited); longer acting than neostigmine

AUC, area under the plasma concentration versus time curve; i.v., intravenous.

29

Non-steroidal anti-inflammatory drugs

Prostaglandins, inflammation and pain

Eicosanoids (meaning that the molecule contains 20 carbon atoms and has double bonds) are members of a family of related polyunsaturated fatty acids derived from the fatty acid precursor arachidonic acid. The family of derivatives includes prostaglandins, thromboxanes and leukotrienes. Arachidonic acid is synthesised in the liver from linoleic acid, which is derived from dietary constituents particularly vegetable oils, for example sunflower oil. Eicosanoids of a different type are also formed from eicosapentaenoic acid (also 20 carbon atoms long), which can be derived from oily fish; in platelets, the type of thromboxane generated from this precursor is less pro-aggregatory than that produced from arachidonic acid (Ch. 11). The prostanoids (generically defined as prostaglandins and thromboxanes) and leukotrienes are local hormones, which are generally synthesised and catabolised close to their site of action.

Prostaglandins are synthesised by oxygenation and ring closure of arachidonic acid, controlled by a rate-limiting cyclo-oxygenase (COX) that occurs as two isoenzymes: COX-1 and COX-2. The products of this reaction are unstable intermediates known as cyclic endoperoxides. Specific enzymes, which differ from cell to cell, convert these intermediates to various prostaglandins (Fig. 29.1). The products of the COX pathway, therefore, differ among various tissues, reflecting the diverse nature of their actions and the individual requirements of each cell type.

The second route for arachidonic acid metabolism is via the lipoxygenase pathway to produce leukotrienes (Fig. 29.1). These are also involved in the inflammatory process by enhancing vascular permeability (leukotrienes C_4, D_4 and E_4) and through chemotactic attraction of leucocytes (particularly leukotriene B_4; see also Ch. 12).

As a broad generalisation, the two forms of COX appear to have different purposes: COX-1 is a constitutive enzyme that is localised mainly to the endoplasmic reticulum. It is produced in the resting state by many cells and contributes to the regulation of several homeostatic processes such as renal blood flow, gastric cytoprotection and platelet aggregation. COX-2, by contrast, is an inducible enzyme, localised to the nuclear envelope in greater concentration than the endoplasmic reticulum. COX-2 is normally present in cells in only

305

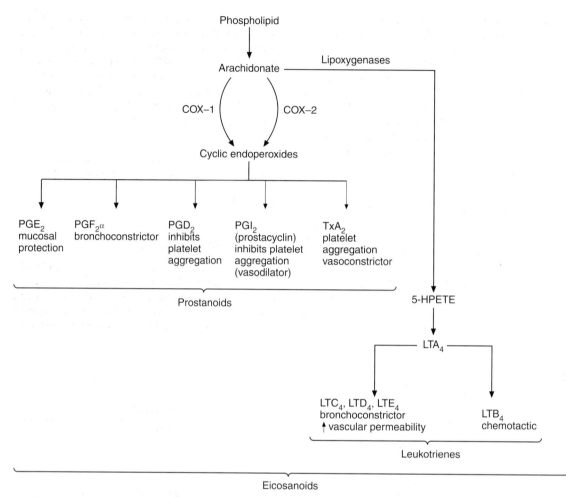

Fig. 29.1
The arachidonic acid cascade. Arachidonic acid can be utilised by cyclo-oxygenase (COX) 1 or 2 to form prostanoids (prostaglandins and thromboxanes). They have a variety of actions depending upon the site of formation and the amount formed. Other properties are shown in Table 29.2. Generally COX-1 results in transient formation of low 'house-keeping' amounts of prostanoids for physiological purposes. COX-2 stimulated by inflammatory cytokines etc. gives rise to high maintained concentrations of prostanoids resulting in pathological events. However, some studies now suggest that COX-2-generated prostaglandins may actually be involved in healing processes. PG, prostaglandin; Tx, thromboxane; HPETE, hydroperoxyeicosatretraenoic acid; LT, leukotrienes.

Table 29.1

Inflammatory mediators acting on nociceptors[a]

Action	Mediator
Direct coupling to membrane receptors	Hydrogen ions
	ATP
	5HT
Mediated by intracellular second messengers	Bradykinin (B_2 receptors).
	Cytokines (e.g. IL-1, IL-6, IL-8 TNF-α)
	Eicosanoids (prostaglandins, LTB_4, LTD_4)
	Histamine (H_1 receptors)
	5HT ($5HT_1$ receptors)

ATP, adenosine trisphosphate; 5HT, 5-hydroxytryptamine; IL, interleukin; LT, leukotriene; TNF, tumour necrosis factor.
[a]Prostaglandin E_2 can sensitise the nociceptive sensory nerves to the actions of many of these mediators.

low amounts but is expressed in endothelial cells, macrophages, synovial fibroblasts, mast cells, chondrocytes and osteoblasts, and many other cell types, in response to elevated cytokine concentrations, for example in inflammation, and in other pathological processes. COX-2 is the enzyme responsible for generation of most of the inflammatory prostaglandins, but in some situations COX-1 is also involved.

The actions of the formed prostaglandins and thromboxanes depend upon the pathological situation, whether they are generated by the COX-1 or COX-2 isoenzyme and whether they are formed in excessive amounts. For example, prostaglandin E_2 (PGE_2) is generated in low physiological amounts by COX-1 in gastric tissues and is important for gastrointestinal mucosal integrity. The potent thromboxane TXA_2 is generated by COX-1 in platelets and is important for platelet aggregation to prevent blood loss during blood vessel damage (Ch. 11). However, platelet aggregation induced by TXA_2 can also contribute to thrombus formation in ischaemic heart disease. In processes of inflammation and repair there is generation of excess amounts of prostaglandins

via elevated COX-2 expression, and this can contribute to the inflammation and pain. In particular, PGE_2 when generated in large amounts produces vasodilation, increased vascular permeability and sensitises pain fibre nerve endings to the stimulant action of bradykinin and 5-hydroxytryptamine (5HT) and other mediators (Table 29.1). A comparison of the major actions of prostaglandins is shown in Table 29.2.

Non-steroidal anti-inflammatory drugs

Mechanism of action

The non-steroidal anti-inflammatory drugs (NSAIDs) share a common mode of action, by inhibition of COX-1 and/or COX-2. Different NSAIDs have different relative effects on the two isozymes. Inhibition of COX reduces the generation of prostaglandins but does not affect the

Table 29.2
Actions of major prostaglandins and leukotrienes[a]

Tissue	Effect	Eicosanoid
Platelets	↑ Aggregation	TXA_2
	↓ Aggregation	PGI_2, PGD_2
Vascular smooth muscle	Vasodilation	PGI_2, PGE_2, PGD_2
	Vasoconstriction	TXA_2
Other smooth muscle	Bronchodilation	PGE_2
	Bronchoconstriction	PGD_2, PGF_2, TXA_2, LTC_4, LTD_4, LTE_4
	GI tract (contraction/relaxation, depends on muscle orientation)	PGF_2, PGE_2, PGI_2, PGD_2
	Uterine contraction	PGE_2, PGF_2
Vascular endothelium	Increased permeability	LTC_4, LTB_4
	Potentiates histamine/bradykinin	PGE_2, PGI_2
Neutrophils/macrophages	Chemotaxis	LTB_4
Gastrointestinal mucosa	Reduced acid secretion	PGE_2, PGI_2
	Increased mucus secretion	PGE_2
	Increased blood flow	PGE_2, PGI_2
Nervous system	Inhibition of noradrenaline release	PGD_2, PGE_2, PGI_2
	Endogenous pyrogen in hypothalamus	PGE_2
	Sedation, sleep	PGD_2
Endocrine/metabolic	Secretion of ACTH, GH, prolactin, gonadotrophins	PGE_2
	Inhibition of lipolysis	PGE_2
Kidney	Increased renal blood flow	PGE_2, PGI_2
	Antagonism of ADH	PGE_2
	Renin release	PGI_2, PGE_2, PGD_2
Pain	Potentiates pain through bradykinin, 5HT	PGE_2, PGD_2
Temperature	Pyretic in hypothalamus	PGE_2

ACTH, adrenocorticotrophic hormone; ADH, antidiuretic hormone; GH, growth hormone; 5HT, 5-hydroxytryptamine; LT, leukotriene; PG, prostaglandin; TX, thromboxane.
[a]Prostaglandins, thromboxanes and leukotrienes are predominantly local hormones synthesised and catabolised close to their sites of action. The actions and unwanted effects of the NSAIDs can largely be explained by inhibition of the formation of the prostaglandins and thromboxanes.

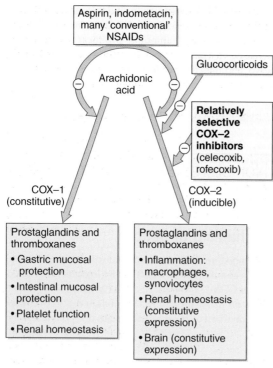

Fig. 29.2
Non-steroidal anti-inflammatory drugs (NSAIDs) and cyclo-oxygenase (COX) 1 and 2 isozymes. Many 'conventional' NSAIDs inhibit COX-1 and COX-2. Selective COX-2-inhibiting NSAIDs may show the advantage of a lower gastrointestinal side-effect profile. However, COX-2 is widely distributed and may be constitutively expressed in some areas, e.g. kidney. Inhibition with long-term treatment may affect renal function.

production of leukotrienes. Indeed, leukotriene production can increase as a result of diversion of arachidonic acid into the lipoxygenase pathway.

A unifying concept explaining the actions of all NSAIDs simply by the extent to which they inhibit COX-1 or COX-2 is not possible at present. However, some general comments can be made (Fig. 29.2).

Selective COX-2 inhibition

- The analgesic actions of NSAIDs appear to result from inhibition of COX-2.
- NSAIDs that inhibit COX-2 selectively (celecoxib, rofecoxib, meloxicam) appear to have useful anti-inflammatory actions and have fewer gastrointestinal damaging actions (COX-1-dependent gastroprotection) when compared with 'conventional' non-selective NSAIDs (Table 29.3). However, this view may turn out to be too simplistic, as recent data suggest that COX-2-generated prostaglandins may also contribute to gastric mucosal integrity and damage repair.
- Highly selective COX-2 inhibitors have little effect on platelet TXA_2 (COX-1-dependent) and therefore do not affect aggregation. These drugs may be better tolerated by patients with clotting disorders.
- In mice that have been bred to be genetically deficient in COX-2, there is significantly higher incidence of renal damage compared with normal animals.

Selective COX-1 inhibition

- Selective COX-1 inhibition reduces platelet aggregation. Aspirin (acetylsalicylic acid) is 150 times more effective at inhibiting COX-1 than COX-2. This is undesirable in patients with clotting disorders but beneficial in some disease states (Ch. 11).
- COX-1 inhibition predisposes to damage to the gastric mucosa. Doses of aspirin sufficient to have anti-inflammatory effects by inhibition of COX-2, therefore, cause gastric damage because the doses required to inhibit the mainly COX-2-mediated inflammatory processes must have significant inhibitory effects on COX-1.

COX-2 versus COX-1 inhibition

Although selective COX-2 inhibitors are likely to spare the gastrointestinal tract, it is too early to say that they

Table 29.3
The level of gastrointestinal disturbance in relation to the ability of NSAIDs to inhibit cyclo-oxygenase (COX) 1 and 2 isoenzymes

Gastrointestinal disturbance	Drug	COX-1:COX-2 inhibitory ratio
High	Indometacin	0.02
	Aspirin	0.006
Low	Ibuprofen	0.07
	Meloxicam	1.25
	Celecoxib	375
	Rofecoxib	?

This table indicates the approximate level of gastrointestinal disturbance and the comparative in vitro ratio of each drug to inhibit COX-1 and COX-2. For example, celecoxib is 375 times more effective for the inhibition of COX-2 than COX-1 whereas aspirin is 160 times more effective for the inhibition of COX-1 than COX-2. The level of gastrointestinal disturbance is clearly low for highly selective COX-2 inhibitors; ibuprofen, which is intermediate in its selectivity for COX-2:COX-1, also causes a relatively low incidence of unwanted effects.

will be advantageous in all patients, particularly those at high risk of gastrointestinal haemorrhage. The effect of long-term COX-2 inhibition requires careful study (Fig. 29.2).

Classification

Figure 29.3 shows the principal types of NSAIDs. They can be classified according to their mechanisms of action:

- rapid, reversible, competitive inhibitors (most NSAIDs)
- time-dependent, reversible, competitive inhibitors (e.g. indometacin, flurbiprofen, diclofenac)
- time-dependent, irreversible inhibitors (salicylate derivatives).

Most NSAIDs produce a reversible conformational change in COX. The irreversible inactivation produced by aspirin involves acetylation of the enzyme and is 150 times more effective for inhibiting COX-1 than COX-2. Other molecules show varying degrees of selectivity for COX-2. Meloxicam and more especially celecoxib and rofecoxib are agents with particularly high COX-2 selectivity (Table 29.3).

Paracetamol

Paracetamol is traditionally included under the banner of NSAIDs although it is, in reality, a simple analgesic without anti-inflammatory activity. This lack is probably because it has a different mode of action to NSAIDs.

Hydroperoxides are generated from the metabolism of arachidonic acid by COX and exert a positive feedback to stimulate COX activity. This feedback is blocked by paracetamol, thus indirectly inhibiting COX, particularly in the brain (this action is analgesic and antipyretic but does not reduce peripheral inflammation).

Actions and effects of NSAIDs

The properties and actions of some commonly used analgesic drugs are compared in Table 29.4. The anti-inflammatory, analgesic and antipyretic effects of NSAIDs are produced by complex modulation of inflammatory mediators. Inhibition of COX and, therefore, reduced prostaglandin production is an important, but not exclusive, mechanism by which this is achieved (Fig. 29.2).

Analgesia. This is largely a peripheral action at the site of pain and is most effective when the pain has an inflammatory origin. It is largely achieved through inhibition of COX-2 and reduced production of prostaglandins in inflamed or injured tissues. Some NSAIDs also decrease leukotriene production by leucocytes (e.g. indometacin, diclofenac) although this is probably not a major mode of action. A small component of the analgesic action of all NSAIDs is reduction of prostaglandin production in the pain pathways of the central nervous system (CNS), such as in the thalamus. This is the main site of action of paracetamol. Other central mechanisms have also been proposed, including reduced 5HT production or interference with the excitatory amino acid

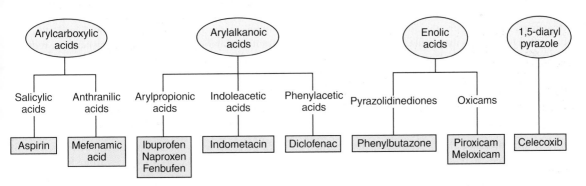

Fig. 29.3
Classification of non-steroidal anti-inflammatory drugs with selected drug examples.

Table 29.4
Properties of some commonly used analgesic drugs

	Aspirin (moderate doses)	Paracetamol	Indometacin	Ibuprofen	Celecoxib
Analgesic	++	++	+	+	+
Anti-inflammatory	+	−	+++	+	+
Antipyretic	+	+	+	+	+
Gastrointestinal bleeding	+	−	+	low	low

NMDA (*N*-methyl-D-aspartate; Ch. 4) in spinal cord pain pathways.

Anti-inflammatory effect. This is partly related to reduced peripheral prostaglandin synthesis. NSAIDs also affect several other inflammatory processes un-related to their effects on prostaglandins. For example, they probably reduce harmful superoxide free radical generation by neutrophils. They may also uncouple G-protein-regulated processes in the cell membrane of inflammatory cells. This would reduce cell responsiveness to a variety of agonists released by damaged tissues. (Paracetamol does not act on peripheral tissues, and has no anti-inflammatory action.)

Antipyretic effect. Fever is reduced through hypothalamic prostaglandin inhibition. Circulating pyrogens enhance prostaglandin production in the hypothalamus, which depresses the response of temperature-sensitive neurons. NSAIDs do not affect normal body temperature.

Reduction of platelet aggregation. This action is mediated by reduced platelet TXA_2 synthesis.

Pharmacokinetics

Most NSAIDs are weak acids that undergo some gastric absorption by pH partitioning (Ch. 2). This explains the relatively high drug concentration in gastric mucosal cells. However, most absorption occurs from the larger surface area of the small bowel. Enteric-coated formulations can be used to reduce release of drug in the stomach and limit direct exposure of the gastric mucosa. Some compounds, such as nabumetone, are formulated as inactive prodrugs (Ch. 2) to limit direct exposure of the gastric mucosa to active drug. These are converted (usually in the liver after absorption) to an active metabolite.

Absorption of NSAIDs from the gut is usually fairly rapid from conventional formulations, but the compounds differ widely in their elimination half-lives. Short-acting drugs require frequent dosing to maintain continuous therapeutic effect, although synovial fluid concentrations in joint disease fluctuate less than the plasma concentrations. Modified-release formulations are widely used to reduce dosing frequency during long-term treatment.

Some NSAIDs can be given by the intramuscular route for rapid onset of analgesia, or rectally to achieve a prolonged action and to avoid direct gastric irritation. Transcutaneous delivery was introduced with the intention of providing high local drug concentrations while attempting to minimise systemic unwanted effects. However, once the drug has penetrated the skin it is widely distributed and this route has no advantage for reducing systemic toxicity.

In the circulation, most NSAIDs are extensively bound to albumin. Competition for these binding sites can occur with other acidic protein-bound drugs, such as warfarin (Ch. 11).

Many NSAIDs undergo hepatic metabolism to inactive compounds. Aspirin (acetylsalicylic acid) is initially converted to an active metabolite, salicylic acid, and finally inactivated by conjugation. The latter process is saturable at higher doses and the metabolism of salicylate then changes from first-order to zero-order elimination kinetics (Ch. 2). This has important implications for aspirin overdose (Ch. 53). Piroxicam undergoes enterohepatic cycling, which contributes to its long half-life. Paracetamol is metabolised mainly by conjugation, but toxic metabolites can be formed that in overdose lead to significant hepatic destruction (Ch. 53).

Unwanted effects

Most unwanted effects arise from the non-selective inhibition of prostaglandin synthesis throughout the body. They are usually dose related. Since paracetamol does not inhibit peripheral prostaglandin synthesis, it does not cause these problems.

Gastrointestinal effects

Dyspepsia, gastric irritation and gastric ulceration are the most frequent unwanted effects. They are thought to occur principally as a result of inhibition of mucosal production of PGE_2 and PGI_2. PGE_2 has several actions that confer cytoprotection in the stomach (Ch. 33). The acidic nature of NSAIDs and their local concentration in gastric mucosal cells enables them to decrease the surface hydrophobicity of the mucus gel layer, reducing its barrier effect. Uncoupling of cellular oxidative phosphorylation by the drugs increases mucosal permeability, with consequent back-diffusion of H^+, which is trapped in the mucosal epithelium and leads to cyto-toxicity. Inhibition of prostaglandin generation reduces mucosal blood flow, which probably enhances cytotoxicity by producing tissue hypoxia and local free radical generation. NSAIDs accumulate within the mucosal cells by direct absorption of the drug from the gastric lumen and also by systemic delivery of the drug to the gastric mucosa. Consequently, rectal administration or the use of a prodrug will reduce but not eliminate the risk of gastric damage. Occult blood loss from the bowel is increased during regular treatment with NSAIDs and the risk of overt gastrointestinal bleeding is greater. (Management of NSAID-induced gastric damage is considered in Ch. 33.) COX-2-selective inhibitors have fewer gastric unwanted effects, but their long-term safety in patients with previous gastric ulceration is unknown.

Rectal administration can also result in local irritation and bleeding.

Both COX-1 and COX-2 inhibitors can exacerbate inflammatory bowel disease (Ch. 34).

Renal effects

Prostaglandins are involved in the maintenance of renal blood flow and have additional effects on the renal tubule that promote natriuresis. NSAIDs can produce a reversible decline in renal function, with a rise in serum creatinine and salt and water retention leading to oedema. The problem is more common if renal function is already impaired (as is often the case in the elderly), if other nephrotoxic drugs are used concurrently or in the presence of heart failure or cirrhosis.

Salt retention

Salt retention can occur even without renal insufficiency. This can exacerbate heart failure or further raise blood pressure in the hypertensive patient. In addition, the efficacy of drug treatments for these conditions (e.g. diuretics, ACE (angiotensin-converting enzyme) inhibitors, β-blockers) is blunted by NSAIDs (Ch. 14). The relative contribution of COX-1- and COX-2-generated prostaglandins to the maintenance of renal function is, as yet, unclear. Consequently, it is not known if selective COX-2 inhibitors will produce less disturbance of renal function.

Hypersensitivity

Hypersensitivity reactions occasionally produce asthma, urticaria, angioedema and rhinitis. Aspirin can precipitate asthma in a subgroup of sensitive asthmatics, through inhibition of PGE_2 production in the lung, with diversion of arachidonic acid towards leukotriene C_4 synthesis (Ch. 12). Patients with nasal polyps and known allergic disorders appear to be most susceptible. Selective COX-2 inhibitors may have less potential to induce asthmatic attacks in NSAID-sensitive individuals.

Other unwanted effects

Other unwanted effects are unrelated to prostaglandin inhibition and are relatively specific for individual compounds:

- aspirin produces tinnitus in toxic doses; overdose of aspirin can be particularly hazardous (Ch. 53)
- indometacin causes CNS unwanted effects such as dizziness, drowsiness and confusion, particularly in the elderly
- skin reactions can occur, especially with fenbufen
- phenylbutazone can produce bone marrow aplasia; its use is now restricted to patients with ankylosing spondylitis, for which it is particularly effective
- paracetamol causes hepatic damage and renal failure in overdose (Ch. 53); otherwise unwanted effects of paracetamol are rare.

Indications for NSAIDs

NSAIDs are indicated for pain relief, particularly for:

- inflammatory conditions affecting joints, soft tissues, etc.
- postoperative pain

- renal colic
- headache
- dysmenorrhoea.

Other indications

NSAIDs are also used

- as an antipyretic in febrile conditions
- to achieve closure of a patent ductus arteriosus in a neonate where patency may be inappropriately maintained by prostaglandin production (these drugs should not be given to a pregnant mother in the third trimester to avoid premature closure of the ductus)
- for primary dysmenorrhoea; stimulation of the uterus by prostaglandins can be responsible for the pain in this condition
- for modest reduction of menstrual blood loss in menorrhagia (excessive blood loss at menstruation)
- prevention of vascular occlusion by inhibition of platelet aggregation (especially low-dose aspirin (Ch. 11)
- reduction in colonic polyps and cancer (COX-1 and COX-2 inhibitors)
- recent studies suggest NSAIDs may reduce the progression of Alzheimer's disease.

Osteoarthritis

Osteoarthritis is the clinical manifestation of joint degeneration that results from loss of articular cartilage and becomes more common with increasing age. Most osteoarthritis is idiopathic (when it can be localised or generalised) but a small proportion is secondary to other conditions such as joint injury or chondrocalcinosis. It is not known whether the initiating factors originate in the articular cartilage or subchondral bone. The integrity of articular cartilage is determined by the structural protein type II collagen, which also binds other macromolecules that contribute to bone stability. Proteoglycan is the other major component and comprises a hydrophilic aggregate macromolecule called aggrecan containing a hyaluronan protein core with chondroitin and keratan sulfate chains. Aggrecan is involved in load dispersal.

The integrity of articular cartilage depends on the balance of production and resorption of the cartilage matrix by embedded chondrocytes. Synthesis of cartilage is determined by several growth factors, such as insulin-like growth factor 1 and transforming growth factor β. Degradation is by matrix metalloproteinases such as collagenases, gelatinase and stromelysin, which degrade both cartilage proteins. These enzymes are synthesised by chrondrocytes in response to stimulation by interleukin 1. It is not known whether the osteoarthritis is caused by increased degradation or decreased synthesis of cartilage.

Loss of cartilage matrix leads to disruption of the cartilage, with swelling and fissuring of the surface. Subchondral bone becomes increasingly vascular and new bone is laid down. There is recent evidence that stiffening of subchondral bone, with less effective shock absorption, may be the initiating factor for cartilage loss, which is enhanced by production of metalloproteinases in bone cells. The evidence for an inflammatory component in the destructive process is equivocal, but many patients will have an inflammatory component at some stage of the disease, with synovial inflammation particularly adjacent to the damaged cartilage.

The cardinal symptom of osteoarthritis is pain during physical activity, which is most pronounced with use of the affected joint, and relieved by rest. Pain also occurs at rest with advanced disease. Stiffness may be troublesome for short periods after rest. Various joints can be involved, particularly the distal interphalangeal joints of the fingers and the carpometacarpal joint of the thumb. Large joints such as the knee, hip, elbow and shoulder are often asymmetrically affected.

Management of osteoarthritis

Treatment currently remains symptomatic. Non-pharmacological therapy such as weight loss, exercise and physical therapy are often useful. If pain is troublesome, simple analgesics should usually be considered as first-line treatment. NSAIDs may be helpful for inflammatory episodes or if paracetamol is ineffective. In vitro studies suggest that some NSAIDs may accelerate the loss of articular cartilage in osteoarthritis. Clinical studies are inconclusive, but avoidance of powerful NSAIDs is probably desirable. Intra-articular or periarticular injection of a corticosteroid (Ch. 44) can provide short-term symptomatic relief in osteoarthritis, even if there is little clinical evidence of joint inflammation. Corticosteroids inhibit proinflammatory mediators in synovial tissue, such as interleukin 1 and tumour necrosis factor α. Long-term management of osteoarthritis may eventually require surgical joint replacement. Compounds under development, particularly metalloproteinase inhibitors and interleukin 1 receptor antagonists, may in future offer the possibility of prevention of cartilage degeneration or even promote regeneration.

FURTHER READING

NSAIDs

Bjorkman DJ (1998) The effect of aspirin and nonsteroidal anti-inflammatory drugs on prostaglandins. *Am J Med* 105(suppl 1B), 8S–12S

Cashman JN (1997) The mechanisms of action of NSAIDs in analgesia. *Drugs* 52(suppl 5), 13–23

Frölich JC (1997) A classification of NSAIDs according to the relative inhibition of cyclooxygenase isoenzymes. *Trends Pharmacol Sci* 18, 30–34

Jouzeau J-Y, Terlain B, Abid A et al. (1997) Cyclo-oxygenase isoenzymes. *Drugs* 43, 563–582

Lichtenstein DR, Wolfe M (2000) COX-2-selective NSAIDs. *JAMA* 284, 1297–1299

Lipsky PE (1999) The clinical potential of cyclooxygenase-2 specific inhibitors. *Am J Med* 106(suppl 5B), 515–575

McCarthy D (1998) Nonsteroidal anti-inflammatory drug-related gastrointestinal toxicity: definitions and epidemiology. *Am J Med* 105(suppl 5A), 3S–9S

Peterson WL, Cryer B (1999) COX-1-sparing NSAIDs – is the enthusiasm justified? *JAMA* 282, 1961–1963

Simon LS (1999) Role and regulation of cyclooxygenase-2 during inflammation. *Am J Med* 106(suppl 5B), 37S–42S

Singh G (1998) Recent considerations in nonsteroidal anti-inflammatory drug gastropathy. *Am J Med* 105(suppl 1B), 31S–38S

Vane JR (1998) Mechanism of action of nonsteroidal anti-inflammatory drugs. *Am J Med* 104(suppl 4A), 2S–8S

Osteoarthritis

Creamer P, Hochberg MC (1997) Osteoarthritis. *Lancet* 350, 503–509.

Perrot S, Menkes C-J (1996) Nonpharmacological approaches to pain in osteoarthritis. *Drugs* 52(suppl 3), 21–26.

Wollheim FA (1996) Current pharmacological treatment of osteoarthritis. *Drugs* 52(suppl 3), 27–38.

Self-assessment

In the following questions the first statement, in italics, is true. Are the accompanying statements also true?

1. *Two isoenzymes, cyclooxygenase (COX) 1 and 2 are involved in the synthesis of prostaglandins and thromboxanes.*

   a. COX-2 is an inducible enzyme.
   b. Prostaglandin E_2 does not cause pain itself but enhances the activity of algesic substances such as bradykinin.
   c. All non-steroidal anti-inflammatory drugs (NSAIDs) inhibit COX-1 and COX-2 isoenzymes with equal potency.
   d. Paracetamol is a potent analgesic and anti-inflammatory agent.

2. *Gastrointestinal complications are the most common unwanted effects of NSAIDs*

   a. NSAIDs reduce gastric blood flow.
   b. Aspirin and warfarin can be safely administered concurrently.

3. *The prostaglandin E_1 analogue misoprostol, if administered with NSAIDs, reduces their potential to cause gastric damage.*

   a. Small daily doses of aspirin can compromise renal function.
   b. The elderly have a greater risk of gastrointestinal adverse events when given NSAIDs.
   c. Ibuprofen is an effective first-choice NSAID in severe rheumatoid arthritis.
   d. Aspirin is a good choice of analgesic therapy for patients with asthma.

4. *Celecoxib and rofecoxib cause fewer gastrointestinal symptoms because they are highly selective COX-2 inhibitors.*

   a. Celecoxib is useful for the inhibition of platelet aggregation in patients with myocardial infarction.
   b. Celecoxib is an antipyretic.

The answers are provided on page 618.

Self-assessment questions

Non-steroidal anti-inflammatory drugs (NSAIDs)

Drug	Half-life (h)	Elimination	Comment
NSAIDs			All drugs given orally (unless otherwise stated); many of the drugs are carboxylic acid derivatives which are eliminated as acyl glucuronides
Aceclofenac	–	Metabolism	Oxidation in liver by CYP2C9 is the major pathway; a minor hydrolytic pathway results in bioactivation by forming diclofenac
Acemetacin	1	Metabolism	Prodrug of indometacin, with high bioavailability and quantitative conversion to indometacin
Aspirin	0.25	Rapid hydrolysis	Salicylic acid is an active metabolite (half-life 3–20 h)
Azapropazone	13–17	Renal (?)	Clearance correlates with creatinine clearance
Dexketoprofen	1–3	Metabolism	Isomer of ketoprofen
Diclofenac	1–2	Metabolism	Given orally, rectally, by deep i.m. injection or i.v. infusion; oral bioavailability is about 60%
Diflunisal	8–12	Metabolism	Major route is conjugation with glucuronic acid (phase II)
Etodolac	6–7	Metabolism	Oxidation (phase I) and conjugation (phase II)
Fenbufen	10–17	Metabolism	Prodrug, oxidised to active metabolites
Fenoprofen	1–3	Metabolism	Oxidation (phase I) plus conjugation (phase II)
Flurbiprofen	2–6	Metabolism + renal	Given orally or rectally; about 25% eliminated unchanged by the kidneys
Ibuprofen	2	Metabolism + renal	About 10% eliminated unchanged by the kidneys
Indometacin (indomethacin)	3–5	Metabolism + renal	Given orally or rectally; half-life may vary from 1 to 16 h
Ketoprofen	1–3	Metabolism	Given orally, rectally or by deep i.m. injection; glucuronidation (phase II) is the major route of elimination
Ketorolac	5–6	Renal + metabolism	Used in postoperative pain; given orally or by i.m. or i.v. injection; renal is major route (60% of dose) of elimination
Mefenamic acid	3–4	Metabolism	Metabolites are known to be inactive
Meloxicam	12–20	Metabolism	COX-2-selective compound; given orally or rectally; COX-2-selective activity is for the parent drug (metabolites are inactive)
Nabumetone	16–27 (metabolite)	Metabolism	Undergoes complete first-pass metabolism by hydrolysis of methyl ester group to yield an active naphthylacetic acid derivative
Naproxen	12–15	Metabolism	Given orally or rectally; metabolised by oxidation and conjugation to inactive products
Phenylbutazone	49–142	Metabolism	Metabolised by oxidation and formation of a C-glucuronide (very rare reaction)
Piroxicam	30–60	Metabolism + renal	Given orally, rectally or by deep i.m. injection; renal excretion accounts for about 10% of dose (99% protein binding minimises glomerular filtration of the drug)
Rofecoxib	17	Metabolism	COX-2-selective compound; reduced in cytosol to inactive metabolites
Sulindac	7–8	Metabolism + renal	Prodrug for active thioether metabolite, which is formed by reduction in the liver and lower bowel
Tenoxicam	44–100	Metabolism	Given orally or by i.m. or i.v. injection; metabolites are known to be inactive
Tiaprofenic acid	2–4	Metabolism	Oxidised by P450 (little other information available)
Tolfenamic acid	2	Metabolism	Metabolites are eliminated in bile
Related drugs			
Benorylate	<0.1	Hydrolysis	Ester of paracetamol and acetylsalicylic acid, absorbed intact and hydrolysed rapidly in blood and liver
Paracetamol (acetaminophen)	3–4	Metabolism	Most metabolised by conjugation (phase II); minor oxidation pathway leads to hepatotoxicity

COX, cyclo-oxygenase; i.m., intramuscular, i.v., intravenous.

Drug compendium

30

Rheumatoid arthritis and other inflammatory arthritides

Rheumatoid arthritis is an inflammatory condition of unknown cause. Autoimmune processes contribute to the maintenance of the condition, but it is uncertain whether it is initiated by autoimmune phenomena or infection. The primary process is infiltration of the synovium around the joint with lymphoid cells, formation of new blood vessels and a proliferation of the synovial membrane. The synovium subsequently invades and destroys joint cartilage and bone. Other forms of inflammatory arthritis do not usually produce erosive changes in periarticular bone or marked joint destruction.

The chronic inflammatory process is initiated by T-lymphocytes, then cellular proliferation and cytokine production in the synovial membranes sustain the condition. The cytokines are produced by macrophages and fibroblasts, and of these tumour necrosis factor α (TNFα) is prominent. This pattern differs from most other immune-mediated diseases. TNFα appears to orchestrate the recruitment of inflammatory cells such as leucocytes by increasing the expression of adhesion molecules (integrins) on leucocytes and vascular endothelial cells. The integrins also interact with basement membrane or matrix proteins such as fibronectin to induce angiogenesis. Antibodies form to the collagen exposed in the damaged cartilage. Complexes of collagen antibody with IgM rheumatoid factor (autoantibodies reactive with IgG) in the cartilage may act as chemoattractants to the inflammatory cells in invasive synovial tissue. The end result is irreversible destruction of cartilage and erosion of periarticular bone.

The symptoms of rheumatoid arthritis appear gradually in most patients and usually involve the proximal interphalangeal joints of the fingers, metacarpophalangeal joints and wrists. Other joints such as the ankles and hips may be involved later. The affected joints are warm, swollen and painful. Stiffness is troublesome, particularly in the morning, as a result of an increase in extracellular fluid in and around the joint. Systemic disturbance is common, including general fatigue and malaise, while extra-articular manifestations such as vasculitis and neuropathy can occur.

Second-line drugs for rheumatoid arthritis

Non-steroidal anti-inflammatory drugs (NSAIDs) provide symptomatic relief but do not alter the long-term

315

progression of joint destruction in rheumatoid arthritis (Ch. 29). A diverse group of compounds may reduce the rate of progression of joint erosion and destruction, leading to improvement both in symptoms and in the clinical and serological markers of rheumatoid arthritis activity. The mechanisms by which they achieve this are poorly understood, but long-term depression of the inflammatory response is probably important even though these compounds have little or no direct anti-inflammatory effect. They all have a slow onset of action, with most producing little improvement until about 3 months after starting treatment. However, it is still unclear whether they modify the long-term outcome of the disease. For this reason, second-line drugs is the term preferred to the alternative disease-modifying drugs.

Gold

Examples: sodium aurothiomalate, auranofin

Mechanism of action

The precise mechanism by which gold acts is unknown, and it has been suggested that the oral and parenteral forms could act differently. A popular concept is that gold is taken up by mononuclear cells and inhibits their phagocytic function. This will reduce the release of inflammatory mediators and inhibit inflammatory cell proliferation. Production of other factors involved in inflammation may also be inhibited, such as complement and free radicals.

Oral gold (auranofin) has a rather slower onset of action than intramuscular gold and is less efficacious, but it much better tolerated.

Pharmacokinetics

The parenteral form of gold (sodium aurothiomalate) is given by deep intramuscular injection. An initial test dose is given to screen for acute toxicity (see below) followed by injections at weekly intervals to gradually achieve a therapeutic concentration in the tissues. Subsequently a smaller dose is used to maintain remission. Oral gold is taken daily. Gold binds readily to albumin and several tissue proteins and accumulates in many tissues such as the liver, kidney, bone marrow, lymph nodes and spleen. Accumulation also occurs in the synovium of inflamed joints. Elimination is largely by the kidney, and to a lesser extent by biliary excretion. Gold has a half-life of several weeks, probably as a result of its extensive tissue binding.

Unwanted effects

The unwanted effects can be serious and all but the most minor effects should lead to immediate cessation of treatment:

- oral ulceration
- proteinuria owing to membranous glomerulonephritis: proteinuria can develop after several weeks of treatment sometimes progressing to nephrotic syndrome; recovery can take up to 2 years following drug withdrawal
- blood disorders, especially thrombocytopenia but also agranulocytosis and aplastic anaemia
- skin rashes
- Diarrhoea: common with oral gold.

Prevention and management of unwanted effects

Urine should be checked for protein and a blood count obtained before each injection of gold, and regularly during oral therapy. Major complications may require chelation of gold with dimercaprol or penicillamine (Ch. 53) to increase its elimination. Corticosteroids can be helpful to treat blood dyscrasias. Gold should not be used if there is a history of renal or hepatic disease, blood dyscrasias or severe skin rashes. If stomatitis, a pruritic rash, neutropenia, thrombocytopenia or significant proteinuria (>1 g in 24 h) develop, gold should be stopped.

Penicillamine

Mechanism of action and uses

Modulation of the immune system is believed to underlie the action of penicillamine. The precise details are uncertain but may include reduced production of immunoglobulins, reduction in the number of activated lymphocytes and stabilisation of lysosomal membranes in inflammatory cells. Penicillamine has not been shown to slow the progression of joint erosions.

Penicillamine can chelate many metals. This is probably of little relevance to its use in arthritis, but has given the drug a role in the management of poisonings (Ch. 53) and in Wilson's disease, a genetically determined illness that is associated with copper overload.

Pharmacokinetics

Pencillamine is well absorbed from the gut, although oral iron supplements substantially reduce its absorption. The half-life is short but there is tight binding of drug to plasma and tissue proteins. Penicillamine is partially metabolised but is also excreted unchanged in the urine. Doses should be increased gradually to reduce the incidence of unwanted effects.

Unwanted effects

Unwanted effects occur frequently and are responsible for about 30% of patients stopping treatment. Many unwanted effects resemble those of gold:

- nausea, vomiting, abdominal discomfort and rashes (often with fever), especially early in treatment

- loss of taste is common but may resolve despite continued treatment
- oral ulceration
- proteinuria, which is caused by immune complex glomerulonephritis and is dose related; nephrotic syndrome can occur
- blood disorders, especially thrombocytopenia but also neutropenia or, rarely, aplastic anaemia.

Regular monitoring of urine protein and blood counts should be carried out during treatment.

Antimalarials

Examples: chloroquine, hydroxychloroquine

The antimalarial drugs are believed to reduce T-lymphocyte transformation and chemotaxis. Their weakly acidic nature permits their uptake into cells in a nonionised form. Having entered the lysosomes inside the cell, the acidic environment traps and concentrates the drug in its ionised state. The phagocytic properties of macrophages depend on acidification of their lysosomes for digestion of engulfed protein. Antimalarial drugs appear to slightly increase the pH inside the lysosome, which changes the processing of peptide antigens and alters the subsequent presentation of antigen on the cell surface. The consequence is a reduction in cellular expression of 'self' peptides, but an intact expression of exogenous peptides. Thus, the interaction between T helper cells and antigen-presenting macrophages responsible for joint inflammation is reduced, with a reduction in the inflammatory response. The major toxic effect of antimalarial drugs is on the retina, although at the low doses that are now recommended they are relatively safe. Annual specialist monitoring of the eyes is still recommended by some rheumatologists. The pharmacokinetics and unwanted effects of these drugs are considered in Chapter 51.

Sulfasalazine

The action of sulfasalazine in arthritis is poorly understood. It is hydrolysed in the colon to 5-aminosalicylic acid (which is believed to contribute little to the antirheumatic action) and to sulfapyridine. The latter moiety probably acts by reducing absorption of antigens from the colon that promote joint inflammation.

High doses of sulfasalazine are required for the treatment of rheumatoid arthritis, which often produce gastrointestinal upset. This can be minimised by increasing the dose slowly and by using an enteric-coated formulation. Other problems include oligospermia (therefore sulfasalazine should be avoided in males who have not completed their family) and blood dyscrasias. Sulfasalazine is discussed more fully in Chapter 34.

Leflunomide

Mechanism of action and uses

Leflunomide is an isoxazole derivative that binds to dehydroorotate dehydrogenase, an enzyme involved in the synthesis of pyridines. This reduces uridine diphosphate (UTP) levels and pyrimidine synthesis in lymphocytes and other rapidly dividing cells. The activity of tyrosine kinase in cells is also reduced by leflunomide. The result is suppression of immunoglobulin production and reduced adhesion of inflammatory cells.

The place of leflunomide compared with other disease-modifying antirheumatic drugs remains to be established. It is being investigated in other disorders, including psoriasis and various autoimmune diseases.

Pharmacokinetics

Leflunomide is a prodrug. It is well absorbed from the gut and converted in the liver to its active metabolite, which has a very long half-life of 15–18 days. The metabolite is excreted via the bile and kidney.

Unwanted effects

Unwanted effects include:

- gastrointestinal upset
- allergic reactions, especially rash
- alopecia
- reversible abnormalities of liver function.

Immunosuppressive drugs

Several drugs with immunosuppressive actions have been shown to be effective in rheumatoid arthritis. These include:

- antimetabolites: methotrexate, azathioprine (Ch. 52)
- alkylating agents: cyclophosphamide, chlorambucil (Ch. 52)
- ciclosporin (Ch. 39).

Antibodies against tumour necrosis factor

Examples: etanercept, infliximab

Mechanism of action and uses

Etanercept is a fusion protein consisting of two recombinant p75 TNF receptors, fused to the Fe portion of human immunoglobulin (IgG$_1$). It binds to TNFα and TNFβ and reduces the activity of TNFα in promoting inflammation. It is also undergoing trials for inflammatory bowel disease.

Infliximab is a chimeric monoclonal murine antibody that neutralises TNFα. It also inhibits production of other inflammatory cytokines, such as interleukin-6, reduces inflammatory cell infiltration into inflamed areas and reduces expression of cellular adhesion molecules. It does not neutralise TNFβ.

Etanercept is given by twice weekly subcutaneous injection. Its half-life is long at about 5 days. Its route of elimination is at least partly via the kidneys.

Infliximab is given by intravenous injection and has a very long half-life of 10–14 days. Its route of elimination is not well understood. Infliximab is also discussed in Chapter 34.

Unwanted effects

Etanercept produces mild injection site reactions and upper respiratory tract symptoms, e.g. rhinitis.

Infliximab produces fever, chills, pruritis or urticaria after infusion in about 15% of patients. It also causes dyspnoea or headache.

Other antibodies

Clinical trials with inhibitors of interleukin 2 are also taking place.

Management of rheumatoid arthritis and other inflammatory arthritides

NSAIDs (Ch. 29) are the mainstay of symptomatic drug treatment. Physical aids such as splinting and bed rest are important for acute episodes. The choice of NSAID is arbitrary, with considerable variation in individual responses to different drugs. Propionic acid derivatives are often used first; they are somewhat weaker than other classes but generally have fewer unwanted effects. More powerful drugs such as indometacin are used when others fail to control symptoms. About 60% of patients can be expected to respond to the first-choice agent and most can be controlled by one of the NSAIDs. Predicting which drug will be most effective is currently impossible. Morning stiffness is often disabling in inflammatory arthritis: this is helped by giving a late evening dose of an NSAID with a long half-life, a modified-release formulation of a compound with a short half-life or an NSAID suppository. Topical NSAIDs applied over the affected joint(s) are not recommended.

Inflammatory arthritides other than rheumatoid arthritis (the seronegative spondylarthritides) do not usually progress to extensive erosive arthritis with joint destruction. By contrast, progressive joint damage is common in rheumatoid arthritis. For this reason, second-line drugs are often used early in rheumatoid arthritis. Indications for these agents include

- the prevention of erosive damage
- the suppression of persistent inflammation that fails to respond to 6 months of treatment with NSAIDs
- patient intolerance to NSAIDs
- a high titre of rheumatoid factor or extra-articular manifestations of rheumatoid disease.

Second-line drugs are almost always used in combination with NSAIDs, particularly in the first few weeks of treatment, since they do not have significant anti-inflammatory action and require 2–3 months before an effect is established. There is no consensus for choice among second-line drugs. Sulfasalazine is often chosen for its low toxicity but methotrexate is probably the most effective agent. Gold (despite a suggestion that it may increase mortality) and penicillamine are also widely accepted as second-line drugs, while immunomodulators other than methotrexate are generally reserved as third-line agents. Cytotoxic drugs, especially cyclophosphamide, appear to be particularly useful for the management of extra-articular manifestations of rheumatoid disease, such as vasculitis, pericarditis or pleurisy.

The role of corticosteroids in rheumatoid arthritis has been controversial. Intra-articular injections are used for individual inflamed joints (especially knee and shoulder). In active disease, short courses of oral prednisolone or pulse therapy with intravenous methylprednisolone (Ch. 44) can produce a rapid onset of effect before second-line drugs work. In early rheumatoid disease, a small dose of oral prednisolone in combination with a second-line drug has been shown to reduce disease progression.

Increasingly, combinations of second-line drugs are being used as standard therapy. An example is low-dose corticosteroids with sulfasalazine and methotrexate. Such combinations appear to be more effective than single agents given alone.

Leflunomide is a new second-line drug that is likely to be used when other more established agents fail to work or are poorly tolerated. Anti-TNF agents are reserved for patients who fail to respond to more conventional therapies.

FURTHER READING

Inflammatory arthritis

Buckley CD (1997) Treatment of rheumatoid arthritis. *Br Med J* 315, 236–238

Cash JM, Klippel JH (1994) Second-line drug therapy for rheumatoid arthritis. *N Eng J Med* 330, 1368–1375

Choy EHS, Scott DL (1997) Drug treatment of rheumatic disease in the 1990s. *Drugs* 53, 337–348

Fox DA (2000) Cytokine blockade as a new strategy to treat rheumatoid arthritis *Arch Int Med* 160, 437–444

Fox R (1995) Antimalarial drugs. Mechanisms of action in autoimmune diseases and prospects for drug development. *Clin Immunother* 4, 219–234

Jackson CG, Williams HJ (1998) Disease modifying antirheumatic drugs. *Drugs* 56, 337–344

Langford CA (1998) Use of cytotoxic agents and cyclosporine in the treatment of autoimmune disease. Part I. Rheumatological and renal diseases. *Ann Intern Med* 128, 1021–1028

Smith JM (2001) Anti-TNF agents for rheumatoid arthritis. *Br J Pharmacol* 51, 201–208

Self-assessment

In the following questions, the first statement, in italics, is true. Are the following statements also true?

1. *Second-line antirheumatic drugs are commonly also called disease-modifying antirheumatic drugs (DMARDs) or slower acting antirheumatic drugs (SAARDs).*

   a. Non-steroidal anti-inflammatory drugs (NSAIDs) reduce the symptoms of rheumatoid disease and retard the progress of the disease.
   b. If penicillamine does not lead to clinical benefit within 6 months it should be stopped.

2. *When tolerated, intramuscular gold is an effective drug for achieving remission in rheumatoid arthritis but unwanted effects limit tolerability.*

   a. Gold can be given by intramuscular or oral routes.
   b. Intramuscular gold can cause proteinuria

3. *Methotrexate or sulfasalazine are often chosen as initial second line therapy for rheumatoid arthritis partly because of their rapid onset of action (4–6 weeks methotrexate, 8–12 weeks sulfasalazine).*

   a. During methotrexate therapy, folic acid is contraindicated.

   b. The combination of sulfapyridine and 5-amino salicylic acid (sulfasalazine) is more effective than either component alone.
   c. Methotrexate has relatively fewer unwanted effects compared with most other second-line drugs for rheumatoid arthritis.

4. *Sulfasalazine can scavenge toxic oxygen metabolites produced by neutrophils, and this may contribute to its effect in rheumatoid arthritis.*
   Combination therapy with second-line drugs should not be used in rheumatoid arthritis.

5. *A major role of corticosteroids is to bridge the gap between starting treatment and the onset of action of the second line treatments for rheumatoid arthritis.*

   a. Intra-articular injections of corticosteroids slow progression of erosions.
   b. Prolonged treatment with high doses of corticosteroids can cause adrenal atrophy.

6. *Ciclosporin is valuable when used in combination with methotrexate in very active early rheumatoid disease.*
   The antimalarials chloroquine and hydroxychloroquine are of little benefit in the treatment of rheumatoid arthritis.

The answers are provided on page 618.

Second-line drugs used to treat rheumatoid arthritis

Drug	Half-life	Elimination	Comment
Auranofin	17–25 days	Renal + faecal (unabsorbed)	Given orally; 13–33% absorbed
Aurothiomalate (sodium salt)	250 days	Renal + faecal	Given by deep intramuscular injection
Azathioprine	3–5 h	Metabolism	Metabolism to 6-mercaptopurine represents a bioactivation process
Chlorambucil	1–2 h	Metabolism	Extensive oral absorption
Chloroquine	30–60 days	Metabolism	Complete absorption; massive tissue distribution (200 l kg^{-1})
Cyclophosphamide	4–10 h	Metabolism + renal	
Ciclosporin	27 h	Metabolism	A lipid-soluble peptide oxidised by CYP3A4
Hydroxychloroquine	18 days	Metabolism	Extensive oral absorption
Methotrexate	8–10 h	Metabolism	Variable and incomplete oral absorption (25–95%): a fraction of the dose shows tissue retention as polyglutamates
Penicillamine	1–6 h	Metabolism + faecal + renal	Incomplete oral absorption
Sulfasalazine			
Parent drug	3–11 h	Reductive metabolism	About 20–30% absorbed in small intestine; reduced to active metabolites
Sulfapyridine	6–17 h	Metabolism	Acetylated and oxidised in liver; cause of many unwanted effects
5-Aminosalicylate	4–10 h	Metabolism + renal + faecal	Acetylated in colonic wall and liver; poor absorption from colon
Etanercept	5 days	Protein clearance	Given by subcutaneous injection twice weekly
Infliximab	9.5 days	Protein clearance	Given by infusion; prolonged duration of action (weeks)
Leflunomide	2 weeks (AM)	Metabolism	Once daily oral dosage; converted to active metabolite (AM)

Gout

The pathophysiology of gout

Uric acid is a relatively insoluble derivative of the nucleic acid purine bases guanine and adenine (Fig. 31.1). If the plasma concentration of uric acid is high it can crystallise as monosodium urate in tissues, which initiates an inflammatory response; in brief, phagocytic cells are attracted to the tissue where they internalise the crystals. This initiates an immune response, with the release of proteolytic and lysosomal enzymes that enhance tissue inflammation and destroy cartilage, damaging the joint. Deposition of uric acid crystals in joints produces an extremely painful acute arthritis with repeated attacks of gout. In some patients, chronic urate deposits (tophi) are found in tendon sheaths and soft tissues.

Uric acid is normally eliminated by the kidney. It is filtered at the glomerulus and then reabsorbed from the proximal tubule. Subsequently, there is considerable distal tubular secretion with a small amount of reabsorption at the same site. Excess uric acid can be deposited in the interstitium of the kidney or form stones in the renal calyces. Both mechanisms will produce progressive renal damage.

Hyperuricaemia results from:

- overproduction of uric acid: from excessive cell destruction (e.g. lymphoproliferative or myeloproliferative disorders, especially during their

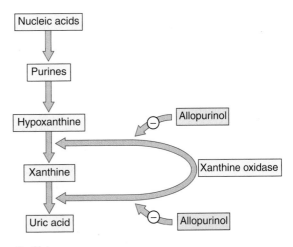

Fig. 31.1
The pathway for production of uric acid and the sites of action of allopurinol.

treatment; Ch. 52), inherited defects that increase purine synthesis, high alcohol intake
- reduced renal excretion: renal failure and drugs that reduce tubular secretion of uric acid (e.g. most diuretics, low-dose aspirin and lactate formed from alcohol).

There are two reasons to consider drug treatment:

- treatment of an acute attack
- reduction of plasma uric acid concentration for prophylaxis against recurrent attacks.

Treatment of gout

Acute gout

For acute attacks, non-steroidal anti-inflammatory agents (NSAIDs; Ch. 29) are the treatment of choice, especially indometacin, but aspirin should be avoided as it can increase plasma urate at some concentrations. Colchicine is usually reserved for patients intolerant of NSAIDs. Intra-articular injection of corticosteroid can be very effective, but oral corticosteroids, for example prednisolone (Ch. 44), are reserved for resistant episodes of gout. Efforts should always be made to identify and remove precipitating causes.

Colchicine

Mechanism of action

Colchicine was originally used as an antimitotic agent. It is believed to act in gout by reducing production of chemotaxins and, therefore, inhibiting leucocyte migration into inflamed tissue. Colchicine also depolymerises proteins in leucocyte microtubules by forming a complex with tubulin in the cell. This interferes with transport into lysosomes of material phagocytosed by leucocytes. Colchicine has a specific anti-inflammatory effect in the gouty joint and has no effect in other forms of inflammatory arthritis.

Pharmacokinetics

Colchicine is poorly absorbed from the gut and partially excreted unchanged in the urine and bile. Some hepatic metabolism also occurs. The initial half-life of colchicine is very short but enterohepatic circulation prolongs its action. It is usually given every 2 h until symptomatic relief is achieved or unwanted effects occur. Pain relief usually begins after about 18 h and is maximal by 48 h.

Unwanted effects

Gut toxicity caused by inhibition of mucosal cell division produces abdominal pain, vomiting and diarrhoea. These effects are common and are often dose limiting.

Prevention of gout attacks

To prevent gout, the serum uric acid concentration should be reduced to less than 3.6 mmol l⁻¹ although it may be necessary to go below 3.0 mmol l⁻¹ to reabsorb gouty tophi. Prophylactic treatment should usually be life-long, since recurrence of gout or tophi frequently occurs if treatment is stopped. Short-term treatment is possible when allopurinol is used for prophylaxis during cytotoxic chemotherapy.

Allopurinol is given for prophylaxis after recurrent attacks of acute gout have been resolved, for chronic deposition of urate in the tissues (tophi) or for uric acid-induced renal damage. It is also given prophylactically before cytotoxic chemotherapy, when tissue breakdown generates large amounts of uric acid. Allopurinol should not be used during an acute attack of gout and cover with a low dosage of an NSAID should be provided during the first 2 months of treatment. Uricosuric drugs are reserved for patients who do not tolerate allopurinol but should be avoided if there is renal damage.

Allopurinol

Mechanism of action

Allopurinol is an analogue of hypoxanthine and competitively inhibits the enzyme xanthine oxidase, thereby reducing uric acid formation and concentration in tissues (Fig. 31.1). Although plasma xanthine and hypoxanthine concentrations increase, they do not crystallise because of their greater water solubility. Xanthine and hypoxanthine are also available for reincorporation into the purine metabolic cycle, and by a feedback mechanism this decreases de novo purine formation.

Pharmacokinetics

Allopurinol is well absorbed from the gut and converted in the liver to a long-acting active metabolite, oxypurinol (alloxanthine). Both compounds are excreted by the kidney. The half-life of oxypurinol is long.

Unwanted effects

- There is an increased risk of acute gout during the first few weeks of treatment. This may be caused by fluctuations in plasma uric acid, perhaps through reabsorption from tissue deposits.
- Allergic reactions, especially rashes. These can be particularly serious in patients with renal impairment.
- Drug interactions: allopurinol inhibits the metabolism of the cytotoxic drugs mercaptopurine and azathioprine (Ch. 52), which are metabolised by xanthine oxidase.

Uricosuric agents

Examples: probenecid, sulfinpyrazone

Mechanism of action

The uricosuric drugs compete with uric acid for reabsorption from the distal renal tubule. Low doses preferentially inhibit tubular secretion of uric acid, which can raise plasma uric acid levels. There is a risk of precipitation of uric acid crystals in the kidney, particularly during the early stages of treatment, which can be prevented by maintaining a high fluid intake and an alkaline urine (using potassium citrate or sodium bicarbonate). Aspirin and other salicylates should not be given with uricosurics since small doses of these drugs inhibit tubular uric acid secretion.

Pharmacokinetics

Both probenecid and sulfinpyrazone are well absorbed from the gut and eliminated partly by metabolism and partly by renal excretion. Their half-lives are intermediate.

Unwanted effects

- Gastrointestinal upset.
- Renal uric acid deposition. Deterioration of renal function can occur if there is pre-existing impairment.
- Probenecid reduces urinary elimination of several drugs, for example penicillins, cephalosporins (Ch. 51), NSAIDs (Ch. 29), sulfonylureas (Ch. 40).

FURTHER READING

Emmerson BT (1996) The management of gout. *N Engl J Med* 334, 445–451

Snaith ML (1995) Gout, hyperuricaemia, and crystal arthritis. *Br Med J* 310, 521–524

Star VL, Hochberg MC (1993) Prevention and management of gout. *Drugs* 45, 212–222

Self-assessment

1. Case history question

A 56-year-old male awakes in the night with sudden severe pain in his first metatarsophalangeal joint which lasted for a week. Over the next few months, he had similar acute episodes of pain in his ankles and knees, as well as his big toe. He had hypertension but no other vascular disease. The GP suspected gout and referred him to a specialist.

a. What treatment should the GP institute for the acute attacks prior to the specialist diagnosis?

b. What test could the rheumatologist do to confirm the suspected diagnosis?

The diagnosis of gout was confirmed.

c. What is the cause of gout?
d. Which drugs would you prescribe and what are the mechanisms by which the drugs act for acute attacks?
e. What would you prescribe for prophylaxis to reduce recurrent attacks and how do these agents act?
f. What might be the consequences of inadequate treatment of this patient?

The answers are provided on page 619.

Self-assessment questions

Drugs used for gout

Drug	Half-life (h)	Elimination	Comments
Allopurinol	0.5–2	Metabolism + renal	High oral bioavailability; eliminated by metabolism to oxipurinol and unchanged in urine (about 10%); oxipurinol is biologically active and although less potent than allopurinol it has a longer half-life (10–40 h) and accumulates on repeated dosage
Colchicine	0.2–1(?)	Renal + metabolism	Good oral absorption; rapidly eliminated from plasma but the reported half-life may reflect the distribution phase, because the half-life in leucocytes is about 60 h
Probenecid	4–17	Metabolism + renal	Complete oral bioavailability; eliminated by hepatic oxidation, glucuronic acid conjugation and by renal excretion (5–10%); the oxidised metabolites are uricosuric
Sulfinpyrazone	4–5	Metabolism	Good oral absorption; metabolised at the SO group to an inactive sulfone (SO_2) and a sulfide (S) analogue (which inhibits platelet aggregation); also metabolised by oxidation and formation of a C-glucuronide (a rare reaction)

THE GASTROINTESTINAL SYSTEM

Nausea and vomiting

Nausea and vomiting

Vomiting is initiated by the vomiting centre in the brain-stem. Efferent connections activate the vasomotor, respiratory and salivatory centres in the medulla. The fundus and body of the stomach relaxes and the pylorus contracts. The lower oesophageal sphincter relaxes and retrograde contraction occurs in the small intestine; these factors provoke vomiting. The afferent trigger to the vomiting centre comes from several sources (Fig. 32.1). An important input is from the chemoreceptor trigger zone (CTZ) in the 4th ventricle, which lies outside the blood–brain barrier. Many drugs produce vomiting by an action on the CTZ (Box 32.1) although stimulation of chemoreceptors in the gut after oral administration may also be important. Vomiting can result from the summation of several inputs, for

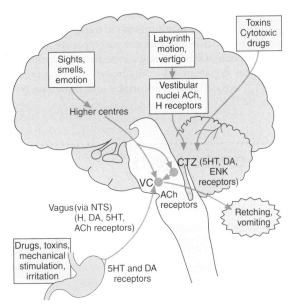

Fig. 32.1
Some of the neuronal pathways and receptors involved in the control of nausea and vomiting. The receptors utilised underpin the mechanisms of action of the anti-emetic drugs. This scheme partly explains why some types of nausea and vomiting are better treated by particular anti-emetics acting at specific receptors. H, histamine type 1 receptor; ACh, muscarinic receptor; 5HT, 5-hydroxytryptamine type 3 and type 4? receptor; ENK, enkephalin receptor; DA, dopamine receptor; NTS, nucleus tractus solitarius; CTZ, chemoreceptor trigger zone; VC, vomiting centre.

Box 32.1

Drugs that produce a high incidence of nausea and vomiting

Allopurinol
Antibiotics (oral use)
Bromocriptine
Cytotoxic agents (especially cisplatin, cyclophosphamide,
   doxorubicin, nitrosoureas)
Digoxin
Gold
Iron (oral use)
Levodopa
Non-steroidal anti-inflammatory drugs
Estrogens (oral use)
Opiate analgesics
Penicillamine
Sulfasalazine
Theophylline

example the genesis of postoperative nausea and vomiting. This frequently occurs in the first 24 h after anaesthesia and surgery; it is provoked by inhalational rather than intravenous anaesthesia, more often by abdominal, ophthalmic or ear, nose and throat procedures, by the use of opioid analgesics and by postoperative pain, hypotension and gastric stasis. After surgery, several sub-emetic stimuli may summate to trigger vomiting.

Several neurotransmitter receptor types are involved in activation of the vomiting centre and CTZ including those for dopamine (D_2), 5-hydroxytryptamine type 3 ($5HT_3$), acetylcholine (muscarinic) and histamine (H_1) (Fig. 32.1).

Anti-emetic agents

Antimuscarinic agents

Examples: hyoscine, promethazine, cyclizine

Mechanism of action and clinical use

Hyoscine (scopolamine) works solely as an antimuscarinic drug (Ch. 4) while some drugs originally developed as antihistamines such as promethazine and cyclizine (Ch. 38) or dopamine receptor antagonists, for example prochlorperazine (see below), also have antimuscarinic activity. Muscarinic receptors are involved in the visceral afferent input from the gut to the vomiting centre and the vestibular nuclei, part of the pathway from the labyrinth to the CTZ. Hyoscine is used for the treatment of motion sickness and postoperative vomiting, promethazine and cyclizine are usually used for treating motion sickness or vomiting caused by vestibular disease. Promethazine is also used to treat vomiting in pregnancy since it appears to be free from teratogenic effects.

Pharmacokinetics

Hyoscine is available for parenteral or transdermal use. Oral absorption is poor. It is partially metabolised in the liver and has an intermediate half-life.

Unwanted effects

Unwanted effects are:

- typical antimuscarinic actions (Ch. 4)
- sedation.

Dopamine receptor antagonists

Examples: metoclopramide, domperidone, prochlorperazine.

Mechanism of action and clinical use

Domperidone, metoclopramide and the antipsychotic drugs block dopamine D_2 receptors and inhibit dopaminergic stimulation of the CTZ (Fig. 32.1).

The pharmacology of the antipsychotic drugs is discussed in Ch. 21; their ability to block dopamine and muscarinic receptors contribute to their anti-emetic effects. Anti-emetic doses of antipsychotic drugs are generally less than one-third of those used to treat psychoses.

Domperidone acts solely by dopamine receptor blockade. This is also an important mechanism for metoclopramide at usual oral doses. However, metoclopramide has enhanced efficacy at high dosages, which are usually given intravenously to treat the vomiting induced by cytotoxic agents such as cisplatin, as then it also acts as a $5HT_3$ receptor antagonist. Metoclopramide also has anti-emetic actions on the gut, increasing the tone of the gastro-oesophageal sphincter and enhancing both gastric emptying and small intestinal motility. These actions may be a result of indirect cholinergic stimulation following from stimulation of the $5HT_4$ receptor subtype in the enteric nervous system.

Dopamine receptor antagonists are mainly used to reduce vomiting induced by drugs and surgery. Antipsychotic drugs, such as the phenothiazine, prochlorperazine, can be used to treat vestibular disorders and motion sickness, probably as a result of their antimuscarinic activity. Pure dopamine receptor antagonists are ineffective in motion sickness.

Pharmacokinetics

Metoclopramide is well absorbed orally and is also available for parenteral use. It is eliminated mainly by metabolism in the liver and has a short half-life. Domperidone is also well absorbed orally but undergoes extensive first-pass metabolism in the gut wall and liver; it can also be given rectally by suppository. Domperidone has an intermediate half-life. Unlike metoclopramide, it only crosses the blood–brain barrier to a limited extent.

Unwanted effects

Central nervous system (CNS) unwanted effects are produced by metoclopramide and the antipsychotics but, to a lesser extent by domperidone (as a result of lower CNS penetration).

- Acute and chronic extrapyramidal effects from dopamine receptor blockade in the basal ganglia (see also Ch. 24) can lead to acute dystonias (especially in children and young adults), akathisia and a parkinsonian-like syndrome.
- Galactorrhoea caused by hyperprolactinaemia can result from pituitary dopamine receptor blockade.
- Drowsiness can occur, mainly with high doses of metoclopramide.

5HT$_3$ receptor antagonists

Example: ondansetron.

Mechanism of action and clinical use

The 5HT$_3$ receptor antagonists block the 5HT$_3$ receptors in the CTZ and in the gut (Fig. 32.1). They are particularly effective against vomiting induced by highly emetogenic chemotherapeutic agents used for treating malignancy (e.g. cisplatin; Ch. 52) and postoperative vomiting that is resistant to other agents. They are also used when the consequences of vomiting could be particularly deleterious, for example after eye surgery.

Pharmacokinetics

Oral absorption is rapid and intravenous and rectal suppository formulations are available. The drugs are extensively metabolised in the liver and have short-half lives.

Unwanted effects

- Headache is common.
- Constipation can occur, probably caused by 5HT$_3$ receptor blockade in the gut.

Cannabinoids

Example: nabilone

Mechanism of action and clinical use

Nabilone, a synthetic derivative of tetrahydrocannabinol (an active substance in marihuana; Ch. 54), is effective in combating sickness induced by cytotoxic drugs; it must be given before chemotherapy is started. The mechanism is uncertain, but it may involve inhibition of cortical activity and anxiolysis; cannabinoid receptors are found in several areas of the CNS.

Pharmacokinetics

Nabilone is absorbed from the gut. It is metabolised in the liver and has an intermediate half-life.

Unwanted effects

- Dysphoric reactions with hallucinations and disorientation are most disturbing to older patients. This may be reduced by concurrent use of prochlorperazine (see dopamine receptor antagonists).
- Sedation, dry mouth and dizziness are common.

Corticosteroids

Dexamethasone and methylprednisolone are weak antiemetics. However, they produce additive effects when given with high dose metoclopramide or with a 5HT$_3$ receptor antagonist such as ondansetron. High doses of dexamethasone can be given intravenously before chemotherapy with subsequent oral doses to prevent delayed emesis. The mechanism of action is unknown but may involve reduction of prostaglandin synthesis. The pharmacology of corticosteroids is discussed in Chapter 44.

Benzodiazepines

Benzodiazepines have no intrinsic anti-emetic activity. They are given orally or intravenously to sedate and produce amnesia before cancer chemotherapy. They are especially useful if the patient has previously experienced vomiting with a cytotoxic treatment, since anticipatory nausea and vomiting are then common with subsequent courses. Benzodiazepines are discussed in Chapter 20.

Management of nausea and vomiting

Anti-emetics are used in a number of situations where nausea and vomiting can be problematic (Table 32.1).

Drug-induced vomiting

It is sometimes necessary to use drugs which carry a high risk of inducing nausea and vomiting (Box 32.1).

Table 32.1
Common indications for various anti-emetic agents

Cause of vomiting	Treatment
Motion sickness	Hyoscine, cyclizine, promethazine
Postoperative vomiting	Hyoscine, metoclopramide, domperidone, prochlorperazine ondansetron (reserved for resistant vomiting)
Drug-induced vomiting	Prochlorperazine, metoclopramide, cyclizine (particularly for opioid-induced vomiting)
Cytotoxic drug-induced vomiting	Prochlorperazine, metoclopramide (especially high doses), nabilone, ondansetron Adjunctive treatments, e.g. corticosteroids, benzodiazepines
Pregnancy-induced vomiting	Promethazine, metoclopramide, pyridoxine

Cyclizine, prochlorperazine or metoclopramide are often effective for opioid-induced vomiting.

More problematic are the highly emetogenic agents used for cancer treatment. For moderately emetogenic treatment, prochlorperazine or high-dose metoclopramide can help. Nabilone is sometimes effective for more refractory vomiting. Dexamethasone is particularly useful for control of delayed nausea, with a $5HT_3$ receptor antagonist such as ondansetron reserved for resistant patients.

For highly emetogenic chemotherapy, a $5HT_3$ receptor antagonist, alone or in combination with dexamethasone, is valuable in achieving control in up to 80% of patients.

Anticipatory vomiting prior to cycles of chemotherapy is most effectively prevented by including a benzodiazepine with the chemotherapy regimen from the start of treatment to produce amnesia.

Postoperative vomiting

Metoclopramide or prochlorperazine are often used to treat postoperative vomiting. If vomiting is severe, or if it carries high risk for the patient (e.g. after eye surgery), then a $5HT_3$ receptor antagonist such as ondansetron is particularly effective.

Motion sickness

Hyoscine and cyclizine are often used to treat motion sickness with promethazine as an alternative. Muscarinic unwanted effects or drowsiness may be troublesome with all these agents.

Vomiting in pregnancy

Vomiting in pregnancy can be troublesome and there is a natural desire to avoid drugs whenever possible. Some clinicians advocate a trial of the vitamin pyridoxine or of ground ginger in this situation. Psychotherapeutic counselling or hypnotism may also be considered, since psychological abnormalities are a frequent trigger. If drugs are necessary, promethazine is the treatment of choice, with metoclopramide as an alternative.

Vertigo

Vertigo is a hallucination of motion, usually perceived as spinning, which is generated in the vestibular system of the inner ear. There are several causes of vertigo, (Box 32.2). The mechanism of vertigo is often poorly understood. Treatment is empirical and involves modulation of neurotransmitters and receptors involved in vestibular sensory pathways. The transmitters that may be involved are:

- glutamate, acting through N-methyl-D-aspartate (NMDA) receptors
- acetylcholine, acting through muscarinic M_2 receptors
- gamma-aminobutyric acid (GABA), acting through $GABA_A$ and $GABA_B$ receptors
- histamine, acting through H_1, H_2 and H_3 receptors
- noradrenaline (norepinephrine) and dopamine, involved in central modulation of vestibular sensory transmission.

Ménières disease is one of the conditions for which the pathogenesis is better understood. It usually presents with intermittent vertigo and associated signs of vagal disturbance such as pallor and sweating. Sensorineural deafness often develops in the later stages. Several contributory causes have been proposed including genetic

---

Box 32.2

Causes of vertigo

Ménières disease
Benign positional vertigo
Migraine
Vestibular neuronitis
Multiple sclerosis
Brainstem ischaemia
Temporal lobe epilepsy
Cerebellopontine angle tumours

predisposition, anatomical abnormalities in the middle ear and various immunological, vascular or viral precipitatory insults.

Drugs for treatment of vertigo

Antimuscarinic agents. Vestibular suppression can be achieved with agents such as hyoscine. Central anticholinergic activity is important and the mechanism of action may be similar to that involved in the treatment of motion sickness.

Antihistamines (histamine H_1-receptor blocker). These are widely used for treatment of vertigo, for example diphenhydramine, cyclizine and promethazine (Ch. 38).

Cimetidine. This drug, which also has some calcium antagonist properties, probably acts mainly via histamine H_2 receptors (Ch. 33). The action of H_2 receptor blockers is believed to be in the CNS.

Histamine receptor agonists. The use of betahistine to treat vertigo illustrates a paradox: that both histaminergic and antihistamine drugs can be effective. Betahistine is an analogue of L-histidine, the metabolic precursor of histamine. It is a partial agonist at postsynaptic histamine H_1 receptors and an antagonist at presynaptic H_3 receptors, which facilitates histaminergic neurotransmission. Betahistine may also have specific effects on vestibular cells. It is metabolised to an active derivative in the liver which has a long half-life. The main unwanted effects are headache and nausea.

Dopamine receptor antagonists. Several antipsychotic drugs are used in vertigo, mainly to treat the associated nausea.

Management of vertigo

Many forms of vertigo are brief and self-limiting. Acute vertigo, such as that caused by viral vestibular neuronitis, is often treated with anti-emetic agents until vestibular compensation occurs, usually encouraged by maintaining activity.

Benign paroxysmal positional vertigo responds poorly to drugs and is most effectively treated by vestibular exercises. Ménières disease is often treated initially with sedative drugs such as promethazine, cinnarizine or prochlorperazine. Modification of the endolymph production in the inner ear with diuretics such as furosemide (frusemide) or hydrochlorothiazide (Ch. 14) is often attempted for chronic symptoms, although evidence of efficacy is lacking. Betahistine is often coprescribed with a diuretic. For persistent symptoms, the vestibular apparatus can be ablated, for example, using local delivery of gentamicin (Ch. 51), which is toxic to the inner ear. Surgical treatment is also used for refractory disease.

Several drugs can cause dizziness or a sensation similar to vertigo. Examples include antihypertensive agents, vasodilators and antiparkinsonian agents. A more serious degree of vestibular damage can be produced by aminoglycosides such as gentamicin (Ch. 51) and loop diuretics such as furosemide (frusemide) (Ch. 14). This type of vestibular toxicity can be reversible.

FURTHER READING

Gregory RE, Ettinger DS (1998) 5-HT$_3$ receptor antagonists for the prevention of chemotherapy-induced nausea and vomiting. *Drugs* 55, 173–189

Mitchelson F (1992) Pharmacological agents affecting emesis. Parts I & II. *Drugs* 43, 295–315, 443–463

Rascol O, Hain TC, Brefel C et al. (1995) Antivertigo medications and drug-induced vertigo. *Drugs* 50, 777–791

Saeed SR (1998) Diagnosis and treatment of Ménières disease. *Br Med J* 316, 368–372

Veyrat-Foller C, Farinotti R, Palmer JL (1997) Physiology of chemotherapy-induced emesis and anti-emetic therapy. *Drugs* 53, 206–234

Self-assessment

In questions 1 and 2, the first statement, in italics, is true. Are the accompanying statements also true?

1. *Nausea and vomiting can be caused by a number of different stimuli that may require different drugs to treat them.*

   a. Toxins need to cross the blood–brain barrier to cause vomiting by stimulating the chemoreceptor trigger zone.
   b. Some antihistamines can be used for motion sickness.

2. *Dopamine antagonists such as metoclopramide used as anti-emetics can cause extrapyramidal movement abnormalities, particularly in the elderly.* Metoclopramide decreases intestinal motility.

3. Case history question

A 35-year-old man is diagnosed with non-Hodgkin's lymphoma requiring many sessions of treatment with combined cytotoxic therapy, including cyclophosphamide, vincristine and prednisolone.

   a. Is the patient likely to experience nausea and vomiting?

Nausea and vomiting started several hours after each course of treatment and continued for 4 to 5 days.

   b. What planned anti-emetic treatment prior to the first course of chemotherapy could be beneficial?
   c. How do the treatments you have chosen work?

The patient became very distressed by the severity of the nausea and vomiting and developed intense nausea and vomiting prior to the administration of the chemotherapeutic agents.

   d. What treatment could be given?

The answers are provided on page 619.

Anti-emetic agents

Drug	Half-life (h)	Elimination	Comments
Antimuscarinics			
Hyoscine (scopolamine)	8	Metabolism	Give orally for motion sickness; radiolabelled studies indicate very poor oral absorption (< 10%); hydrolysed to inactive product
Antihistamines			
Cinnarizine	3	Metabolism	Given orally but very variable absorption; numerous metabolites which are eliminated in the urine and faeces
Cyclizine	20	Metabolism	Given orally; few data are available; demethylated metabolite has no activity
Dimenhydrinate	–	Metabolism	Given orally; is a prodrug for diphenhydramine (which has a half-life of about 3–9 h; oral dosage is about 70% as effective as intravenous dosage in forming diphenhydramine
Meclozine	?	?	Given orally; no relevant data are available
Promethazine	7–14	Metabolism	Given orally; low bioavailability (25%); bile is a major route of elimination of the (inactive) metabolites.
Dopamine receptor antagonists			
Chlorpromazine	8–35	Metabolism	Given orally, rectally or by deep intramuscular injection; oral bioavailability is variable (4–70%); more than 100 metabolites have been identified with wide interpatient variability
Domperidone	12–16	Metabolism	Given orally or rectally; low bioavailability (about 15%); oxidised in liver to metabolites excreted in urine and faeces
Metoclopramide	3–5	Metabolism + renal	Given orally or by intramuscular injection or intravenous injection over 1–2 min; oral bioavailability is variable (40–100%); eliminated by *N*-sulfation (a rare reaction) and renal excretion
Perphenazine	9	Metabolism	Given orally; low oral bioavailability (30–40%); undergoes extensive hepatic metabolism
Prochlorperazine	6–7	Metabolism	Given orally, rectally or by deep intramuscular injection; variable absorption of oral doses
Trifluoperazine	14 (7–18)	Metabolism	Given orally; oral bioavailability has not been defined; numerous metabolites formed
$5HT_3$ antagonists			
Granisetron	4 (3–9)	Metabolism (+ some renal)	Given orally or by intravenous injection or infusion; oral bioavailability is 40–70%; metabolised by CYP3A4 with wide interindividual variability in kinetics
Ondansetron	3	Metabolism	Given orally, rectally, by intramuscular injection or by slow intravenous infusion; oral bioavailability is good (60%); oxidised in liver by CYP3A4 plus CYP2D6 (but no in vivo difference in kinetics between extensive and poor metabolisers of debrisoquine)
Tropisetron	6–7	Metabolism	Given by slow intravenous injection or infusion followed by oral dosage; metabolised by CYP2D6 and poor metabolisers show an increased incidence of side-effects
Cannabinoids			
Nabilone	?	Metabolism	Given orally; few data available
Corticosteroids			See Chapter 44
Benzodiazepines			See Chapter 20

Dyspepsia and peptic ulcer disease

The spectrum of disease

Dyspepsia is the term used for a group of symptoms that arise from the upper gastrointestinal tract. They include heartburn, abdominal pain or discomfort, belching and nausea. Dyspepsia can occur alone or it can be associated with a number of upper gastrointestinal disorders.

Peptic ulcer disease

Peptic ulceration can occur in the stomach or duodenum. Characteristic features include epigastric pain (relieved by antacids or by food), nocturnal pain and vomiting. Peptic ulcer disease is more common in males and in smokers, and there is often a family history of the disorder. It is also more common in people who use non-steroidal anti-inflammatory drugs (NSAIDs; Ch. 29) or who have a heavy alcohol intake. Women more often have gastric rather than duodenal ulceration. Symptoms are a poor guide to the location of an ulcer, although patients with gastric ulcer may have pain that is made worse by food and they are more likely than those with duodenal ulcer to have weight loss, anorexia and nausea. Ulcers are known to require the presence of both acid and peptic activity for their occurrence(Fig. 33.1). However, gastric ulcers are often associated with breakdown of the

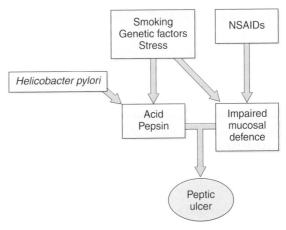

Fig. 33.1
Factors predisposing to peptic ulceration. NSAIDs, non-steroidal anti-inflammatory agents.

protective functions of gastric mucosa, in association with normal or reduced acid secretion, whereas duodenal ulceration is usually accompanied by excess acid secretion. The reasons for this are only now starting to be understood (see below). Duodenal ulceration is characteristically a relapsing disorder even after successful healing. A proportion of patients who present with peptic ulcer symptoms, especially over the age of 45 years, will have a gastric cancer. Investigation by endoscopy above this age is important since drug treatment can produce symptomatic improvement in patients with early gastric cancer.

Helicobacter pylori and peptic ulceration

Helicobacter pylori (*H. pylori*) is present in the mucosa of about 40% of individuals in the UK and up to 90% in other countries. Only a small percentage of infected individuals develop helicobacter-associated disease. It is, however, an acknowledged risk factor for gastritis, peptic ulcer, gastric cancer and mucosa-associated lymphoid tissue (MALT) lymphoma. Infection with *H. pylori* is seen in 95% of patients with gastric ulcer and 80% of those with duodenal ulcer. *H. pylori* survives in a microaerophil environment. It is able to survive brief exposure to acid conditions by producing ammonia from urea, as the organism contains a high concentration of the enzyme urease. A multitude of factors determine whether an individual acquires the infection and whether it becomes associated with peptic ulcer or gastric cancer. If *H. pylori* infection is confined to the antral mucosa it causes excess acid secretion, which may result in duodenal ulcers. If it occupies the corpus or corpus and antral mucosa (pangastritis) normal or decreased acid secretion occurs and this appears to be associated with gastric ulcers and eventually gastric cancer. *H. pylori* causes inflammation and production of several damaging substances including ammonia and inflammatory cytokines. Some strains of *H. pylori* are more virulent than others. If *H. pylori* is not eradicated, about 80% of gastric and duodenal ulcers will re-occur within a year. If *H. pylori* is eradicated, the recurrence rate is low.

Gastro-oesophageal reflux disease

Gastro-oesophageal reflux disease (GORD) can produce heartburn, pain or difficulty on swallowing and regurgitation of gastric contents into the mouth. If associated with oesophagitis, there may be more prolonged chest pain and chronic bleeding. Reflux is produced by a low basal pressure in, or transient relaxation of, the lower oesophageal sphincter in the absence of swallowing. This allows gastric acid, pepsin and bile to come into contact with the vulnerable epithelium of the oesophagus. Reflux often co-exists with abnormal oesophageal peristalsis, which reduces clearance of refluxed material. Up to 50% of symptomatic patients have no apparent oesophagitis at endoscopy, whereas severe oesophagitis can produce few symptoms, unless complications such as stricture or anaemia arise.

Control of gastric acid secretion and mucosal protection

Acid secretion into the cannaliculi of gastric parietal cells is caused by the activity of a membrane-bound proton pump which exchanges K^+ and H^+ across the cell membrane (H^+/K^+-ATPase). Hydrogen ions are obtained from carbonic acid (H_2CO_3) using carbonic anhydrase and HCO_3^- enters the plasma in exchange for Cl^-. Chloride ions are then secreted into the stomach lumen with H^+ via a symport carrier. The activity of the proton pump is controlled by several mediators including histamine, gastrin and acetylcholine (Fig. 33.2).

Gastric mucosal cells are protected against acid digestion by several mechanisms. These include:

- secretion of a barrier of adherent mucus gel from the cells
- secretion of bicarbonate into the mucus layer
- intrinsic resistance of the cell membranes to hydrogen ion back-diffusion
- high mucosal blood flow, which removes H^+ from the mucosa and provides additional bicarbonate
- the phospholipid hydrophobic barrier.

Many of these protective functions are dependent on the synthesis of prostaglandins (PG), especially PGE_2 and PGI_2 (Ch. 29), by gastric mucosal cells.

Drugs for treating dyspepsia and peptic ulcer

Antisecretory agents

It is only necessary to raise intragastric pH above 3 for a few hours in the day to promote healing of most ulcers. The duration of acid suppression will then determine the rate of healing but not the eventual proportion of healed ulcers. Rapid healing requires acid suppression

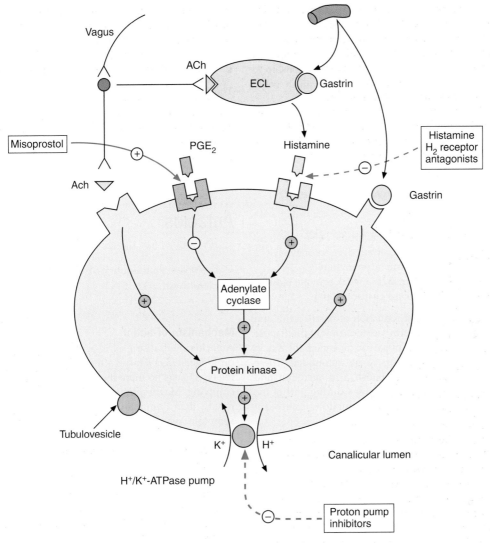

Fig. 33.2
Control of gastric acid secretion. Acid secretion from the parietal cell is stimulated by acetylcholine (ACh), histamine and gastrin. Gastrin and ACh also reinforce acid secretion by causing the release of histamine from the enterochromaffin like cells (ECL) which lie close to the parietal cells in the gastric pits. Prostaglandin E_2 (PGE$_2$) reduces acid secretion. The sites of action of the main drugs used to inhibit acid secretion from the parietal cell are shown. There are no useful inhibitors of gastrin action and the muscarinic receptor inhibitor, pirenzipine, is no longer available in the UK.

for a minimum of 18–20 h per day. Several classes of drug have antisecretory actions.

Proton pump inhibitors

Examples: omeprazole, lansoprazole, pantoprazole, rabeprazole

Mechanism of action

Since the proton pump is the final common pathway for acid secretion in gastric parietal cells, inhibition of the pump can almost completely block acid secretion (Fig. 33.2). Proton pump inhibitors are irreversible inhibitors of H$^+$/K$^+$-ATPase, and the return of acid secretion is dependent on the synthesis of new enzyme. Acid production is inhibited by about 90% for approximately 24 h with a single dose.

Pharmacokinetics

Omeprazole is a prodrug that is unstable in acid. It is, therefore, given as an enteric-coated formulation. The parent drug is a weak base and is concentrated in the acid environment of the secretory canaliculi of the gastric parietal cell. Activation then occurs by protonation of the compound. Absorption is variable and incomplete, although it improves with repeated dosing. Elimination is by hepatic metabolism. Omeprazole has a short plasma half-life but, because of the irreversible mechanism of action, the half-life of the drug bears no relationship to the duration of action. Lansoprazole has much better initial absorption than omeprazole.

Unwanted effects

Proton pump inhibitors have a number of unwanted effects:

- gastrointestinal upset, for example epigastric discomfort, nausea and vomiting, diarrhoea.
- headache
- skin rashes
- omeprazole induces the cytochrome P450 system in the liver but has few important drug interactions apart from with warfarin or phenytoin (Ch. 2); lansoprazole, by contrast, is a weak enzyme inducer
- long-term use may cause gastric atrophy.

Concern that substantial reduction of gastric acid, and the associated rise in gastrin secretion, might predispose to an increased incidence of gastric cancer (cf. the risk in pernicious anaemia) appears to be unfounded. These drugs do not completely abolish acid secretion and intragastric pH can still fall below 4 during part of the day. Proton pump inhibitors have a modest suppressant effect on *H. pylori*.

Histamine H$_2$ receptor antagonists

Examples: cimetidine, ranitidine

Mechanism of action

Histamine H$_2$ receptor antagonists act competitively on gastric parietal cells. They reduce basal acid secretion and pepsin production and prevent the increase that occurs in response to a number of secretory stimuli. They reduce acid secretion by about 60% (Fig. 33.2).

Pharmacokinetics

Absorption of cimetidine and ranitidine from the gut is almost complete but both undergo first-pass metabolism. Elimination is mainly by renal excretion for cimetidine, and partially by metabolism. A greater proportion of ranitidine is eliminated by metabolism. The half-lives are short.

Unwanted effects

Unwanted effects of histamine H$_2$ receptor antagonists include:

- diarrhoea

- headache
- confusion in the elderly
- gynaecomastia with cimetidine, because of an antiandrogen effect
- inhibition of hepatic cytochrome P450s (cimetidine).

Therapeutic doses of cimetidine, but not ranitidine, inhibit the hepatic cytochrome P450s enzyme complexes. This creates the potential for important drug interactions with compounds such as warfarin, phenytoin, tolbutamide and theophylline (Ch. 2).

Antacids

Examples: aluminium hydroxide, magnesium trisilicate

Mechanism of action

Antacids neutralise gastric acidity. They have a more prolonged effect if taken after food; if used without food the effect lasts no more than an hour because of gastric emptying. Magnesium salts neutralise acid much more rapidly than aluminium salts. Antacids quickly produce symptom relief in ulcer disease, but large doses are required to heal ulcers. Most are relatively poorly absorbed from the gut. Liquids work more rapidly, but tablets are more convenient to use.

Unwanted effects

- Constipation can occur with aluminium salts and diarrhoea, with magnesium salts. Mixtures may have less effect on stool consistency.
- Systemic alkalosis can occur with very large doses.
- In advanced renal failure, requiring dialysis, retention of absorbed aluminium may contribute to metabolic bone disease and encephalopathy.
- Drug interactions: aluminium salts can bind other drugs and reduce their absorption, for example NSAIDs and tetracycline.

Alginic acid

Alginic acid is an inert substance. It is claimed that it forms a raft of high pH foam which floats on the gastric contents and that alginic acid will protect the oesophageal mucosa during reflux. All proprietary preparations combine alginic acid with an antacid which is probably responsible for much of the clinical effect.

Cytoprotective agents

Sucralfate

Mechanism of action
Sucralfate is an aluminium salt of sucrose octasulfate. It dissociates in an acid environment to its anionic form which binds to the ulcer base and creates a protective barrier to pepsin and bile and inhibits the diffusion of gastric acid. Sucralfate also stimulates the gastric secretion of bicarbonate and prostaglandins. It is not absorbed from the gut.

Unwanted effects
Constipation can occur with sucralfate.

Bismuth salts

Example: tripotassium dicitratobismuthate

Mechanism of action
Bismuth salts precipitate in the acid environment of the stomach and then bind to glycoprotein on the base of an ulcer. The resulting complex adheres to the ulcer and has similar local effects to sucralfate. Bismuth salts also suppress *H. pylori*, which may contribute to ulcer healing. Used alone it produces long-term eradication of *H. pylori* infection in 20% of patients. Bismuth is also available as a combination product with ranitidine (as ranitidine bismuth citrate).

Unwanted effects
- Blackened stools can occur.
- Absorption of bismuth chelates from the gut is minimal, but in severe renal failure the inability to excrete the small amounts of absorbed bismuth could produce encephalopathy.

Because of the small risk of accumulation of bismuth, courses are usually limited to a maximum of 6 weeks.

Prostaglandin analogues

Example: misoprostol

Mechanism of action
Misoprostol is an analogue of prostaglandin E_1 (Ch. 29) and has several potentially useful actions including:

- increased gastric mucus production
- enhanced duodenal bicarbonate secretion
- increased mucosal blood flow, which aids buffering of H^+ that diffuses back across the mucosa
- inhibition of gastric acid secretion.

Misoprostol has both a direct effect on gastric acid secretion and it also reduces endogenous histamine release. The overall effect of misoprostol is to limit the damage caused by agents such as acid and alcohol to superficial mucosal cells. It is most widely used to reduce NSAID-induced gastric damage.

Pharmacokinetics
Misoprostol is well absorbed from the gut but undergoes extensive first-pass metabolism. The half-life is very short (20 min) and elimination is mainly by hepatic metabolism.

Unwanted effects
Unwanted effects of misoprostol include:

- diarrhoea and abdominal cramps caused by a local effect on gut motility (fairly common)
- uterine contractions, therefore avoid in pregnancy
- menorrhagia and postmenopausal bleeding.

Carbenoxolone

Mechanism of action
Carbenoxolone is a synthetic derivative of a constituent of liquorice. It has a steroid structure and enhances the synthesis of gastric mucus perhaps by stimulating prostaglandin secretion. This increases the protective barrier in the stomach against acid and peptic digestion. It is rarely used since the advent of newer ulcer-healing agents.

Pharmacokinetics
Absorption from the gut is almost complete. The major route of elimination is the liver and the half-life is long.

Unwanted effects
Aldosterone-like actions (because of the steroid structure) on the kidney produce salt and water retention and hypokalaemia. Hypertension or heart failure can result from the fluid retention.

Prokinetic drugs

Example: metoclopramide

Mechanism of action
Metoclopramide is a dopamine receptor-blocking agent that is fully discussed in Chapter 32. Peripherally it enhances gastric motility by stimulating acetylcholine

release or sensitising receptors. The effect is to hasten gastric emptying and to increase gastro-oesophageal sphincter tone.

Pharmacokinetics
Metoclopramide is rapidly absorbed and bioavailability is 80%. It crosses the blood–brain barrier.

Unwanted effects
Unwanted effects of metoclopramide include:

- sedation
- extrapyramidal effects, increased prolactin and aldosterone release.

Management of dyspepsia and peptic ulcer disease

Most patients with dyspepsia do not have significant underlying disease (i.e. non-ulcer dyspepsia). In all cases, efforts should be made to remove causative agents, for example smoking, excess alcohol or NSAIDs. For persistent symptoms, antacids provide symptomatic relief. Younger patients (especially under 45 years of age) who do not have associated features, such as anaemia, weight loss, dysphagia, early satiety or persistent vomiting, are often treated without initial investigation. A histamine H_2 receptor antagonist or proton pump inhibitor should not be given for more than about 6 weeks in the absence of a confirmed diagnosis. Investigation should be carried out if symptoms fail to respond within 2 weeks or recur after stopping treatment. Accurate diagnosis can usually be obtained by gastroduodenoscopy although more specialised tests may be required in some patients.

Confirmed peptic ulceration

Eradication of *H. pylori* is first-line treatment in peptic ulcer and combinations of acid inhibitors and antibiotics are given. Proton pump inhibitors produce the fastest rate of healing (over 90% of ulcers heal in 4 weeks). Histamine H_2 receptor antagonists usually give symptomatic relief for both gastric and duodenal ulcers within a week, but healing of the ulcer is much slower requiring up to 8 weeks for duodenal ulcer or 12 weeks for gastric ulcer. Other agents such as colloidal bismuth and sucralfate will heal ulcers in a similar proportion of patients but are less often used since they do not improve symptoms as quickly. If *H. pylori* infection is identified and eradicated, this enhances ulcer healing and reduces relapse so that maintenance therapy with

acid suppressing drugs is often unnecessary for uncomplicated ulcers. If *H. pylori* is not eradicated 80% of ulcers will re-occur within a year whereas following successful eradication this is less than 20%.

Eradication of *H. pylori*

This is a rapidly progressing field of research, and new indications for eradication have been recently proposed (Box 33.1). Several eradication regimens are used: the highest eradication rates involve treatment with high dosage of a proton pump inhibitor combined with two antibiotics (to minimise resistance) given for 1 to 2 weeks (Box 33.2). Such regimens can have a significant incidence of unwanted effects. The incidence of resist-

---

Box 33.1

Indications for eradication of *Helicobacter pylori*

Recommended
Proven peptic ulcer
Low-grade mucosa-associated lymphoid tissue (MALT) gastric lymphoma
Severe gastritis
After resection of early gastric cancer

Suggested
Functional dyspepsia
Family history of gastric cancer
Non-steroidal anti-inflammatory drug (NSAID) therapy

Box 33.2

Eradication regimens for *Helicobacter pylori*

1. Proton pump inhibitor (PPI), for example omeprazole or lansoprazole, combined with two antimicrobials either metronidazole or tinidazole plus amoxicillin or clarithromycin for 7 to 10 days (eradication rate 70–90%).
2. Original triple therapy was colloidal bismuth with two antimicrobials chosen from metronidazole or tinidazole plus clarithromycin amoxycillin or tetracycline for 14 days (eradication rates can vary from 50–90% and compliance may be poor).
3. Ranitidine bismuth citrate plus clarithromycin or amoxicillin plus metronidazole or tinidazole for 7 days (eradication rate 70–98%).
4. In resistant cases *quadruple therapy* is used. PPI + colloidal bismuth plus metronidazole or tinidazole plus amoxicillin tetracycline or clarithromycin for 7 days (eradication rate 93–98%).

ance to metronidazole (up to 50% in some places) and clarithromycin is increasing, and guidance is required on resistance in a particular geographical location. Resistance to amoxicillin is also developing. Resistance to tinidazole is currently lower than to metronidazole. Maintenance therapy with acid-suppressant treatment is only required if symptoms continue despite eradication of *H. pylori* and after exclusion of more serious conditions.

Mucosa-associated lymphoid tissue lymphoma

An uncommon tumour of gut lymphoid tissue is the mucosa-associated lymphoid tissue (MALT) lymphoma, which is associated with *H. pylori* infection. In a small number of patients, eradication has brought about regression of the tumour.

Peptic ulceration associated with non-steroidal anti-inflammatory drugs

If the provoking agent such as NSAIDs cannot be withdrawn then ulcers will often heal if an ulcer healing agent is coprescribed. Continued use of NSAIDs can slow ulcer healing by histamine H_2 receptor antagonists, but probably not by proton pump inhibitors. Eradication of *H. pylori* infection is recommended, although this may not eliminate ulcer risk. The prostaglandin analogue misoprostol provides effective prophylaxis against gastric ulceration or its recurrence. Antisecretory agents and misoprostol protect equally well against recurrent duodenal ulceration. Careful patient selection is recommended before prophylaxis against ulceration is given in the absence of symptoms. Those at higher risk are the elderly, smokers, alcohol users and patients with a history of previous ulceration.

Gastro-oesophageal reflux disease

Initial measures against GORD include avoidance of tight clothing, smoking, alcohol and caffeine and encouraging weight loss. Raising the head of the bed by 15 cm at night can be helpful. For mild persistent symptoms, reduction of gastric acid with antacids, with or without the addition of an alginate to provide a mechanical barrier, is often helpful. Proton pump inhibitors are the most effective treatment for severe resistant or relapsing GORD. They will rapidly ease symptoms and heal oesophagitis in up to 85% of patients by 8 weeks. Failure to heal with a proton pump inhibitor often indicates biliary rather than acid reflux. However, long-term treatment may result in atrophy of the body of the stomach. Histamine H_2 receptor antagonists often relieve troublesome symptoms but may not produce mucosal healing; heartburn is relieved in up to 50% of patients after 4 weeks, but oesophagitis only heals in about 20%. Better response rates can often be achieved by using these drugs at high dosages, which will produce healing in 70–80% of patients by 8 to 12 weeks.

An alternative approach is to enhance oesophageal motility with a prokinetic drug such as metoclopramide. This drug encourages normal peristalsis in the upper gastrointestinal tract and produces similar symptomatic relief to histamine H_2 receptor antagonists. However, metoclopramide has not been shown to heal oesophagitis.

Patients with symptoms of oesophageal reflux often suffer relapse. Intermittent therapy with healing agents, or use of an alginate after healing, often controls recurrent symptoms. More severe disease requires continuous drug treatment. Long-term use of a proton pump inhibitor is the most effective treatment for severe or resistant reflux disease; histamine H_2 receptor antagonists are useful for prophylaxis after treatment of mild oesophagitis. About 60% of patients will only need a low maintenance dose after healing has occurred.

Surgery to prevent reflux is usually reserved for younger patients with persistent symptoms. It is often performed laparoscopically.

FURTHER READING

Agréus L, Talley N (1997) Challenges in managing dyspepsia in general practice. *Br Med J* 315, 1284–1288

Barbezat GO (1998) Recent advances: Gastroenterology. *Br Med J* 316, 125–128

de Boer WA, Tytgaat GNJ (2000) Treatment of *Helicobacter pylori* infection. *Br Med J* 320, 31–34

Fisher RS, Parkman HP (1998) Management of non-ulcer dyspepsia. *N Engl J Med* 339, 1376–1381

Pope CE (1994) Acid-reflux disorders. *N Engl J Med* 331, 656–660

Richardson P, Hawkey CJ, Stack WA (1998) Proton pump inhibitors. *Drugs* 56, 307–335

Scheiman J (1998) Agents used in the prevention and treatment of nonsteroidal anti-inflammatory drug-associated symptoms and ulcers. *Am J Med* 105(suppl 5A), 32s–38s

Soll AH (1996) Medical treatment of peptic ulcer disease. *JAMA* 275, 622–629

Self-assessment

In questions 1–6, the first statement, in italics, is true. Are the accompanying statements also true?

1. Helicobacter pylori *infection induces a spectrum of consequences. Some infected individuals have persistently reduced acid secretion, whereas others may have enhanced acid secretion.*

   a. *H. pylori* infection is found in the duodenum in persons with duodenal ulcers.
   b. Recurrence of duodenal ulcers following healing with proton pump inhibitors (PPIs) is approximately 20% over a year if *H. pylori* is not eliminated.
   c. *H. pylori* is a risk factor for the development of certain types of gastric cancer.
   d. Gastric acid inhibits bacterial growth.
   e. There is little risk of *H. pylori* developing resistance to antimicrobial treatment.
   f. Omeprazole is a prodrug.
   g. Histamine acts on H_1 receptors on the parietal cell to stimulate acid secretion.
   h. Vagal stimulation of the parietal cell increases acid secretion.

2. *An unwanted effect of antacids containing magnesium salts is diarrhoea.*
   Antacids do not heal peptic ulcers.

3. *Therapeutic doses of cimetidine, but not ranitidine, can potentiate the effects of other drugs by inhibiting hepatic cytochrome P450 enzymes.*

   a. Ranitidine causes gynaecomastia.
   b. Cimetidine reduces acid secretion by more than 90%.
   c. The active metabolite of omeprazole is a reversible inhibitor of the H^+/K^+-ATPase proton pump.

4. *Proton pump inhibitors are converted to their active form at acid pH.*

   Omeprazole inhibits the cytochrome P450 system in the liver.

5. *Misoprostil helps prevent mucosal damage by non-steroidal anti-inflammatory drugs (NSAIDs).*

   a. Prostaglandin E_2 reduces gastric mucosal blood flow.
   b. Misoprostil causes constipation.
   c. Histamine H_2 receptor antagonists and proton pump inhibitors are not useful for treatment of ulcers induced by NSAIDs.

6. *Proton pump inhibitors are first-line drugs in the treatment of gastro-oesophageal reflux disease.*

   Metoclopramide increases the rate of gastric emptying and raises lower oesophageal sphincter tone.

7. Case history question

   A 47-year-old man is a newly appointed headmaster of a large comprehensive school and he is experiencing some difficulties with the increasing demands of the job. He has increased his smoking from 5 to 20 cigarettes a day and he drinks 10 units of alcohol a week. He has a varied, good diet. He has suffered intermittently from dyspepsia for some years, taking proprietary antacids when required. His symptoms have now increased and the pain is causing him to wake most nights. He has bought a supply of ranitidine from the local chemist without consultation with the pharmacist. Following 2 weeks of treatment his symptoms were successfully relieved and he was symptom-free for 3 months. His symptoms then returned and he took a further treatment with ranitidine for 2 weeks. He was symptom-free for a further month but when symptoms returned again he consulted his GP.

   a. Why have his symptoms returned?
   b. Would his symptoms have been less likely to return following a short course of a proton pump inhibitor?
   c. What should be the GP's course of action?
   d. Why do some patients infected with *H. pylori* develop gastric ulcer and some duodenal ulcers?
   e. What eradication therapy for *H. pylori* should be given, and is a proton pump inhibitor beneficial when given with antimicrobial therapy?

   The eradication therapy given was 7 days with omeprazole, metronidazole and clarithromycin. The patient was symptom-free for 6 weeks but then his symptoms returned.

   f. What are the possible reasons for the return of the symptoms?
   g. What treatment could be given?

   The answers are provided on pages 619–621.

Drugs used for dyspepsia and peptic ulcer disease

Drug	Half-life (h)	Elimination	Comments
Antisecretory agents			
Omeprazole	1	Metabolism	PPI; metabolised by CYP2C19; poor metabolisers have plasma AUC values 20-fold higher than fast metabolisers; no data available on plasma concentration–response relationship; induces cytochrome CYP1A2
Lanzoprazole	1.3–1.7	Metabolism	PPI; weak correlation between blood levels and response, but local concentrations are of greater importance; induces cytochrome P450 enzymes
Pantoprazole	0.7–1.4	Metabolism	PPI; about 20% hepatic first-pass metabolism; unlike omeprazole does not induce cytochrome P450 enzymes
Rabeprazole	1–2	Metabolism	PPI; induces cytochrome P450 less than omeprazole; limited *H. pylori* inhibition
Cimetidine	1–3	Renal	Histamine H_2 receptor antagonist; incomplete absorption; cleared by renal tubular secretion; weak relationship between blood levels and therapeutic response; inhibits cytochrome P450 enzymes
Famotidine	3–4	Renal + biliary	Histamine H_2 receptor antagonist; incomplete absorption; weak relation between blood levels and response; does not affect cytochrome P450 enzymes
Nizatidine	1.5–1.6	Renal + metabolism	Histamine H_2 receptor antagonist; blood levels correlate with response, but wide interpatient variability in concentration–effect relationship; does not affect cytochrome P450 enzymes
Ranitidine	2–3	Renal + metabolism	Histamine H_2 receptor antagonist; bioavailability about 50%; cleared by renal tubular secretion and oxidation; no effect on cytochrome P450 enzymes
Cytoprotective agents			
Carbenoxolone	8–20	Metabolism	Systemic levels correlate with hypokalaemia, but not with the therapeutic response; eliminated in bile as a glucuronide
Misoprostol	0.3 (acid)	Metabolism	Misoprostol is a methyl ester of misoprostol acid; misoprostol per se is not detectable in blood after oral dosage, because of essentially complete first-pass metabolism to misoprostol acid
Sucralfate	–	–	Minimal absorption (2% or less); no data on the fate of absorbed material (the high polarity would probably result in rapid renal excretion)
Tripotassium dicitrato-bismuthate	–	–	Minimal absorption; absorbed bismuth is eliminated slowly in the urine
Prokinetic drugs			
Metoclopramide	3–5	Metabolism + renal	Major route of metabolism is by the (unusual) formation of an *N-* sulfate
Antacids	–	–	Antacids include aluminium hydroxide, magnesium trisilicate, hydrocalcite (mixed aluminium/magnesium preparation) and sodium carbonate; produce local effects within the stomach; their absorption and systemic fates are not of therapeutic importance
Alginic acid	–	–	Produces local effects within the stomach
Antimicrobials			See Chapter 51
Dimeticone	–	None	Antifoaming agent indicated for infantile colic; polysiloxane, which is chemically inert; excreted in faeces with minimal absorption

AUC, area under the curve for plasma concentration versus time; PPI, proton pump inhibitor.

34 Inflammatory bowel disease

Crohn's disease and ulcerative colitis are chronic inflammatory disorders of the gastrointestinal tract, together termed inflammatory bowel disease. Their aetiology is unknown although there is genetic predisposition and both conditions can occur in the same families. Hypotheses for increased risk in susceptible individuals include infective agents, local ischaemia and an altered immune state. Cigarette smoking increases the risk of Crohn's disease but slightly decreases the risk of ulcerative colitis. Patients can experience periods of relapse and remission over many years

Ulcerative colitis is a disorder that is confined to the mucosa and submucosa and in which inflammation is usually restricted to the large bowel. The extent of the colonic involvement varies but the rectum is always involved and mucosal inflammation is continuous, not patchy. Symptoms include bloody diarrhoea, fever and weight loss. Ulcerative colitis can be associated with extracolonic manifestations such as uveitis, sacroileitis and various skin disorders.

Crohn's disease is a transmural granulomatous condition that can involve any part of the gut. The bowel involvement is discontinuous and segmental, often sparing the rectum. Fistula formation, small bowel strictures and perianal disease such as abscesses and fissures are common. Clinical features of colonic involvement include diarrhoea, abdominal pain and fatigue. Involvement of more proximal parts of the gut produces various symptoms depending on the site of the disease, and diarrhoea need not be present. Crohn's disease must be differentiated from cytomegalovirus colitis.

Treatment of both types of inflammatory bowel disease is intended to induce and maintain remission and the drugs used for these two conditions are broadly similar. Crohn's disease is, however, less responsive to some of the widely used drugs especially when it involves the small intestine.

Drugs for inflammatory bowel disease

Aminosalicylates

Examples: sulfasalazine, mesalazine, olsalazine, balsalazide

Mechanism of action and effects

The active anti-inflammatory constituent of all the aminosalicylates is 5-aminosalicylic acid (5-ASA). The various products are formulated to deliver the active agent in a variety of ways. Sulfasalazine was the first aminosalicylate shown to be effective in treating inflammatory bowel disease. Colonic flora cleave sulfasalazine into its constituent parts, 5-ASA and sulfapyridine. Sulfapyridine is probably responsible for many of the unwanted effects of this drug. 5-ASA can also be given without the sulfapyridine component (mesalazine). The mechanisms of action of aminosalicylates are not clear, but they may involve inhibition of leucocyte chemotaxis by reducing cytokine formation, reduced free radical generation and inhibition of the production of inflammatory mediators (such as prostaglandins, thromboxanes, leukotrienes and platelet-activating factor). Aminosalicylates can be useful for achieving remission but are mainly used for reducing the relapse rate in ulcerative colitis and less reliably in Crohn's colitis.

Pharmacokinetics

Sulfasalazine is partially absorbed from the gut intact but most reaches the colon where it undergoes reduction by gut bacteria to sulfapyridine and 5-ASA. Sulfapyridine and about 20% of the 5-ASA are absorbed from the colon, and then metabolised in the liver. Both have intermediate half-lives in the circulation. Mesalazine must be given as an enteric-coated or modified-release formulation to limit absorption from the small bowel. Olsalazine is a formulation of two 5-ASA molecules joined by an azo bond. It is not absorbed from the upper gut and 5-ASA is released after splitting of the azo bond by the colonic flora. Balsalazide is a prodrug in which 5-ASA is linked to a carrier molecule (4-amino-benzoyl-β-alanine) by an azo bond which is cleaved by bacterial azo reduction in the large bowel.

Mesalazine and sulfasalazine can be given rectally (by suppository or enema) for distal disease in the colon.

Unwanted effects

Unwanted effects caused by sulfapyridine are:

- headache, nausea, vomiting
- blood dyscrasias, especially agranulocytosis (these have also been reported with 5-ASA alone)
- oligospermia
- rashes.

Those caused by 5-ASA are:

- nausea, diarrhoea, abdominal pain
- skin rashes including urticaria
- nephrotoxicity (this is an unusual complication: 5-ASA can cause chronic interstitial nephritis and renal impairment).

Corticosteroids

Examples: prednisolone, hydrocortisone, budesonide

Corticosteroids (Ch. 44) are very effective for inducing remission in patients with active inflammatory bowel disease. There is little evidence that they prevent relapse when used at doses that do not produce major unwanted effects. Newer corticosteroids formulated for topical use, such as budesonide (see also Ch. 44), have limited systemic unwanted effects and are useful alternatives to the older drugs. Topical treatment with liquid or foam enemas or suppositories is used for localised rectal disease, but oral or parenteral administration is needed for more severe or extensive disease.

Tumour necrosis factor α antibody

Example: infliximab

Mechanisms and uses

Infliximab is the first monoclonal antibody to be approved for the treatment of Crohn's disease. It inhibits the binding of tumour necrosis factor-α (TNF-α) to its receptors. This probably reduces proinflammatory cytokine (e.g. interleukins 1 and 6; IL-1, IL-6) production, leucocyte migration and infiltration, neutrophil and eosinophil activation. An infusion of infliximab can induce remission in Crohn's disease for up to 3 months. Long-term safety and efficacy have not yet been established. Intermittent administration with gaps of several weeks may reduce the severity of the disease. (Infliximab is also discussed in Ch. 30 under its role in arthritis.) There are few unwanted effects.

Pharmacokinetics

Infliximab is administered intravenously. The elimination half-life is about 9.5 days. Etanercept, a TNF-α inhibitor approved for arthritis is undergoing trials in inflammatory bowel disease.

Immunosuppressives

Azathioprine (and less often 6-mercaptopurine) is useful in some cases of active inflammatory bowel disease and may enable corticosteroid doses to be reduced. They are slow acting, requiring months of treatment for full effectiveness. Ciclosporin, mycophenolate moxetil and methotrexate are also being evaluated for Crohn's disease, but they appear to be less effective than azathioprine. Details of these drugs are found in Ch. 39.

Antimicrobials

Metronidazole (Ch. 51) is moderately effective in some cases of Crohn's disease, although the mechanism of action is uncertain. Data are emerging for similar benefit from other antimicrobials such as clarithromycin and ciprofloxacin.

Management of inflammatory bowel disease

Ulcerative colitis

If the disease is limited to the rectum or left side of the colon (distal colitis) rectal drug delivery is often successful. For mild symptoms, topical mesalazine or corticosteroid can be used. Foam enemas or suppositories will treat inflammation up to 12–20 cm, while liquid enemas are effective up to 30–60 cm (i.e. to the splenic flexure). An oral aminosalicylate is an alternative approach for more severe disease. Oral corticosteroids may be necessary to induce remission, with gradual dosage reduction when control is achieved to minimise unwanted effects. Once symptoms are quiescent, maintenance treatment with topical mesalazine or an oral aminosalicylate is usually necessary. Indicators of disease severity are shown in Box 34.1.

More extensive colitis will respond to an oral aminosalicylate if symptoms are mild to moderate, but the response can take 6 to 8 weeks. Oral corticosteroids induce remission more quickly. Non-steroidal anti-inflammatory drugs (NSAIDs) and probably both non-selective and selective cyclo-oxygenase 2 (COX-2) inhibitors (Ch. 29), can exacerbate symptoms in severe colitis, while opioids (Ch. 35) should be used with care for treatment of diarrhoea in extensive colitis since they can precipitate the life-threatening complication toxic megacolon.

Severe colitis requires intensive fluid and electrolyte replacement, with initial avoidance of food. Anaemia should be corrected by transfusion and parenteral nutrition may be necessary. Large doses of parenteral corticosteroid should be given. Broad-spectrum antimicrobials to include cover for anaerobes (e.g. metronidazole combined with cefuroxime) are usually added, although there is no good evidence that antibiotics are beneficial. Failure to respond to this treatment usually indicates a need for colectomy.

Immunosuppressives are usually reserved for refractory colitis, or they are used as corticosteroid-sparing agents if the patient has disease that requires long-term corticosteroid use for control.

Crohn's disease

The mainstay of medical treatment for active Crohn's disease is corticosteroid therapy, usually with prednisolone orally. This can be combined with metronidazole to treat concomitant small bowel bacterial overgrowth. Maintenance corticosteroid therapy does not reduce the risk of relapse, and every effort should be made to withdraw the drug once disease activity has been controlled. Immunosuppressant drugs such as azathioprine may be useful to aid this process especially in chronically active Crohn's disease where corticosteroid dependence occurs in 40–50% of patients.

Disease confined to the distal colon can respond to topical therapy with a corticosteroid; an oral aminosalicylate such as sulfasalazine can also be useful. An elemental diet has produced similar results to corticosteroid therapy in active Crohn's disease.

Surgery may be necessary for disease refractory to medical therapy. Intestinal obstruction can require bowel resection, or abcesses may need drainage. A defunctioning ileostomy to 'rest' the bowel may allow active inflammation to settle with medical therapy in refractory disease.

Infliximab, an antibody against TNF-α, has been successfully used to induced remission in Crohn's disease that is resistant to conventional therapy.

Box 34.1

Indicators of severity of ulcerative colitis

More than 6–10 stools per day
Fever
Tachycardia
Anaemia
Nausea, vomiting
Abdominal tenderness
Abdominal distension with high-pitched bowel sound
Rebound tenderness and reduction in bowel movements
(toxic megacolon)

FURTHER READING

Elson CO (1996) The basis of current and future therapy for inflammatory bowel disease. *Am J Med* 100, 656–662

Ghosh S, Shand A, Ferguson A (2000) Ulcerative colitis. *Br Med J* 320, 1119–1123

Hanauer SB (1996) Inflammatory bowel disease. *N Engl J Med* 334, 841–847

Longford CA, Klippel JH, Balow JE et al. (1998) Use of cytotoxic agents and cyclosporine in the treatment of autoimmune disease. Part 2: Inflammatory bowel disease, systemic vasculitis and therapeutic toxicity. *Ann Intern Med* 129, 49–58

Rampton DS (1999) Management of Crohn's disease. *Br Med J* 319, 1480–1485

Travis SPL, Jewell DP (1994) Salicylates for ulcerative colitis – their mode of action. *Pharmacotherapy* 63, 135–161

Self-assessment

In questions 1 and 2, the first statement, in italics, is true. Are the accompanying statements also true?

1. *Treatment for inflammatory bowel disease can be with 5-aminosalicylic acid (5-ASA), which is different from the constituent of aspirin (acetylsalicylic acid).*

   a. The active constituent of sulfasalazine is 5-aminosalicylic acid.
   b. Mesalazine (5-ASA) can be given rectally.

2. *The aetiology of inflammatory bowel disease is unknown.*

   a. Cigarette smoking increases the risk of Crohn's disease.
   b. Mesalazine is equally useful in the treatment of Crohn's disease involving the colon or the small bowel.
   c. Corticosteroids are effective for maintaining remission in ulcerative colitis.
   d. Immunosuppressives such as azathioprine are ineffective for the treatment of Crohn's disease.

3. Case history question

> A 35-year-old man presents with a 3-week period of frequent diarrhoea with mucus but no blood in the stool. Stool analysis for infective agents was negative. Sigmoidoscopy indicated gross thickening of the mucosa with no significant friability. Changes were present in restricted areas (skip lesions) with intervening normal mucosa. Histology was diagnostic of Crohn's disease and investigation suggested that the condition was confined to the sigmoid colon and rectum.

   a. What is the cause of Crohn's disease?
   b. How would the patient be treated initially?
   c. How do corticosteroids act in Crohn's disease?
   d. How should the corticosteroid be given, and why?
   e. Why should the corticosteroid dosage be reduced slowly at the end of treatment?
   f. How can remission be maintained in this patient?
   g. Is it likely that this patient will become corticosteroid dependent, and what alternative therapies can be given to try to reduce this?

The answers are given on page 621.

Drugs used in inflammatory bowel disease

Drug	Half-life (h)	Elimination	Comment
Aminosalicylates[a]			
Balsalazide	–	Metabolism	Converted to 5-aminosalicylate in colon
Mesalazine (5-aminosalicylate)	0.5–1.0	Metabolism + renal + faecal	Poorly absorbed from gut; may be more effective than sulfasalazine in the presence of diarrhoea because there is no requirement for reduction by the gut flora
Olsalazine	1	Metabolism + renal + faecal	Only 3% absorbed in upper intestine; bacterial azoreduction generates 5-aminosalicylate which is partly absorbed and excreted in urine as parent drug and acetyl metabolite
Sulfasalazine	3–11 (parent drug)	Reductive metabolism	About 20–30% absorbed in small intestine; reduced to active metabolites
	6–17 (sulfapyridine)	Metabolism	Acetylated and oxidised in liver; cause of many unwanted effects
	4–10 (5-aminosalicylate)	Metabolism + renal + faecal	Acetylated in colonic wall and liver; poor absorption from colon
TNFα antibodies			
Infliximab	9.5 days		Monoclonal antibody against tumour necrosis factor α. No evidence of accumulation on repeated infusion
Corticosteroids (budesonide, hydrocortisone and prednisolone)			see Chapter 44
Immunosuppressives			
Azathioprine	3–5	Metabolism	Metabolism to 6-mercaptopurine represents a bioactivation process
Ciclosporin	27	Metabolism	A lipid-soluble peptide oxidised by CYP3A4
Antibiotics			
Metronidazole	6–9	Metabolism + some renal	May be useful in patients who fail to respond to sulfasalazine

[a]The elimination half-life of the absorbed drug is not related to the amount at the site of action

35 Constipation, diarrhoea and irritable bowel syndrome

Constipation

Humans normally defecate with a frequency from once every 2 days (sometimes less in women) to three times a day. Maintenance of 'regular' bowel habits is a preoccupation of Western societies, best achieved by increasing dietary fibre. Nevertheless, laxative drugs are widely prescribed or taken without prescription, and they are frequently abused.

Constipation is the passage of hard, small stools less frequently than the patient's own normal function. It is often associated with straining. There are many causes (Box 35.1). Symptoms of constipation include mild abdominal discomfort and distension, similar to those of irritable bowel syndrome (see below).

Underlying organic disease should be excluded when there is persistent constipation or if there has been a recent change in bowel habit.

Laxatives

The mechanisms of action of common laxatives are shown in Figure 35.1.

Bulking agents

Bulking agents include various polysaccharides: wheat bran, ispaghula husk, sterculia (or the synthetic alternative methylcellulose), which are not broken down by

---

Box 35.1

Causes of constipation

Diet low in fibre or fluid
Disease, for example colonic cancer, myxoedema, hypercalcaemia
Iatrogenic (drug-induced), for example opioid analgesics, antimuscarinic agents, antacids, Ca^{2+} antagonists
Slow gut transit, especially in young women
Immobility
Hypotonic colon in the elderly or following chronic laxative abuse

---

OSMOTIC LAXATIVES

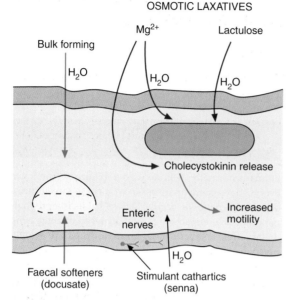

Fig. 35.1
Sites of action of the major types of laxative drug.

digestive processes. They have several mechanisms of action:

- a hydrophilic action causing retention of water in the gut lumen, which expands and softens the faeces
- stimulation of colonic mucosal receptors by the increased bulk, promoting peristalsis
- proliferation of colonic bacteria, which further increases faecal bulk
- sterculia also contains polysaccharides that are broken down to fatty acids and have an osmotic effect.

After ingestion, bulking agents take at least 24 h to work. A liberal fluid intake is important to lubricate the colon and minimise the risk of obstruction. Bulking agents are useful for establishing a regular bowel habit in patients with chronic constipation, diverticular disease and irritable bowel syndrome, but they should be avoided if the colon is atonic or there is faecal impaction. Unwanted effects include a sensation of bloating, flatulence or griping abdominal pain. Regular fibre intake may also be of benefit for diarrhoea.

Osmotic laxatives

Magnesium salts and lactulose are most frequently used. Magnesium salts are poorly absorbed, osmotically active solutes, which increase the small and large bowel luminal fluid volume. They may also stimulate chole-cystokinin release from the small intestinal mucosa, which enhances intestinal secretions and motility. These actions result in more rapid transit of gut contents into the large bowel, where distension promotes evacuation within 3 h. About 20% of ingested magnesium is absorbed and has central nervous system (CNS) and neuromuscular-blocking activity if it is retained in the circulation in large enough amounts, for example in renal failure.

Lactulose is a semisynthetic disaccharide of fructose and galactose. In the bowel, bacterial action releases fructose and galactose which ferment to lactic and acetic acids. These are osmotically active and also lower intestinal pH, which favours overgrowth of selected colonic flora. The proliferation of ammonia-producing bacteria is inhibited, which is useful in the treatment of hepatic encephalopathy. Lactulose can take more than 24 h to take effect.

Sodium acid phosphate is an osmotic preparation that is given as an enema or suppository, usually as bowel preparation before local procedures or surgery.

Irritant and stimulant laxatives

Important examples are senna, bisacodyl, danthron and sodium picosulfate. They act by largely unknown mechanisms, probably stimulating local reflexes through myenteric nerve plexuses in the gut. This enhances gut motility and reduces reabsorption of water and electrolytes. They are useful for more severe forms of constipation, but tolerance is common with regular use and they can produce abdominal cramps. Given orally, they stimulate defecation after about 6 to 12 h.

Senna has the most gentle purgative action of this group. Given orally, it is hydrolysed by colonic bacteria to release irritant anthracene glycoside derivatives, sennosides A and B. Bisacodyl can be given orally, or rectally for a more rapid action in 15–30 min; it undergoes enterohepatic recirculation. Sodium picosulphate is a powerful irritant and is used to prepare the bowel for surgery or colonoscopy. Danthron is a stimulant that is carcinogenic at high doses in animals; its use in human should, therefore, be limited to elderly or terminally ill patients. It is available as co-danthramer, a combination with the surface wetting agent poloxamer '188', and as co-danthrusate, a combination with the mildly stimulant agent docusate (see below).

Chronic use of any of these compounds may lead to progressive deterioration of normal colonic function with eventual atony (cathartic colon) possibly by damaging the myenteric plexus.

Lubricants and stool softeners (emollients)

Docusate sodium has detergent properties which may soften stools by increasing intestinal fluid secretion; it also has stimulant activity but overall it is a relatively ineffective compound. It is given rectally, or orally in combination with danthron (co-danthrusate). Arachis oil or glycerol can be given rectally or liquid paraffin, orally. Glycerol, used as a suppository, is a gentle method for stimulating colonic activity and provoking evacuation. Liquid paraffin is not recommended since it impairs the absorption of fat soluble vitamins; it can cause anal seepage and accidental inhalation produces lipoid pneumonia.

Management of constipation

For short-term use, a stimulant laxative such as senna or bisacodyl orally can be taken at night to give a morning bowel action. Senna, magnesium salts or docusate appear to be safe in pregnancy. Bisacodyl or glycerol suppositories will give a more rapid effect. Co-danthramer or co-danthrusate are suitable for elderly or terminally ill patients with opioid-induced constipation.

For long-term treatment of constipation, dietary modification, supplemented by bulking agents is recommended. Lactulose is useful as a second-line agent and specifically to treat constipation in patients with hepatic encephalopathy.

Diarrhoea

Severe acute diarrhoea is usually a result of gastrointestinal infection, and it can be the consequence of both reduced absorption of fluid and an increase in intestinal secretions. Viral gastroenteritis is a common cause in children but bacteria are more often responsible in adults. Traveller's diarrhoea is a particularly common problem because of exposure of the traveller to organisms which they have not encountered before. Common causes include enterotoxin-producing *Escherichia coli*, *Clostridium jejuni* and *Salmonella* and *Shigella* species. Parasites such as *Giardia lamblia*, *Cryptosporidium species* and *Cyclospora cayetanesis* are less commonly involved. Diarrhoea may result from local release of bacterial enterotoxins which have a variety of actions on gut mucosal cells, including stimulation of intracellular AMP, which causes excess Cl^- secretion into the bowel.

Drugs can also produce diarrhoea, most often magnesium salts (see above), cytotoxic agents (Ch. 52) and α- and β-adrenoceptor-blocking drugs (Chs. 5 and 6). Broad-spectrum antimicrobials often produce diarrhoea by altering colonic flora (Ch. 51). Occasionally this is associated with pseudomembranous colitis caused by overgrowth of toxin-producing *Clostridium difficile* in the bowel.

Chronic diarrhoea requires full investigation for non-infectious causes such as carcinoma of the colon, inflammatory bowel disease or coeliac disease.

Drugs for diarrhoea

Opioids

Opioids act as antimotility drugs and allow greater time for fluid absorption from gut contents. The antimotility action of opioids is probably a result of binding to μ- and possibly κ-receptors in the myenteric plexus of the intestinal wall (Ch. 19). This enhances segmental contractions, inhibits propulsive movements of the gut, and prolongs transit time of intestinal contents. Widely used examples are codeine, loperamide and diphenoxylate. Most have short half-lives. Loperamide has an intermediate half-life giving it a longer duration of action. It also has a more rapid onset of action and it is more selective for the gut, partly because of a high first-pass metabolism which limits systemic absorption. Loperamide has additional antimuscarinic activity that also inhibits peristalsis. Other antimuscarinic drugs have too many unwanted effects to be clinically useful for this indication. Unwanted effects of opioid drugs are discussed in Chapter 19.

Adsorbent agents

Kaolin, chalk, ispaghula and methylcellulose are adsorbents which are relatively ineffective in the treatment of diarrhoea. They may act by adsorbing toxins from microorganisms.

Treatment of diarrhoea

Hydration. In acute infective diarrhoea this is the most important aspect. Replacement of Na^+, glucose and K^+ is as important as fluid replacement. Intravenous fluid may be necessary, but a high oral fluid intake, which can be with specially formulated oral rehydration solutions, is often sufficient. Fluid and electrolyte balance are particularly important in children.

Antidiarrhoeal drugs. Opioids are useful for mild-to-moderate diarrhoea. They should be avoided in patients with dysentery, when prolonging contact of the organism with the gut mucosa can be detrimental. In young children, severe abdominal distention caused by ileus can occur with opioids and again it is recommended that they are not used.

Traveller's diarrhoea. This can be prevented in people travelling to high-risk areas by antimicrobial prophylaxis. Co-trimoxazole or ciprofloxacin are most often recommended (Ch. 51) depending on the area to which the person is travelling. Alternatively, the antimicrobial can be taken at the first sign of illness, and it will usually shorten the duration of the attack to less than 24 hours.

Antimicrobial-induced diarrhoea. Stopping the provoking drug usually leads to rapid resolution. In prolonged, severe cases, when pseudomembranous colitis is suspected or *Clostridium difficile* toxin has been detected in the stool, treatment with oral metronidazole or vancomycin (Ch. 51) should be given.

Inflammatory bowel disease. In this case, diarrhoea should be treated by management of the underlying condition (see Ch. 34).

Irritable bowel syndrome

Irritable bowel syndrome (IBS) is characterised by abdominal pain and alterations in bowel habit, varying from diarrhoea to constipation, for which no cause can be identified. It is said to occur in 15% of the population. Abdominal pain can often be relieved by defecation, but there is a sensation of incomplete evacuation and mucus is passed per rectum. Ill-defined patterns of dysmotility throughout the gut have been reported. A strong psychological component is also evident. Drug therapy should form only part of the treatment, supplemented by counselling and psychological support. Constipation can be treated with bulking agents and diarrhoea, with an opioid. Some patients will also respond favourably to alterations in diet, antispasmodic agents or short courses of benzodiazepines (Ch. 20) or tricyclic anti-depressants (Ch. 22).

Drug treatment

Antispasmodic agents

Examples: mebeverine, dicycloverine (dicyclomine), propantheline.

Mechanism of action

Antispasmodic agents have both antimuscarinic and, in the case of mebeverine and dicycloverine (dicyclomine), direct antispasmodic properties (possibly by phospho-diesterase inhibition). They can relieve gut spasm and the associated pain. Propantheline also inhibits gastric emptying.

Pharmacokinetics

Oral absorption of mebeverine and dicycloverine (dicyclomine) is good and the compounds are metabolised in the liver. The half-lives are short. Propantheline is a poorly absorbed quaternary amine; most is hydrolysed in the bowel.

Unwanted effects

The unwanted effects of antispasmodic agents are mainly antimuscarinic actions (Ch. 4).

5-Hydroxytryptamine receptor agonists and antagonists

Examples: alosetron, tagaserod

Alosetron and tagaserod are newly introduced drugs acting on 5-hydroxytryptamine (5HT) receptors, which are ubiquitous in the gastrointestinal tract. Their long-term safety and efficacy and precise mechanisms of action have yet to be established. Alosetron is an antagonist of $5HT_3$ receptors and has some beneficial effect in diarrhoea-predominant IBS; it appears to be particularly beneficial in women. Tagaserod is a partial agonist at $5HT_4$ receptors and is effective in the treatment of constipation-predominant IBS. Further studies on these compounds will be required before their position in the treatment of IBS is established.

FURTHER READING

Maxwell PR, Medall MA, Kumar D (1997) Irritable bowel syndrome. *Lancet* 350, 1691–1695

Fallon M, O'Neill B (1997) ABC of palliative care: constipation and diarrheoa. *Br Med J* 315, 1293–1295

McFarlane XA, Morris AI (1997) Faecal incontinence and constipation. *J R Coll Physicians Lond* 31, 487–492

Farthing MJG (1998) New drugs in the management of the irritable bowel syndrome. *Drugs* 56, 11–21

Self-assessment

In the following questions, the first statement, in italics, is true. Are the accompanying statements also true?

1. *Regulation of gastrocolonic motility involves the central nervous system, the enteric nervous system and gastrointestinal hormones.*

   a. Defecation once every 3 days in the absence of any organic disease requires investigation.
   b. The majority of cases of 'simple' constipation can be treated by life-style changes.
   c. Chronic intake of senna causes progressive hyperactivity of colonic motility.

2. *A drug history is important in investigation of patients with chronic constipation or diarrhoea.*

   a. Antacids containing aluminium salts can cause constipation.
   b. All laxatives act to stimulate bowel movements within 3 to 6 h.

3. *The causes of diarrhoea are many but can be largely of psychological origin in some patients.*

   a. In infants (< 2 years) infectious diarrhoea is mainly caused by bacteria.
   b. Pseudomembranous colitis may result from the use of broad-spectrum antimicrobial drugs.
   c. The use of antidiarrhoeal agents may increase the residence of enteroinvasive bacteria in the gut.

4. *In industrial countries, the use of antimicrobials to treat acute episodes of diarrhoea is rarely necessary.*

   a. There is little resistance among *Vibrio cholera* strains to tetracycline.
   b. Oral rehydration powders must be reconstituted with water to give a hypertonic solution.

The answers are provided on pages 621–622.

Drugs used in constipation and diarrhoea

Drug	Half-life (h)	Elimination	Comment
Constipation			
Bulk and osmotic laxatives	–	–	Act through their lack of absorption; uptake and systemic disposition is not relevant to their therapeutic effects (bran, ispaghula husk, sterculia, lactitol, lactulose, magnesium salts and rectal phosphates or sodium citrate); bulking agents may affect the absorption of nutrients and minerals
Gut stimulants			May undergo significant absorption and produce adverse systemic effects, for example danthron and oxyphenisatin produce liver damage; senna compounds such as sennoside are degraded by the gut microflora and produce local effects; bisocodyl undergoes variable, but extensive, absorption and is excreted as a glucuronide
Diarrhoea			
Adsorbants	–	–	Kaolin acts because of its lack of oral absorption
Codeine	3–4	Metabolism	Codeine is oxidised to morphine (about 5%) by CYP2D6
Diphenoxylate	2–3	Metabolism + bile	Given as co-phenotrope (co-formulation with atropine)
Loperamide	10–12	Metabolism	Main effect is from the parent drug prior to absorption; metabolites retain antidiarrheal activity
Morphine	1–5	Metabolism	Used in combination with kaolin for short-term treatment of diarrhoea; eliminated by conjugation with glucuronic acid

36

Liver disease

Acute and subacute liver failure

The syndrome of acute or subacute liver failure is said to be present if a patient develops encephalopathy within 12 weeks of the onset of jaundice. It arises from a number of insults to liver cells, principally viral infection (such as hepatitis B) or the toxic effects of drugs and chemicals. In the UK, paracetamol poisoning is the most common cause (Ch. 53).

Presenting symptoms are often non-specific with malaise, nausea and abdominal pain. As the syndrome progresses, signs of impairment of brain function occur with initial confusion followed by drowsiness and coma. These clinical features reflect increased central nervous system (CNS) neuroinhibition, caused by endogenous toxins that the liver fails to remove, and alterations in neurotransmitter synthesis.

Management

N-Acetylcysteine should be given if paracetamol was the precipitant (Ch. 53) and it may be useful in other forms of acute liver failure through beneficial effects on microcirculatory haemodynamics. Other management is supportive and includes:

- prevention and management of bacterial and fungal infection
- treatment of cerebral oedema by mechanical ventilation and infusion of mannitol (Ch. 14)
- treatment of shock, often with norepinephrine (Ch. 7)
- prevention of hypoglycaemia with intravenous dextrose
- artificial support for renal failure with haemofiltration or haemodialysis.

For many patients, liver transplantation is necessary.

Chronic hepatic encephalopathy

Many chronic liver diseases predispose patients to the neuropsychiatric disturbance known as chronic hepatic encephalopathy. The clinical features are similar to those occurring in acute liver failure.

357

Management

There are three main management methods.

- Lactulose (Ch. 35) can be given orally to reduce absorption of neurotoxins by decreasing intestinal transit time and increasing nitrogen fixation by colonic bacteria.
- Oral antimicrobials such as neomycin or metronidazole (Ch. 51) reduce bacterial ammonia production in the colon. Neomycin is less favoured because of its potential to cause nephrotoxicity and ototoxicity, even though little is absorbed from the gut.
- Supplements of branched-chain amino acids can be given.

Variceal haemorrhage

Gastro-oesophageal varices are large venous communications between the oesophagus and proximal stomach that arise from portal hypertension. They are found in 70% of patients with cirrhosis and they carry a high risk of haemorrhage, from which mortality is high.

Management

Management of gastro-oesophageal varices may be surgical or with drugs.

- Repletion of blood volume can be carried out with colloid solution or, preferably, whole blood. Impaired coagulation and thrombocytopenia are common findings in advanced liver disease and transfusion of platelet concentrates and fresh frozen plasma may be necessary.
- Endoscopic variceal injection with sclerosants is successful in up to 95% of patients.
- Balloon tamponade of the bleeding point achieves control in 80–90% of patients. It is usually used to treat rebleeding after endoscopic sclerosant therapy.
- Vasopressin (Ch. 43) produces splanchnic vasoconstriction, which can reduce bleeding from varices. However, systemic vasoconstriction causes ischaemic complications in up to 50% of patients. It is therefore little used, although co-administration of the vasodilator glyceryl trinitrate (trinitroglycerin; Ch. 5) may reduce the systemic complication rate.
- Octreotide (Ch. 43) is more effective than vasopressin for stopping haemorrhage. It works by reducing portal venous pressure and, therefore, flow in the splanchnic circulation and varices. It is successful in up to 65% of patients and is mainly used when sclerosant therapy is not immediately available.

Autoimmune liver disease

There are three principal forms of autoimmune liver disease: autoimmune hepatitis, primary biliary cirrhosis (PBC) and the less common primary sclerosing cholangitis. The pathogenesis of these diseases is poorly understood, but the occurrence of autoimmune phenomena (such as circulating autoantibodies) and histological evidence of immunogically competent cells in the inflammatory infiltrate in the liver has encouraged the use of immunosuppressant treatments.

Management

There are several therapeutic options for autoimmune liver disease.

- Corticosteroid therapy, usually with prednisolone (Ch. 44), induces remission in 80% of patients with autoimmune hepatitis, but it is relatively ineffective in PBC.
- Azathioprine (Ch. 39) has a corticosteroid-sparing action in autoimmune hepatitis and it may improve survival in PBC.
- Ciclosporin or tacrolimus (Ch. 39) are occasionally effective for PBC but rarely needed for autoimmune hepatitis.
- Ursodeoxycholic acid is the only drug licensed for use in PBC. This is a bile acid that is produced by bacterial oxidation of chenodeoxycholic acid. It retards progression of the disease by a cytoprotective effect (by reducing nitric oxide synthesis), immune modulation and suppression of the cytotoxic effect of other bile acids. The main unwanted effect is diarrhoea.
- Liver transplantation is necessary for end-stage disease in all autoimmune liver disease, and it has good long-term results.

Chronic viral hepatitis

There are three hepatic viral infections that can cause chronic hepatitis: hepatitis B virus (HBV), hepatitis C virus (HCV) and hepatitis delta virus (HDV). The end result of the chronic inflammation produced by any of these viruses is cirrhosis.

Management

The only effective treatment for inducing remission in chronic viral hepatitis is interferon alfa. There is no role for this drug in treatment of acute hepatitis B infection, which usually resolves spontaneously. The viral reverse transcriptase inhibitor lamivudine (Ch. 51) has recently been used in chronic hepatitis B infection to reduce liver inflammation and fibrosis. Treatment is usually continued for at least 1 year. Tribavirin is sometimes used with interferon alfa for treatment of hepatitis C infection.

Interferon alfa

Mechanism of action and effects

Interferons are glycoproteins produced by various cells in response to bacterial or viral infections. Interferon alfa is produced by leucocytes; it is a cytokine with a complex mechanism of action. Interferons bind to cell surface receptors and stimulate production of enzymes in the host cell that inhibit viral mRNA translation by host ribosomes. This inhibits viral replication. The long-term remission rate in viral hepatitis is between 20 and 40%.

Pharmacokinetics

Interferon alfa is given by subcutaneous injection daily or three times a week for 4–6 months. It has a short half-life. Generally the recombinant product interferon alfa-2b is used. It differs from the natural product by having a methionine in position 23 and by not being glycosylated.

Unwanted effects

● Immediate effects are almost universal and include headache, myalgia, fever and rigors, usually

occurring 4–6 h after injection. Tolerance occurs with repeated use.
● Delayed effects include fatigue, headache, myalgia and anorexia.

Tribavirin

Mechanism of action and use

Tribavirin (ribavirin) is a synthetic nucleoside analogue with activity against some RNA and DNA viruses. It inhibits viral RNA and protein synthesis, and it increases the production of antiviral cytokines. It has little effect on viral replication when used alone, but it enhances the efficacy of interferon alfa against hepatitis C virus by about threefold.

It is used orally in combination with subcutaneously administered interferon alfa for synergistic benefit in initial treatment of chronic hepatitis C virus infection or for relapse after initial treatment with interferon alfa alone. Tribavirin is also used by inhalation for the treatment of respiratory syncitial virus bronchiolitis.

Pharmacokinetics

Tribavirin is well absorbed rapidly from the gut but undergoes some first-pass metabolism in the liver. It is metabolised in the liver and partially excreted unchanged by the kidney. Its half-life is about 11 days.

Unwanted effects

Unwanted effects include:

● accumulation in red cells leads to haemolysis
● nausea
● dyspnoea

FURTHER READING

Hoofnagle JH, Di Bisceglie AM (1997) The treatment of chronic viral hepatitis. *N Engl J Med* 336, 347–356

Koff RS (1999) Advances in the treatment of chronic viral hepatitis. *JAMA* 282, 511–512

Krawitt EL (1996) Autoimmune hepatitis. *N Engl J Med* 334, 897–903

Malik AH, Lee WM (2000) Chronic hepatitis B virus infection: treatment strategies for the next millennium. *Ann Intern Med* 132, 723–731

Mas A, Rodés J (1997) Fulminant hepatic failure. *Lancet* 349, 1081–1085

McCormack G, McCormick PA (1999) A practical guide to the management of oesophageal varices. *Drugs* 57, 327–335

Neuberger J (1997) Primary biliary cirrhosis. *Lancet* 350, 875–879

Riordan SM, Williams R (1997) Treatment of hepatic encephalopathy. *N Engl J Med* 337, 473–479

Self-assessment

1. Case history question

> Mr S a 61-year-old publican presented 'feeling as though I am 9 months' pregnant'. His abdominal swelling was caused by ascites, which was drained. A liver biopsy was performed, which showed micronodular cirrhosis. He commenced treatment with oral spironolactone.

  a. Was this a good choice of diuretic?

> He remained well on this regimen for 5 years but continued to imbibe large quantities of alcohol. He re-presented as an emergency having had a haematemesis and melaena. At the time he was slightly jaundiced and demonstrated signs of encephalopathy. In addition, there was gynaecomastia and testicular atrophy. The liver edge was palpable 8 cm below the right costal margin. Investigations showed a bilirubin of 27 mmol l^{-1} (normal <17), an albumin of 30 g l^{-1} (normal 32–50) and a gastroscopy which, performed under sedation with intravenous diazepam, revealed oesophageal varices.

  b. What evidence is there to indicate diminished hepatic reserve in this patient?
  c. In what way(s) will the pharmacodynamics and pharmacokinetics of diazepam be altered in this patient? Was diazepam a good choice?
  d. What alterations to dosage of diazepam might be necessary when compared with its use in patients without liver disease?

> It has been shown that the incidence of rebleeding from oesophageal varices can be reduced by the oral administration of propranolol (by reducing portal venous pressure).

  e. What effect is this man's liver disease likely to have on the pharmacodynamics and pharmacokinetics of propranolol? Specifically in what way will the free fraction of the drug in plasma be affected; how will its bioavailability be influenced and what, if any, will be the effects on the drug's half-life?
  f. Patients with hepatic cirrhosis are often treated with colestyramine and/or lactulose. How do these drugs work and what benefits are produced?
  g. What would you use for pain relief in a patient with established liver cirrhosis?

The answers are provided in pages 622–623.

Drugs used in liver disease

Drug	Half-life	Elimination	Comments
Interferon alfa	3–4 h	Metabolism	Given by subcutaneous, intramuscular or intravenous injection; peak levels appear 4–8 h after subcutaneous or intramuscular injection; taken up by kidney and catabolised
Tribavirin (ribavirin)	7–21 days	Metabolism + renal	Given orally; oral bioavailability is 50%; metabolised by hydrolysis of ribosyl group from triazole moiety, which is then excreted in urine; very slowly cleared from erythrocytes and tissue compartments (shorter half-lives are reported after single doses)

37

Obesity

Obesity is defined as a body mass index (BMI) above $30 \, kg \, m^2$, compared with the ideal range of $18.5–24.9 \, kg \, m^2$. A BMI of $25–29.9 \, kg \, m^2$ is considered overweight. A simpler measure of obesity is the waist–hip ratio (WHR), which should not exceed 1.0 in men or 0.95 in women. Recent data suggest that waist circumference above 102 cm in males or 88 cm in females may be equally predictive of increased risk of obesity-related disease. Weight gain after the age of 20 years is more predictive of increased risk than obesity in childhood.

The health consequences of obesity are considerable (Table 37.1). Weight loss reduces the associated morbidity, but it can be difficult to achieve and to maintain. The prevalence of obesity is increasing in the Western world; it varies from less than 10% in the Netherlands to about 50% in some parts of Eastern Europe. In the UK, it is currently about 15%.

Pathogenesis

Obesity results when energy input exceeds output, usually determined by the balance between energy intake and exercise, or muscular work. Obesity usually develops gradually, and small imbalances are all that is required for progressive weight gain. Several genetic factors regulating weight have been identified. Among these is a gene that encodes for the hormone leptin, which is produced only by adipose tissue. Leptin acts as a signal to specific hypothalamic receptors to indicate the degree of filling of adipocytes and to induce the sensation of satiety. Leptin inhibits the hypothalamic appetite-stimulating neurotransmitter neuropeptide Y. Leptin also increases the expression of corticotrophin-releasing factor, which decreases appetite. Circulating concentrations of leptin are usually high in obesity, but genetic abnormalities of the leptin system predisposing to obesity are probably rare. Several other neurotransmitters and hormones are known to influence appetite: 5-hydroxytryptamine (5HT, serotonin), dopamine, cholecystokinin and insulin inhibit while endogenous opioids, noradrenaline and glucocorticoids stimulate appetite.

At present, too little is known about the central modulation of satiety to develop safe and effective drugs acting at this level.

Table 37.1
Adverse health consequences of obesity

Metabolic consequences	Clinical consequences
Hypertension	Coronary artery disease (BMI >29 increases risk fourfold)
Hyperlipidaemia (raised very low density lipoproteins, reduced high density lipoproteins)	Non-insulin-dependent diabetes mellitus (BMI >35 increases risk 40-fold)
	Stroke
Hyperuricaemia	Osteoarthritis
Insulin resistance	Sleep apnoea
	Large bowel and endometrial cancer (BMI >30 increases risk two to fivefold)
	Low self-esteem

BMI, body mass index.

Drugs for treatment of obesity

Pancreatic lipase inhibitors

Example: orlistat

Mechanism of action

By blocking pancreatic lipase, orlistat reduces triglyceride digestion and thus, energy intake from dietary fat. It achieves sustained weight loss when used as an adjunct to dietary restriction and exercise.

Pharmacokinetics

Orlistat is minimally absorbed after oral administration and an effect on energy intake is seen after 24–48 h. The half-life of the absorbed fraction of orlistat is short.

Unwanted effects

Unwanted effects of orlistat include:

- gastrointestinal upset, including faecal soiling
- reduced absorption of fat-soluble vitamins.

Methylcellulose

Methylcellulose is sometimes used to provide bulk in the gut but there is little supportive evidence of its benefit in obesity.

Catecholaminergic drugs

Example: phentermine

Mechanism of action

Phentermine stimulates the release of noradrenaline in the central nervous system. Noradrenaline acts on the hypothalamus to produce appetite suppression. Rapid recurrence of weight gain often follows withdrawal of the drug.

Pharmacokinetics

Phentermine is well absorbed from the gut and has an intermediate half-life. Elimination is by both metabolism and renal excretion.

Unwanted effects

Phentermine is not recommended for routine treatment of obesity. The licence for phentermine was recently temporarily withdrawn by the European Commission but the Medicines Commission in the UK has reinstated its licence. It can be associated with pulmonary hypertension. A previously available catecholaminergic drug, fenfluramine, was withdrawn in 1997 because of an association with valvular heart disease.

Other unwanted effects of phentermine include:

- dry mouth
- euphoria, insomnia, restlessness and hallucinations: tolerance to these effects usually develops within 2 weeks
- dependence: because of its central stimulatory actions, the use of the drug is restricted to a recommended maximum of 12 weeks.

Phenylpropanolamine

Phenylpropanolamine is a centrally acting sympathomimetic stimulant present in many over-the-counter obesity and cold remedies. Voluntary withdrawal of this drug has been called for in the USA because of an association between its consumption and haemorrhagic stroke.

Fluoxetine

The SSRI antidepressant fluoxetine (Ch. 22) causes weight loss, but it is not licensed for this use.

Management of obesity

The cornerstone of management of obesity is to reduce energy intake by 500–600 kcal below daily requirements. Fat is 'energy dense' and should be particularly restricted. However, dietary restriction alone is usually inadequate and increased exercise combined with diet is more effective than either alone. Exercise need not be vigorous, provided it is maintained long term; walking or cycling is usually enough if performed daily. Behaviour modification is essential for long-term compliance with treatment.

Drug treatment should be restricted to individuals with obesity who fail to respond to the above measures. In the morbidly obese (BMI >40 kg m^2) surgery to restrict the size of the stomach (gastroplasty) or wiring the jaw to reduce solid food intake have been used. Existing treatments for obesity can be expected to produce weight loss of about 10–15%, which is often enough to ameliorate the obesity-related metabolic disorders and their accompanying clinical manifestations.

FURTHER READING

Anon (1998) Executive summary of the clinical guidelines on the identification, evaluation and treatment of overweight and obesity in adults. *Arch Intern Med* 158, 1855–1867

Björntorp P (1997) Obesity. *Lancet* 350, 423–426

Kernan WN, Viscoli CM, Brass LM, et al. (2000) Phenylpropanolamine and the risk of hemorrhagic stroke. *N Engl J Med* 343, 1826–1832

Rosenbaum M, Leibel RL, Hirsch J (1997) Obesity. *N Engl J Med* 337, 396–407

Wilding J (1997) Obesity treatment. *Br Med J* 315, 997–1000

Yanovski JA, Yanovski SZ (1999) Recent advances in basic obesity research. *JAMA* 282, 1504–1506

Self-assessment

Are the following statements true or false?

1. Drug treatment for obesity should be restricted to those who fail to lose weight by other means, for example diet and exercise.

2. Courses of appetite-suppressant drugs are virtually all followed by a rebound in weight gain.

3. Centrally acting appetite suppressants inhibit the effects of noradrenaline.

4. The centre that controls appetite is in the posterior pituitary.

5. Leptin is a peptide produced in muscle cells that inhibits appetite.

The answers are given on page 623.

Drugs used in obesity

Drug	Half-life (h)	Elimination	Comments
Methylcellulose	–	Not absorbed	Taken before meals to produce a sense of satiety; preparations that swell should be taken carefully with water to avoid oesophageal obstruction; little evidence to support efficacy
Orlistat	1–2	Metabolism	Taken before, during or immediately after a meal; negligible absorption (about 1%) and low systemic exposure in clinical use; action is local within the intestine; no significant effects on the absorption of other drugs; systemic disposition is not important
Phentermine	19–24	Renal	Taken in the morning; eliminated in the urine with a shorter half-life (about 8 h) at low urine pH (basic drug); licence temporarily withdrawn but reinstated in 2000

THE IMMUNE SYSTEM

38

Antihistamines and allergic disease

Atopy, allergic disorders and anaphylaxis

Atopic individuals produce specific IgE when exposed to common environmental allergens such as house dust mite, grass pollen or animal dander. Many atopic people also have allergic disease such as asthma, hayfever and eczema although the two are not invariably associated. All allergic reactions arise from type 1 hypersensitivity reactions with activation of mast cells and basophils by antigens, release of preformed mediators and synthesis of new mediators (Fig. 39.1).

Allergic reactions to antigens vary in severity. At the most severe end of the spectrum is anaphylaxis, a systemic allergic reaction, which is life threatening because of respiratory obstruction and/or hypotension. Severe anaphylactic reactions can occur within minutes of exposure to the allergen. There are several causes of anaphylaxis (Box 38.1). Drugs can also act directly on mast cells to release mediators without the involvement of IgE. Such reactions are called anaphylactoid, and they present in the same way as true anaphylaxis. If the allergen exposure is via systemic injection then hypotension and shock will predominate. Foods are more likely to cause facial and laryngeal oedema with prominent respiratory problems. Of the mediators released from mast cells, histamine is particularly important, but tryptase, prostaglandin D$_2$ and leukotrienes (LTB$_4$ and LTC$_4$) also contribute.

Box 38.1

Causes of anaphylaxis

Foods: especially peanuts, tree nuts, fish, shellfish, eggs, milk

Drugs: especially penicillin, intravenous anaesthetic agents, aspirin and other non-steroidal anti-inflammatory drugs, intravenous contrast media, morphine

Bee and wasp stings

Latex rubber

Histamine as an autacoid

Histamine is a heterocyclic amine that functions as a local hormone (autacoid). It is found in mast cells, particularly in tissues that come into contact with the outside world, for example skin, lungs and gut, where it forms part of the tissue defence mechanisms. It is also present in circulating basophils where it may have a similar role. Histamine is found also in enterochromaffin-like cells in the stomach where it participates in acid secretion (Ch. 33) and in the brain where it acts as a neurotransmitter (Ch. 4).

Histamine is synthesised in mast cells and basophils from dietary histidine by decarboxylation. After release from the cells it is rapidly metabolised. Its effects are mediated by three distinct types of receptor known as H_1, H_2 and H_3. In general, the H_1 receptors are involved in the 'defensive' actions of histamine. Gastric acid secretion is mediated by H_2 receptors, and H_3 receptors are involved in neurotransmission, possibly in the autonomic nervous system and in itch and pain perception.

Allergic reactions involve the action of histamine at H_1 receptors. The following reactions are major effects of H_1 receptor stimulation.

- Increased capillary permeability can produce oedema. This can lead to urticaria, angioedema and laryngeal oedema. The consequent loss of circulating blood volume contributes to hypotension.
- Capillary and venous dilation can produce marked hypotension. In the skin histamine contributes to the weal and flare response; an axon reflex via H_1 receptors is responsible for the spread of vasodilation or flare from the oedematous weal.
- Smooth muscle contraction can occur, especially bronchiolar and intestinal.
- Skin itching is provoked, in combination with kinins and prostaglandins; histamine also produces pain.

Histamine H_1 receptor antagonists (antihistamines)

Examples:

'older' histamines: chlorphenamine (chlorpheniramine), promethazine

'non-sedating' antihistamines: terfenadine, fexofenadine, astemizole, cetirazine, loratadine, mizolastine

Mechanisms of action and effects

The antihistamines are selective for histamine H_1 receptors (H_2 receptor antagonists are not called antihistamines). Most are competitive antagonists, except astemizole, which binds tightly to the receptor and produces non-competitive inhibition. Antihistamines suppress many of the vascular effects of histamine.

Some compounds have other actions that can be used therapeutically, for example the older compounds have marked sedative effects (e.g. chlorphenamine (chlorpheniramine), promethazine) or antimuscarinic effects, which suppress nausea in motion sickness (e.g. promethazine; Ch. 32).

Newer ('non-sedating') antihistamines such as terfenadine, astemizole, fexofenadine, loratadine and mizolastine do not have sedative or anticholinergic actions. Cetirazine has some sedative effects. The newer agents also reduce mediator release from basophils and mast cells by inhibiting either Ca^{2+} influx or intracellular Ca^{2+} release.

Pharmacokinetics

Antihistamines are well absorbed from the gut and most are metabolised in the liver to active compounds with long half-lives. Astemizole undergoes extensive first-pass metabolism, but its active metabolites have a very long half-life of more than 7 days, giving the drug a very long duration of action. Like most drugs with very long half-lives its onset of effect is slow (over 5 days) unless a loading dose is given (Ch. 2). Astemizole is metabolised by the cytochrome P450 system (CYP3A4). Cetirizine undergoes little hepatic metabolism, and it is mainly eliminated by the kidney. It has an intermediate half life. Intravenous chlorphenamine (chlorpheniramine) is available for medical emergencies. Several topical formulations of antihistamines exist, including a nasal spray for allergic rhinitis, skin preparations for insect stings (but see unwanted effects) and eyedrops for allergic conjunctivitis.

Unwanted effects

- Sedation or fatigue can occur (not with astemizole, fexofenadine, loratadine, mizolastine).
- Appetite stimulation occurs with astemizole.
- Dry mouth can occur with older drugs that have antimuscarinic effects.
- Topical antihistamines for use on the skin should be avoided because hypersensitivity reactions are common.
- Ventricular arrhythmias, particularly torsade de pointes, can occur with high doses of terfenadine or astemizole because of K^+ channel blockade. This occurs particularly if they are used in combination with imidazole antifungal agents (e.g. itraconazole) or macrolide antimicrobials (e.g. erythromycin), which complete for the enzyme CYP3A4 in the liver

(Ch. 2). The active metabolite of terfenadine, fexofenadine maintains the antihistamine activity without the arrhythmogenic activity.

Management of allergic disorders

Anaphylaxis

This is a medical emergency and requires rapidly acting treatments. The patient should be laid flat with the feet raised if there is hypotension. Epinephrine (adrenaline) should be given intramuscularly and doses repeated every 10 min until the patient is stable. Patients known to have allergies that cause anaphylaxis can carry a pre-loaded epinephrine (adrenaline) syringe for emergencies, accompanied by detailed instructions on its appropriate use. Intravenous epinephrine (adrenaline) is only given if there is profound shock, and then in a very dilute solution with close cardiac monitoring.

Once epinephrine (adrenaline) has been given, late relapse can be prevented by intramuscular or slow intravenous infusion of chlorphenamine (chlorpheniramine) and hydrocortisone (Ch. 44). Oxygen should be given in high concentration and if there is marked bronchospasm an inhaled β-adrenoceptor agonist such as salbutamol (Ch. 12). This can be particularly useful if the patient is taking a β-blocker, when epinephrine (adrenaline) may be less effective on the airway. If there is persistent hypotension, then intravenous fluid (a colloid such as gelatin or dextran if possible, crystalloid such as saline if a colloid is unavailable) should be given rapidly.

Seasonal and perennial rhinitis

The symptoms of rhinitis include nasal obstruction, sneezing, itching and inflammation of the lining of the nose. These result from increased glandular secretion with nasal obstruction, mucous rhinorrhea and afferent nerve stimulation, which causes itching and sneezing. Allergies can cause both perennial (usually house dust mite) or seasonal rhinitis (pollens and moulds). The allergic response also makes individuals more susceptible to the effects of non-specific irritants such as tobacco smoke or changes in temperature. Rhinitis also has several non-allergic causes, including acute infection or chronic sinus infection. Aspirin can produce rhinitis (as well as asthma (Ch. 12)) in sensitive subjects, probably by enhancing leukotriene generation. Prolonged use of nasal decongestants such as the α_1-adrenoceptor agonist oxymetazoline can also cause rhinitis. Less frequent causes include β-blockers (Ch. 5) and angiotensin-converting enzyme (ACE) inhibitors (Ch. 6).

Oral antihistamines are useful for reducing itching, sneezing and rhinorrhea, but they are less effective for nasal obstruction. They can also be useful if there is associated allergic conjunctivitis. Topical antihistamines (such as azelastine or levocabastine) are also available for use in the nose. For more severe allergic rhinitis, a topical intranasal corticosteroid (Ch. 44) is the treatment of choice, providing relief from most symptoms. Topical sodium cromoglycate or nedocramil (Ch. 12) are useful in atopic subjects but they are less effective than antihistamines or topical corticosteroids. The antimuscarinic drug ipratropium bromide (Ch. 12) can also be used topically for relief of rhinorrhea. Nasal decongestants have a role early in treatment, but they should not be given long-term because of the risk of rebound nasal congestion. Oral corticosteroids are reserved for the most severe symptoms. If drugs fail, then surgery to remove nasal polyps, to reduce the size of the inferior turbinates or to correct a deviated nasal septum may be helpful.

Urticaria

Acute urticarial reactions often occur to the same allergens that cause anaphylaxis. Antihistamines are the treatment of choice, with an oral corticosteroid (Ch. 44) for more severe episodes.

Chronic urticaria can be provoked by physical factors such as cold, sun, stroking the skin (dermographism) or exercise, or it can be caused by urticarial vasculitis in association with connective tissue diseases such as systemic lupus erythematosus. In the absence of an obvious provoking factor, the cause is autoimmune caused by IgG autoantibodies to the IgE receptors on mast cells and basophils. Antihistamines can be useful to suppress the itch from urticaria, but often they have little effect on the weal. Corticosteroids (Ch. 44) may be needed in high dosage for severe symptoms, but long-term use should be avoided. Immunosuppression with ciclosporin (Ch. 39) has been used successfully in some patients with severe autoimmune urticarias.

Allergic conjunctivitis

Topical treatment is usually successful (see Ch. 50).

Contact and atopic eczema

Contact and atopic eczemas are considered in Ch. 49.

Asthma

Although asthma often has an allergic component, antihistamines have little or no role. The management of asthma is considered in Chapter 12.

FURTHER READING

Ewan PW (1998) Anaphylaxis. *Br Med J* 316, 1442–1445

Greaves MW, Sabroe RA (1998) Allergy and the skin 1 – urticaria. *Br Med J* 316, 1147–1150

Mackay IS, Durham SR (1998) Perennial rhinitis. *Br Med J* 316, 917–920

Mattila KJ, Paakkari I (1999) Variations among non-sedating antihistamines: are there real differences? *Eur J Clin Pharmacol* 55, 85–93

Parikh A, Scadding GK (1997) Seasonal allergic rhinitis. *Br Med J* 314, 1392–1395

Slater JW, Zechnich AD, Haxby DG (1999) Second-generation antihistamines. *Drugs* 57, 31–37

Self-assessment

In questions 1 and 2, the first statement, in italics, is true. Are the accompanying statements also true?

1. *Antihistamines such as fexofenadine and loratadine are non-sedating.*

   a. Fexofenadine is associated with electrocardiograph (ECG) changes.
   b. Antihistamines reduce acid secretion from the parietal cell.
   c. Fexofenadine reduces the release of histamine from mast cells.

2. *The allergic response in mast cells from atopic individuals can cause the release of leukotrienes, histamine and prostaglandins from sensitised mast cells.*

   a. Corticosteroids are ineffective for treating allergic rhinitis.
   b. Histamine is the only mediator that causes symptoms in rhinitis.

3. Case history question

   > A 15-year-old boy visited his doctor with his mother complaining of repeated episodes of rhinorrhoea, nasal congestion, sneezing, itching eyes over a 6-month period, starting soon after they bought a cat. His symptoms are interfering with his school work. He has no history of asthma but his mother is asthmatic. Otherwise he has been fit and healthy over the last year and has taken no medication.

   a. What is the likely diagnosis?

   > A skin test reaction showed him to be responsive to cat dander and house dust mite.

   b. What treatment would you give?

   The answers are provided on page 623.

Antihistamines

Drug	Half-life (h)	Elimination	Comments
Non-sedating antihistamines			All drugs given orally only
Acrivastine	2	Renal + metabolism	Limited kinetic data available; renal excretion of unchanged drug accounts for 60% of an oral dose indicating high bioavailability; about 15% converted to an active metabolite which has a half-life of 4 h
Cetirizine	9	Renal	Complete bioavailability; clearance is about 50% of glomerular filtration rate, but drug is highly protein bound (93%) indicating the possibility of active tubular secretion; very slight metabolism
Fexofenadine	14	Renal	Oral bioavailability has not been defined; about 1% only is metabolised (by CYP3A4); it is the active metabolite of terfenadine
Loratadine	10	Metabolism	Oral bioavailability (about 10%) increased by food; it is a prodrug which undergoes extensive first-pass metabolism by CYP3A4 and CYP2D6 to an active metabolite which has a half-life of 28 h
Mizolastine	15	Metabolism	Oral bioavailability is about 70%; active metabolites have not been detected
Terfenadine	See fexofenadine	Metabolism	Essentially complete first-pass metabolism to the active metabolite, fexofenadine; negligible blood concentrations of parent drug after oral dosage; inhibition of first-pass metabolism by CYP3A4 linked to adverse cardiac effects (torsade de pointes)
Sedating antihistamines			
Alimemazine (trimeprazine)	4–7	Renal + metabolism	Given orally; minor metabolic pathways include *S*-oxidation and *N*-dealkylation (which produces an active metabolite)
Azatadine	9	Metabolism + renal	Given orally; few data available; excreted in urine unchanged and as a conjugate
Brompheniramine	25	Metabolism + renal	Given orally; main route of elimination is as inactive metabolites; bioavailability has not been well defined (probably about 50%) but it is reduced by food
Chlorphenamine (chlorpheniramine)	22	Renal + metabolism	May be given orally or by subcutaneous, intramuscular or slow intravenous injection; renal excretion is more important than metabolism; bioavailability is high (>80%)
Clemastine	21	Metabolism	Given orally; metabolised by oxidation; oral bioavailability is 40% (earlier data indicated a half-life of 4–6 h)
Cyproheptadine	1–4	Metabolism	Given orally; eliminated by oxidative metabolism; few kinetic data are available; duration of action is about 12 h
Diphenhydramine	3–9	Metabolism	Given orally; oral bioavailability is 40–60%; oxidised to a polar carboxylic acid (possibly by CYP2D6)
Diphenylpyraline	32	Metabolism	Given orally; few kinetic data available
Doxylamine	10	Metabolism	Given orally; metabolic fate has not been defined in humans
Hydroxyzine	20–30	Metabolism	Given orally; metabolised to cetirizine (which then has a formation rate limited half-life similar to hydroxyzine)
Mequitazine	45	Metabolism	Given orally; few kinetic data available
Pheniramine	16–19	Metabolism + renal	Given orally; approximately equal amounts in urine as unchanged drug and oxidised (*N*-dealkyl) metabolite
Promethazine	7–14	Metabolism	Given orally, by deep intramuscular injection, or by slow intravenous infusion; low oral bioavailability (25%); bile is the major route of elimination of the (inactive) metabolites
Triprolidine	3	Metabolism	Given orally; well absorbed but bioavailability has not been defined; undergoes extensive oxidative metabolism in animals; fate in humans has not been defined (but only 1% is excreted unchanged in urine)

The immune response and immunosuppressive drugs

Biological basis of the immune response[a]

The immune system is highly complex and the elucidation of many of its main aspects has been one of the triumphs of biomedical research.

Natural and adaptive immunity

Natural (innate) immune defences include:

- Physicochemical barriers to infection (impermeable skin and mucous membranes, low pH in stomach, mucociliary escalator in airway, antibacterial agents in skin and tear secretions, e.g. lysozyme)
- Non-specific mechanisms (alternative pathway of complement activation, stimulation of phagocytosis by bacterial cell wall lipopolysaccharides, activation of mast cells by tissue damage).

Adaptive immune responses are superimposed upon the innate mechanisms. They are evolutionarily more recent and depend on their exquisite specificity in recognising 'non-self' molecules, usually foreign proteins, either via the production of specific antibodies or via cell-mediated immunity. Examples include:

- classical (antibody-dependent) pathway of complement activation, leading to non-specific lysis of bacterial cells
- antibody-dependent activation of resident leucocytes (mast cells and macrophages), leading to recruitment of further phagocytes (neutrophils, monocytes) and phagocytosis of pathogens in an acute inflammatory response
- Antibody-dependent cytolysis of virally infected cells.

Humoral immunity

Both innate immunity and adaptive immunity involve complex networks of soluble humoral components and

---

[a] We are grateful to Dr Anthony Sampson, who wrote this section.

cellular components. In adaptive immunity, the production of specific antibodies to a foreign protein is initiated by recognition of the antigen by immunoglobulin (Ig) molecules on the surface of a specific clone of B-lymphocytes. These are derived from a few of the millions of clones (cell lines) of B-cell precursors each of which has surface Ig directed towards the specific foreign molecule (clonal selection; Fig. 39.1a). Alternatively, fragments of antigens are presented to B-cells by antigen-presenting cells (APC), including macrophages, dendritic cells in the lung, and Langerhans cells in the skin. The antigen fragment is presented within the cleft of major histocompatibility complex (MHC) type II molecules on the APC surface. After contact with its specific antigen, the B-cell clone undergoes repeated gener-

ations of cell division (clonal proliferation); some of the daughter cells become memory cells that allow a more rapid B-cell response in later encounters with the antigen (Fig. 39.1b). Once proliferated, the specific B-cell clone becomes susceptible to cytokines from activated T-helper (Th) lymphocytes. Antigen-presenting cells also express antigen fragments associated with MHC II that are recognised by Th-cells via a specific T-cell receptor (TCR), which recognises the antigen, the MHC II molecule, and several costimulatory molecules. Supported by interleukin (IL)-1 from the APC, the Th-cell undergoes clonal proliferation. This is perpetuated over numerous cell divisions by IL-2 from the Th-cells themselves. Activated Th-cells produce a number of cytokines including interleukins that convert B-cells

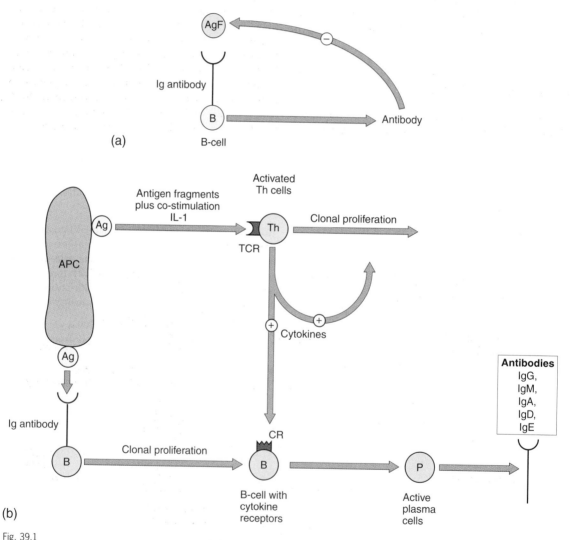

Fig. 39.1
(a) In **adaptive immunity** there is production of specific antibodies to a foreign protein (AgF) after recognition of AgF by a selected group of B-cells carrying surface immunoglobulin (Ig) directed specifically towards AgF.
(b) Antigen fragments can also be presented to B-cells by an antigen-presenting cell (APC). This results in B-cell clonal proliferation. Antigen fragments are also presented to T-cells via a T-cell receptor (TCR) that recognises the antigen. T-cells undergo clonal proliferation, produce interleukins (IL) and stimulate B-cells to produce antibodies (IgG, IgM, IgA, IgD and IgE). Th, T helper cell; P, plasma cell; Ag, antigen; CR, cytokine receptor.

into active plasma cells that secrete antibodies of the IgG, IgM, IgA, IgD, and IgE classes.

The immunoglobulin molecule contains two identical heavy chains that are distinctive to the Ig class (gamma, mu, alpha, delta, and epsilon) linked to two light chains (kappa or lambda) by disulfide bonds. High concentrations of monomeric IgG are found in the plasma and in tissue spaces. IgM circulates as pentamers linked by J chains, while IgA is secreted onto mucosal surfaces as dimers linked by a segment of its receptor termed the secretory piece. IgD may be involved in early-life processing of B-cells. IgE is important in immune responses to intestinal parasites and also in allergic hypersensitivity reactions such as hay fever and asthma. On encountering an antigen, the primary immune response consists of IgM, replaced later by IgG. On a further encounter with the antigen, the secondary immune response occurs sooner and consists of large amounts of of IgG produced by long-lived B memory cells.

Cell-mediated immunity

Not all adaptive immune responses involve antibodies. Cell-mediated immunity is involved in responses to viral infection, graft rejection, chronic inflammation, and tumour immunity (Fig. 39.2).

Virally infected host cells express fragments of viral proteins as antigens in association with MHC I molecules on the cell surface. These can be recognised by specific TCRs on the surface of cytotoxic T-cells (Tc), which can kill the virus-infected host cell.

Delayed hypersensitivity also occurs. This aspect of cell-mediated immunity involves the regulation by antigen-specific T-lymphocyte clones of 'non-specific' inflammatory cells, including macrophages, neutrophils, eosinophils, and basophils. Following recognition of antigens associated with MHC class II on the APC, Th-cells proliferate under the influence of IL-2, and secrete a number of cytokines that regulate leucocyte proliferation, recruitment and activation. The type of response is determined by the profile of cytokines secreted. A subset of Th cells called Th1-cells secrete interferon-γ (IFN-γ) to activate macrophages, which in turn secrete IL-8 and other neutrophil chemoattractants. This leads to macrophage/neutrophil-dependent inflammation, associated with immune responses to persistent infections such as tuberculosis. In contrast, cytokines derived from Th2-cells promote Type 4 hypersensitivity reactions (e.g. asthma; see below).

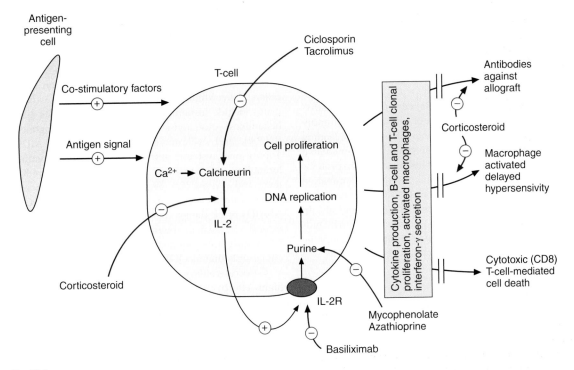

Fig. 39.2
Aspects of cell-mediated immunity. This shows in simplified form some steps in T-cell activation following antigen presentation to the T-cell receptor and subsequent events that may contribute to the aspects of the immune response in cell-mediated immunity. Drugs used as immunosuppressives (red arrows) act at the sites shown. Corticosteroids act at many sites (Ch. 44). IL-2, interleukin 2; IL-2R, interleukin 2 receptor.

Unwanted immune reactions

Inflammation and immunity are essential to protect the host against pathogenic and other damage, but excessive, inappropriately prolonged or misdirected immune responses may cause disease, including hypersensitivity reactions, graft rejection and autoimmune diseases.

Hypersensitivity reactions

Hypersensitivity reactions were classified by Gell and Coombs.

Type 1 (acute, immediate). This includes hay fever and acute asthma. IgE molecules on the surface of mast cells and basophils are cross-linked by harmless antigens (allergens such as pollens, house-dust mites) leading to synthesis and/or release of inflammatory mediators. These include cysteinyl-leukotrienes, prostaglandins, histamine, platelet-activating factor, proteases and cytokines.

Type 2 (cytotoxic). Cell surface antigens, including microbial proteins and drug molecules haptenised onto cell surfaces, trigger binding of IgG and IgM antibodies (opsonisation), leading to activation of complement (classical pathway) and cytolysis of the target cell. Examples include destruction of red cells after incompatible blood transfusion and haemolytic anaemia caused by binding of some drugs to host cells.

Type 3 (complex-mediated). Soluble antigens react with excess circulating antibodies to form complexes that precipitate in small blood vessels, causing vasculitis and organ damage. Serum sickness from foreign serum is a systemic type 3 reaction, while the Arthus reaction is a local response to an injected antigen (e.g. non-human insulins).

Type 4 (cell-mediated, delayed type hypersensitivity). Inappropriate regulation of cell-mediated immunity may cause damaging chronic inflammation, leading to fibrosis and granuloma formation. Cell-mediated immunity misdirected against harmless foreign proteins (allergens) can lead to chronic allergic inflammation (asthma, hay fever, eczema), or cause contact sensitivity in the skin to haptenising metals and chemicals. In allergy, a subset of T-cells (Th_2) secrete cytokines including IL-4, IL-5 and IL-13, which promote eosinophilic inflammation and overproduction of IgE by B-cells.

Transplant rejection

In blood transfusion, rejection occurs because non-self antigens on red blood cells (ABO system) trigger type 2 hypersensitivity reactions in the recipient. In immunodeficient patients, transfused T-cells react against recipient antigens (graft-versus-host reactions). For organ transplants, host-versus-graft reactions between foreign MHC molecules (human leucocyte antigens,

HLA) must be reduced by HLA tissue typing. Rejection involves destruction of the graft by B-cells, T-cells, and macrophages, and it can be immediate (days), acute (weeks), or chronic (years).

Autoimmunity

Autoimmune diseases are caused by a failure of tolerance of the immune system to 'self' molecules; the immune system therefore reacts against host tissues. Numerous mechanisms cause autoimmune diseases, including viral infection of host cells, binding of drug molecules to host cells (e.g. penicillin), antigens shared between host cells and microbes, and sequestered antigens liberated by cell damage. Examples include haemolytic anaemia, diabetes, Addison's disease, rheumatoid arthritis, myasthenia gravis, systemic lupus erythematosus and thyroiditis.

Immunopharmacology principles

The immune system presents a large number of potential molecular targets for therapeutic intervention. Present drugs tend to be non-specific immunosuppressants with a range of adverse effects; recombinant DNA and monoclonal antibody technologies may allow the development of immunomodulatory drugs that block specific immune interactions.

Inflammatory mediators released by leucocytes can be blocked by antagonists at their receptors on target cells, or by inhibiting their synthesis. Antimediator drugs include histamine H_1 receptor antagonists (antihistamines), cysteinyl-leukotriene receptor antagonists (LTRA), and cyclo-oxygenase inhibitors (NSAIDs). Topical and systemic antihistamines (e.g. terfenadine, loratadine, cetirizine) are used in the control of hay fever and eczema (Ch. 38), while oral LTRAs (montelukast, zafirlukast) are used in asthma (Ch. 12). Oral NSAIDs block the synthesis of prostaglandins and are extensively used in rheumatoid arthritis (Chs 29 and 30). Future antimediator drugs may include cytokine antagonists that block IL-4 or IL-5 receptors.

Corticosteroids (e.g. dexamethasone, prednisone) are highly effective anti-inflammatory drugs that can be used systemically to suppress type 4 hypersensitivity reactions, autoimmune diseases (e.g. rheumatoid arthritis) and graft rejection (Ch. 44). Cushingoid unwanted effects are a drawback with systemic treatment; they are used topically for inflammatory skin disease and by inhalation for asthma (e.g. beclomethasone, fluticasone; Ch. 12). Corticosteroids modulate transcription of genes encoding pro-inflammatory cytokines (granulocyte–macrophage colony-stimulating factor, IL-1, IL-2, IL-4, IL-5, IL-8) and cellular adhesion molecules. Hence, they reduce the proliferation of lymphocytes, eosinophils and monocytes in the bone marrow and prevent their recruitment to the inflammatory site.

Other immunosuppressants include azathioprine and methotrexate, which act as antimetabolites preventing the synthesis of DNA in lymphocytes (and other rapidly dividing cells). Alkylating agents including cyclophosphamide have also been used in rheumatoid arthritis. Gold compounds may suppress phagocytosis or interfere with complement activation (Ch. 30).

The most effective immunosuppressant is ciclosporin, which binds to immunophilins (cyclophilin) in T-cells and prevents activation of calcineurin and subsequent production of cytokines involved in T-cell clonal proliferation, particularly IL-2. Ciclosporin may also kill opportunistic infective bacteria in immunosuppressed patients. Together with corticosteroids, ciclosporin is front line therapy to prevent transplant rejection, but nephrotoxicity is a major drawback.

Passive immunity describes the transfer of humoral immunity by injection of immunoglobulins (gammaglobulins) taken from an immunised human or animal, and also the transfer of IgG across the placenta and in maternal colostrum in neonates. An extension of this concept is to use the high specificity of antibodies to block critical molecular interactions in the immune system, such as the binding of an antigen to its specific B-cell or T-cell receptors. Mouse monoclonal antibodies against the antigen or receptor can be 'humanised' by recombinant DNA technology to replace the mouse Fc portion with human Fc portion so that the therapeutic antibody does not itself trigger an immune response. Humanised chimeric monoclonal antibodies that neutralise IgE can prevent mast cell degranulation following allergen exposure for several weeks after a single injection.

Immunosuppressive drugs

In addition to the drugs discussed in this chapter, others such as glucocorticoids, methotrexate and cyclophosphamide are also used for their immunosuppressive properties in various disease states. Methotrexate and cyclophosphamide have immunosuppressive properties at doses much lower than those required to treat malignancy (Ch. 52). These drugs are more fully discussed in other chapters as indicated in the text. Immunosuppressive drugs are widely used in many diseases, examples of which are rheumatoid arthritis, psoriasis, inflammatory bowel disease. Their benefit is both through modulation of the immune system and in some cases through their anti-inflammatory properties.

Calcineurin inhibitors

Examples: ciclosporin, tacrolimus

Ciclosporin

Mechanism of action

Ciclosporin is a fungal cyclic peptide which inhibits Th-cells. It binds in the cell cytoplasm to a receptor called cyclophilin, leading to inhibition of the enzyme calcineurin phosphatase. Activated calcineurin, which is produced in response to an antigenic signal at TCRs, dephosphorylates nuclear factor of activated T-cells, which enters the cell nucleus and binds to the IL-2 promoter region. By inhibiting activation of calcineurin, ciclosporin inhibits expression of the nuclear regulatory proteins and T-cell activation genes that code for IL-2 transcription following T-cell activation and inhibits the maturation of cytotoxic T-cells. There is a lesser suppression of IFN-γ production, which suppresses the expression of major histocompatibility antigens on macrophages. Ciclosporin also stimulates production of tumour growth factor β (TGF-β). This may help to prevent acute rejection, but long-term it could increase the risk of chronic rejection.

Pharmacokinetics

Oral absorption of the standard formulation of ciclosporin is variable and incomplete, requiring initial dispersion by bile salts. For this reason a microemulsion formulation has been developed. This emulsifies when it comes into contact with water in the gut increasing the surface area for absorption, which then becomes independent of bile production. After absorption, ciclosporin selectively concentrates in some tissues including liver, kidney, several endocrine glands, lymph nodes, spleen and bone marrow. Extensive metabolism by cytochrome P450 occurs in the liver and the half-life is long. Trough plasma drug concentration monitoring is important to guide dosage for optimal effectiveness and to minimise toxicity; monitoring is needed less frequently if the microemulsion formulation is taken.

Unwanted effects

- Nephrotoxicity almost always occurs. Acute effects include intrarenal vasoconstriction that may persist and contribute to long-term sequelae, which include interstitial fibrosis and tubular atrophy. The decline in renal glomerular function is usually reversible but permanent renal impairment can result. Induction of TGF-β may be a contributory factor.
- Hypertension, often associated with fluid retention, occurs in up to 50% of patients. It usually responds to standard antihypertensive drug treatment.

- Convulsions can occur, most frequently if corticosteroids are given concurrently. They often occur in association with hypertension and are more common in children.
- Tremor can occur.
- Hypertrichosis (excessive hair growth) and gum hypertrophy are common.
- Gastrointestinal disturbance including anorexia, nausea and vomiting.
- Hyperlipidaemia can occur.
- Drug interactions can be severe and caution should be taken when ciclosporin is used with other nephrotoxic drugs such as aminoglycoside antimicrobials (Ch. 51). Drugs that induce liver cytochrome P450 (Ch. 2) can reduce the plasma concentration of ciclosporin to subtherapeutic levels.

Tacrolimus

Mechanism of action and effects

Tacrolimus inhibits calcineurin and T-cell proliferation in a similar manner to ciclosporin, after binding to a receptor protein called FK-binding protein-12. Unlike ciclosporin, tacrolimus does not stimulate production of TGF-β. Tacrolimus also enhances transformation of the glucocorticoid receptor, which may contribute to a corticosteroid-sparing effect.

Pharmacokinetics

Tacrolimus is more water soluble than ciclosporin and undergoes more predictable though poor absorption from the gut compared with the standard formulation of ciclosporin. It has an intermediate half-life and is metabolised by the liver.

Unwanted effects

These are similar to ciclosporin except that tacrolimus causes less hypertension, hirsutism or gum hyperplasia. Other effects that are more common with tacrolimus include:

- diabetes
- pleural and pericardial effusions
- cardiomyopathy in children, who should be monitored by echocardiography.

Interleukin-2 receptor antibodies

Example: Basiliximab

Basiliximab is a chimaeric monoclonal antibody that binds to the α-subunit of the IL-2 receptor, and prevents T-cell proliferation. It is usually given in combination with a corticosteroid and ciclosporin in allogenic renal transplantation.

Pharmacokinetics

Basiliximab is given by intravenous infusion immediately before and again 4 days after surgery. It has a long half-life of about 10 days.

Unwanted effects

None reported.

Antiproliferative agents

Examples: mycophenolate mofetil, azathioprine

Mycophenolate mofetil

Mycophenolate mofetil inhibits the enzyme inosine monophosphate (IMP) dehydrogenase, which is involved in the conversion of IMP to xanthine monophosphate. Inhibition of this enzyme depletes the cell of guanine nucleotides and inhibits cellular DNA synthesis. Lymphocytes rely on de novo purine nucleotide synthesis, unlike neutrophils, which can re-use preformed guanine released from the breakdown of nucleic acids (the salvage pathway). Mycophenolate mofetil is, therefore, more specific for inhibition of lymphocyte function.

A further action of mycophenolate mofetil involves inhibition of smooth muscle proliferation in arterial walls. This may also be important in reducing graft rejection as a consequence of obliterative arteriopathy.

Pharmacokinetics

Mycophenolate mofetil is an ester of mycophenolic acid. It is almost completely absorbed from the gut, and cleaved rapidly to the acid derivative after absorption. Elimination is via hepatic metabolism. The half-life of the active acid metabolite is long, and inhibition of IMP dehydrogenase activity is prolonged after a single dose.

Unwanted effects

- Gastrointestinal upset is very common, including nausea, diarrhoea and abdominal cramps. Tolerance to these symptoms often occurs.
- Bone marrow suppression can occur resulting in leucopenia and anaemia.
- Opportunistic infections may be increased, especially with cytomegalovirus.

Azathioprine

Mechanism of action

Azathioprine is widely used for immunosuppression. Most of the effects of azathioprine result from cleavage to the active derivative 6-mercaptopurine (Ch. 52). Both cell- and antibody-mediated immune reactions are suppressed. Effects on the immune response include impaired synthesis of immunoglobulins by B-lymphocytes, and inhibition of the infiltration of mononuclear cells into inflamed tissue. These arise from the antimetabolite action of 6-mercaptopurine, which interferes with purine biosynthesis, thus impairing DNA synthesis in the S-phase of the cell cycle (Fig. 52.1).

Pharmacokinetics

Oral absorption is almost complete. Azathioprine is a prodrug, and its metabolism in the liver produces active compounds. The half-life is short.

Unwanted effects

- Bone marrow suppression with dose-dependent leucopenia can occur. Regular monitoring of the white cell count is essential.
- There is a small risk of carcinogenicity, especially lymphomas.
- There is increased susceptibility to infection, often with 'opportunistic' organisms.
- Gastrointestinal disturbances can occur, especially nausea and vomiting.
- Alopecia can occur.
- Drug interactions: the most important interaction is with allopurinol (Ch. 31); allopurinol inhibits the enzyme xanthine oxidase, which is involved in the metabolism of azathioprine. The dose of azathioprine should be reduced by 75% if the drugs are used together.

Immunosuppression in organ transplantation

The immune response and its place in the rejection of a transplanted organ is a complex process. In general terms, rejection starts to occur when the recipient T-cells recognise foreign antigens from the transplant presented by antigen presenting cells. This recognition results in the T-cell producing the cytokine IL-2 which is a prime stimulant for T-cell clonal proliferation and further cytokine production. For this to occur optimally, a poorly understood co-stimulatory signal from the antigen presenting cell is also required. (Without the co-stimulatory signal the T-cell may undergo apoptosis). Graft destruction then occurs as increased generation of B-cells, cytotoxic T-cells and monocyte/macrophages results in antibody production against the graft, lysis of cells and delayed hypersensitivity responses. Not all these responses need to occur. Immunosuppressive drugs act at the steps of T-cell activation, proliferation and cytokine production (Fig. 39.2).

Effective immunosuppression has improved the early survival of kidney, liver, heart and lung transplants. However, suppression of acute rejection is more effective than prevention of chronic rejection, which responds poorly to immunosuppressive therapy. Regimens for immunosuppression vary among units and according to the immunogenicity of the transplanted tissue. Combination therapy with a corticosteroid, calcineurin inhibitor and an antiproliferative agent is usually used. For kidney transplantation, triple therapy often with the corticosteroid prednisolone (Ch. 44) azathioprine and ciclosporin is widely employed. Acute rejection can be reduced by treatment with the IL-2 receptor antibody basiliximab. With such regimens, more than 80% of kidney grafts will survive beyond one year. Only half of those that fail are lost from rejection and the rest from thrombosis. Progressive graft loss continues after the first year with only 50–60% of grafts surviving at 10 years. Most of these late graft losses are as a result of chronic vascular rejection. If this occurs, increasing the dosages of the primary immunosuppressive drugs may help. There is interest in the possibility that drugs such as tacrolimus or mycophenolate mofetil may reduce the incidence of chronic rejection. Late acute rejection is a less common problem. It can sometimes be overcome by high-dose corticosteroid or the use of anti-lymphocytic globulin (although the use of these is associated with an increased risk of opportunistic infection and long-term malignancy). Tacrolimus can also be used successfully as a rescue treatment during late episodes of acute rejection.

In contrast to renal transplants, pancreatic transplants are more immunogenic and quadruple immunosuppressive regimens are widely used. Induction treatment with antilymphocytic globulin is then followed by ciclosporin, azathioprine and a corticosteroid. Mycophenolate mofetil is sometimes substituted for azathioprine or tacrolimus for ciclosporin. Despite these treatments, 5-year graft survival is only about 60% and the risk of post-transplant infection is high.

Triple immunosuppressive therapy is used for heart (50% 10-year survival), heart–lung (30% 10-year survival), liver (70% 10-year survival) and intestinal (40–50% 3-year survival), transplants. Tacrolimus is often included in these regimens.

Immunosuppression in other disorders

Immunosuppression therapy is used in several diseases in which an autoimmune component may contribute to the pathogenesis. These include various connective tissue diseases such as vasculitis or systemic lupus erythematosus, certain types of glomerulonephritis, chronic active hepatitis, psoriasis, Crohn's disease and some haematological disorders. Drugs may be given alone or in combination. Those most widely used include corticosteroids, azathioprine, methotrexate and cyclophosphamide (Ch. 52). Ciclosporin and mycophenolate mofetil have also been studied in disorders such as asthma, inflammatory bowel disease and psoriasis, with some success.

FURTHER READING

Denton MD, Magee CC, Sayegh MH (1999) Immunosuppressive strategies in transplantation. *Lancet* 353, 1083–1091

Suthanthiran M, Strom TB (1994) Renal transplantation. *N Engl J Med* 331, 365–376

Self-assessment

In questions 1–3, the first statement, in italics, is true. Are the accompanying statements also true?

1. *Ciclosporin, tacrolimus and corticosteroids decrease maturation of cytotoxic T-cells by suppressing interleukin-2 transcription.*

   a. Ciclosporin does not cause bone marrow suppression.
   b. With ciclosporin administration, careful assessment of renal function is required.

2. *Immunosuppression induced by glucocorticoids involves their effects on T-cells and inflammation.*
   Tacrolimus enhances transformation of the glucocorticoid receptor.

3. *Using smaller doses than for cancer chemotherapy, drugs such as cyclophosphamide, methotrexate and azathioprine are immunosuppressant.*
   Azathioprine suppresses antibody-mediated immune responses.

4. Case history question

   A 35-year-old woman is about to receive her second kidney transplant. The previous transplant lasted 5 years but, despite immunosuppression with prednisolone and ciclosporin, it was eventually rejected.

   a. How might you reduce the chances of acute rejection of the second transplant?
   b. What are the long-term risks of combination chemotherapy with corticosteroids, tacrolimus and azathioprine?

   The answers are provided on page 623.

Immunosuppressive drugs[a]

Drug	Half-life	Elimination	Comment
Azathioprine	3–5 h	Metabolism	Oral or intravenous dosage; converted to active metabolite, 6-mercaptopurine, which is converted to nucleoside and uric acid analogues (therefore interaction with allopurinol)
Basiliximab	7–11 days	Metabolism	Monoclonal antibody given by intravenous infusion; binding to interleukin-2 receptor alpha chain maintained for 1 to 2 weeks after dosage; usually given with ciclosporin or corticosteroid immunosuppressives
Ciclosporin	27 h (10–40)	Metabolism	Oral or intravenous dosage; oral bioavailability is 40%; lipid-soluble cyclic peptide metabolised by CYP3A4 in liver and gut wall to at least 25 metabolites some of which retain biological activity
Daclizumab	20 days	Metabolism	Monoclonal antibody given by intravenous infusion; normally given every 2 weeks for a total of 5 doses; usually given with ciclosporin or corticosteroid immunosuppressives
Mycophenolate mofetil	18 h (as MPA)	Metabolism	Oral or intravenous dosage; very rapidly hydrolysed (within minutes) to the active form mycophenolic acid (MPA); oral and intravenous doses undergo essentially quantitative conversion to MPA; MPA is eliminated as a glucuronide conjugate
Tacrolimus	9 h (4–41)	Metabolism	Oral or intravenous dosage; metabolised by CYP3A4 in liver and gut wall; low bioavailability combined with low systemic clearance indicate that it undergoes extensive first-pass metabolism in the gut wall but not the liver; metabolites are mostly inactive

[a]Immunostimulants are covered in Chapter 52 (Cancer chemotherapy). See also the inflammatory arthritides (Ch. 30).

Drug compendium

THE ENDOCRINE SYSTEM AND METABOLISM

40

Diabetes mellitus

Control of blood glucose

Glucose occupies a central position in metabolism as the predominant substrate for energy production. Cells receive their supply of glucose from blood, and control mechanisms ensure that blood glucose concentrations remain within narrow limits. Glucose enters the blood by absorption from the gut and from breakdown of stored glycogen in the liver. At physiological concentrations it leaves the blood almost entirely by active transport into the cells; in most tissues this transfer is dependent on the action of the polypeptide hormone insulin.

Insulin is a protein which is rapidly secreted from the beta cells of the islets of Langerhans in the pancreas in response to a small rise in blood glucose; its secretion is inhibited by a fall in blood glucose. Insulin consists of two peptide chains, A and B, connected by two disulfide bridges. The secretion of insulin is biphasic in response to a rise in plasma glucose (both the actual concentration and the rate of change). **Phase one** of release occurs within seconds, and lasts for only a few minutes. This consists of release of stored hormone. **Phase two** is more gradual and is partly due to synthesis of new insulin. Glucose stimulates insulin production by elevation of intracellular ATP concentrations in the pancreatic beta cell. This leads to closure of inward rectifier K^+_{ATP} channels in the cell membrane, and reduced membrane K^+ permeability. The islet cell therefore depolarises and voltage-dependent Ca^{2+} channels in the cell membrane open. Calcium ion influx into the cell triggers exocytosis of insulin granules. In addition to glucose, many other factors influence insulin secretion (Fig. 40.1).

All peripheral tissues express specific cell surface receptors for insulin which are linked to the enzyme tyrosine kinase (Ch. 1). On activation of these receptors the glucose transporter (Glut 4) is translocated to the cell surface, allowing glucose uptake. Insulin therefore promotes active transport of glucose into the cell, particularly in skeletal muscle, accompanied by potassium. In the liver, insulin inhibits the conversion of amino acids to glucose (gluconeogenesis), promotes glucose storage as glycogen, and inhibits the breakdown of glycogen (glycogenolysis). The overall effect is to increase glycogen stores. Insulin reduces plasma free fatty acids and increases adipocyte triglyceride storage. It does this by preventing triglyceride breakdown in fat by inhibiting lipases. It also increases circulating hydrolysis of

Endogenous stimulants of insulin secretion
Glucose
Amino acids
Fatty acids
Vagal effects
Glucagon
Cortisol
Gastrin
Secretin

Inhibitors of insulin secretion
Sympathetic effects,
somatostatin

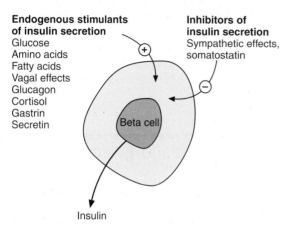

Beta cell

Insulin

Fig. 40.1
Some physiological factors controlling insulin secretion.

triglycerides from lipoproteins by enhancing lipoprotein lipase. Glucose entry into lipocytes provides glycerol phosphate for esterification of fatty acids.

The effects of insulin on protein metabolism include increased amino acid transport into muscle and enhanced protein synthesis, and inhibition of the catabolism of amino acids in the liver. The effects on different tissues are summarised in Table 40.1.

Table 40.1
Metabolic effects of insulin

Liver	Increased glucose storage as glycogen
	Decreased protein catabolism
	Increased protein synthesis
Muscle	Increased protein synthesis
	Increased glycogen synthesis
	Increased glucose uptake
	Increased amino acid uptake
Adipose tissue	Increased triglyceride storage
	Increased triglyceride synthesis
	Decreased lipolysis

Several hormones naturally inhibit the anabolic action of insulin, particularly on carbohydrate metabolism. These include glucagon, growth hormone, cortisol and catecholamines (Fig. 40.1). Most of these hormones are released in stressful situations that require the breakdown of glycogen reserves for energy.

Diabetes mellitus

Failure to secrete sufficient insulin to maintain a normal level of blood glucose results in diabetes mellitus. The condition is diagnosed when the fasting plasma glucose concentration exceeds 7 mmol l^{-1}. The long-term consequences include increased risk of the development of vascular and neuropathic disease (Table 40.2) . Two patterns of diabetes mellitus are recognised: type 1 and type 2.

Type 1 (or insulin-dependent) diabetes mellitus; IDDM

Type 1 diabetes represents a severe deficiency of insulin production and usually presents in youth. There is destruction of pancreatic beta cells, sometimes as part of an autoimmune process although the cause in many cases is unknown. The clinical picture reflects the failure of glucose uptake into cells in sufficient quantities to maintain energy production and anabolic metabolism. Patients are tired and unwell, lose weight, develop polyuria and polydipsia, and are prone to ketoacidosis because of breakdown of fatty acids and amino acids in the liver.

Table 40.2
Complications of diabetes

Complication	Consequences
Microvascular	
Nephropathy	Microalbuminuria, macroalbuminuria, renal failure
Retinopathy	Background retinopathy, proliferative retinopathy with blindness
Peripheral neuropathy	Loss of peripheral sensation
	Pain, ulceration
Autonomic neuropathy	Impotence
	Gastrointestinal disturbance
	Orthostatic hypotension
Macrovascular	
Cardiovascular disease	Hypertension
	Ischaemic heart disease
Cerebrovascular disease	Stroke

Type 2 (or non-insulin-dependent) diabetes mellitus; NIDDM

Type 2 diabetes, which usually presents later in life, is the consequence of a relative deficiency of insulin. It accounts for about 85% of cases of diabetes in the western world. In type 2 diabetes, phase one of insulin secretion is absent, and phase two is slowed. Overall, maximum insulin release is reduced by up to 50%, particularly in non-obese patients with type 2 diabetes in whom reduced insulin secretion is more important than tissue insulin resistance. More often type 2 diabetics are overweight, which increases cellular resistance to insulin in the liver and peripheral tissues. Type 2 diabetics do not usually become ketotic. Sufficient glucose enters cells to permit adequate energy production for most situations. The main problem is excess glucose outside the cells rather than a shortfall inside.

Insulins and insulin analogues

When endogenous insulin production is severely impaired, it must be replaced by therapeutic administration of insulin. Normal insulin secretion from the pancreas is into the portal circulation and is strictly related to metabolic needs. Sixty per cent of insulin released from the pancreas is extracted by the liver before reaching the systemic circulation. Therapeutic delivery of insulin is to the systemic circulation, and the relationship to metabolic needs can only be approximated by the dosages used and their timing in relation to meals.

Natural insulin formulations

Insulins for therapeutic administration used to be extracted from either cattle or pig pancreas. Bovine insulin differs chemically from human insulin in three amino acid residues, and porcine in one, but their action is very similar to human insulin. Recombinant DNA technology has allowed in vitro manufacture of insulin with the same structure as human insulin and these preparations are superseding those of animal origin. All current insulin preparations have a low content of impurities that caused problems in the past.

Pharmacokinetics

Insulin must be given parenterally as it is digested in the gut. Subcutaneous injection is used for routine treatment, and intravenous infusion for emergency situations. The half-life of insulin in plasma is very short (about 8–16 min), and to avoid the need for frequent injections during maintenance treatment, the absorption of insulin from injection sites must be prolonged. Insulin is formulated either in a soluble preparation or is complexed with a substance to delay absorption from the injection site (Table 40.3). After subcutaneous injection, the maximum plasma concentration of soluble insulin is achieved about 2 hours later, compared to minutes after intravenous injection. To limit the increase in plasma glucose concentration generated by a meal, subcutaneous insulin must be given at least 30 minutes before eating. The action of intravenous soluble insulin lasts less than an hour and is mainly terminated by degradation in the kidney. Continued absorption from a subcutaneous injection site prolongs the duration after injection to about 5 hours.

Recommended subcutaneous injection sites include upper arms, thigh, buttocks or abdomen. Absorption is faster from the abdomen than from the limbs, although strenuous exercise can increase absorption from the limbs.

To generate intermediate or long-acting insulin, it is complexed with:

Protamine: to create the intermediate-acting isophane insulin. This can be given as a ready mixed preparation with soluble insulin (biphasic isophane insulin). The ratio of soluble to isophane insulin in biphasic insulin varies from 10:90, through 20:80; 30:70, 40:60 to 50:50.

Zinc: to create the intermediate/long-acting insulin zinc suspension.

Protamine and zinc: to create the long-acting protamine zinc insulin. This is now rarely used since it binds with soluble insulin if given in the same syringe. Insulin molecules form dimers in solution. In the presence of zinc these complex into hexamers. The size of these molecular aggregates determines the rate of diffusion from the site of injection. Such complexes act as modified-release formulations for subcutaneous administration (Table 40.3).

Unwanted effects

- The main problem is an excessive action producing hypoglycaemia. Neuroglycopenia with confusion and coma can occur. Treatment is by intravenous injection of 50% glucose if the patient is unconscious or oral glucose if not. Glucagon (see below) can be given intramuscularly to the unconscious patient if venous access is not available, followed by a sugary drink on waking. Hypoglycaemia can usually be avoided by careful matching of meals, exercise and insulin. All patients taking insulin should carry a card with details of their treatment. Although most diabetics get warning symptoms of hypoglycaemia, some do not and are prone to sudden and severe hypoglycaemic coma. This can occur after transfer from animal to human insulin.

Table 40.3
Comparisons among insulins following subcutaneous administration

Type	Onset of action (h)	Peak activity (h)	Duration (h)	
Insulin formulations				
Neutral (regular or soluble)	0.5	1–3	7	Short-acting
Isophane	1	2–6	20	Intermediate/long-acting
Zinc	2	6–14	22	Long-acting
Protamine–zinc	4	12–24	30	Long-acting
Insulin analogues				
Insulin lispro	0.25 min	0.5–0.75	2–5	Short-acting
Insulin glargine	1	5	15–30	Long-acting

- Rebound hyperglycaemia can occur after an episode of hypoglycaemia, especially at night (Somogyi effect). This results from the compensatory release of hormones such as adrenaline, cortisol, glucagon and growth hormone. It can produce ketonuria, leading to a mistaken belief that too little insulin has been given.
- Animal insulins produce circulating antibodies, although this is less common with current highly-purified preparations. These could diminish the activity of the insulin (insulin resistance) or produce local reactions (lipoatrophy) at injection sites.
- Insulins can cause local fat hypertrophy at the injection site; rotating the site of injection reduces this.

Insulin analogues

Examples: insulin lispro, insulin glargine

Mechanism of action and effects
The insulin analogues are chemical modifications of naturally occurring insulin that remain monomeric in solution. Insulin lispro has two changes in the amino acids at the C-terminal end of the polypeptide B chain, sterically hindering its ability to form dimers. These changes have no effect on the binding of the molecule to cellular insulin receptors. Insulin glargine also has two amino acid changes (involving glycine and arginine, hence the name). This makes the molecule more soluble at acid pH, and less soluble at physiological pH. Insulin glargine precipitates after subcutaneous injection, slowly redissolves and is then absorbed.

Pharmacokinetics
Compared to standard soluble insulin, absorption of insulin lispro from a subcutaneous injection site occurs faster and leads to an earlier and high peak plasma concentration. The duration of action is also shorter at almost 3 hours. There is a reduced frequency of hypoglycaemia compared to soluble insulin because of the shorter duration of action. Insulin lispro must be given just before a meal. It can be mixed with long-acting standard insulins and is available as a biphasic formulation with insulin lispro protamine in a 25:75 ratio. Insulin glargine is slowly and uniformly absorbed after injection, and avoids plasma insulin peaks. The onset of action is about 1 hour, with maximum effect at 5 hours and duration of 15–30 hours.

Unwanted effects
Unwanted effects are similar to those of other insulins.

There is no reported excess of immunogenic reactions compared to standard insulin.

Therapeutic regimens for insulin

The choice of regimen for insulin administration depends on the age, life style, circumstances and preference of the patient. Options include:

Single daily injections before breakfast or at bedtime: used mainly for the few elderly patients who require insulin and in whom long-term complications of diabetes are less relevant. An intermediate or long-acting insulin is used which can be combined with a short-acting one to optimise control.

Twice daily injections before breakfast and evening meal: suitable for patients who have a reasonably stable pattern of activity and eating habits. Short and intermediate-acting insulins are combined, either in fixed ratios provided by the manufacturers, or in varying ratios according to individual requirements. Fixed ratios vary from 10% short with 90% intermediate-acting to a 50% mixture of each component.

Multiple injections before breakfast and evening meal and at bedtime, sometimes with a further injection before the midday meal: increasingly used in younger, active patients who require more flexibility in their life style. Short-acting insulin is given before meals and the amount adjusted for the size of the meal. Administration can be facilitated by the use of portable 'pen-injectors'. A longer-acting insulin can be added at breakfast in a three-times daily regimen and is used alone in the evening to ensure a 'background' effect of insulin throughout the 24 h.

Intravenous infusion: used for patients in ketoacidotic crises, in labour, during and after surgery or at other times when the patient's usual routine cannot be adhered to. Short-acting insulin is infused in 5% dextrose solution with added potassium chloride (unless the patient is hyperkalaemic).

Intraperitoneal. Patients being treated for chronic renal failure by continuous ambulatory peritoneal dialysis can add their insulin to the dialysis fluid. This is the only therapeutic regimen in which insulin has direct access to the portal circulation.

Oral hypoglycaemic drugs

The main sites of action of oral hypoglycaemic drugs are shown in Figure 40.2.

Sulfonylureas

Examples: tolbutamide, chlorpropamide, glibenclamide, gliclazide

Mechanism of action
Sulfonylureas act mainly by increasing the release of insulin from the pancreatic beta cells in response to stimulation by glucose (Fig. 40.2). This is achieved by inhibition of K^+_{ATP} channel activity in the cell membrane (see 'Control of blood glucose' above). The receptor for sulfonylureas is a regulator of the potassium channel proteins. Sulfonylureas also increase glucose utilisation in peripheral tissues by mechanisms that are independent of the action of insulin. This may be caused by stimulation of glucose transport across the cell membrane and activation of cellular enzymes that enhance non-oxidative metabolism of glucose in fat and muscle cells.

Pharmacokinetics
Sulfonylureas are structurally related to sulfonamides. They are absorbed rapidly (although the rate of absorption is reduced when taken with food), are highly protein bound, and are metabolised by the liver. Chlorpropamide depends partly on the kidney for its elimination. The very long half-life of chlorpropamide (about 2 days) may lead to accumulation and its use in the elderly is dangerous. Tolbutamide and gliclazide have intermediate half-lives; glibenclamide has a longer duration of action than would be predicted from its short plasma half-life owing to selective concentration in pancreatic islet cells.

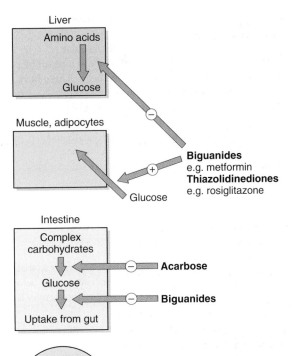

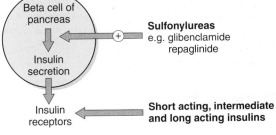

Fig. 40.2
The actions of oral hypoglycaemic drugs and insulin.

Compounds with a short duration of action are usually preferred when starting treatment with a sulfonylurea to minimise the risk of hypoglycaemia.

Unwanted effects
- Gastrointestinal disturbance.
- Excessive (and particularly nocturnal) hypoglycaemia is most frequent with the longer-acting drugs, especially if there is concurrent hepatic or renal impairment.
- Weight gain is almost inevitable unless dietary restrictions are observed.
- Sensitivity reactions include skin rashes and, rarely, blood dyscrasias (in common with most sulfonamides; see Ch. 51).
- Chlorpropamide increases renal sensitivity to antidiuretic hormone and can produce water retention with dilutional hyponatraemia.
- Chlorpropamide often produces flushing when alcohol is taken, owing to inhibition of aldehyde dehydrogenase (Ch. 54).

- Sulfonylureas should be avoided in patients with acute porphyria.
- Sulfonylureas may increase cardiovascular mortality in type 2 diabetes, possibly as a result of inhibition of K^+_{ATP} channels in the heart. These have a cardioprotective role in ischaemic tissue, preventing cell depolarisation to conserve intracellular energy stores. Inhibition of the channels may lead to enhanced cell death and arrhythmias in patients with ischaemic heart disease (see Ch. 5). However, recent evidence has failed to confirm the original concerns about cardiovascular mortality.

Repaglinide

Mechanism of action

The mechanism of action of repaglinide is similar to that of sulfonylureas, but it binds to a distinct site on the beta cell. Its place in therapy compared to sulfonylureas is not yet established.

Pharmacokinetics

Repaglinide is rapidly and well absorbed from the gut, and is given immediately before a meal. It is extensively metabolised in the liver to inactive metabolites and has a short half-life.

Unwanted effects

- Hypoglycaemia
- Gastrointestinal upset including nausea, vomiting, abdominal pain, diarrhoea or constipation
- Hypersensitivity reactions with rashes and urticaria.

Biguanides

Example: metformin

Mechanism of action and effects

Metformin does not affect insulin secretion; it reduces hepatic gluconeogenesis and also limits glucose absorption from the gut and facilitates its uptake in peripheral tissue. The mechanisms involved remain unclear. Metformin can also suppress appetite, which is useful in overweight patients, and when used alone it does not cause hypoglycaemia. An additional benefit is improvement in the adverse plasma lipid profile found in diabetes; metformin raises high-density lipoprotein cholesterol and reduces triglycerides (Ch. 48). The action of metformin is complementary to that of sulfonylureas.

Pharmacokinetics

Metformin is well absorbed from the gut and excreted unchanged by the kidney. It has a short half-life.

Unwanted effects

- Gastrointestinal upset, including anorexia, nausea, abdominal discomfort and diarrhoea, which are usually short-lived.
- Inhibition of pyruvate metabolism encourages lactate accumulation. In situations that lead to an increase in anaerobic metabolism (e.g. shock with hypoxaemia), lactic acidosis can result. This is more common in the presence of cardiac, renal or hepatic impairment.

Thiazolidinediones

Example: rosiglitazone

Mechanisms of action and effects

Thiazolidinediones have no effect on insulin secretion and are referred to as 'insulin sensitisers'. They enhance glucose utilisation in peripheral tissues, especially adipocytes, and may also suppress gluconeogenesis in the liver by inhibition of the enzyme fructose-1,6-bis-phosphatase. The effect is mediated through binding to the nuclear peroxisome proliferator-activated receptor (PPAR-γ). Stimulation of this receptor enables it to interact with the retinoid X receptor (RXR) in the nucleus and enhances the expression of genes that control adipocyte differentiation. As a result, adipose tissue more readily takes up fatty acids from the blood. Reduced availability of fatty acids to muscle improves insulin sensitivity. Rosiglitazone is relatively selective for fat cells in muscle tissue. In addition to reducing the plasma glucose concentration, rosiglitazone also improves diabetic dyslipidaemia. It decreases plasma triglyceride and increases HDL cholesterol concentrations due to increased lipolysis of triglycerides in VLDL. However, other lipoprotein markers of atherogenesis may be adversely affected, for example increases in the plasma concentrations of LDL cholesterol and lipoprotein (Ch. 48).

Pharmacokinetics

Rosiglitazone is well absorbed from the gut and is metabolised in the liver. It has a short half-life. The mechanism of action involves gene transcription and therefore the onset of action is gradual, over 6–8 weeks.

Unwanted effects

- Fluid retention leading to oedema, probably secondary to peripheral vasodilation
- Aggravation of obesity because of fat cell differentiation.

Glucosidase inhibitors

Example: acarbose

Mechanism of action and effects

Carbohydrate digestion in the bowel involves several enzymes that sequentially degrade complex polysaccharides such as starch into monosaccharides such as glucose. Initial digestion of carbohydrates in the gut lumen is carried out by amylases from the saliva and pancreas. The final digestion of oligosaccharides is carried out by β-galactosidases (including lactase) and various α-glucosidase enzymes (such as maltase, isomaltase, glucoamylase and sucrase which hydrolyses the disaccharide, sucrose) in the small intestinal brush border. Acarbose competes with dietary oligosaccharides for α-glucosidase enzymes, and has a higher affinity for these enzymes. Binding to the enzymes is reversible, so that digestion and absorption of glucose after a meal is slower than usual but not prevented. As a result, the postprandial peak of blood glucose is reduced and blood glucose concentrations are more stable through the day. Acarbose has no effect on insulin secretion or its tissue action.

Pharmacokinetics

Oral absorption of acarbose is very poor. Only about 2% of the active parent drug reaches the circulation. Inactive metabolites are formed in the gut lumen by enzymic degradation. About one-third of the oral dose is absorbed as inactive metabolite and most of this is excreted in the faeces.

Unwanted effects

Gastrointestinal effects include flatulence, abdominal distension and diarrhoea owing to fermentation of unabsorbed carbohydrate in the bowel. These effects are dose-related and often transient.

Drugs to increase plasma glucose levels

Glucagon

Mechanism of action and use

Glucagon is a polypeptide that is synthesised by the alpha cells of the pancreatic islets of Langerhans. It binds to specific hepatocyte receptors and activates membrane-bound adenylate cyclase. The consequent increase in intracellular cyclic AMP leads to inhibition of glycogen synthetase. This blocks the effect of insulin on hepatocytes and mobilises stored liver glycogen. Glucagon is used to raise blood glucose in severe hypoglycaemia.

Pharmacokinetics

Glucagon must be given by intramuscular or intravenous injection, and acts in 10–20 min. It is degraded rapidly by enzymes in the blood stream, liver and kidney.

Unwanted effects

- Nausea and vomiting
- Very occasionally allergic reactions.

Management of type 1 diabetes

The aim of treatment is to maintain a plasma glucose concentration as close to normal as possible. The most dramatic complication of untreated type 1 diabetes is diabetic ketoacidosis (Fig. 40.3) which can lead to coma if it is severe. Systemic infection or dietary indiscretion can precipitate ketoacidosis in a treated type 1 diabetic. Apart from treatment of any precipitating cause, the management of ketoacidosis includes:

- Restoration of extracellular volume: hyperglycaemia leads to an osmotic diuresis with excessive urinary salt and water loss. Replacement by physiological (0.9%) saline is essential.
- Potassium replacement: the osmotic diuresis results in excessive urinary potassium loss. Potassium is also shifted from cells into extracellular fluid in exchange for hydrogen ions in the ketoacidotic state. Correction of the extracellular acidosis reverses this shift and can produce profound hypokalaemia. Once the patient has a good urine flow, intravenous potassium supplements are usually required.
- Intravenous insulin until the ketosis is abolished and the plasma glucose is below 15 mmol l^{-1}.

The metabolic acidosis will usually correct with treatment of the hyperglycaemia and fluid replacement. Intravenous sodium bicarbonate is occasionally required if the arterial pH is less than 7.0.

Maintenance treatment of type 1 diabetes should include an appropriate diet with a regulated carbohydrate intake distributed throughout the day. Excess dietary saturated fat should be avoided. The complications of type 1 diabetes can be reduced by close control of the blood sugar concentration using insulin in an appropriate regimen (see above).

The success of the chosen approach can be monitored by measurement of the blood sugar concentrations, often carried out on a finger-prick blood specimen using a blood glucose reagent strip. If peak or trough blood glucose estimations are outside an acceptable range, the insulin regimen should be adjusted, although this should not be done more than once or twice a week. Long-term control of diabetes is usually assessed by the plasma concentration of glycosylated haemoglobin (HbA$_1$ or the specific fraction HbA$_{1c}$). A high concentration is a good marker for the risk of developing

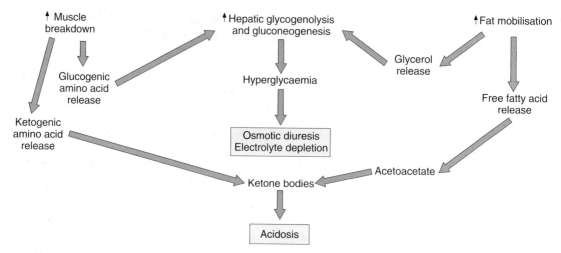

Fig. 40.3
Pathophysiology of diabetic ketoacidosis.

microvascular and neuropathic complications. An HbA$_{1c}$ level greater than 7% carries a higher risk of complications (upper limit of normal 6.0%). For HbA$_1$ the highest risk is at a concentration greater than 8.7% (upper limit of normal 7.5%).

Hyperglycaemia leads to formation of glycosylation end products, which may be promotors of vascular and neurological damage.

Management of type 1 diabetes in special situations

- Close attention to diabetic control is important in pregnancy since poor control will affect the fetus, leading to increased intrauterine and perinatal mortality.
- At times of intercurrent illness, the dose of insulin will need to be increased, guided by blood sugar monitoring, to counteract the hyperglycaemic action of hormones released during stress reactions.
- During and after surgery, soluble insulin should be given in 5% dextrose solution by intravenous infusion, dosage being guided by the blood glucose concentrations. Subcutaneous insulin can be restarted when the patient is able to eat and drink.

Management of type 2 diabetes

The mainstays of treatment are life-style and dietary modifications. As for type 1 diabetes, close control of the

blood sugar concentration in type 2 diabetes reduces the risk of microvascular complications, although the effect on macrovascular complications such as myocardial infarction is less convincing.

More than 75% of newly diagnosed type 2 diabetics are obese. Weight reduction not only improves blood glucose levels but also reduces other cardiovascular disease risk factors. Dietary advice should include:

- reducing energy intake if obese (an average weight loss of 18 kg is required to control blood sugar)
- eating small regular meals
- ensuring that more than half the total energy intake is from carbohydrates
- total fat contributing less than 35% of total energy intake
- encouraging high-fibre foods and limiting sucrose and alcohol intake.

This should be combined with advice to exercise regularly and stop smoking as appropriate. Non-obese patients often require early treatment with an oral hypoglycaemic agent, usually a sulfonylurea. For obese patients, life style and dietary advice should initially be encouraged, with use of metformin if this fails. Combination therapy with a sulfonylurea and metformin can be useful if a single drug is insufficient to reduce the blood glucose concentration. Within three years of onset, 50% of patients will need combination therapy to achieve glycaemic control. Failure of oral treatment usually implies 'beta-cell exhaustion', and up to 30% of type 2 diabetics require insulin with or without an oral hypoglycaemic drug.

Acarbose is of limited value in those patients demonstrating postprandial hyperglycaemia. It may be most effective in early diabetes when there is still sufficient insulin secretion for it to influence glycaemic control.

The role of drugs such as rosiglitazone remains to be determined.

Of crucial importance in type 2 diabetes is intensive management of other risk factors for cardiovascular disease. In particular, intensive control of raised blood pressure with a β-blocker or ACE inhibitor reduces both microvascular and macrovascular complications. Evidence for superiority of ACE inhibitor therapy compared to a β-blocker is inconclusive. Treatment of the abnormal atherogenic plasma lipid profile that is common in type 2 diabetes has been less fully studied, but if the calculated 10-year risk of cardiovascular disease is greater than 30%, treatment should be started. Once a diabetic patient has developed coronary artery disease, intensive lipid lowering with a statin (Ch. 48) will reduce the risk of subsequent myocardial infarction or death.

Future developments in the management of diabetes

Several new approaches to the management of diabetes are being studied. These include inhaled or oral insulin formulations which could dramatically change the convenience of therapy for diabetics, and increase the use of insulin in type 2 diabetes.

The amylin agonist pramlintide is under development for reducing postprandial hyperglycaemia. Amylin acts like insulin to lower plasma glucose, and is deficient in diabetes.

A variety of drugs are being investigated for the treatment of diabetic complications. These include aldose reductase inhibitors that reduce the conversion of glucose into sorbitol, which damages tissues, and aminoguanidine which inhibits ACE formation and may reduce diabetic nephropathy.

FURTHER READING

Clark CM, Lee DA (1995) Prevention and treatment of the complications of diabetes mellitus. *N Engl J Med* 332, 1210–1217

Day C (1999) Thiazolidinediones: a new class of antidiabetic drug. *Diabet Med* 16, 179–192

DeFronzo RA (1999) Pharmacologic therapy for Type 2 diabetes mellitus. *Ann Intern Med* 131, 281–303

Fagan TC, Sowers J (1999) Type 2 diabetes mellitus. Greater cardiovascular risks and greater benefits of therapy. *Arch Intern Med* 159, 1033–1034

Haffner SM (1998) Management of dyslipidemia in adults with diabetes. *Diabetes Care* 21, 160–178

Holleman F, Hoekstra JBL (1997) Insulin Lispro. *N Engl J Med* 337, 176–183

Mogensen CE (1998) Editorial: Combined high blood pressure and glucose in type 2 diabetes: double jeopardy. *Br Med J* 317, 693–696

Scheen AJ (1997) Drug treatment of non-insulin-dependent diabetes mellitus in the 1990s. *Drugs* 54, 355–368

Scheen AJ, Lefebvre PJ (1998) Oral antidiabetic agents. *Drugs* 55, 225–236

Schoonjons K, Auwerx J (2000) Thiazolidinediones: an update. *Lancet* 355, 1008–1010

Self-assessment

In questions 1–4 the first statement, in italics, is true. Are the accompanying statements also true?

1. *Oral hypoglycaemic drugs (sulfonylureas, biguanides, thiazolidinediones, acarbose) are only used in type 2 diabetes and act by different mechanisms to control glucose levels.*

   a. Glibenclamide is the drug of choice in patients who have no insulin secretion.
   b. Sulfonylureas should be administered in conjunction with a dietary regimen, particularly in obese patients.
   c. Glibenclamide can cause hypoglycaemia, particularly in the elderly, and should be used very cautiously in these patients.

2. *Hyperglycaemia results from uncontrolled glucose output from the liver and reduced uptake of glucose into muscle and other tissues.*

   a. The oral hypoglycaemic drugs metformin and gliclazide can be administered together.

3. *Untreated diabetes during pregnancy results in increased intrauterine and perinatal mortality.*

   a. Oral hypoglyaemics given to a pregnant mother can cause hypoglycaemia in the fetus and are normally substituted with insulin in pregnancy.
   b. Sulfonylureas should not be given together with the antimicrobial trimethoprim in diabetic patients.

4. *Different formulations of insulin are available that have varied peak effects and duration of action.*

   a. Insulin lispro has a longer duration of action than isophane insulin.

5. Case history question

> A 35-year-old teacher, Mr JH, was admitted to hospital as an emergency. He had developed a sore throat a week previously. His GP prescribed penicillin, but the soreness persisted and Mr JH noticed profuse white spots on the back of his throat. He drank fluids copiously and passed more urine than usual. Two days before admission he began to vomit. The day before admission be became drowsy and confused. He had lost approximately 2 stones in weight, despite eating more than usual. A great uncle had diabetes mellitus. Mr JH was clinically dehydrated and ketones could be smelt on his breath. Results of measurements on plasma indicated that this patient had diabetic ketoacidosis.

   a. The patient has diabetes mellitus. Which type of diabetes does he have?
   b. What is the significance of his sore throat?
   c. Is it significant that his great uncle suffered from diabetes mellitus?
   d. Explain his polydipsia and polyurea.
   e. What should be the immediate treatment of this patient and why should treatment be rapidly instituted?
   f. After the patient has recovered, what general advice should be given about diet?
   g. Mr JH is a '3 meals a day' man whose only exercise was walking a mile to work and back each day. Although insulin regimens vary widely, suggest a possible regimen for this patient and the types of insulin that could be given.
   h. How long before meals should subcutaneous injection of regular insulin be given?
   i. In addition to glucose levels, what other indicator can be measured to indicate good control in diabetes?
   j. Mr JH became more active, joined a health club and met a partner who liked to party. His eating became more irregular with hurried meals. His glycaemic control deteriorated. What alterations to his insulin regimen may be helpful?

The answers are provided on pages 623–624.

Drugs used for diabetes mellitus (all drugs, apart from insulin formulations and glucagon, are given orally)

Drug	Half-life (h)	Elimination	Comments
Insulins			
Soluble insulin Insulin aspart Insulin lispro	See text	Metabolism	Normally given by subcutaneous injection; the onset and duration of action depends on the formulation used, e.g. insulin zinc suspension, isophane insulin, protamine zinc insulin; biphasic insulin lispro and biphasic isophane insulin *Soluble insulin* is a sterile solution of bovine, porcine or human insulin *Insulin aspart* is a recombinant human insulin analogue in which two amino acids are reversed *Insulin lispro* is a recombinant human insulin analogue in which two amino acids are reversed
Insulin glargine	See text	Metabolism	*Insulin glargine*, unlike insulin lispro, has a longer duration of action than soluble insulin
Sulfonylureas			
Chlorpropamide	25–60	Metabolism + renal	Complete oral bioavailability; eliminated by oxidative metabolism (not CYP2D6) to inactive metabolites and by renal excretion (about 20%)
Glibenclamide	2–4	Metabolism	Complete oral bioavailability; metabolised in liver to active hydroxy metabolites that have a longer duration of action than the parent drug (one study has reported a terminal half-life for the parent drug of 10 hours); CYP2D6 not involved in metabolism
Gliclazide	6–14	Metabolism (+ renal)	Variable absorption between patients, probably linked to differences in first-pass metabolism; eliminated largely by oxidative metabolism in the liver with 10% excreted unchanged
Glimepiride	5–9	Metabolism	Complete bioavailability; oxidised by P450 to hydroxy and carboxy metabolites, the former of which retains activity; drug clearance increases at low creatinine clearance (probably because of decreased plasma protein binding)
Glipizide	2–4	Metabolism	Complete oral bioavailability; oxidised in the liver to inactive hydroxy metabolite
Gliquidone	17	Metabolism	Complete oral bioavailability; eliminated in bile as metabolites formed by oxidation and conjugation; parent compound responsible for most of activity
Tolazamide	7	Metabolism (+ renal)	Good absorption; eliminated largely (85%) by metabolism to five products which are inactive or of low activity
Tolbutamide	4–37 (mean = 7)	Metabolism	Complete oral bioavailability; about 1 in 500 patients has severely impaired metabolism of tolbutamide; metabolised by CYP2C9/10 (note – it was originally thought that tolbutamide was metabolised by the same isoenzyme as mephenytoin but this is now known to be CYP2C19); single allelic variant of CYP2C9 may be responsible for the rare impaired metabolism
Biguanides			
Metformin	2–4	Renal	Oral bioavailability is 50–60% owing to incomplete absorption; eliminated largely unchanged by renal tubular secretion
Other hypoglycaemics			
Acarbose	3	Renal	α-Glycoside hydrolase inhibitor; negligible oral absorption (1–2%); main action is in the intestinal tract; the systemic disposition data given are largely irrelevant to therapeutic use
Guar gum	Not relevant	Not relevant	Inhibits glucose absorption

continued

Drug compendium

Drugs used for diabetes mellitus (all drugs, apart from insulin formulations and glucagon, are given orally) *(continued)*

Drug	Half-life (h)	Elimination	Comments
Other hypoglycaemics (continued)			
Repaglinide	1	Metabolism	Good oral bioavailability (60%); eliminated by CYP3A4 oxidation to metabolites that are eliminated in the faeces
Rosiglitazone	3–4	Metabolism	Not currently licensed in UK; complete oral bioavailability; oxidised by CYP2C8 to hydroxy and demethylated metabolites
Glucagon			
Glucagon	5–10 min	Metabolism	Given by subcutaneous, intramuscular or intravenous injection; rapidly and extensively degraded by liver and kidneys
Treatment of chronic hypoglycaemia			
Diazoxide	28	Renal (+ metabolism)	Used for chronic hypoglycaemia due to islet cell hyperplasia or tumour and *is not used* for acute hypoglycaemia; non-diuretic analogue of thiazides; good oral bioavailability; eliminated largely by glomerular filtration; long half-life is due to high protein binding (90%)

The thyroid and control of metabolic rate

Thyroid function

The term 'basal metabolism' refers to the energy-utilising chemical processes of the body at rest. Its rate is controlled by the thyroid hormones, L-thyroxine (T_4) and triiodothyronine (T_3), which stimulate tissue oxygen consumption. This creates a drain on energy reserves such as glycogen and fat, but thyroid hormones also promote gluconeogenesis with consequent wasting of tissues that supply the substrate for glycogen formation such as muscle and bone. Thyroid hormones interact with the sympathetic nervous system, in particular enhancing the effects of β-adrenoceptor stimulation (Ch. 4).

T_3 and T_4 are synthesised in the thyroid gland. Inorganic iodine is trapped with great avidity by the gland by an enzyme-dependent process, oxidised and attached to tyrosine. The combination of two di-iodinated tyrosine molecules or one di-iodinated molecule with one mono-iodinated tyrosine molecule forms T_4 and T_3. The enzyme thyroxine peroxidase is important both in the initial oxidation and the final combination steps (Fig. 41.1).

Synthesis and release of thyroid hormones are controlled by the anterior pituitary hormone, thyrotrophin (thyroid-stimulating hormone, TSH). This in turn is controlled by the hypothalamus which secretes thyrotrophin-releasing hormone (TRH). Circulating T_3 and T_4 exert a negative feedback on both the hypothalamic and pituitary hormones (Fig. 41.2).

Circulating thyroid hormones are highly protein-bound (particularly T_4, of which less than 0.1% is free), mostly to thyroxine-binding globulin (TBG). Only the free fraction of hormone can bind to specific cell receptors. The thyroid secretes mainly T_4 and a small amount of T_3. Most T_3 is derived from peripheral deiodination of T_4 by the enzyme thyroxine 5' deiodinase, which is found in the liver, kidney and brain. T_3 is much more biologically active than T_4, but its half-life in the circulation is about 1.5 days compared to about 7 days for T_4. Elimination of T_3 and T_4 is by conjugation, mainly in the liver.

The cellular actions of thyroid hormone are largely caused by interaction of T_3 with nuclear receptors. These receptor–T_3 complexes act as nuclear transcription factors which interact with DNA and either inhibit or stimulate genes depending on the tissue involved.

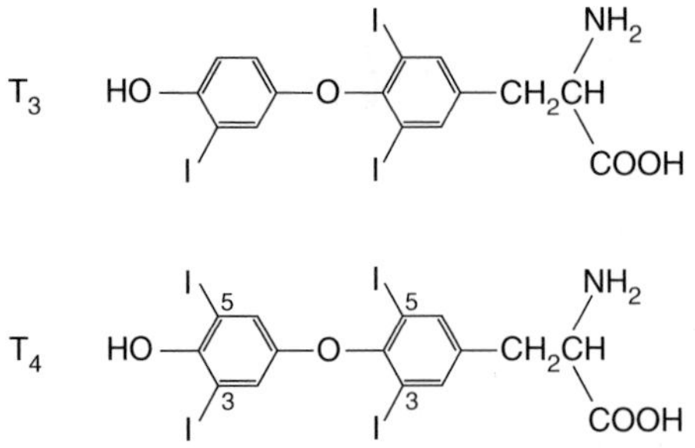

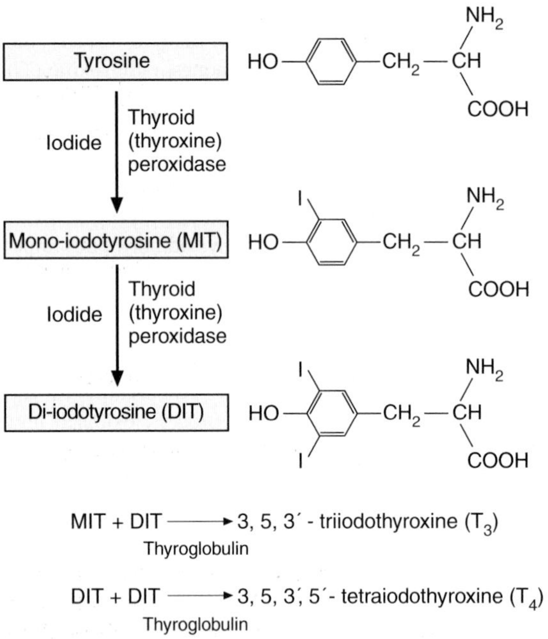

T_3 HO—⬡—O—⬡—CH_2CH—NH_2 / COOH

T_4 HO—⬡—O—⬡—CH_2CH—NH_2 / COOH

| Tyrosine |

HO—⬡—CH_2—CH—NH_2 / COOH

Iodide | Thyroid (thyroxine) peroxidase

| Mono-iodotyrosine (MIT) |

HO—⬡—CH_2—CH—NH_2 / COOH

Iodide | Thyroid (thyroxine) peroxidase

| Di-iodotyrosine (DIT) |

HO—⬡—CH_2—CH—NH_2 / COOH

$$\text{MIT + DIT} \longrightarrow 3, 5, 3' \text{ - triiodothyroxine } (T_3)$$
Thyroglobulin

$$\text{DIT + DIT} \longrightarrow 3, 5, 3', 5' \text{ - tetraiodothyroxine } (T_4)$$
Thyroglobulin

Fig. 41.1
The sequence of the synthesis of thyroid hormones.
Peroxidation of iodide occurs after its incorporation into thyroglobulin, the colloidal substance that fills the lumen of the thyroid follicles.

Hyperthyroidism

The commonest form of hyperthyroidism (thyrotoxicosis) is Graves disease, an autoimmune condition in which thyroid-stimulating IgG binds to thyrotrophin receptors on thyroid cells and initiates signal transduction. In many patients there is also an immunologically mediated inflammatory reaction in the extrinsic muscles of the eyes causing swelling and the characteristic exophthalmos. Toxic multinodular goitre and thyroid adenomas (toxic nodule) are less common causes of hyperthyroidism, except in areas of iodine deficiency. Symptoms of hyperthyroidism, which include weight loss, palpitation, sweating, nervousness and tremor, are in part mediated by excess β-adrenoceptor stimulation. Signs are often less marked in the elderly.

Drugs for treatment of hyperthyroidism

Thionamides

Examples: carbimazole, propylthiouracil

Mechanism of action
Thionamides inhibit thyroxine peroxidase, and therefore synthesis of thyroid hormone (Fig. 41.2). The long half-life of T_4 means that changes in the rate of synthesis take 4–6 weeks to lower circulating T_4 and T_3 concentrations to normal. In patients with autoimmune thyroid disease these drugs also appear to have an immuno-suppressive effect, reducing the levels of thyrotrophin receptor-stimulating antibody. This may explain their ability to produce long-term remissions.

Pharmacokinetics
Carbimazole is the drug of choice; it is almost completely absorbed from the gut and rapidly converted by first-pass metabolism to the active derivative methimazole. Methimazole has a short half-life and is excreted mainly in the urine. Propylthiouracil has only about one-tenth of the activity of methimazole and has a short half-life due to rapid liver metabolism. It is usually reserved for patients intolerant of carbimazole. Although the anti-thyroid drugs have short half-lives, they accumulate in the thyroid which extends their duration of action.

Unwanted effects
- Gastrointestinal upset, especially nausea and taste disturbance.
- Allergic rashes. There is incomplete cross-sensitivity between carbimazole and propylthiouracil.
- Bone marrow suppression, especially agranulocytosis. A severe sore throat with fever is often the presenting complaint, and should be immediately reported by the patient. The onset is sudden and routine blood counts are unhelpful. The risk is higher with propylthiouracil. The blood count usually recovers about 3 weeks after drug withdrawal.
- Placental transfer and secretion in breast milk can produce neonatal hypothyroidism, but propylthiouracil does not transfer in large enough quantities to cause problems. Nevertheless, small doses should be used in these situations.

β-Adrenoceptor antagonists (β-blockers)

β-Blockers are fully described in Chapter 5. β-Blockers act on the target tissues to modulate the additive effects of

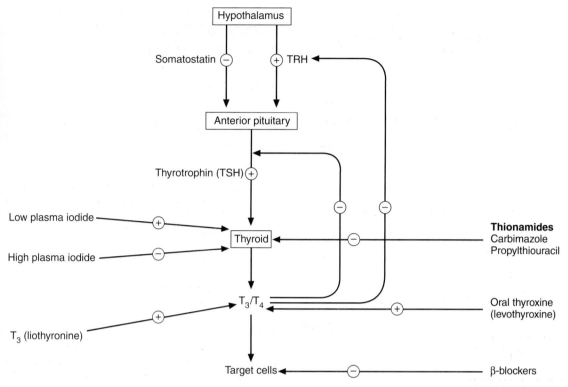

Fig. 41.2
Control of thyroid hormone synthesis and release and sites of action of drugs acting on the thyroid. TRH = thyrotrophin-releasing hormone. Thyrotrophin (TSH, thyroid-stimulating hormone) is inhibited by circulating levels of T_3 and T_4. Drugs used are shown in red.

thyroid hormones and β-adrenoceptor stimulation. They have immediate effects on symptoms such as anxiety, palpitation and tremor but do not alter the rate of thyroid hormone synthesis or secretion.

Management of hyperthyroidism

Carbimazole is the drug of choice for Graves' hyperthyroidism, and initially treatment should be continued for 12–24 months. There is some evidence that relapse rates are lower after longer treatment periods. It is usual to start treatment with a high dosage for 4–6 weeks, then to gradually reduce the dosage every 4–6 weeks, provided the serum T_4 concentration is within the normal range. Treatment is continued with the lowest possible dose that controls the serum T_4. Exophthalmos associated with Graves disease responds poorly to treatment. Severe thyroid eye disease can be helped by treatment with oral prednisolone if antithyroid treatment is not improving the condition. β-Blockers are particularly useful for symptomatic relief during the early period of treatment with carbimazole.

Approximately 50% of patients with Graves disease have a single episode which is cured by drug treatment. Those who relapse will usually do so repeatedly and most are offered definitive treatment by either a subtotal thyroidectomy (for a large goitre) or a therapeutic dose of radioactive iodine (^{131}I). Both may eventually produce hypothyroidism, delayed by several months or years. The theoretical risk of cancer or leukaemia following radioiodine treatment has not been substantiated in clinical studies.

Before surgery, patients are usually given oral potassium iodide for up to 2 weeks. Iodides inhibit thyroxine synthesis and release and, importantly, reduce the vascularity of the hyperplastic thyroid gland. Alternatively, initial treatment with carbimazole can be given to achieve a euthyroid state.

Before radioiodine treatment, patients should be stabilised with carbimazole to reduce the risk of a thyroid crisis immediately after isotope treatment. However, antithyroid drug treatment must be stopped 3–4 days before radioactive iodine is given or it will prevent uptake of the iodine by the thyroid cells. β-Blockers can be useful in this period to prevent symptomatic relapse. Carbimazole can be restarted 2–4 days after radioiodine to cover the few weeks before radioiodine is fully effective. Following radioiodine treatment, permanent hypothyroidism can occur; up to one year after treatment the incidence is determined by the initial dose, thereafter the risk is 2–3% annually.

A toxic nodule can be removed surgically but radioactive iodine is extremely effective since the isotope is taken up only by the abnormal tissue (the remainder is suppressed by the absence of thyrotrophin in the circulation). Multinodular toxic goitres are usually treated by radioiodine. Carbimazole is unsuitable as sole treatment for these conditions, since spontaneous remission does not occur.

Hypothyroidism

Hypothyroidism is usually caused by primary thyroid failure, and the low circulating T_4 concentration is accompanied by a raised plasma thyrotrophin concentration. Autoimmune thyroiditis is the commonest cause, but hypothyroidism is occasionally congenital or can follow treatment for hyperthyroidism by surgery or radioiodine. Rarely, hypothyroidism can be secondary to pituitary or hypothalamic failure, when the circulating thyrotrophin concentrations will be low. Drug therapy with lithium (Ch. 22) or amiodarone (Ch. 8) can produce hypothyroidism. Typical symptoms of hypothyroidism are non-specific and include lethargy, slowing of mental processes, cold intolerance, weight gain, constipation or menorrhagia. Severe hypothyroidism (myxoedema) produces marked coarsening of the facial appearance and may ultimately lead to a hypothermic, comatose state.

Management of hypothyroidism

Standard treatment is with oral thyroxine (levothyroxine, T_4) although its absorption is incomplete and variable. Sufficient T_3 will be formed by peripheral deiodination of T_4, but the proportion of circulating T_3 is usually lower than normal. Therefore, circulating levels of T_4 will often need to be higher than those in healthy subjects to obtain a satisfactory response. In some patients, particularly those with ischaemic heart disease, a rapid increase in metabolic activity with thyroxine replacement can cause excessive cardiac stimulation. Thyroxine should, therefore, be introduced gradually, starting with a small dose. Owing to the long half-life, steady-state plasma concentrations will not be achieved with a constant dose of thyroxine for about 5 weeks.

The adequacy of T_4 replacement therapy is best monitored by measurement of the serum thyrotrophin concentration 4–6 weeks after a change in dose of thyroxine. When the thyrotrophin concentration is within the normal range, the plasma T_4 will usually be slightly high or in the upper part of the normal range.

Treatment with triiodothyronine (T_3 liothyronine) is usually reserved for intravenous use in patients with severe hypothyroidism (myxoedema coma) when its potency, more rapid effect and shorter half-life allow more rapid attainment of a therapeutic blood concentration.

FURTHER READING

Dayan CM, Daniels GH (1996) Chronic autoimmune thyroiditis. *N Engl J Med* 335, 99–107

Lazarus JH (1997) Hyperthyroidism. *Lancet* 349, 339–343

Lindsay RS, Toft AD (1997) Hypothyroidism. *Lancet* 349, 413–417

Weetman AP (1997) Hypothyroidism: screening and subclinical disease. *Br Med J* 314, 1175–1178

Weetman AP (2000) Graves' disease. *N Engl J Med* 343, 1236–1248

Woeber KA (2000) Update on the management of hyperthyroidism and hypothyroidism. *Arch Intern Med* 160, 1076–1071

Self-assessment

In questions 1 and 2 the first statement, in italics, is true. Are the accompanying statements also true?

1. *Manufacture and secretion of T_3 and T_4 are controlled by thyrotrophin and plasma iodide.*

   a. Most circulating T_3 and T_4 are bound to albumin.
   b. Thyroxine (T_4) has a long residence time in the body.
   c. At target cells T_4 is converted to T_3 which then binds to specific DNA-linked receptors.
   d. Hyperthyroidism will be made worse by iodine administration.

2. *Severe hypothyroidism causes 'myxoedema' in adults and cretinism in children; its origins are immunological.*

   a. Therapy with ^{131}I can cause hypothyroidism.
   b. Hypothyroidism is treated with oral thyroxine.
   c. When thyroxine is administered it takes about 5 weeks for steady-state plasma concentrations to be reached.

3. Case history question

> A 45-year-old man suffered from weight loss, palpitations, tremor, anxiety, sweating and eyelid retraction, orbital and ocular inflammation. Blood tests showed increased levels of free and bound T_3 and T_4. A diagnosis of Graves thyrotoxicosis was made. An ECG showed atrial fibrillation.

   a. What is Graves disease?
   b. What other blood tests could be done to confirm this diagnosis?
   c. Why was the free T_3 and T_4 measured?
   d. How could symptoms be controlled?
   e. What drug could be given to control the hyperthyroidism?

> With treatment the patient became euthyroid but relapsed in the following year. A decision was made to treat the patient with ^{131}I.

   f. What treatment should be given before administering the ^{131}I and what are the reasons for this?
   g. How long after treatment would you expect to see benefit?

The answers are provided on page 624.

Thyroid and antithyroid drugs

Drug	Half-life	Elimination	Comments
Thyroid hormones			
Levothyroxine/ thyroxine	6–7 days	Metabolism	Given orally; oral bioavailability is 50–80% (with some variability between brands); metabolised by deiodination in peripheral tissues to T_3 (which has a half-life of 1–2 days).
Liothyronine (L-triiodothyronine)	1–2 days	Metabolism	Given orally or by slow intravenous injection; almost complete oral bioavailability; metabolised by deiodination and conjugation with glucuronic acid and sulfate.
Antithyroid drugs			
Carbimazole	3–5 hours (methimazole)	Metabolism	Given orally; complete absorption with complete presystemic metabolism to the active form methimazole; methimazole is eliminated by metabolism plus some renal excretion.
Iodine and iodide	–	Renal	Given orally; complete oral absorption; incorporated into thyroid hormones; excreted largely in urine.
Propylthiouracil	1–3 hours	Metabolism	Given orally; bioavailability is 50–75% due to poor absorption; the main metabolic route is formation of an *S*-glucuronide.

42

Calcium metabolism and metabolic bone disease

Regulation of calcium metabolism

Calcium ions play a part in a large number of cellular activities, including stimulus–response coupling in striated and smooth muscle, endocrine and exocrine glands. Calcium modulates the action of intracellular cyclic AMP and is a cofactor for numerous intracellular enzymes and for blood clotting. However, more than 98% of Ca^{2+} is in the bones, in the form of hydroxyapatite crystals deposited on the protein matrix of bone which gives it mechanical strength.

Calcium circulates in plasma partly bound to protein and partly in the free ionised (and therefore 'active') form. The free fraction is precisely maintained within narrow limits principally by the actions of parathyroid hormone (PTH) and 1,25-dihydroxy vitamin D_3 (calcitriol). Calcitonin reacts to changing plasma Ca^{2+} concentrations but its effect in overall control of Ca^{2+} homeostasis is less important. Calcium in plasma is in constant flux with Ca^{2+} in the gut, renal tubules and bone. This is illustrated, with the main controlling factors, in Figure 42.1.

PTH is a polypeptide hormone which is the main physiological regulator of Ca^{2+} in blood. Its secretion is stimulated from parathyroid chief cells via the Ca^{2+}-sensing receptor by a reduction of ionised Ca^{2+} in plasma; secretion is inhibited when the concentration rises. PTH binds to receptors on distal renal tubular cells and various cells in bone, generates intracellular cyclic AMP and triggers an influx of Ca^{2+} into the cell. The main effect in the kidney is to inhibit tubular phosphate reabsorption and to promote Ca^{2+} retention. The principal action of PTH in bone is stimulation of resorption by osteoclasts which increases bone turnover, although enhanced osteoblastic activity results in some bone repair. The effect on the kidney occurs within minutes of PTH release, while that on bone begins in 1–2 hours.

Vitamin D has a steroid nucleus. A precursor of active vitamin D, ergocalciferol (vitamin D_2), is absorbed from the gut but, given adequate sunlight, the major source of vitamin D is conversion of 7-dehydrocholecalciferol in the skin to cholecalciferol (vitamin D_3). Therefore, cholecalciferol is really a skin-derived hormone rather than a vitamin, but this source was discovered after the dietary origins. Cholecalciferol is further metabolised to 25-hydroxy D_3 in the liver and

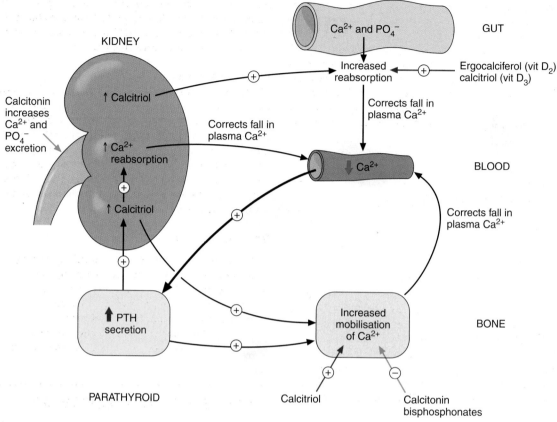

Fig. 42.1

Regulation of calcium metabolism. The primary response to a fall in plasma calcium is to stimulate PTH production from parathyroid. This increases calcitriol (vitamin D_3) formation in the kidney. This in turn increases gut absorption of Ca^{2+}. PTH further increases bone mobilisation of Ca^{2+} to return plasma Ca^{2+} to normal. An increase in plasma Ca^{2+} conversely decreases PTH secretion. Calcitonin, secreted by the thyroid, decreases Ca^{2+} reabsorption from the kidney and decreases bone turnover. Drugs for hypercalcaemia are shown in green. Drugs for hypocalcaemia are shown in red.

then in the kidney to 1,25-dihydroxy D_3 (calcitriol). 1α-hydroxylation is an essential step for activation of vitamin D. PTH stimulates 1α-hydroxylase activity in the kidney. The main effect of vitamin D is to increase the plasma concentration of Ca^{2+} by stimulating its absorption from the gut. It acts via typical steroid receptors in the cell nucleus (Ch. 1), which trigger synthesis of an intracellular Ca^{2+}-binding protein. In the kidney, vitamin D promotes phosphate retention in contrast to the action of PTH. Vitamin D increases osteoclastic activity in bone. 1,25-Dihydroxy vitamin D_3 also inhibits the transcription of the gene coding for PTH. These actions of vitamin D affect Ca^{2+} turnover in bone over periods of days to weeks.

Calcitonin is a peptide secreted by the parafollicular, or C, cells of the thyroid when the Ca^{2+}-sensing receptor detects a rise in plasma Ca^{2+}. The main target cell is the osteoclast, which it inhibits by stimulation of adenylate cyclase, thus reducing bone turnover. Calcitonin also decreases Ca^{2+} and phosphate reabsorption by the kidney.

Hypercalcaemia

The main causes of hypercalcaemia are:

- increased resorption of Ca^{2+} from bone, for example primary hyperparathyroidism, secretion of parathyroid-related hormone by cancer cells, bony metastases. These are the major causes of severe hypercalcaemia
- increased absorption of Ca^{2+} from gut through excessive use of vitamin D
- reduced renal excretion of Ca^{2+}, for example thiazide diuretics (Ch. 14).

Hypercalcaemia occurs when excessive mobilisation of Ca^{2+} into the extracellular space exceeds the capacity to remove it. Chronic moderate hypercalcaemia produces a progressive decline in renal function, formation of renal stones and ectopic calcification (e.g. cornea, blood vessels). Severe hypercalcaemia causes anorexia, nausea, vomiting, constipation, drowsiness and confusion, eventually leading to coma. Hypercalcaemia impairs the ability of the kidney to reabsorb salt and water; in conjunction with vomiting this can lead to depletion of plasma volume and renal failure. When the plasma Ca^{2+} concentration rises above 3.5 mmol l^{-1} (normal usually <2.6 mmol l^{-1}) then urgent treatment is indicated, since sudden death can occur from cardiac arrest.

Antiresorptive drugs for hypercalcaemia

Calcitonin

Mechanism of action and effects
The actions of calcitonin on bone and kidney have been discussed above. Calcitonin begins to act within a few hours of administration with a maximum effect between 12 and 24 hours; however, the hypocalcaemic effect produced by repeated administrations only lasts between 2 and 3 days. Downregulation of calcitonin receptors on osteoclasts then results in a rebound increase in bone resorption, and loss of the clinical response.

Pharmacokinetics
Salmon calcitonin (salcatonin) is now exclusively used, since it is less immunogenic than the earlier preparation of pork calcitonin. It is usually given by intramuscular or subcutaneous injection although intravenous infusion can be used. The half-life is very short at 15 min, and it is broken down to inactive fragments by enzymic degradation in plasma and in the kidney.

Unwanted effects
- Facial flushing occurs in most patients.
- Nausea is common, vomiting can occur.
- Tingling in the hands.
- Unpleasant taste.

Bisphosphonates

> Examples: disodium etidronate, disodium pamidronate, alendronic acid

Mechanisms of action and effects
Bisphosphonates are pyrophosphate analogues that bind to hydroxyapatite crystal in bone matrix and inhibit bone dissolution. They also inhibit osteoclast attachment to bone matrix, and stimulate osteoblasts to produce an inhibitor of osteoclast formation. Following a single intravenous infusion, the plasma Ca^{2+} concentration falls gradually with a maximum effect after about a week, persisting for up to 4 weeks after treatment.

Pharmacokinetics
Bisphosphonates are poorly absorbed from the gut (less than 10% of the ingested dose). Oral formulations are best taken with the stomach empty, to avoid binding by Ca^{2+} in food. A more reliable route is by intravenous infusion. Etidronate and alendronic acid are only available in an oral formulation, pamidronate only for intravenous use. Removal from blood is rapid via the kidney, but their effect is prolonged since they remain bound to calcium salts in bone.

Unwanted effects
- Gastrointestinal disturbance, particularly nausea, abdominal pain and diarrhoea or constipation.
- Alendronic acid can cause severe oesophagitis.
- Pamidronate causes transient pyrexia and influenza-like symptoms after infusion.
- Prolonged use impairs mineralisation of newly formed bone with consequent risk of osteomalacia.

Treatment of hypercalcaemia

When possible the primary cause should be corrected, for example removal of a parathyroid adenoma or treatment of myeloma. Additional measures may include correction of dehydration, enhancing renal excretion of Ca^{2+} and inhibiting bone resorption.

Most patients with severe hypercalcaemia are fluid depleted at presentation. Rehydration with intravenous saline is essential; this also promotes a sodium-linked Ca^{2+} diuresis in the proximal and distal renal tubules. Loop diuretics such as furosemide (frusemide; Ch. 14) increase renal Ca^{2+} elimination but require concurrent use of high volumes of intravenous saline and intensive monitoring of fluid balance for safe use.

A bisphosphonate, especially by intravenous infusion, is the drug treatment of first choice for severe hypercalcaemia. Initial hydration is essential to avoid precipitation of calcium bisphosphonate in the kidney. Oral treatment may be sufficient for less severe hypercalcaemia. Because of the delay in onset of action of the bisphosphonates, calcitonin can be given for an early effect. Glucocorticoids, such as prednisolone (Ch. 44), are effective for lowering Ca^{2+} when vitamin D excess is an important factor, for example in sarcoidosis, for acute treatment of vitamin D overdose or for hypercalcaemia associated with haematological malignancy such as myeloma. Glucocorticoids probably act by reducing the effect of vitamin D on intestinal Ca^{2+} transport, but can take several days to work.

Hypocalcaemia

There are two major underlying causes of hypocalcaemia:

1. deficiency of parathyroid hormone, for example idiopathic hypoparathyroidism, after surgical parathyroid removal
2. deficiency of vitamin D, for example dietary deficiency, limited exposure to sunlight, renal failure (failure of 1α-hydroxylation).

Hypocalcaemia produces neuromuscular irritability with paraesthesiae of the extremities or around the mouth, muscle cramps and tetany. When severe it can produce fits. Chronic hypocalcaemia, especially in congenital hypoparathyroidism, is associated with mental deficiency, fits, intracranial calcification (e.g. choroid plexus) and ocular cataracts.

Drugs for hypocalcaemia

Vitamin D

Examples: ergocalciferol (vitamin D_2), alfacalcidol (1α-hydroxycholecalciferol), calcitriol (1,25-dihydroxycholecalciferol)

Mechanism of action

This is discussed above. A dose-related increase in Ca^{2+} and phosphate absorption from the gut occurs at lower concentrations than those stimulating bone resorption. Ergocalciferol can only be used if 1α-hydroxylation by the kidney is unimpaired.

Pharmacokinetics

The fat-soluble D vitamins are well absorbed orally in the presence of bile. They can also be given intravenously. Conversion of ergocalciferol to active derivatives by the kidney has been discussed above. Both alfacalcidol and calcitriol are active forms of vitamin D. They have short half-lives and are excreted mainly in the bile.

Unwanted effects

- Excessive dosing will produce hypercalcaemia.
- Excretion of vitamin D supplements in breast milk can cause hypercalcaemia in a suckling infant.

Treatment of hypocalcaemia

Mild hypocalcaemia can be treated with oral calcium supplements, taken between meals to avoid binding to dietary phosphate and oxalate which are poorly absorbed. In the absence of reversible pathology such as malabsorption due to coeliac disease, the mainstay of treatment for more severe hypocalcaemia is vitamin D supplements. The few individuals who have vitamin D deficiency from inadequate diet or lack of exposure to sunlight (such as is seen in Asian women in the UK) will respond to small doses of vitamin D. Most causes of hypocalcaemia, however, require much larger doses of vitamin D (usually given as ergocalciferol) to maintain normocalcaemia than those derived from the diet. Oral calcium supplements (as carbonate or citrate salts) are often used with vitamin D for treatment of chronic hypocalcaemia. For patients with severe renal impairment, alfacalcidol or calcitriol should be used.

Parathyroid hormone is not available for replacement therapy and alfacalcidol is given for treatment of hypoparathyroidism. Large doses of ergocalciferol could be used, but carry a risk of excessive dosage leading to hypercalcaemia. Calcitriol is rarely required unless a very rapid onset of action is necessary.

Acute severe hypocalcaemia (sometimes occurring after parathyroidectomy) must be treated with intravenous calcium (as gluconate, gluceptate or chloride salt).

Metabolic bone disease

Osteomalacia

Osteomalacia is the bone disease resulting from failure of adequate bone mineralisation due to lack of vitamin D. Bone pain is prominent and low plasma Ca^{2+} and phosphate concentrations produce muscle weakness. In developing children the bones become distorted (rickets). Treatment is with vitamin D (ergocalciferol) supplements.

Osteoporosis

Osteoporosis is the loss of bone mass due to reduced organic bone matrix, and consequently mineral content, which reduces the mechanical strength of bone. To some extent it is a natural and inevitable part of the ageing process. In females, however, a marked increase in bone loss occurs after the menopause. Other predisposing factors include smoking, heavy alcohol intake and immobility. Osteoporosis in younger patients is associated with trabecular bone loss and predisposes to spontaneous vertebral fractures. In older patients cortical bone is also lost, increasing the risk of traumatic fracture, particularly of the neck of the femur. Sometimes osteoporosis is secondary to other conditions such as corticosteroid therapy (Ch. 44), myeloma, alcoholism or thyrotoxicosis. Once established it is extremely difficult to reverse and emphasis should be placed on prevention where possible.

Prevention of osteoporosis

The major opportunity for preventing osteoporosis is the use of hormone replacement therapy (HRT) with estrogens (Ch. 45) in peri- and postmenopausal women. Unless a hysterectomy has been performed, progestogens must be given as well to prevent endometrial hyperplasia and an increased risk of carcinoma. The duration of treatment with HRT remains controversial because of the slight concern that long-term use may provoke breast cancer. However, 5–10 years of estrogen therapy may be required, and there is uncertainty over whether bone loss accelerates when therapy is stopped.

Oral calcium supplements probably also reduce the risk of vertebral fractures in postmenopausal women; the addition of vitamin D (ergocalciferol) may confer greater benefit.

Raloxifene is a tissue-selective oestrogen receptor modulator which has oestrogenic effects on bone but oestrogen antagonist actions on breast and uterine receptors. It increases bone mineral density but, although it is licensed for prevention of osteoporosis, the effect on fracture risk is unknown. Unwanted effects include hot flushes and venous thromboembolism (Ch. 45).

Treatments for established osteoporosis

The choice of treatment depends on the clinical circumstances. Pain relief is important if there are fractures, but drug treatment to prevent bone loss can reduce the risk of further fractures by up to 50%. Options include:

Hormone replacement therapy (HRT). Unlike drugs that inhibit bone resorption, HRT increases bone mineral density by up to 10% in the first two years of treatment.

Oral bisphosphonates produce an increase in bone density. Most studies have been carried out in postmenopausal women. Oral etidronate, given for 2 weeks at 3-monthly intervals, usually with continuous calcium supplements, increases vertebral bone mineral content, and may reduce fractures. It may also be effective in corticosteroid-induced osteoporosis. Alendronic acid has also been shown to reduce hip and wrist fractures.

Oral fluoride supplements increase bone formation in osteoporotic bone, but also produce a defect in mineralisation of cortical bone. This can be minimised by giving calcium supplements but the ability of fluoride to prevent fractures is unproven.

Salmon calcitonin: given subcutaneously this produces a modest increase in bone mass. Introduction of an intranasal formulation may make this a more attractive treatment in the future.

Calcitriol has proved effective in corticosteroid-induced osteoporosis and can be used as an alternative to a bisphosphonate.

Paget's disease of bone

Paget's disease of bone is a disturbance of bone remodelling characterised by both excessive bone reabsorption by osteoclasts and an increase in formation of poor quality bone. This new bone matrix is non-lamellar woven bone with areas of osteosclerosis, leaving bone that is structurally weakened. Paget's disease mainly affects the skull and long bones. The aetiology is unknown but a slow virus infection may initiate the disease.

About a third of the bone lesions are asymptomatic. Clinical features include bone pain and deformity, nerve entrapment and pathological fractures. Active treatment should be given if symptoms or a risk of complications are identified. Apart from symptomatic measures such as analgesics, two main treatments are used:

Bisphosphonates primarily inhibit bone resorption but long-term use can also impair bone mineralisation and produce osteomalacia by creating secondary hyperparathyroidism. With intermittent treatment (e.g. 6 months out of every 12 months) prolonged remission of symptoms and reduction in complications can be achieved. Oral treatment is usually sufficient, with intravenous treatment reserved for severe disease. Calcium supplements may reduce the risk of osteomalacia.

Calcitonin, by reducing osteoclastic bone resorption, can reduce pain and then improve the structural abnormalities in pagetic bone. Pain relief usually begins within 2 weeks, but treatment may be necessary for several months to improve bone modelling. Approximately 50% of patients will relapse on stopping treatment. Calcitonin is often reserved for initial treatment while awaiting a response to a bisphosphonate.

FURTHER READING

Bushinsky DA, Monk RD (1998) Calcium. *Lancet* 352, 306–311

Delmas PD, Meunier PJ (1997) The management of Paget's disease of bone. *N Engl J Med* 336, 558–566

Eastell R (1998) Treatment of postmenopausal osteoporosis. *N Engl J Med* 338, 736–746

Eastell R, Peel N (1998) Osteoporosis. *J Roy Coll Phys Lond* 32, 14–18

Francis RM (1998) Management of established osteoporosis. *Br J Clin Pharmacol* 45, 95–99

Watters J, Gerrard G, Dodwell D (1996) The management of malignant hypercalcaemia. *Drugs* 52, 837–848

Zahrani AA, Levine MA (1997) Primary hyperparathyroidism. *Lancet* 349, 1233–1238

Self-assessment

In questions 1 and 2 the first statement, in italics, is true. Are the accompanying statements also true

1. *Hypocalcaemia develops when there is a deficiency in PTH or vitamin D or target organs do not respond to these hormones.*

   a. Vitamin D deficiency can lead to hypoparathyroidism.
   b. Calcitonin decreases Ca^{2+} resorption in the kidney.
   c. Bisphosphonates lower blood Ca^{2+} levels rapidly.

2. *The cornerstone of treatment for the prevention of bone loss in postmenopausal women is estrogen replacement.*

   a. Oestrogens maintain bone density by directly enhancing Ca^{2+} absorption from the intestine.
   b. Raloxifene stimulates oestrogen receptors on bone, breast and uterine tissue.

3. Case history question

   > A 25-year-old women with diffuse muscle weakness and bone pain was diagnosed suffering from osteomalacia.

   a. How would you treat this patient?
   b. How do the drugs exert their benefit?
   c. What unwanted effects could occur?

   The answers are provided on pages 624–625.

Drugs used to regulate calcium metabolism and in metabolic bone disease

Drug	Half-life	Elimination	Comments
Calcitonin			
Calcitonin/salcatonin	3–9 min (HC) 12–21 min (SC)	Metabolism	Given by subcutaneous or intramuscular injection or by slow intravenous infusion; peak plasma concentrations are seen 15–45 minutes after subcutaneous injection; rapidly metabolised by the kidney (note, biological effects are prolonged for hours or days); half-life depends on source species (HC, human calcitonin; SC, salmon calcitonin)
Bisphosphonates (all these drugs share similar fates in the body)			
Alendronic acid (alendronate)	11 years (bone)	Renal	Given orally; very low oral bioavailability (<1%) reduced even further by food; the absorbed fraction is eliminated by glomerular filtration; about 40% of an intravenous dose is eliminated and the remainder retained and eliminated very slowly, due to binding to bone
Elodronate (sodium)	2 hours (plasma), years (bone)	Renal	Given orally or by slow intravenous infusion; low but variable oral absorption (2–20%); the absorbed fraction has a fate similar to alendronate; the reported plasma half-life after oral dosage would probably reflect slow absorption (prior to bone deposition and turnover)
Etidronate (disodium)	2–6 hours (plasma), very long (bone)	Renal	Given orally; low absorption (1–9%); about 50% of intravenous dose is eliminated in the urine within 24 hours, but the remainder is retained in bone and elimination is dependent on bone turnover (presumably 11 years as for alendronate, see above)
Pamidronate (disodium)	0.5 hours (plasma), very long (bone)	Renal	Given by slow intravenous infusion; the fate is similar to alendronate (see above) and the half-life given is the distribution from plasma to tissues; the half-life in bone depends on bone turnover (and has been reported to be about 2 years)
Tiludronic acid	Very long (bone)	Renal	Given orally; oral bioavailability is highly variable (between and within patients) and low (about 6%); see alendronate for probable fate in the body
Vitamin D			
Alfacalcidol	3 hours	Metabolism	Given orally or by intravenous injection; 1α-hydroxycholecalciferol; high bioavailability; undergoes side chain oxidation by a 25-hydroxylase to calcitriol which is the active form
Calcitriol	24 hours	Metabolism	Given orally or by intravenous injection; 1α,25-dihydroxycholecalciferol; rapidly and completely absorbed; oxidised to inactive metabolites
Cholecalciferol (vitamin D_3)	Not defined	Metabolism	Given orally or by intravenous injection; high oral bioavailability; oxidised at 25-position to 25-hydroxycholecalciferol, which is oxidised to the active 1,25-dihydroxy compound in the kidney
Dihydrotachysterol	10 hours (?)	Metabolism	Given orally; synthetic analogue of vitamin D_2; peak concentrations are at 4 hours after dosage; few kinetic data available
Ergocalciferol (calciferol; vitamin D_2)	Not defined	Metabolism	Given orally or by intravenous injection; high oral bioavailability; metabolic precursor of cholecalciferol; metabolised to 1,25-dihydroxycholecalciferol

43 Pituitary and hypothalamic hormones

Anterior pituitary and hypothalamic hormones

Thyrotrophin and thyroid releasing hormone are considered in Chapter 42.

Growth hormone

Growth hormone (GH) or somatotropin, is a 191-amino acid peptide that is synthesised in specific cells in the anterior pituitary. Its secretion is controlled by the hypothalamus via a releasing hormone (GHRH; Fig. 43.1) and also modulated by a release-inhibiting hormone (GHRIH or somatostatin). GH is released in pulses repeatedly during both day and night. Like other peptide hormones, GH binds to cell surface receptors and activates adenylate cyclase. It has direct metabolic effects on several tissues; these are anabolic in relation to protein metabolism (especially in skeletal muscle and epiphyseal cartilage) and catabolic in relation to fat. The proliferating effects on epiphyseal cartilage stimulate bone growth. The anabolic effects on muscle and bone are mediated by insulin-like growth factor 1 (IGF-1). IGF-1 is synthesised by the liver in response to GH stimulation and bound to specific proteins in plasma.

Therapeutic use of growth hormone

GH from human cadaveric pituitary origin (which could transmit the prion-mediated Creutzfeldt–Jakob disease) has been replaced since 1985 by biosynthetic GH (somatropin) developed using recombinant DNA techniques. Treatment was initially confined to children with severe GH deficiency (who usually lack GHRH: pituitary dwarfism) to improve linear growth. Patients with idiopathic short stature and those with chronic renal insufficiency or Turner's syndrome are now also receiving GH. To be effective, the hormone must be given before the closure of the epiphyses in long bones.

Pharmacokinetics

GH has a very short half-life of approximately 25 min, so plasma concentrations fluctuate widely. By contrast, concentrations of IGF-1 are much more constant due to its high protein binding. As a consequence, three doses of GH per week give good clinical results, although daily dosing is often used. GH is usually given by subcutaneous injection, although the intramuscular route can be used.

Unwanted effects

- There is a transient insulin-like action which occasionally produces hypoglycaemia.
- If excessive doses are used (as may happen during illicit use by athletes) there is a risk of diabetes mellitus in predisposed individuals.
- Pain at the injection site.

Acromegaly

Acromegaly results from excessive production of GH, almost always by an adenoma in the anterior pituitary which also secretes prolactin in one-third of cases. The clinical features arise from excessive growth of bone and soft tissue. Complex metabolic consequences include insulin resistance with diabetes and hypertension. Occasionally, the tumour extends above the sella turcica causing compression of the optic chiasm. This usually results in a bitemporal hemianopia, progressing eventually to complete loss of vision.

The morbidity and mortality of acromegaly vary according to its severity. Untreated acromegalic patients have a life expectancy approximately half that of individuals without acromegaly, due to an excess incidence of cardiovascular and respiratory disease and carcinoma of the colon. Acromegaly is therefore usually treated actively. Surgery by the trans-sphenoidal route is the usual treatment of choice, sometimes followed by external radiotherapy if the tumour was large. Three groups of patients may be suitable for drug treatment:

1. those in whom an excess of growth hormone persists despite surgery and radiotherapy; after radiotherapy the plasma GH concentration can take 1–2 years to fall
2. those with mild acromegaly
3. the elderly.

Drugs for acromegaly

Bromocriptine

Further details of the dopamine receptor agonist bromocriptine can be found in Chapter 24. In healthy subjects dopaminergic receptor stimulation increases secretion of growth hormone, but in acromegaly there is a paradoxical decrease. The clinical response to bromocriptine is unpredictable, and it is not widely used.

Somatostatin analogues

Example: octreotide

Mechanisms of action and uses

Synthetic derivatives of somatostatin (GHRIH) are both more potent and longer-acting than the native compound. Like somatostatin, they also inhibit the release of gastro-entero-pancreatic peptide hormones, for example insulin, glucagon and gastrin, via specific intestinal receptors which generate intracellular cyclic AMP and promote calcium influx into the cell.

Somatostatin analogues are used before pituitary surgery and for persistent acromegaly after surgery and radiotherapy. Given by subcutaneous injection they reduce GH release and pituitary tumour size. Somatostatin analogues are also used in the management of other endocrine tumours, for example carcinoid tumours (to reduce flushing and diarrhoea), VIPoma (to reduce diarrhoea) and glucagonoma (to improve the characteristic necrolytic rash). Octreotide is also used to stop bleeding from oesophageal varices (Ch. 36).

Pharmacokinetics

Octreotide is given by subcutaneous injection. It has a short half-life but suppresses GH secretion for up to 8 hours. A depot preparation has now been introduced in which octreotide is absorbed onto microspheres and given by deep intramuscular injection. The duration of action of this preparation is about 4 weeks. The depot preparation is used once control has been achieved by the use of the conventional formulation three times daily.

Unwanted effects

- Gastrointestinal upset, especially abdominal pain and diarrhoea, is common. It usually resolves with continued treatment.
- Gallstones, owing to suppression of cholecystokinin secretion with decreased gallbladder motility. The increase in bowel transit time alters colonic flora and makes bile more lithogenic.

Adrenocorticotrophic hormone (ACTH)

ACTH is a straight-chain polypeptide with 39 amino acids, of which the 24 that form the N-terminal are essential for full biological activity. It promotes steroidogenesis in adrenocortical cells by occupying cell surface receptors and stimulating adenylate cyclase. Release of ACTH occurs in response to the hypothalamic peptide corticotrophin-releasing factor (CRF). CRF secretion is pulsatile and has a diurnal rhythm with maximal release in the morning around the time of waking. Other factors, including chemical (e.g. ADH, opioid peptides), physical (e.g. heat, cold, injury) and psychological influences also affect release of CRF. The main inhibitory influence on ACTH release is negative feedback control by circulating glucocorticoids. This occurs at both hypothalamic and pituitary levels. Adrenal androgens, although stimulated by ACTH, play no part in feedback control.

Therapeutic uses of ACTH

ACTH preparations of animal origin have been replaced by a less allergenic synthetic peptide analogue, tetracosactide, which consists of the active N1–24 amino acid section of the ACTH molecule. There are two formulations of tetracosactide:

1. A rapid-acting form that increases steroidogenesis for about an hour and is suitable for tests of adrenocortical function. In patients with suspected adrenal insufficiency, there is a subnormal or no rise of plasma cortisol after intramuscular or intravenous injection.
2. A depot form that is absorbed slowly into the circulation over several hours and can be used as an alternative to exogenous corticosteroid therapy. However, the unpredictable response means that the therapeutic value of this drug is limited. Once absorbed into the circulation, tetracosactide is metabolised rapidly with a half-life of about 10 min.

Unwanted effects
Prolonged use will produce all the features of corticosteroid excess (Ch. 44).

Prolactin

Prolactin is a glycoprotein similar in structure to growth hormone but secreted by distinct cells in the anterior pituitary (Fig. 43.1). The major hypothalamic control mechanism is inhibition by dopamine via D2 receptors on the secretory cells (Ch. 45). The main target tissue for prolactin is the breast, which secretes milk in response to prolactin if it is primed by ovarian hormones. At delivery, the maternal plasma oestrogen concentration falls, and that of prolactin rises. Release of prolactin during suckling may be due to production of a specific prolactin-releasing factor from the hypothalamus, or perhaps in response to thyrotrophin-releasing hormone (TRH). A high plasma concentration of prolactin leads to a failure of Graafian follicle growth and a low oestrogen state in the female. It may also interfere with gonadotrophin release. A high concentration of circulating prolactin is physiological during lactation, and this may explain the relative subfertility of women who are breast feeding.

Hyperprolactinaemia

Persistent hyperprolactinaemia is usually caused by a micro-adenoma of the anterior pituitary or by the action of dopamine receptor antagonist drugs such as phenothiazines (Ch. 21). In younger women hyperprolactinaemia can produce amenorrhoea, infertility and signs and symptoms of oestrogen deficiency (e.g. vaginal dryness and dyspareunia, galactorrhoea and osteoporosis). In men it may cause hypogonadism. The long-acting dopamine receptor agonist bromocriptine (Ch. 24) can be used to suppress prolactin secretion.

Gonadotrophin-releasing hormone (GnRH)

GnRH is a decapeptide that is synthesised in the hypothalamus and controls release of both luteinising hormone (LH) and follicle-stimulating hormone (FSH) from the anterior pituitary (Fig. 43.1). Surface receptors on the secretory cells are induced by repeated stimulation with GnRH, but pulsatile exposure is essential to maintain responsiveness. Tolerance to constant-rate infusions of GnRH is rapid because of downregulation of cell surface receptors. There is negative feedback control via neural pathways and sex steroids.

Synthetic GnRH (gonadorelin)

Synthetic GnRH is available for treatment of female infertility. In women with amenorrhoea due to impaired release of GnRH, repeated pulses of exogenous gonadorelin will often lead to normal pituitary–gonadal function, including a regular menstrual cycle and ovulation. The hormone is usually infused subcutaneously in pulses every 90 minutes (to avoid receptor downregulation) from a portable syringe-driving pump. Unwanted effects include nausea, headaches and abdominal pain.

Gonadorelin (GnRH) analogues

Examples: buserelin, goserelin

Structurally similar to the natural hormone, gonadorelin analogues initially stimulate GnRH receptors, but rapidly promote receptor downregulation which then inhibits further gonadotrophin production. This latter action underlies their clinical use (Ch. 46).

Pharmacokinetics
Buserelin can be given either by subcutaneous injection or by nasal spray. It has a short half-life. Goserelin must be given by subcutaneous injection and is available as an oily depot preparation. Depot formulations inhibit gonadotrophin production for up to 4 weeks after a single injection.

Unwanted effects

- Menopausal effects in women, with hot flushes, sweating, vaginal dryness and sexual dysfunction.
- Orchidectomy-like effects in men, with loss of libido, gynaecomastia, and vasomotor instability.
- Hypersensitivity reactions.
- Osteoporosis with repeated courses.

Clinical uses of gonadorelin analogues

- The main use is to reduce testosterone secretion in men with prostatic cancer to castration levels. An initial rise in testosterone from receptor stimulation can produce tumour 'flare' in the first 1–2 weeks of treatment (Ch. 52). An anti-androgen (Ch. 46) is usually given to counteract this effect.
- Treatment of endometriosis by reducing oestrogen secretion.
- Treatment of advanced breast cancer in women by reducing oestrogen secretion.
- To achieve reduction in endometrial thickness prior to intrauterine surgery.
- Gonadorelin analogues are also used in female patients undergoing preparation for assisted conception by methods such as in vitro fertilisation (IVF). In these patients ovulation is targeted on a particular date. Inhalation of a gonadorelin analogue will 'switch off' natural cyclical menstrual activity. Ovarian stimulation treatment (see Gonadotrophins below) is then begun to achieve maturation of oocytes at the time chosen for egg recovery prior to IVF.

Gonadotrophins

Luteinising hormone (LH) and follicle-stimulating hormone (FSH) are glycoproteins. Release of both hormones from the anterior pituitary is stimulated by pulsatile exposure to gonadotrophin-releasing hormone (GnRH). Negative feedback by inhibin, a hormone of gonadal origin, selectively inhibits FSH secretion. In addition, both gonadotrophins are subject to negative feedback from gonadal steroids, including progesterone (Ch. 45).

In the male, LH acts on specific receptors on the surface of the Leydig cells in the testes and stimulates adenylate cyclase, leading to the production of testosterone. FSH acts in a similar way on the Sertoli cells of the seminiferous tubules, stimulating the formation of a specific androgen-binding protein.

In the female, receptors for FSH and LH are found in granulosa cells of ovarian follicles. FSH is responsible for follicular development. The rising oestradiol concentration in the late follicular phase has a positive feedback effect on secretion of LH, and produces a short-lived surge of LH release. This triggers rupture of the follicle, release of the ovum, and formation of the corpus luteum (Ch. 45). Both FSH and LH, like human chorionic gonadotrophic hormone (hCG) are also produced in large quantities by the placenta during pregnancy.

Gonadotrophins for therapeutic use

FSH and LH are extracted from urine obtained from postmenopausal women (known as human menopausal gonadotrophin: hMG). A purified preparation, urofollitropin, contains FSH only. FSH is also available as a recombinant genetically engineered product known as follitropin. Human chorionic gonadotrophin (hCG) is secreted by the placenta and extracted from the urine of pregnant women. It contains large quantities of LH. Gonadotrophins are given by intravenous or subcutaneous injection.

Clinical uses of gonadotrophins

- Treatment of infertility when deficiency of gonadal stimulation by gonadotrophin is the limiting factor. hMG encourages the development of a single mature Graafian follicle. Release of the ovum is then stimulated by a single large intramuscular injection of hCG.
- Preparation for assisted conception (in vitro fertilisation) involves giving large doses of hCG or hMG to stimulate the maturation of several follicles after preparation with a gonadorelin analogue. These ova are then 'harvested' by aspiration of the follicles.

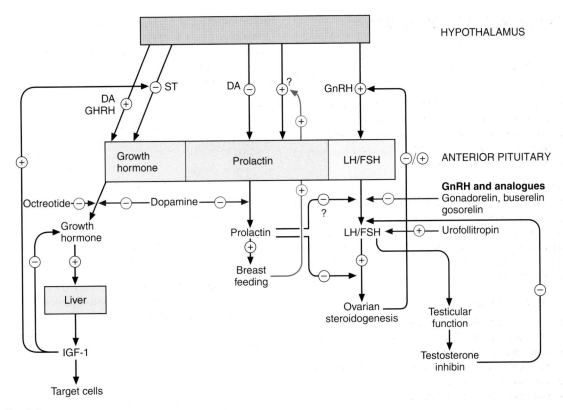

Fig. 43.1
Control mechanisms for the release of growth hormone, gonadotrophins and prolactin from the anterior pituitary. For control of other hormones see Chapter 41 (thyroid) and Chapter 44 (adrenocorticotrophic hormones).

Oestrogens usually have a negative feedback effect on GnRH except in the late follicular phase of the menstrual cycle when the feedback is positive. Gonadorelin is a GnRH analogue. On continued administration it rapidly downregulates the GnRH receptors inhibiting LH/FSH release. The actions of drugs are shown in red. ST = somatostatin; DA = dopamine; IGF-1 = insulin-like growth factor-1; GnRH = gonadotrophin-releasing hormone; ? = regulating hormone not yet established. *Note*: physiologically, dopamine stimulates growth hormone release but paradoxically in acromegaly it inhibits release.

- Male patients with gonadotrophin deficiency require long courses of gonadotrophin injections initially to achieve external sexual maturation and then to maintain satisfactory sperm production. Spermatozoa take 70–80 days to mature, and a year or more of treatment may be needed to achieve optimal response. A combination of hMG and hCG is usually given.

Unwanted effects

- The main risk in women is hyperstimulation of the ovaries which can become grossly enlarged as a result of multiple follicle stimulation, leading to considerable abdominal pain, ascites and even pleural effusions.
- In men the commonest problem is gynaecomastia or oedema with prolonged use.

Posterior pituitary hormones

Vasopressin (antidiuretic hormone, ADH)

Vasopressin is a nonapeptide, sometimes referred to as arginine vasopressin (AVP) because human vasopressin has an arginine residue in position 8. In most pharmacology textbooks it is referred to as antidiuretic hormone (ADH). It is released from neurosecretory cells of the hypothalamus and transported down the axons of the nerve cells that form the pituitary stalk. ADH is stored in the nerve endings in the posterior pituitary and released in response to stimulation of the hypothalamus via osmoreceptors, sodium receptors and volume receptors. ADH has two main target tissues: vascular smooth muscle (via V1 receptors) leading to calcium influx into the cell, and distal tubules of the kidney nephron (via V2 receptors) leading to intracellular cAMP production. In the kidney, ADH facilitates water reabsorption to produce a more concentrated urine. Vasoconstriction sufficient to raise blood pressure only occurs at high blood ADH concentrations. Vasopressin is metabolised in many tissues, including the liver and kidney, and has a very short half-life of about 10 min. It is given therapeutically by subcutaneous or intramuscular injection or by intravenous infusion.

Clinical uses of vasopressin

- Treatment of cranial diabetes insipidus (see below), although the long-acting derivative desmopressin is usually used for maintenance treatment.
- To control bleeding from oesophageal varices in portal hypertension (Ch. 36). Aqueous vasopressin is infused intravenously to produce vasoconstriction.

Desmopressin

ADH has a short duration of action. By deamination of residue 1 and substitution of D-arginine for L-arginine in position 8 the diuretic effect is increased, the pressor effect is reduced and the action is prolonged. The resulting compound, known as des-amino-D-arginine vasopressin (DDAVP or desmopressin), is absorbed through the nasal mucosa and is most conveniently administered by a metered-dose nasal spray. It can also be given by subcutaneous, intramuscular or intravenous injection. An additional action of parenteral desmopressin is to increase clotting factor VIII concentration in blood; this effect can be useful in patients with mild to moderate haemophilia to prevent bleeding.

Like the native hormone, desmopressin is metabolised in the liver and kidney, but has a longer half-life of around 75 min.

Unwanted effects

Unwanted effects include potentiation by drugs that mimic ADH (see treatment of nephrogenic diabetes insipidus, below) producing dilutional hyponatraemia as a result of excess water retention.

Diabetes insipidus

Diabetes insipidus is usually caused by a failure of secretion of ADH in the hypothalamus ('cranial' diabetes insipidus). Tumours, inflammatory conditions and granulomatous conditions such as sarcoidosis, and trauma to the hypothalamus are the main causes. A distinct condition known as nephrogenic diabetes insipidus occurs when the kidney is unresponsive to vasopressin. It results from a hereditary deficiency of renal ADH receptors or arises as a consequence of drug therapy, particularly with lithium (Ch. 22) or the tetracycline demeclocycline. Diabetes insipidus presents clinically with thirst, polyuria and a tendency to high plasma osmolality with an inappropriately low urine osmolality. Vasopressin produces concentrated urine in patients with cranial diabetes insipidus but the response in nephrogenic diabetes insipidus is impaired. Desmopressin is used for the long-term treatment of cranial diabetes insipidus.

Treatment of nephrogenic diabetes insipidus is more difficult. Paradoxically, thiazide diuretics (Ch. 14) can reduce the polyuria, as can carbamazepine (Ch. 23). Chlorpropamide (Ch. 40) is also used, but its acceptability is limited by the risk of hypoglycaemia. Carbamazepine and chlorpropamide are believed to sensitise the renal tubule to the effect of ADH.

Oxytocin

Oxytocin is discussed in Chapter 45.

FURTHER READING

Baylis PH (1998) Diabetes insipidus. *J Roy Coll Phys Lond* 32, 108–111

Bichet DG (1998) Nephrogenic diabetes insipidus. *Am J Med* 105, 431–442

Colao A, Lombardi G (1998) Growth hormone and prolactin excess. *Lancet* 352, 1455–1461

Jennings JC, Moreland K, Peterson CM (1996) In vitro fertilisation. *Drugs* 52, 313–343

Lamberts SWJ, Van der Lely A-J, de Herder WW, Hofland LJ (1996) Octreotide. *N Engl J Med* 334, 246–254

Lamberts SWJ, de Herder WW, Van der Lely A-J (1998) Pituitary insufficiency. *Lancet* 352, 127–134

Monson JP (1998) Adult growth hormone deficiency. *J Roy Coll Phys Lond* 32, 19–22

Vance LE, Mauras N (1999) Growth hormone therapy in adults and children. *N Engl J Med* 341, 1206–1216

Wass JAH, Sheppard MC (1998) New treatments for acromegaly. *J Roy Coll Phys Lond* 32, 113–117

Self-assessment

In questions 1–3 the first statement, in italics, is true. Are the accompanying statements also true?

1. *Growth hormone has anabolic effects in skeletal muscle and epiphyseal cartilage, and catabolic effects in fat cells.*

   a. Somatostatin stimulates growth hormone release.
   b. Somatostatin is produced only from the hypothalamus.
   c. The inhibition of growth hormone release by bromocriptine in patients with acromegaly is paradoxical.
   d. Octreotride is a useful drug for the treatment of acromegaly.

2. *Prolactin is an anterior pituitary hormone that is an essential hormone for milk secretion by the mammary gland; it also contributes to reduced fertility by suppressing steroidogenesis.*

   a. Bromocriptine reduces prolactin secretion.
   b. Continuous administration of analogues of gonadotrophin stimulates sex steroid synthesis.
   c. The gonadotrophin analogue gonadorelin has no clinical use in males.
   d. Gonadorelin is used for the treatment of endometriosis.
   e. Follitropin is a genetically engineered FSH used in preparation for in vitro fertilisation.

3. *Vasopressin is an antidiuretic hormone and acts on the collecting ducts to facilitate water reabsorption. In nephrogenic diabetes insipidus the response to vasopressin is impaired.*

   a. Vasopressin is a peptide.
   b. Nephrogenic diabetes insipidus is a condition in which there is a failure of secretion of vasopressin (antidiuretic hormone).
   c. In nephrogenic diabetes insipidus, thiazide diuretics increase the polyuria.

4. Case history question

   An assessment of a 10-year-old girl with short stature showed that she had abnormally low levels of GHRH and growth hormone.

   a. Is this girl too old to benefit from treatment?
   b. If not, what treatment would you recommend and how would you administer it?
   c. What unwanted effects might occur?

The answers are provided on page 625.

Pituitary and hypothalamic hormones

Drug	Half-life (h)	Elimination	Comments
Anterior pituitary hormones			
Chorionic gonadotrophin	30–35	Metabolism + renal	Given by subcutaneous or intramuscular injection; glycoprotein extracted from the urine of pregnant women; the half-life is longer after subcutaneous or intramuscular injection (30–35 h) because of slow release from the site of injection
Follitropin alfa and beta	24 (alfa), 30–40 (beta)	Metabolism + renal	Given by subcutaneous or intramuscular injection; recombinant human follicle-stimulating hormone
Human menopausal gonadotrophins (menotropins)	7–10 (FSH), 3 (LH)	Metabolism	Given by deep intramuscular injection; contains a 1:1 mixture of pituitary-derived follicle-stimulating hormone (FSH) and luteinising hormone (LH); peak concentrations seen at 4–6 hours after administration; metabolites eliminated in urine
Urofollitropin	15 (rhFSH)	Metabolism (+ renal)	Given by subcutaneous or intramuscular injection; gonadotrophin preparation from human menopausal urine containing FSH but not LH; half-life given is for recombinant human FSH (rhFSH)
Tetracosactide (cosyntropin)	0.2	Metabolism	Corticotropin (ACTH) analogue given by intramuscular or intravenous injection; slower release from intramuscular injection; metabolised by endopeptidases in serum
Anti-oestrogens			
Clomifene (clomiphene)	5 days	Metabolism + bile	Anti-oestrogen given orally; a racemate with the more active isomer (zuclomifene) accumulating over the first few days of treatment; undergoes enterohepatic circulation
Growth hormone			
Somatropin	0.5 (iv)	Metabolism	Given by subcutaneous or intravenous injection; synthetic form of growth hormone (somatotropin); serum half-life after subcutaneous administration (usual route) is 4 hours due to absorption rate limited elimination
Hypothalamic hormones			
Gonadorelin	4 minutes	Metabolism (+ renal)	Given by subcutaneous or intravenous injection; synthetic analogue of luteinising hormone releasing hormone; very short half-life probably reflects tissue uptake and intracellular metabolism
Protirelin	4 minutes (TRH)	Metabolism	Given by intravenous injection; thyrotrophin-releasing hormone; rapidly metabolised by tissues and serum; half-life is for TRH
Sermorelin	1 (GHRH)	Metabolism	Given by intravenous injection; analogue of growth hormone releasing hormone (GHRH); half-life is for GHRH; the release and removal rates of GH after GHRH are about 10 min and 20–30 min respectively
Posterior pituitary hormones and antagonists			
Desmopressin	0.5–2	Metabolism	Given orally, intranasally or by subcutaneous, intramuscular or intravenous injection; analogue of ADH; poor oral bioavailability due to presystemic metabolism; metabolised by liver, kidney and plasma to inactive products
Terlipressin	0.5	Metabolism	Given by intravenous injection; triglycyl prodrug of lysine-vasopressin which is metabolised by hydrolysis to the active form (which then has a formation-rate limited half-life of 0.5 hours)
Vasopressin (argipressin)	5–15 minutes	Metabolism	Given by subcutaneous or intramuscular injection or by intravenous infusion; rapidly metabolised by kidney, liver, brain and placenta
Demeclocycline	10–15	Renal + bile	Given orally; has anti-ADH action possibly due to blockade of renal tubular effects of ADH; oral bioavailability is 66% (due to poor absorption)

44

Corticosteroids (glucocorticoids and mineralocorticoids)

Structure and synthesis of steroid hormones

Steroid hormones constitute a range of compounds synthesised mainly in the adrenal cortex and the gonads. They are derived from cholesterol and share a common nucleus (Fig. 44.1). The natural glucocorticoid, hydrocortisone, and the mineralocorticoid, aldosterone, differ only in their constituents at position 17 and 18. Hydrocortisone has a hydroxyl grouping at position 17 and aldosterone an aldehyde grouping at position 18.

The steroid hormones are produced principally in the adrenal cortex (adrenal corticosteroids) and can be classified according to their effects in relation to hydrocortisone. Their glucocorticoid activity affects carbohydrate and protein metabolism, and their mineralocorticoid activity affects water and electrolyte balance (see below and Table 44.1). There is some overlap in activity of individual molecules, particularly when their structures are similar, for example hydrocortisone (cortisol) has approximately equal glucocorticoid and mineralocorticoid activity. Synthetic steroids are constructed to enhance either the glucocorticoid or mineralocorticoid activity. The other major group of steroid hormones, the sex hormones, are considered in Chapters 45 and 46.

The pathways of steroid hormone synthesis are shown in Figure 44.2.

Glucocorticoid (and to a lesser extent mineralocorticoid) secretion is controlled by the hypothalamic–pituitary–adrenal axis (Fig. 44.3). Elevations in glucocorticoid concentrations feed back and reduce corticotrophin-releasing factor (CRF) release.

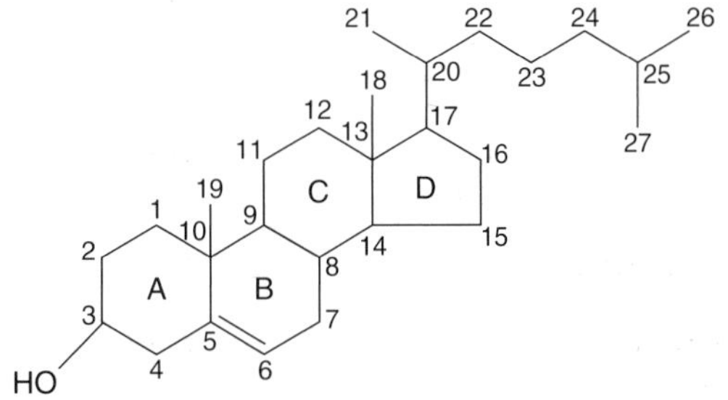

Fig. 44.1
The 'core' structure of steroid hormones is derived from the cholesterol molecule shown. Note: the four rings are each identified by a letter and each carbon atom by a number.

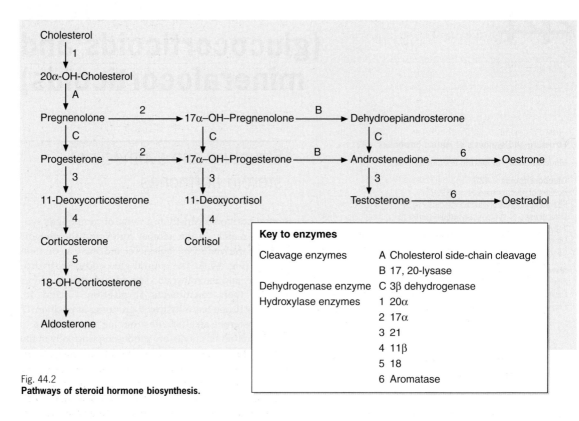

Fig. 44.2
Pathways of steroid hormone biosynthesis.

Table 44.1
Relative glucocorticoid and mineralocorticoid activities of some natural and synthetic steroid hormones

	Glucocorticoid	Mineralocorticoid
Cortisol (hydrocortisone)	1	1
Prednisolone	4	0.8
Dexamethasone	30	Negligible
Betamethasone	30	Negligible
Aldosterone	0	80
Fludrocortisone	10	125

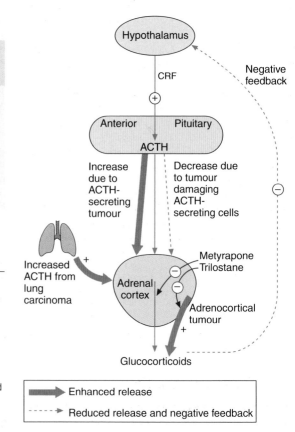

Fig. 44.3
Control of secretion of glucocorticoids and mineralocorticoids. Stimulation by CRF (corticotrophin-releasing factor) and ACTH (adrenocorticotrophic hormone) increases the release of glucocorticoids and mineralocorticoids. The level of corticosteroid in the blood feeds back and negatively controls the release of ACTH. Synthetic glucocorticoids have the same action, suppressing the hypothalamic–pituitary axis. In conditions in which excess corticosteroids are released, e.g. in ACTH-secreting tumours or adrenocortical tumours, steroid synthesis and release can be reduced by drug therapy, shown in red. In patients with tumours that result in hormone-induced reduction in glucocorticoids, synthetic glucocorticoids can be administered.

Mode of action of steroid hormones

All steroid hormones share a common receptor mechanism. The distribution of the various receptors in different tissues gives specificity to each type of steroid hormone and defines its activity. Steroids are protein-bound to circulating binding globulins. They are highly lipophilic and cross the cell membrane by diffusion and enter the nucleus after binding to a specific receptor that is normally associated with heat-shock protein. The steroid–protein complex enters the nucleus and binds to a corticosteroid response element on the target genes. This leads to either increased or decreased transcription of proteins depending on the target cell. Inhibition of transcription is caused by binding of transcription factors such as AP-1 and NFκB. The time taken for modulation of protein synthesis explains why therapeutic doses of glucocorticoids take many hours to have their clinical effect.

Glucocorticoids

Cortisol (also known as hydrocortisone) is the main natural glucocorticoid in humans. It is synthesised in the adrenal cortex in response to ACTH from the anterior pituitary. Receptors for cortisol are found in many tissues, giving it a wide range of actions. Glucocorticoids inhibit transcription of the genes for synthesis of inducible cyclooxygenase (COX-2), the inducible form of nitric oxide synthase and of inflammatory cytokines such as interleukins IL-1, IL-2 and IL-5 and TNFα and many others. T-helper lymphocyte proliferation and B lymphocyte maturation are reduced (Ch. 39). In addition, corticosteroids stimulate production of the intracellular protein lipocortin-1. Lipocortin-1 inhibits phospholipase A_2 and therefore reduces the synthesis of prostaglandins and leukotrienes (Ch. 29). It may also impair leucocyte migration in response to the cytokine IL-1. Other effects of glucocorticoids are probably related to induction of the transcription of several enzymes involved in metabolic control.

Actions of glucocorticoids

Therapeutic doses of glucocorticoids produce a wide range of effects.

Anti-inflammatory actions

The immunological and vascular actions of glucocorticoids confer anti-inflammatory activity. In addition, they inhibit mononuclear cell and neutrophil leucocyte migration and their adhesion to inflamed capillary endothelium. The ability of these inflammatory cells to respond to and destroy phagocytosed microorganisms and to release oxygen free radicals is also reduced. Decreased production of cytokines, including several interleukins and granulocyte-macrophage colony-stimulating factor (GM-CSF) (Ch. 47), contributes to these actions. Production of prostaglandins and leukotrienes is reduced since glucocorticoids indirectly inhibit the synthesis of the enzymes phospholipase A_2 and directly inhibit the synthesis of cyclooxygenase-2 (COX-2) (Ch. 29). Fibroblast activity is also impaired, which reduces tissue repair.

Immunological actions

The main immunological effect is reduced proliferation of T lymphocytes. This is largely due to reduced production of the cytokine IL-2 (Ch. 39).

Metabolic effects

The metabolic effects of glucocorticoids are catabolic in nature. Gluconeogenesis is increased and leads to increased storage of glycogen in the liver and to a lesser extent in muscle. Tissue uptake and utilisation of glucose is impaired. These actions promote hyperglycaemia.

Fat is redistributed from the corticosteroid-sensitive fat stores in the limbs to the corticosteroid-resistant stores in the face, neck and trunk. This action results from enhancement of the lipolytic response to catecholamines.

Protein is degraded to enable synthesis of glucose and to increase the available pool of amino acids, while protein synthesis is inhibited. As a result there is breakdown of tissues, particularly muscle but also in skin and bone, and an overall negative nitrogen balance.

Capillary permeability is decreased, which has a protective effect on blood volume and raises blood pressure. The sensitivity of vascular walls to the vasoconstrictor actions of catecholamines is also enhanced.

Central nervous system effects

Plasma cortisol concentrations rise to a peak at the time of awakening and are lowest during sleep. In general, high circulating concentrations of cortisol are associated with alertness, but severe disturbances of mood may occur with abnormally high levels. Low concentrations produce a feeling of lethargy.

Mineralocorticoid effects

Natural glucocorticoids also have mineralocorticoid activity (see below). Synthetic glucocorticoid compounds are altered structurally to change the relationship between the amount of mineralocorticoid and glucocorticoid activity (Table 44.1).

Pharmacokinetics of glucocorticoids

Both natural and synthetic glucocorticoids are used in clinical practice. They are readily absorbed from the gut. The natural glucocorticoid hydrocortisone binds to corticosteroid-binding globulin and albumin in the blood; it is extensively metabolised in the gut wall and liver. Prednisone is a synthetic glucocorticoid which is effectively a prodrug because most of its activity results from conversion in the liver to prednisolone; the latter compound is preferred in clinical practice. Synthetic glucocorticoids are more potent than hydrocortisone and more slowly metabolised in the liver, giving them a longer duration of action. Substantial amounts are excreted via the kidney. They bind to albumin but not to corticosteroid-binding globulin.

Most glucocorticoids are available in formulations for parenteral use. This does not appreciably shorten the time to onset of action which is delayed by up to 8 h while protein synthesis is modulated intracellularly. Glucocorticoids can also be delivered topically to reduce their systemic actions.

The plasma half-lives of all glucocorticoids are short, but their biological (i.e. effective) half-lives are long (varying from 12 h for hydrocortisone to 2 days for dexamethasone), due to their actions on protein synthesis.

Clinical uses of systemically administered glucocorticoids

Box 44.1 shows some of the uses of systemic glucocorticoids.

Physiological replacement therapy for corticosteroid deficiency. Hydrocortisone or an equivalent synthetic glucocorticoid is given orally twice daily in doses as close as possible to the amount normally secreted by the adrenal cortex. In stressful situations, for example intercurrent infection, the dose must be doubled or tripled. Acute adrenal insufficiency requires immediate treatment with high-dose intravenous hydrocortisone. Conditions that can give rise to corticosteroid deficiency are shown in Box 44.3.

Therapeutic uses. The anti-inflammatory and immunosuppressive effects of glucocorticoids are used for various inflammatory diseases (especially those which are immunologically mediated) and neoplastic conditions, particularly when they involve lymphoid tissue (Box 44.1). Powerful glucocorticoids such as prednisolone with little mineralocorticoid activity are usually chosen.

For uses of ACTH and analogues see Chapter 43.

Box 44.1

Examples of diseases for which systemic glucocorticoid therapy is useful

Replacement therapy in corticosteroid deficiency
Acute inflammatory disease
  Bronchial asthma
  Anaphylaxis and angioedema
  Acute fibrosing alveolitis
Chronic inflammatory disease
  Connective tissue disorders, e.g. systemic lupus erythematosus, polymyositis, vasculitides
  Renal disorders, e.g. glomerulonephritis
  Hepatic disorders, e.g. chronic active hepatitis
  Bowel disorders, e.g. inflammatory bowel disease
  Eye disorders, e.g. posterior uveitis
Neoplastic disease
  Myeloma
  Lymphomas
  Lymphocytic leukaemias
Miscellaneous disorders
  Bell's palsy
  Sarcoidosis
  Organ transplantation

Topical administration of glucocorticoids

Topical use of glucocorticoids can deliver high concentrations to a target site and reduce systemic unwanted effects. However, at higher doses significant absorption into the blood can occur. Examples of the clinical uses of topical corticosteroids are given in Table 44.2.

Unwanted effects of glucocorticoids

Pharmacological doses of glucocorticoids given over long periods will produce the typical features of adrenocortical overactivity (Cushing's syndrome). Unwanted glucocorticoid actions are shown in Box 44.2.

Cushing's syndrome

Cushing's syndrome is characterised by the effects of excess glucocorticoid (see 'Unwanted effects of glucocorticoids' above). There are four causes (Box 44.3).

Table 44.2
Examples of topical corticosteroid administration

Disease	Mode of administration	Chapter
Asthma	Aerosol	12
Vasomotor rhinitis	Aerosol	38
Eczema	Ointment or cream	49
Superficial ocular inflammation	Aqueous solution	50
Ulcerative colitis	Aqueous solution or foam enema	34
Proctitis	Suppository	34
Arthritis	Aqueous solution by intra-articular injection	30

Box 44.2

Unwanted effects of glucocorticoids

- Central obesity with 'buffalo hump', moon face and abdominal striae.
- Loss of supporting tissue in skin with skin atrophy, bruising, and poor wound healing. Local atrophy can be marked at the site of topical steroid application.
- Osteoporosis due to catabolism of protein matrix in the bone and defective mineralisation.
- Proximal (i.e. shoulder and hip girdle) muscle wasting and weakness.
- Hyperglycaemia, which may lead to overt diabetes mellitus (Ch. 40).
- Peptic ulceration due to gastrointestinal prostaglandin inhibition (Ch. 33).
- Mood changes, including euphoria and occasionally psychosis.
- Posterior capsular cataracts in the eye, and exacerbation of glaucoma.
- Increased susceptibility to infection with bacteria, viruses or fungi. Activation of latent infection such as tuberculosis can also occur.
- Growth retardation in children, with reduced linear bone growth and premature epiphyseal closure.
- After long-term treatment, sudden withdrawal can produce an acute adrenal crisis due to suppression of the hypothalamic–pituitary–adrenal axis and adrenal atrophy. Recovery of adrenal responsiveness can take several months. Basal cortisol secretion is restored before maximal responses, leaving patients at risk during stress and intercurrent infection.
- Mineralocorticoid effects (which vary among the different drugs).

Box 44.3

Causes of Cushing's syndrome (corticosteroid excess) and corticosteroid deficiency

Causes of Cushing's syndrome
- Excessive secretion of ACTH by the anterior pituitary (pituitary adenoma) (Cushing's disease)
- Excessive secretion of ACTH from an ectopic source (most commonly carcinoma of the bronchus)
- A tumour of the adrenal cortex secreting predominantly cortisol
- Iatrogenic: administration of glucocorticoid or ACTH in pharmacological doses

Causes of corticosteroid deficiency
- Primary adrenal insufficiency (Addison's disease)
  - autoimmune adrenalitis
  - infections, e.g. tuberculosis, various fungi, opportunistic infections in AIDS
  - metastatic carcinoma
- Secondary adrenocortical failure (deficient ACTH from the anterior pituitary)
  - pituitary tumour
  - sarcoidosis
  - suppression of the hypothalamic–pituitary–adrenal axis by prolonged glucocorticoid treatment at pharmacological doses
- Various enzyme defects in cortisol synthesis (congenital adrenal hyperplasia)

Management of Cushing's syndrome

The definitive treatment for excessive pituitary secretion of ACTH (usually from an adenoma) and for unilateral adrenal tumours is surgery, with subsequent radiotherapy for some pituitary tumours.

Drug treatment to reduce corticosteroid secretion is desirable for several weeks before surgery to reverse the excessive tissue catabolism and correct the metabolic disturbance. This is usually achieved with metyrapone. This drug reduces corticosteroid biosynthesis by competitive inhibition of 11β-hydroxylase (Figs 44.1, 44.2 – enzyme 4). It also inhibits cytochrome P450 in the liver which can produce important drug interactions (Ch. 2). Oral absorption of metyrapone is variable, and extensive metabolism occurs in the liver. Gastrointestinal upset is the main unwanted effect. Trilostane is an alternative to metyrapone, and is a reversible inhibitor of the earlier enzymatic step of 3β-dehydrogenation (Fig. 44.2 – enzyme C).

Ectopic ACTH secretion is not usually amenable to surgical cure but palliative drug treatment with metyrapone can be helpful (Fig. 44.3).

Mineralocorticoids

Aldosterone is the principal mineralocorticoid and is secreted from the zona glomerulosa of the adrenal cortex. Aldosterone secretion is regulated by several factors, of which angiotensin II (Ch. 6), a low plasma Na^+ and a high plasma K^+ are the most important. Angiotensin II acts via specific AT_2 receptors to induce aldosterone release. ACTH has some effect on aldosterone secretion. Receptors for aldosterone are found in fewer tissues than are glucocorticoid receptors; the main target cell is in the distal renal tubule and collecting duct. Aldosterone increases the permeability of the luminal tubular membrane to Na^+ by increasing the number of Na^+ channels. It also stimulates the Na^+/K^+-ATPase pump in the basolateral membrane which leads to active Na^+ reabsorption and loss of K^+ into tubular urine (Ch. 14). Water is passively reabsorbed with Na^+ so that extracellular fluid volume and blood pressure are increased. Target cells for aldosterone contain the enzyme 11β-hydroxysteroid dehydrogenase that degrades glucocorticoids and minimises tissue response to these agents.

Fludrocortisone

Pharmacokinetics
Aldosterone is almost completely inactivated at its first passage through the liver and is therefore unsuitable for oral administration. 9α-Fluorohydrocortisone (fludrocortisone) is a synthetic alternative which is well absorbed from the gut; about 10% escapes first-pass metabolism. The half-life is short due to hepatic metabolism, but its action is prolonged by slow absorption.

Unwanted effects
Excessive Na^+ retention and K^+ loss can occur with pharmacological doses. Hypertension can result; however, the expansion of blood volume stimulates atrial stretch receptors leading to secretion of atrial natriuretic peptide. The resulting natriuresis initiates an 'escape' mechanism which establishes a new equilibrium between Na^+ intake and excretion at a higher blood volume. Consequently, oedema does not usually occur.

Clinical uses of fludrocortisone

- Fludrocortisone is given as replacement therapy for patients with defective aldosterone production. This condition is usually the result of primary adrenal pathology with destruction of all three zones of the cortex (Addison's disease).
- Expansion of blood volume by fludrocortisone can be used to raise blood pressure in postural hypotension resulting from autonomic neuropathy; however, it often produces supine hypertension without fully eliminating the postural fall in blood pressure.

Primary hyperaldosteronism (Conn's syndrome)

Autonomous oversecretion of aldosterone causes hypertension and a hypokalaemic alkalosis. Most cases are caused by an adenoma in the zona glomerulosa of the adrenal cortex and are treated surgically. The remainder are usually the result of hyperplasia of both zonae glomerulosa; these cases are usually less severe clinically and a potassium-sparing diuretic (usually spironolactone) is the treatment of choice (Ch. 14).

FURTHER READING

Ganguly A (1998) Primary aldosteronism. *N Engl J Med* 339, 1828–1834

Lipworth BS (1999) Systemic adverse effects of inhaled corticosteroid therapy. *Arch Intern Med* 159, 941–955

Oelkers W (1996) Adrenal insufficiency. *N Engl J Med* 335, 1206–1212

Self-assessment

In questions 1–4 the first statement, in italics, is true. Are the accompanying statements also true?

1. *Beclomethasone and budesonide penetrate mucosal membranes but have short half-lives systemically, reducing toxic effects.*

   a. Oral fludrocortisone is a useful anti-inflammatory steroid in severe asthma.
   b. Beclomethasone is not used orally.

2. *Corticosteroids take many hours to produce their clinical effect because they act to modify cellular production of proteins*

   a. Hypoglycaemia is common during glucocorticoid administration.
   b. If prolonged administration of prednisolone results in unwanted effects, it is appropriate to withdraw the drug slowly.

3. *Mineralocorticoid secretion is decreased in Addison's disease. Examples are primary adrenal insufficiency (predominantly autoimmune) or secondary insufficiency, e.g. due to a pituitary tumour or following prolonged glucocorticoid treatment.*

   a. Aldosterone secretion is inhibited by angiotensin II.
   b. Aldosterone and cortisol secretion are regulated by ACTH.

4. *Glucocorticoids affect all inflammatory responses caused by infection, chemical or altered immune responses.*

   a. Dexamethasone causes vomiting.
   b. Glucocorticoids delay wound healing.
   c. Before giving an intra-articular injection of glucocorticoid in gout, infection of the joint should be excluded.

5. Case history question

   > A 35-year-old female showed signs of cortisol excess including centripetal obesity, muscle weakness, easy bruising and amenorrhoea.

   a. What are the possible causes?

   > She was not taking corticosteroids, eliminating an iatrogenic cause. Cortisol levels in a 24 h urine were elevated. Plasma ACTH levels were also high.

   b. What do these results indicate?

   > A single high dose of dexamethasone was administered and resulted in only marginal suppression of cortisol.

   c. What does this result indicate?

   > A CT scan and other tests showed an inoperable carcinoma of the bronchus.

   d. What treatment could be given?

The answers are provided on pages 625–626.

Drug compendium

Corticosteroids. The durations of action ('biological half-lives') of corticosteroids greatly exceed their chemical half-lives because of their mechanism of action.

Drug	Half-life	Elimination	Comments
Glucocorticoids			
Betamethasone	35–55	Metabolism	Given orally, topically, by intramuscular or slow intravenous injection or by intravenous infusion; phosphate ester prodrug used for injections; ester prodrugs hydrolysed to betamethasone which is inactivated by metabolism
Cortisone acetate	1–2 (HC)	Metabolism	Given orally; oral bioavailability is 20–90%; rapidly hydrolysed and converted to cortisol (hydrocortisone; HC) which is inactivated by oxidation to cortisone and reduction to tetrahydrocortisol
Deflazacort	1	Metabolism	Given orally; bioavailability not affected by food (absolute bioavailability not defined); hydrolysed to the active 21-desacetyl metabolite (21-hydroxy-compound)
Dexamethasone	2–4	Metabolism	Given orally, by intramuscular or slow intravenous injection or by intravenous infusion; phosphate ester prodrug used for injections; high but variable oral bioavailability possibly due to intestinal CYP3A metabolism; metabolised in the liver by CYP3A4-mediated oxidation to the 6-hydroxy compound
Hydrocortisone (cortisol)	1–2	Metabolism	Given orally, by intramuscular or slow intravenous injection or by intravenous infusion; phosphate ester prodrug used for injections, variable absorption (30–90%) due to first-pass metabolism; metabolised by oxidation to cortisone and reduction to dihydro- and tetrahydro-cortisol
Methylprednisolone	1–3	Metabolism	Given orally, by intramuscular or slow intravenous injection or by intravenous infusion; injectable forms are lipid soluble esters in solvents; high oral bioavailability (80–90%); esters are very rapidly hydrolysed; metabolised in liver and kidney by reduction to 20-hydroxy compound
Prednisolone	2–4	Metabolism	Given orally, topically and by intramuscular injection; injectable form is the acetate ester as an aqueous suspension; high oral bioavailability (70–80%); extensively metabolised but all pathways have not been defined
Triamcinolone	2–5	Metabolism	Given by deep intramuscular injection as an aqueous suspension; metabolised by oxidation
Mineralocorticoids			
Fludrocortisone acetate	0.5	Metabolism	Given orally; low bioavailability (10%) due to first-pass metabolism; hydrolysed to fludrocortisol which is reduced and eliminated as conjugated metabolites

45

Female reproduction

The menstrual cycle

Physiology

The endocrine function of the hypothalamic–pituitary–ovarian axis acts through a series of feedback loops to control the reproductive processes of the menstrual cycle (Fig. 45.1). Following the shedding of the endometrium (days 1–3/5 of the menstrual cycle), a group of follicles in the ovary start to develop and mature under the influence of the gonadotrophic hormones follicle-stimulating hormone (FSH) and luteinising hormone (LH) secreted from the anterior pituitary. The gonadotrophic hormones are in turn under the control of secretion of increased amounts of gonadotrophin releasing hormone (GnRH) secreted from the hypothalamus (Fig. 45.1). The prolonged release of low levels of FSH and LH results in the selection and ongoing maturation of a single Graafian follicle; this is prepared for ovulation at the expense of the remaining antral follicles

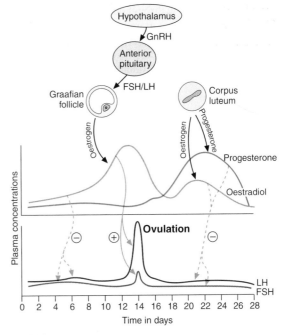

Fig. 45.1
Endocrine control of the menstrual cycle. ⊖ - - -, Negative feedback; ⊕ ——, positive feedback.

which regress. The regression possibly results from the lack of gonadotrophin receptors on the unsuccessful follicles.

The developing Graafian follicle is driven by FSH and LH to convert the androgens produced by thecal cells of the follicle into oestradiol within granulosa cells. Oestrogen secretion from the follicle slowly rises as the follicle matures. In the window of time between the early to mid follicular phase of the menstrual cycle, the modest concentration of oestrogen secreted exerts a negative feedback on both hypothalamic and pituitary gonadotrophin secretions. The low concentrations of progesterone also weakly suppress gonadotrophin secretion in the early follicular phase. Although circulating FSH levels are low, oestradiol enhances the effectiveness of the action of gonadotrophin on the ovary to stimulate further oestradiol synthesis.

In the late follicular phase, a cohort of granulosa cells in the maturing Graafian follicle differentiates under the influence of FSH and starts to express LH receptors. These granulosa cells can then be stimulated by LH to secrete progesterone and are destined to become the corpus luteum. The elevated circulating oestradiol levels in the mid to late follicular phase eventually reach a critical concentration of about 200 pg ml^{-1} for 48 hours. This sustained concentration of estradiol and the relatively rapid rate of increase in oestradiol triggers a switch from a negative feedback to a positive feedback of oestradiol upon the pituitary and hypothalamus. As a result, the midcycle surge of LH and, to a lesser extent FSH, that is essential for ovulation begins.

Following ovulation, the plasma LH levels fall rapidly and remain low throughout the secretory phase. The reason for this is that granulosa cells containing LH receptors proliferate in the corpus luteum and produce increasing concentrations of progesterone; this in turn suppresses LH and FSH production by negative feedback on the hypothalamus and pituitary. Elevated plasma levels of oestrogen arise from oestrogen produced by the corpus luteum. If implantation of a fertilised ovum does not occur, the corpus luteum regresses after about 10 days, possibly under the influence of local synthesis of vasoconstrictor prostaglandin F$_{2\alpha}$, although there is little direct confirmation of this in humans.

From day 1 to late in the menstrual cycle gradually increasing plasma concentrations of oestrogen and progesterone produced as the menstrual cycle progresses result in proliferation and vascularisation of endometrial cells, which are able to secrete a variety of fluids and nutrients aimed at making the endometrium receptive for implantation. The temporal precision of the change in receptivity is critical if successful implantation is to occur. Oestrogens and progesterone cause the endometrium to become oedematous, and glands secrete increasing quantities of amino acids, sugars and glycoproteins in a viscous liquid. At the end of the menstrual cycle the low circulating levels of progesterone and oestrogen present

eventually do not support the endometrium. Deprived of hormonal support, the endometrial spiral arteries go into spasm and the endometrial cells die, producing digestive enzymes. As a consequence of this and other changes, the endometrium is shed during menstruation.

The cervical mucus is also influenced by oestrogen and progesterone concentrations. Under the dominant influence of progesterone cervical mucus is viscid and less penetrable by sperm, whereas at ovulation the high plasma oestradiol concentration results in a thinner, elastic mucus that is easily penetrable by sperm. Progesterone inhibits the motility of the fallopian tube, altering the transport of sperm, and the fertilised or unfertilised oocyte. Excess progesterone may alter the chance of fertilisation occurring or the embryo may reach the uterine cavity when the endometrium is not receptive to implantation. Oestrogens have the opposite action, increasing tubal motility, and may accelerate the transport of the ovum into the uterine cavity.

Pregnancy is accompanied by considerable hormonal changes. The feto-placental unit together produce progressively greater quantities of oestrogen and progesterone which reach the maternal circulation. The placenta also produces human chorionic gonadotrophin (hCG) (Ch. 43) which reaches a peak circulating concentration at about 50–60 days of gestation then falls. hCG stimulates progesterone and oestrogen production from the corpus luteum. The corpus luteum is essential for the maintenance of pregnancy during the first 6–8 weeks, after which placental production of hormones takes over. The increasing placental production of oestrogens, progesterone and human placental lactogen as pregnancy advances results in the development of duct and milk-secreting cells in the breast. The precise balance of sex steroids also contributes to quiescence of the uterus during pregnancy and the onset of labour at term.

Steroidal contraceptives

Oral contraceptives ('the pill') are the most widely used form of contraception and contain either a combination of a synthetic estrogen and a progestogen (a C-19 synthetic progesterone derivative) or a progestogen alone. The failure rate is 0.2–3 pregnancies per 100 women-years of use. The estrogen component of the combined pill is usually ethinylestradiol, but is occasionally mestranol. Over the years the dose of the estrogen component has been reduced and now the majority of so-called 'second-generation' pills (to differentiate them from first-generation pills with a high estrogen content) have 20–30 µg ethinylestradiol, although other concentrations are available (see later). The progestogen component of the second-generation contraceptives is either levonorgestrel or norethisterone which possess progestational but also androgenic activity. Newer progestogens, such as gestodene and desogestrel, with less androgenic acitivity are now widely used. Pills containing these progestogens are referred to as 'third-generation' pills. Other differences and similarities between second- and third-generation contraceptives are discussed later.

Mechanisms of contraception

Elevated circulating levels of synthetic estrogen and progestogen prevent the precise cyclic pattern of hormone-related events seen in the normal menstrual cycle.

- The combination of estrogen and progestogen exerts its contraceptive effect mainly through inhibition of ovulation.
- The estrogen component, and to a lesser extent the progestogen, suppress LH and FSH secretion and follicular development.
- Progestogen produces asynchronous development of the endometrium with stromal thinning which makes it less receptive to implantation. Fallopian tube motility is increased by estrogens and decreased by progestogens; this may affect fertility by altering the rate of transport of the gamete.
- Progestogen alters cervical mucus, making it thicker and less copious, and thereby creating an

environment more hostile to sperm penetration. With the oral progestogen-only pill ovulation is inhibited in only about 25% of women. Contraception must therefore rely upon the other actions of the hormone (Fig. 45.2).

Combined oral contraceptive

Monophasic preparations

Monophasic preparations contain fixed amounts of estrogen and progestogen. They are taken daily for the first 21 days of the menstrual cycle followed by 7 days without contraceptive. Twenty-eight day packs ('every day' preparations) are available which, to improve compliance, include an inactive substance such as lactose during the 7 contraceptive-free days. The 'combined oral contraceptive pill' refers to preparations that usually contain 20–30 μg ethinylestradiol. High-strength pills are also available containing 50 μg ethinylestradiol or mestranol. There are several different formulations of the combined oral contraceptive pill which contain variable amounts of either second- or third-generation progestogen (depending upon the progestational potency of the progestogen used). Preparations are also available that contain different amounts of the same progestogen, but the dose is kept constant throughout

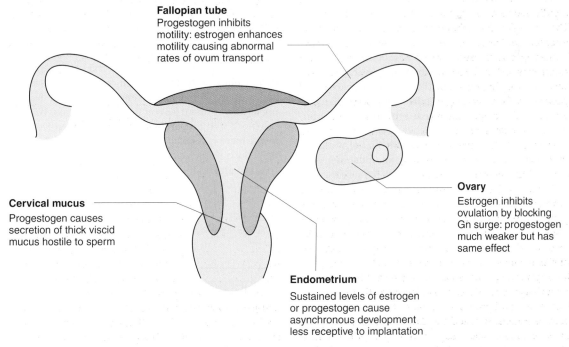

Fallopian tube
Progestogen inhibits motility: estrogen enhances motility causing abnormal rates of ovum transport

Cervical mucus
Progestogen causes secretion of thick viscid mucus hostile to sperm

Ovary
Estrogen inhibits ovulation by blocking Gn surge: progestogen much weaker but has same effect

Endometrium
Sustained levels of estrogen or progestogen cause asynchronous development less receptive to implantation

Fig. 45.2
The contraceptive actions of the synthetic estrogen and progestogen in the contraceptive pill. Gn, gonadotrophin LH and FSH.

the menstrual cycle; for example, Microgynon 30® contains 150 μg levonorgestrel and Ovran 30® 250 μg levonorgestrel. In some women it may be necessary to change the formulation to reduce minor unwanted effects such as breakthrough bleeding or weight gain during the menstrual cycle. The androgenic or anti-androgenic properties possessed by different progestogens may influence the suitability of an individual preparation for a particular woman.

Biphasic and triphasic preparations

Biphasic and triphasic preparations are designed to mimic more closely the changes in sex hormone concentrations that occur during the natural menstrual cycle. The total steroid intake through the cycle is no less than with monophasic preparations. Several preparations are available, all of which contain ethinylestradiol in combination with either norethisterone or levonorgestrel. In most preparations, the ethinylestradiol dose is kept constant as in the monophasic pills, although in some it is stepped up from days 7 to 12. Progestogen doses are increased once (biphasic) or twice (triphasic) as the menstrual cycle proceeds. Biphasic and triphasic preparations containing second- or third-generation progestogens are available.

Oral and injectable progestogen-only contraceptive

Oral progestogen

The progestogen-only pill is particularly useful for women in whom the administration of estrogen is considered to be undesirable, for example if there is a history of thromboembolic disorders (see below). It is as effective as combined pills containing 30 μg of ethinylestradiol although some reports say that pregnancy rates are slightly higher. Tablets containing levonorgestrel, norethisterone or ethynodiol are given continuously, without a break, and must be taken within 3 h of the usual time every day. Because the dose of progestogen is low, bleeding does occur at approximately monthly intervals but may be irregular. Breakthrough bleeding occurs in up to 40% of women; this is much higher than with the combined oral contraceptive. Some women become amenorrhoeic. Ectopic pregnancy may be increased in women taking the progestogen-only pill, due to impaired tubal transport, but its occurrence is extremely rare.

Injectable progestogen

Intramuscular injection of a progestogen, either medroxyprogesterone acetate or norethisterone, can provide contraception for up to 8–12 weeks. Ovulation is reliably inhibited, unlike with the oral progestogen-only contraceptives, and therefore there is a low incidence of ectopic pregnancy. Its effect is fully reversible but there is a high incidence of amenorrhoea when its use is stopped.

Subcutaneous implants of progestogens

Progestogens such as levonorgestrel can be released from polydimethylsiloxone (silicone) capsules. The subdermal implants of 6 capsules require surgical insertion and provide contraception for up to 5 years. Unwanted effects are the same as those experienced with the progestogen-only oral contraceptive but, since first-pass metabolism is avoided, lower doses of progestogen are needed.

Progestogen-containing intrauterine contraceptive device

Copper intrauterine contraceptive devices (IUCD) with a levonorgestrel releasing system from a silicone reservoir provide effective contraception with reduced menstrual blood loss compared with IUCDs that do not contain a progestogen. The progestogen is released from the device for a period of 3 years.

Efficacy of hormonal contraception

When taken according to the recommended schedule, the failure rate for the combined oral contraceptive is 0.2%. Failure of the progestogen-only pill is age-related and is up to 5% in young women, falling with decreasing fertility to about 0.3% at the age of 40 years. With the combined oral preparations contraceptive protection is lost if there is a delay of more than 12 h in taking the daily dose. In such circumstances the missed pill should be taken and additional contraceptive measures should be used for 7 days. With the progestogen-only contraceptive, if there is a delay of only 3 h or more after the normal time of taking the pill, other contraceptive precautions should be taken for 2–3 days.

Emergency postcoital ('morning-after') contraceptive

Two products are approved for use in the UK. The first contains 50 μg ethinylestradiol and 250 μg levonorgestrel. Two tablets are taken as soon as possible after unprotected intercourse but not later than 72 h after. A further two tablets are taken exactly 12 h after the first dose. Nausea is a frequent adverse effect occurring in up to 40% of patients; vomiting can occur and an antiemetic (Ch. 32) may be needed. Absorption takes 2 h; vomiting after this time will not affect the efficacy of treatment. The mechanism of action may be to accelerate transport of the fertilised ovum so that it reaches the uterine cavity before the endometrium is receptive. The treatment is successful in at least 95% of cases. This preparation may be available over-the-counter in the near future.

The second preparation contains progestogen only and requires two doses of 750 μg each of levonorgestrel given 12 hours apart. This method is said to be successful in 85% of expected pregnancies. Unwanted effects of nausea and vomiting occur but are lower than with the estrogen-containing preparation. This preparation is available without prescription.

Pharmacokinetics of contraceptive steroids

The synthetic estrogens, like the naturally occurring oestradiol-17β, are well absorbed orally but are less rapidly degraded and undergo a variable amount of enterohepatic recycling. There is considerable interindividual variation in plasma levels of estrogen and progestogens after ingestion of the combined oral contraceptive pill. Progesterone itself is inactive orally because of extensive hepatic metabolism.

The pharmacokinetics of individual synthetic estrogens and progestogens vary widely and data on ethinylestradiol and norethisterone only are summarised.

Ethinylestradiol is absorbed rapidly from the gut and peak plasma levels are reached in 1 h. It undergoes considerable first-pass metabolism and has an intermediate half-life (Ch. 2). Enterohepatic circulation of ethinylestradiol is responsible for maintaining effective plasma concentrations with low-dose formulations. Norethisterone is rapidly and completely absorbed from the gut and also undergoes extensive first-pass metabolism in the intestinal wall and liver. Peak plasma concentrations occur after 1–3 h, and it has an intermediate half-life.

Unwanted effects

Both estrogen and progestogen have a number of minor and major unwanted effects but the incidence of the major effects, although important, is relatively low:

Thromboembolism. The incidence of venous thromboembolic disease is increased by taking the combined oral contraceptive. The risk is independent of age or parity. The mechanism is complex but includes procoagulant activity from increased production of clotting factors X and II and decreased production of the protective antithrombin (Ch. 11). Fibrinolysis is impaired and reduced prostacyclin generation enhances platelet aggregation (Ch. 11). The risks associated with these changes are greatest in women who smoke, since smoking increases the risk of thrombogenesis. The baseline risk of venous thromboembolism in women of reproductive age is 5 or less per 100 000. In women taking second-generation pills it is 15 per 100 000 and in those taking pills containing gestodene and desogestrel (third-generation) it is 30 per 100 000. The risk in pregnancy is 60 per 100 000. It is still controversial whether the small increased risk of the third-generation pills is genuinely different from that of second-generation pills and it is now considered insufficiently secure to advise a change in oral contraceptive usage.

Ischaemic heart disease and stroke. Analysis of data in women largely taking the second-generation pills has indicated that there is no significantly increased risk of myocardial infarction for women who are non-smokers, irrespective of age. With third-generation pills containing gestodene or desogestrel it has recently been suggested that there may be less risk of arterial disease compared with second-generation pills. It is certain, however, that there is an increased risk of myocardial infarction and cerebrovascular disease in women taking the combined oral contraceptive who smoke and particularly those over the age of 35 years. Older smokers who also use the combined oral contraceptive have a six- to ten-fold increase in risk. This may be the result of adverse changes in the plasma lipoprotein profile when a combined preparation is used (see below). However, this mechanism is speculative, and it has been suggested that enhanced thrombogenesis rather than premature atherogenesis is responsible for the excess cardiovascular effects. If older women use the combined contraceptive pill, then the lowest possible dose of estrogen should be given. Whether a second- or third-generation progestogen should be advised is not clear. In older non-smokers mortality from cardiovascular disease associated with use of the oral contraceptive is approximately doubled.

Increase in blood pressure. A small increase in blood pressure is frequently found during use of the combined oral contraceptive but a significant rise can occur in about 5% of previously normotensive women; regular monitoring of blood pressure is important. A rise in blood pressure occurs in up to 15% of women with pre-existing hypertension. The mechanism is probably an increase in plasma renin activity (Ch. 6) produced by estrogen and to a lesser extent progestogen. Blood pressure may remain elevated for some months after the combined contraceptive is stopped.

Cancer. Oral contraceptives reduce the risk of endometrial and ovarian cancers, but the effect on the incidence of cervical cancer is uncertain. Recent evidence suggests that there is little or no effect. Despite numerous studies the question of an association between combined oral contraceptives and breast cancer remains unresolved; any risk is, however, small.

Nausea, mastalgia, depression, headache and provocation of migraine can occur. They are probably related to the estrogen content of the pill and can often be minimised by prescribing contraceptives with a low estrogen content.

Breakthrough bleeding occurs frequently in some women while in others withdrawal bleeding fails to occur. Gestodene-containing pills or triphasic preparations probably give the best cycle control. Amenorrhoea after stopping the combined contraceptive can last beyond a few months in about 5% of women and a small number can experience amenorrhoea for more than a year. A history of irregular periods before taking the pill increases the chance of prolonged amenorrhoea.

Metabolic effects. Estrogens alone increase protective plasma HDL cholesterol but their combination with progestogens in the second-generation pills reduces HDL cholesterol possibly due to the effect of the progestogen component (see also Ch. 48). These factors, together with impaired glucose tolerance, hyperinsulinaemia, and clotting factor changes, have been implicated in the genesis of cardiovascular disease. Some of the changes relate to the dose of estrogen used and these have been addressed by lowering the estrogen concentration and modifying the progestogen content. The concerns about the estrogen component of the contraceptive pills and cardiovascular disease are difficult to equate with the in vitro effects of estrogens which increase vascular prostacyclin and nitric oxide synthesis, inhibit platelet adhesion and suppress smooth muscle cell proliferation. Estrogens also reduce cholesterol accumulation in the arterial walls of cholesterol-fed animals. Some progestogens such as norethisterone and medoxyprogesterone acetate may oppose the beneficial effects of estrogens on the arterial wall. With the second-generation pills, the induced metabolic changes are thought to have little impact if individuals with pre-existing cardiovascular disease or older smokers are excluded from analyses. The third-generation pills containing gestodene and desogestrel probably do increase plasma triglycerides but, unlike the progestogens in the second-generation pills, elevate HDL cholesterol. Although the latter could be advantageous, the effect may be illusory as there is little evidence that the second-generation pills promote atherosclerosis. There is also little evidence for a lesser effect of gestogene or desogestrel on carbohydrate metabolism when compared with levonorgestrel.

Increased skin pigmentation can occur in some women given estrogens. The androgenic progestogens can sometimes cause or aggravate hirsutism and acne or produce weight gain. In patients with hyperandrogen-aemia, the third-generation pills would be preferred as gestogene and desogestrel have little androgenic activity.

Effects on the liver are occasionally seen. Cholestatic jaundice can be produced by progestogens, and estrogens increase the risk of gallstones.

Drug interactions

Drugs that alter the metabolism of oestrogen may cause a reduction in the efficacy of the combined pill which may result in breakthrough bleeding and contraceptive failure. Contraception failure may also occur in patients treated with anticonvulsants (e.g. barbiturates or phenytoin) or rifampicin which induce liver cytochrome P450 enzymes (Ch. 2), and some antibiotics, for example ampicillin (Ch. 51), which alter the gut flora and thereby decrease the enterohepatic circulation of the oestrogen. A pill containing 50 μg of ethinylestradiol should be used if these drugs are given long-term, and alternative methods of contraception should be used for the duration of a course of antimicrobials and for 7 days after (4 weeks in the case of rifampicin).

Non-contraceptive uses of the combined oral contraceptive

The combined contraceptive can be used:

- to reduce excessive blood loss from menorrhagia
- to reduce the pain of dysmenorrhoea
- to treat premenstrual tension
- to treat endometriosis

Hormone replacement therapy (HRT)

Treatment with estrogens during the peri- and postmenopausal period is often advocated to try to reverse the effects of oestrogen deficiency. Benefits of HRT include:

Relief of symptoms. These include vasomotor instability (hot flushes and night sweats), and altered sexual and urinary function. Vasomotor instability results from resetting of the hypothalamic temperature set-point so that it perceives that the body is warmer than it is. Vasodilation and sweating result in an attempt to disperse heat. The mechanism is uncertain but may be due to high concentrations of gonadotrophic hormones. Loss of connective tissue in the vagina and trigone of the bladder underlies many of the other problems. Other postmenopausal symptoms such as irritability and depression are less certainly related to oestrogen deficiency.

Prevention of long-term effects of oestrogen withdrawal. Bone loss leading to osteoporosis (Ch. 42) and an increased susceptibility to fracture occur after the menopause. Cardiovascular and cerebrovascular disease are also increased. The cause of the increased cardiovascular disease is uncertain. Unfavourable changes in lipids may be part of the explanation, due to a reduced HDL_2 cholesterol subfraction and increased LDL cholesterol (Ch. 48). However, an independent effect of oestrogen in reducing plasma fibrinogen (a factor in thrombogenesis) may be more important.

Unopposed oestrogens (i.e. without progestogen) in postmenopausal women reduce the risk of cardiovascular disease and stroke by about 50%, and it appears that combined estrogen/progestogen preparations also offer protection. Oestrogen receptors are found on the cells of the arterial wall, and stimulation decreases arterial resistance and increases vessel compliance which may also be important.

Oral administration

If treatment is given for more than a few weeks to a woman who has a uterus, then progestogen treatment is also needed for 12 days each calendar month or continuously if withdrawal bleeding is to be avoided. The majority of oral preparations contain the natural estradiol-17β as the oestrogen although the synthetic estrogen, mestranol, is also available. Preparations with conjugated equine oestrogens are also available. The progestogen used is synthetic norethisterone or levonorgestrel. Oral estrogen replacement will also reduce the symptoms of postmenopausal estrogen deficiency although relief may take up to 3 months. Treatment for symptom relief probably should be given for at least 6 months to perimenopausal women, after which withdrawal can be attempted to see if symptoms have spontaneously resolved. The duration of treatment for the prevention of osteoporosis (between 5 and 10 years) is discussed in Chapter 42.

Another approach to management of menopausal problems is to give oral tibolone, a synthetic molecule with combined weak oestrogenic, progestogenic and andogenic properties. Tibolone reduces the risk of withdrawal bleeding and progestogenic unwanted effects (see below). Taken continuously, it reduces postmenopausal symptoms and prevents bone loss. Vaginal bleeding can occur in women who still produce some endogenous oestrogen and therefore tibolone is usually reserved for patients who are at least one year postmenopausal.

Raloxifene is a newer selective oestrogen-receptor modulator with tissue specificity. This drug has oestrogen-receptor agonist effects on bone and liver but not on the breast and reproductive tissues. It is, therefore,

reserved for reduction of the risk of osteoporosis and does not reduce menopausal vasomotor symptoms.

Vaginal application

Estrogen cream (usually estradiol-17β) or pessaries can be used to treat vaginal atrophy and dyspareunia and can relieve perimenopausal urinary symptoms such as frequency and dysuria. Considerable systemic absorption occurs with some formulations, and oral progestogen may be needed. Creams or pessaries are used daily for 2–3 weeks initially and then applied twice weekly for as long as required.

Subcutaneous implants

Estradiol can be surgically implanted as pellets which release drug for up to 6 months. The major use for this option is when compliance is poor, perhaps because of nausea with oral estrogen. Oral progestogen must also be given for 10–12 days each month if the woman has a uterus, and continued for up to 2 years after stopping estrogen to prevent vaginal bleeding from persistent high estrogen levels.

Transdermal administration

A variety of patch-delivered steroids are available. In some preparations, estrogen alone is delivered by patches twice weekly for 2 weeks followed by patches for 2 weeks delivering estrogen plus progestogen. In some regimens, progestogen is delivered orally while continuing with the patch-delivered estrogen. Patches delivering continuous estrogen plus progestogen (norethisterone) are also available. Avoidance of first-pass metabolism means that a lower dose of progestogen can be used transdermally, which might reduce unwanted effects. Estradiol gels applied twice daily are also available and require 12 days progestogen per month in women with a uterus.

Unwanted effects

- Breakthrough bleeding can be troublesome, but regular withdrawal bleeds during the cycle are common and may be preceded by symptoms of premenstrual tension.
- Breast pain and abdominal or leg cramps due to the estrogen or progestogen component.

- Nausea and vomiting, most commonly with ethinylestradiol.
- Depression, irritability, loss of energy and poor concentration due to progestogen.
- The effect of short-term use of HRT on the risk of breast cancer is very low. For longer-term administration there is an increased risk. Taking HRT for 10 years leads to a 35% increase in the risk of developing breast cancer. This needs to be considered alongside evidence that between the ages of 65 and 74 a woman has a 6% risk of dying from ischaemic heart disease but a 1% risk of dying from breast cancer. It appears that HRT does not increase the risk of dying from breast cancer and may, in fact, improve the prognosis. This appears to be because if breast cancer does develop it is less severe.
- Increased risk of other cancers such as endometrial hyperplasia, which can be prevented by the use of progestogens.

Benefits and risks of hormone replacement therapy

The benefits and risks of hormone replacement therapy are highly individual for the patient. Overall, there is reduced mortality in women who use hormones post-menopausally compared with non-users; the benefits, however, appear to diminish with the length of time of use. The major reason for benefit in recent users is the decrease in death from coronary heart disease. However, although it is clear that women with a high risk of coronary heart disease benefit from hormone replacement therapy, it is unclear whether protection is afforded to women who have already developed coronary heart disease. Although there is some suggestion that progesterone may reduce those effects, at least in vitro, it does appear that cardiovascular protection is afforded equally by combined therapy, as well as with estrogens alone.

Hormone replacement therapy also clearly reduces the risk of osteoporotic fractures (Ch. 42).

The debate continues about which women should be offered hormone replacement therapy and the length of time for which they should take it. The future may be brighter, with limitations on the length of time for which women should take hormone replacement therapy while supplementing its use with other non-steroidal and non-medicinal treatments.

The onset and induction of labour

The aetiology of the induction of labour in women is still uncertain (Fig. 45.3). The actual onset may be multi-

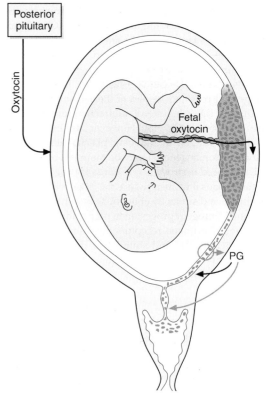

Fig. 45.3
Induction of labour. Prostaglandin (PG) is synthesised by the amnion and the decidua and can act to stimulate the uterus and soften the cervix. Although PG and fetal and maternal oxytocin may be involved in the processes of labour, their role in the initiation of labour is uncertain.

factorial in nature and it is probable that prostaglandins, oxytocin, progesterone, oestrogen and corticosteroids are among the agents involved.

Prostaglandins

Prostaglandin $F_{2\alpha}$ and E_2 have many actions that could contribute to labour. They are synthesised by the cells of the amnion and decidua. The levels of these prostaglandins increase progressively in the amniotic fluid during labour and have been shown to be elevated before the discernible onset of labour. The uterine sensitivity to prostaglandins increases at term when it is approximately 10-fold higher than in earlier pregnancy. The contractility of the uterus during labour commences at the uterotubular junction and progresses through the body of the uterus to the cervix, thus promoting efficient labour. This type of contractile pattern, which is not seen in early pregnancy, is caused by prostaglandins and oestrogens promoting the synthesis of gap junctions. These are specialised connections between the smooth muscle cells allowing excitatory impulses to pass between cells. Only in uterine muscle cells that are rich in gap junctions can the 'right type' of uterine contractility occur and result in efficient progress of labour. The progesterone-dominated uterus has few gap junctions. Prostaglandins also increase gap junctions and increase the synthesis of oxytocin from the posterior pituitary. Prostaglandin E_2 softens the cervix, an essential prerequisite for the smooth passage of labour. Indometacin has been used experimentally to inhibit preterm labour in limited trials. The concern in using indometacin is its ability to close the ductus arteriosus prematurely in the fetus by inhibiting prostaglandin synthesis. Prostglandin E_2 also increases the synthesis of oxytocin from the posterior pituitary.

Oxytocin

Oxytocin is a peptide produced by the posterior pituitary. It has a marked uterotonic action at term but is much less effective earlier in pregnancy. The reason for this is that there is a marked increase in the expression of uterine oxytocin receptors from about 35 weeks of pregnancy onwards. Oxytocin levels in the maternal circulation do not increase during labour until the second stage. There are, interestingly, higher levels of oxytocin in the fetal circulation than in the mother during labour. Inhibitors of the oxytocin receptor have been produced and limited data suggest partial usefulness in the inhibition of preterm labour.

Steroid hormones

Oestrogens and progesterone both increase during pregnancy, and overall the actions of oestradiol promote uterine contractility while those of progesterone diminish it. There is, however, little evidence to suggest that progesterone concentrations fall prior to the onset of labour; it has been suggested that this may occur at a uterine level but may not be reflected in the maternal circulation. Oestradiol increases the number of uterine oxytocin receptors and increases oxytocin release from the posterior pituitary. It increases gap junctions, and fundal dominance of uterine contractility is increased by an effect on the functional pacemaker at the uterotubular junction. Oestradiol increases the synthesis of prostaglandins and increases the sensitivity of the uterus to their effects. Oestradiol also has a softening effect on the cervix. In contrast, progesterone decreases gap junctions and diminishes pacemaker activity. It also decreases the sensitivity of the uterus to oxytocin and prostaglandins.

Drugs used for inducing labour

Oxytocin and prostaglandins are the only drugs used to induce labour.

Oxytocin

Oxytocin is used for the induction of labour and to augment contractions in inadequate labour. It is given by slow intravenous infusion to induce labour. The concentration given depends upon the response of the patient: the aim is to produce regular coordinated contractions at intervals of approximately 1½–2 minutes with complete relaxation between contractions. Oxytocin is an effective uterine stimulant in women at term, and labour will usually proceed well if the cervix is partially dilated and softened prior to its use. Inappropriately high concentrations of oxytocin can cause hypertonus in which the uterus does not relax between contractions and fetal distress can occur. As labour progresses and the woman's 'endogenous' induction mechanisms come into play the concentration of oxytocin may need to be reduced. Following delivery, postpartum haemorrhage can be reduced by increasing the concentration of oxytocin or giving oxytocin combined with ergometrine intramuscularly (syntometrine) (see below). Oxytocin, unlike prostaglandins, does not soften the cervix and is now often used after intravaginal prostaglandin has been given for this purpose (see below). Oxytocin in high doses has a weak antidiuretic activity as it is related to vasopressin (Ch. 43).

Prostaglandins

Prostaglandin (dinoprostone) causes contractions of both the non-pregnant and the pregnant uterus. Like oxytocin, in correct doses it can produce contractions that are indistinguishable from spontaneous labour. Prostaglandins have the advantage, however, of softening the cervix. Thus, they can be used for induction of labour before term. Dinoprostone (prostaglandin E_2) is given as vaginal tablets, pessaries or gels for induction of labour or for priming of the uterus prior to rupture of membranes and induction by oxytocin. Insertion of dinoprostone suppositories is frequently accompanied by uterine contractions; in some women it will only result in cervix softening whereas others will go into labour. Extra-amniotic and intravenous prostaglandin E_2 is now far less commonly used for induction of labour. Prostaglandin $F_{2\alpha}$ (dinoprost) is rarely used.

Carboprost (15-methyl $PGF_{2\alpha}$) is used for reduction of postpartum haemorrhage (see below) but not for induction of labour. Gemeprost (a PGE_1 analogue) is used for the induction of abortion (see below) and is not licensed for labour induction.

Prostaglandins are also given for the induction of labour in women after intrauterine death of the fetus.

Unwanted effects

- Hypertonus
- Gastrointestinal disturbances, particularly diarrhoea.

Postpartum haemorrhage

Following delivery of the baby, postpartum haemorrhage can be reduced by increasing the concentrations of oxytocin being administered or by giving the prostaglandin analogue, carboprost. This causes marked hypertonic concentration of the uterus and compresses intrauterine blood vessels. Ergometrine can be given together with oxytocin or alone for the reduction of postpartum haemorrhage. It should not be used for induction of labour as it causes hypertonic contractions of the uterus and fetal distress. The action of ergometrine on the uterus is partially through α-adrenoceptors and it, therefore, also produces vasoconstriction which limits haemorrhage.

Pharmacokinetics

Ergometrine can be given intramuscularly or intravenously.

Unwanted effects

- Vomiting
- Peripheral vasoconstriction.

Induction of abortion

Prostaglandins are widely used for the induction of abortion. In the *second trimester* their use results in fewer complications than dilatation and curettage or other surgical techniques. Prostaglandin E_2 (dinoprostone), given most commonly by the extra-amniotic route, or gemeprost (prostaglandin E_1 analogue), given by the intravaginal route, are used for the medical induction of late therapeutic abortion. The mechanism of action of these drugs is to produce prolonged uterine contraction. Gemeprost is also given as a pessary to ripen and soften the cervix prior to surgical abortion.

Mifepristone

Mechanism of action and uses

Mifepristone is a potent antiprogestogen and antiglucocorticoid. It is an increasingly important drug used for the termination of early and mid-trimester pregnancy given in combination with the prostaglandin E_1 analogue, gemeprost. In early pregnancy, up to 63 days of gestation, mifepristone is given as a single dose followed 36–48 hours later by gemeprost. The same technique is used for late termination of pregnancy. The action of mifepristone is to significantly reduce the interval from induction to abortion after the prostaglandins are given, by virtue of its antiprogestogenic actions.

Mifepristone also has a softening effect on the uterine cervix and can be used for cervical ripening prior to the induction of labour at term, although it is not licensed in the UK for this purpose.

Since mifepristone has an antiglucocorticoid activity, it can be used in the treatment of Cushing's syndrome (Ch. 44).

Pharmacokinetics

Mifepristone is orally absorbed and metabolised slowly by the liver generating an active metabolite. The half-life is, therefore, long.

Unwanted effects

Unwanted effects include nausea, vomiting and abdominal pain.

Uterine relaxants and preterm labour

Prematurity is the largest cause of neonatal morbidity, and mortality and we are very poor at preventing it.

β_2-Adrenoceptor agonists

Examples: terbutaline, ritodrine, salbutamol

β_2-Stimulants inhibit uterine contractility in the short term, enabling treatment with corticosteroids to enhance lung maturation (Ch. 13).

Overall analysis has shown that the use of β_2-adrenoceptor agonists has not improved fetal morbidity or mortality. They have been administered intravenously, or by inhaler or by slow infusion pumps. They are generally only effective for inhibiting preterm labour for about 48 hours. Unwanted effects include fetal and maternal tachycardia (see also Ch. 12).

Other agents for preterm labour

Magnesium sulfate is widely used in the USA for treating women in preterm labour. It may work by inhibiting Ca^{2+} availability. It is as effective as β_2-adrenoceptor agonists. Unwanted effects are minor.

Limited studies have also claimed effectiveness for calcium channel antagonists, indometacin and oxytocin receptor antagonists, although their effectiveness is mainly short-term and studies are generally too small to allow firm conclusions.

Uterine and vaginal infection is also thought to be an important risk factor for preterm labour in a subgroup of women, and some data have demonstrated the effectiveness of antimicrobials in delaying delivery.

Dysmenorrhoea

Primary dysmenorrhoea (pain associated with menstruation) is of unknown aetiology; many explanations have been proposed including uterine hyperactivity, prostaglandin or leukotriene generation and excessive production of vasopressin. Excess prostaglandin concentrations have been measured in endometrial curettings. A variety of non-steroidal anti-inflammatory drugs have been used for the relief of dysmenorrhoea including ibuprofen, indometacin and mefenamic acid. All NSAIDs are useful for the relief of primary dysmenorrhoea, with approximately 70% of patients being relieved of their symptoms. However, there are differences among the NSAIDs which are poorly understood and the efficacy in dysmenorrhoea does not seem to be simply related to their analgesic activity.

The combined oral contraceptive and the progestogen-only pill are effective in reducing symptoms of dysmenorrhoea. Small studies also suggest that calcium channel antagonists and β_2-adrenoceptor agonists have some beneficial effect.

Menorrhagia

Excessive menstrual blood loss is a common gynaecological problem. Menstrual loss can be reduced variably by NSAIDs (Ch. 29), and numerous different NSAIDs have been used. They are administered only during the time of menstruation. The combined oral contraceptive and the progestogen-only contraceptives can also reduce excessive menstrual loss. For the progestogen-only pill to be useful, it has to be administered for 3 weeks at a fairly high dose. A more effective way of administering the progestogen is from an intrauterine contraceptive device, where reduction in blood loss of up to 90% can be expected within a 12 month period.

The antifibrinolytic agent, tranexamic acid (Ch. 11), can also reduce blood loss by up to 50%. Its effect is rapid in onset and therapy is only required during the menstruation period. Unwanted effects are gastrointestinal upsets and headaches.

FURTHER READING

Chamberlain G, Zander L (1999) Induction. *Br Med J* 318, 995–998

Clinical Synthesis Panel on HRT (1999) Hormone replacement therapy. *Lancet* 354, 152–155

Greendale GA, Lee NP, Arriola ER (1999) The menopause. *Lancet* 353, 571–580

Mendelsohn ME, Karas RH (1999) The protective effects of estrogen on the cardiovascular system. *N Engl J Med* 340, 1801–1811

Mitlak BH, Cohen JF (1999) Selective estrogen receptor modulators. *Drugs* 57, 653–663

Norwitz ER, Robinson JN, Shallis JRG (1999) The control of labor. *N Engl J Med* 341, 660–666.

O'Brien PA (1999) The third generation oral contraceptive controversy. *Br Med J* 319, 795–796

Prentice A (1999) Medical management of menorrhagia. *Br Med J* 319, 1343–1345

Self-assessment

In the following questions the first statement, in italics, is true. Are the accompanying statements also true?

1. *The mid-cycle surge in LH and FSH is essential for ovulation to occur.*

   a. Oestrogen has a negative feedback effect on LH and FSH secretion from the anterior pituitary throughout the follicular phase.
   b. The elevated level of progesterone in the secretory phase is under the control of gonadotrophins.

2. *Progesterone causes cervical mucus to be viscous and hostile to the passage of sperm. This is an important contraceptive action of the oral progestogen-only pill.*

   a. The oral progestogen-only pill inhibits ovulation in 90% of women.
   b. Both oestrogen and progesterone inhibit the motility of the fallopian tube, altering the rate of transport of sperm and the oocyte.
   c. The functioning corpus luteum is essential for the maintenance of pregnancy for about the first 6–8 weeks following implantation.

3. *The second generation of combined contraceptives refers to those that have low concentrations of ethinylestradiol and generally either levonorgestrel or norethisterone as the progestogenic component. The third generation of combined contraceptives contains the progestogens gestodene or desogestrel.*

   a. There is little to choose between the different progestogens in contraceptive pills in terms of their androgenic activity.
   b. The combined oral contraceptives administered in a biphasic or triphasic pattern result in the overall administration of less estrogen and progestogen.
   c. Plasma concentrations of administered ethinylestradiol are reduced because ethinylestradiol undergoes substantial first-pass metabolism.
   d. With the combined oral contraceptive pill and the progestogen-only pill, effective protection may be lost if there is a delay of more than 12 h in taking the daily dose.

4. *The antimicrobials rifampicin and ampicillin can lower the effective concentrations of ethinylestradiol in the plasma.*

   a. Antiepilepsy drugs such as carbamazepine can reduce the plasma concentrations of estrogens and progestogens.

5. *There is no significant increased risk of myocardial infarction irrespective of age in women who are non-smokers taking the combined contraceptive pill.*

   a. Mortality from venous thromboembolism is increased in women who smoke, particularly those over the age of 35 years.
   b. The second- and third-generation oral contraceptives can decrease glucose tolerance.

6. *In women who have not had a hysterectomy, unopposed estrogen treatment can result in endometrial hyperplasia and an increased risk of endometrial cancer.*

   a. Postmenopausal women taking continuous therapy containing both estrogen and protestogens do not experience breakthrough bleeding.
   b. Estrogens and progestogens can be given by skin patches to reduce the level of first-pass metabolism.
   c. Raloxifene is a selective estrogen receptor modulating agent.
   d. Tibolone reduces bone loss in postmenopausal women.

7. *Unlike oxytocin, the prostaglandins have a softening effect on the cervix.*

   a. Oxytocin is preferred to prostaglandins for the induction of labour in a patient at 34 weeks' gestation.
   b. Progesterone increases the number of gap junctions in the uterus.
   c. Natural prostaglandins are produced from the posterior pituitary during labour.

8. *For the induction of abortion, mifepristone should be given 24–48 h before the administration of prostaglandins.*

   a. Prostaglandins given for the induction of labour do not produce hypertonic uterine activity.
   b. Ergometrine can be used for the induction of labour.

9. *Non-steroidal anti-inflammatory drugs are used in treating dysmenorrhoea.*

   a. The combined oral contraceptive is ineffective for relieving the symptoms of dysmenorrhoea.

10. *β_2-adrenoceptor agonists do not reduce fetal mortality or morbidity in preterm labour.*

    a. Magnesium sulfate inhibits uterine motility.

The answers are provided on pages 626–627.

Drugs acting on the female reproductive system

Drug	Half-life (h)	Elimination	Comments
Estrogens			
Conjugated estrogen equine	–	Metabolism	Given as sulfate conjugates of 10+ equine estrogens; absorbed intact and after hydrolysis; excreted as sulfate conjugates
Estradiol	1	Metabolism	Metabolised to estrone, which undergoes P450 oxidation
Estradiol valerate	–	Metabolism	Assumed to be a prodrug for estradiol
Ethinylestradiol	8–24	Metabolism	Oxidation plus direct conjugation with glucuronic acid and sulfate
Mestranol	8–24	Metabolism	>50% is converted to ethinylestradiol
Progestogens			
Desogestrel	30	Metabolism	P450 oxidation in gut wall and liver
Dydrogesterone	6	Metabolism	Oxidation, plus reduction to 2α-dihydro analogue (which retains activity)
Gestodene	18	Metabolism	Undergoes oxidation plus reduction reactions; oxidation of ethynyl ($-C{\equiv}CH$) side chain causes 'suicide inactivation' of CYP3A4
Hydroxyprogesterone hexanoate	2–11	Metabolism	Activity is due to the hexanoate (caproate) ester; hydroxyprogesterone is almost without activity
Levonorgestrel	8–30	Metabolism	Reduction plus oxidation followed by conjugation
Medroxyprogesterone acetate	30	Metabolism	Oxidation and reduction reactions to give 26 essentially inactive metabolites
Norethisterone	5–12	Metabolism	Major route is reduction of unsaturated A ring, and ketone to a saturated 3-hydroxymetabolite
Norethisterone acetate	–	Hydrolysis	Prodrug of norethisterone
Norgestimate	–	Metabolism	Active metabolites include the 17-deacetyl compound ($t\frac{1}{2} = 16$–17 h), the 3-keto analogue and levonorgestrel
Norgestrel	See levonorgestrel		
Progesterones used primarily for endometriosis			
Danazol	3	Metabolism	Antigonadotropic effects are due to parent drug
Gestrinone	27	Metabolism	Oxidation to less active products which are excreted as conjugates
Gonadorelin	4 minutes	Metabolism+renal	Complex peptide given by intravenous injection (half-life may reflect tissue distribution and binding at therapeutic doses rather than excretion and metabolism)
Gonadorelin analogues			
Buserelin	3–6 minutes	Metabolism+excretion	Complex peptide (see above concerning half-life)
Goserelin	4	Metabolism	Complex peptide; metabolised by cell peptidases
Leuprorelin acetate (Leurprolide)	3	Metabolism	Complex peptide; metabolised by proteases
Nafarelin	4	Metabolism	Slow hydrolysis; inactive metabolites have long half-lives (85 h)
Triptorelin	3	Metabolism	(Kinetic data are for male subjects)
Drugs used for menopausal vagal symptoms/osteoporosis			
Raloxifene	28	Metabolism	Undergoes extensive first-pass conjugation with glucuronic acid and enterohepatic recycling
Tibolone	Unknown	Metabolism	Reduction of 3-keto group, and isomerisation

continued

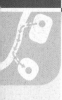

Drugs acting on the female reproductive system *(continued)*

Drug	Half-life (h)	Elimination	Comments
Antiestrogens (induce gonadotropin release)			
Clomiphene	? days	Metabolism	Clomiphene exists as 2-isomers of which the Z (*cis*) is active and the E (*trans*) is inactive; Z-isomer is eliminated more slowly and is detectable in plasma one month after treatment
Drugs used to treat mastalgia (see also bromocriptine and danazol)			
Gamolenic acid	–	Metabolism	Rapidly metabolised to dihomogammalenolenic acid and incorporated into membranes and lipid metabolism
Prostaglandins and oxytocics			
Carboprost	–	–	No published kinetic data
Dinoprostone (PGE$_2$)	30 seconds	Metabolism	Dehydrogenation
Ergometrine	2	Metabolism	Massive interindividual variability after oral dosage
Gemeprost	–	Metabolism	Systemic half-life not known; very rapidly hydrolysed (within minutes) and subsequently oxidised
Oxytocin	2–10 minutes	Metabolism	Rapid metabolism via reduction of the intramolecular disulfide bond followed by peptidase hydrolysis
Drugs used for effects on ductus arteriosus			
Alprostadil (PGE$_1$)	30 seconds	Metabolism	Maintains patency; metabolised by dehydrogenation
Indometacin	3–5	Metabolism	Causes closure; metabolised by conjugation and oxidation
Drugs used primarily for therapeutic abortions			
Mifepristone	12–72	Bile+metabolism	Undergoes extensive enterohepatic recycling
Myometrial relaxant drugs			
Ritodrine	15–20	Metabolism	Conjugation with sulfate and glucuronic acid
Salbutamol (albuterol)	3–5	Metabolism+renal	Conjugation with sulfate
Terbutaline	14–18	Metabolism+renal	Conjugation with sulfate

46

Androgens and anabolic steroids

Androgens

Naturally occurring androgens are 19-carbon steroids synthesised in the adrenal cortex and gonads. They have characteristic actions on the reproductive tract and other tissues as well as an anabolic effect on metabolism. A number of synthetic androgenic steroids have been developed. When the predominant action of these molecules is anabolic rather than on reproductive tissues the substance is described as an 'anabolic steroid'. Although there are a few medical uses for such compounds, they have achieved notoriety because of their abuse by athletes to enhance muscle development.

Testosterone is the most powerful and major androgen secreted by the Leydig cells of the testis when stimulated by the gonadotrophin luteinising hormone (Ch. 43). The adrenal cortex, stimulated by ACTH, releases a greater proportion of dehydroepiandrosterone and androstenedione (Fig. 44.2).

Testosterone

Actions of testosterone
The actions of testosterone are in part due to its metabolite dihydrotestosterone. The latter is produced in the prostate, skin and reproductive tissues by the action of the enzyme 5α-reductase. Dihydrotestosterone has a higher affinity for the androgen receptor than testosterone. Actions include:

- Sexual differentiation in the fetus.
- Sexual development of the male testis, penis, epididymis, seminal vesicles and prostate at puberty, and maintenance of these tissues in the adult.
- Spermatogenesis in the adult.
- Stimulation and maintenance of sexual function and behaviour.
- Metabolic actions. Testosterone is a powerful anabolic agent producing a positive nitrogen balance with an increase in the bulk of tissues such as muscle and bone. In the skin sebum production is increased, which can provoke acne. Growth of axillary, pubic, facial and chest hair is stimulated. In the liver, testosterone increases the synthesis of several proteins including clotting factors, but decreases high-density lipoprotein (HDL) synthesis

(Ch. 48). Testosterone also induces several liver enzymes including steroid hydroxylases.

- Haematological actions. Testosterone stimulates production of erythropoietin by the kidneys leading to a higher haemoglobin concentration in men than women.

Pharmacokinetics

Oral preparations. Testosterone is well absorbed from the gut but is almost completely degraded by first-pass metabolism in the gut wall and liver. Esterification to form 17-β hydroxyl derivatives creates a hydrophobic compound. Of these, testosterone undecanoate is absorbed via lacteals into the lymphatic system, thus avoiding hepatic metabolism. It can, therefore, be given orally.

Testosterone esters for depot injection. The most popular form of replacement therapy for hypogonadal men is a regular intramuscular injection of a testosterone ester in oily solution. Testosterone is absorbed gradually after ester hydrolysis at the site of injection. Examples include testosterone enanthate and testosterone propionate.

Transdermal delivery. A patch containing testosterone can be used to treat hypogonadism. It is usually applied to the back, abdomen, upper arm or thigh, rotating the site daily to avoid skin irritation.

Subcutaneous implant. A pellet of crystalline testosterone provides a reservoir for gradual absorption of testosterone into the systemic circulation for up to 4 months. A minor surgical procedure is necessary, and therefore this method of delivery is rarely used.

Circulating androgens are bound largely to a specific transport protein, sex hormone binding globulin (SHBG), which has a greater affinity for androgens than for oestrogen.

Unwanted effects

- In hypogonadal adolescents, initial nitrogen retention and a spurt in linear growth is followed by premature epiphyseal closure and short stature. A short course can be used for treatment of delayed puberty without inducing epiphyseal closure.
- Conversion to oestrogens by aromatase results in gynaecomastia in some patients (Fig. 44.2).
- Suppression of gonadotrophin release with diminished testis size and reduced spermatogenesis. Hypogonadal men will not regain fertility while taking androgens.
- Increased risk of prostate cancer.
- Cholestatic jaundice.

Clinical uses of testosterone

- The main clinical use for testosterone is as replacement therapy for primary hypogonadism in adult males.
- It can be used briefly in constitutionally delayed puberty even in the absence of hypogonadism.

- Androgens are occasionally beneficial in some forms of aplastic anaemia for promoting erythropoiesis.

Danazol

Mechanism of action

Danazol is an androgen derivative described as an 'impeded' androgen. It has little androgenic effect on peripheral tissues and is not convertible to an estrogen. Its main property is feedback inhibition of gonadotrophin and gonadotrophin-releasing hormone secretion.

Pharmacokinetics

Danazol is well absorbed orally, metabolised in the liver and has a short half-life.

Unwanted effects

Unwanted effects are mainly a consequence of the weak androgenic activity (see testosterone) and include nausea, skin reactions and mood changes.

Clinical uses of danazol

- To reduce gonadal activity in endometriosis, menorrhagia and premenstrual syndrome (particularly when mastalgia is a problem). It can produce a hypogonadal state, therefore treatment often cannot be prolonged.
- Long-term management of hereditary angioedema.

Anabolic steroids

Examples: nandrolone, stanozolol

Anabolic steroids are most frequently encountered as drugs of abuse to improve athletic performance. In medical practice there are few indications for these compounds with little evidence for efficacy. Stanozolol is given orally and nandrolone as an ester by intramuscular injections in a depot formulation.

Unwanted effects

- Androgenic effects may be troublesome in women.
- Stanozolol can cause cholestatic jaundice and liver tumours after long-term use.

Clinical uses

Nandrolone: the promotion of erythropoiesis in aplastic anaemias, or for the itching of chronic biliary obstruction in palliative care.

Stanozolol: for hereditary angioedema and for the vascular manifestations of Behçet's disease.

Abuse of anabolic steroids

The ability of androgens to promote an increase in muscle mass has led to their abuse to improve physical performance by athletes, weightlifters and body-builders. Often several different androgens are used for prolonged periods, perhaps with a brief 'drug-free' period. Abused compounds include testosterone, nandrolone, stanozolol and others licensed only for veterinary use. The consequences of abuse include:

- weight gain from muscle hypertrophy and fluid retention
- acne in adolescent and young men
- decreased testicular size and reduced sperm count
- hepatotoxicity with cholestasis, hepatitis or occasionally hepatocellular tumours
- atherogenic changes in the plasma lipids with a rise in plasma LDL cholesterol and a fall in HDL cholesterol (Ch. 48); this may predispose to premature vascular disease
- psychological disturbance including changes in libido, increased aggression and psychotic symptoms.

Antiandrogens

Cyproterone acetate

Mechanism of action

Cyproterone acetate, a 21-carbon steroid, is a progestogen, a weak glucocorticoid (Ch. 44), and at high doses has an inhibitory action on peripheral androgen receptors. Its progestational activity includes feedback inhibition of gonadotrophin secretion.

Pharmacokinetics

Cyproterone acetate is well absorbed orally, metabolised in the liver and has a long half-life of 2 days.

Unwanted effects

- Antiandrogenic effects, for example gynaecomastia.
- Inhibition of spermatogenesis.
- Reduction in libido and potency in males.
- Hepatotoxicity with long-term use causing hepatitis and occasionally hepatic failure.

Flutamide

Mechanism of action

Flutamide is a relatively pure antiandrogen without significant glucocorticoid or progestogenic actions.

Pharmacokinetics

Flutamide is well absorbed orally, metabolised in the liver and has a short half-life. The major metabolite 2-hydroxyflutamide is more active than the parent compound.

Unwanted effects

- Antiandrogenic effects, for example gynaecomastia.
- Gastrointestinal upset.
- Insomnia.

Clinical uses of antiandrogens

- The main use of antiandrogens is in the initial treatment of carcinoma of the prostate, usually in conjunction with a gonadorelin analogue (Chs 43, 45).
- Cyproterone acetate is used in male sexual offenders as 'chemical castration'.
- In females, cyproterone acetate can be given for manifestations of hyperandrogenisation such as acne and hirsutism which occur in polycystic ovary syndrome.

5α-Reductase inhibitors

Example: finasteride

Mechanism of action and effects

5α-Reductase is an enzyme associated with androgen-dependent target cells. It is responsible for the conversion of testosterone to dihydrotestosterone (DHT) which is the hormone responsible for prostatic growth. In the adult male finasteride can produce regression of benign prostatic hypertrophy and improve the symptoms of prostatism (Ch. 15).

FURTHER READING

Bagatell CJ, Bremner WJ (1996) Androgens in men – uses and abuses. *N Engl J Med* 334, 707–714

Franks S (1998) Polycystic ovary syndrome. *J Roy Col Phys Lond* 32, 111–113

Rittmaster RS (1994) Finasteride. *N Engl J Med* 330, 120–125

Self-assessment

In the following questions the first statement, in italics, is true. Are the accompanying statements also true?

1. *Mature men with androgen deficiency may have decreased libido, impotence, reduced muscle mass and reduced body hair.*

    a. Testosterone cannot be given orally.
    b. Testosterone alone cannot stimulate spermatogenesis.
    c. Nandrolone causes less virilisation than androgens in women.

2. *The antiandrogen cyproterone acetate is used as an adjunct to the treatment of prostate cancer and hirsutism.*

    a. Antiandrogens can cause gynaecomastia.

The answers are provided on page 627.

Drug	Half-life	Elimination	Comment
Androgens			
Danazol	3 hours	Metabolism	Clinical uses are *not* related to its weak androgenic activity (see text); given orally; metabolites are inactive
Mesterolone (methyltestosterone)	3 hours	Metabolism	Given orally; eliminated as glucuronides and sulfate conjugates; oral bioavailability is 50%
Testosterone and esters	See comments	Metabolism	Given orally (as undecanoate), by intramuscular injection (as enanthate or propionate), as an implant (as testosterone) or as patches (as testosterone); testosterone per se is inactive orally; testosterone is very rapidly cleared from blood and the different dosage methods act as 'sustained-release' preparations that maintain blood testosterone concentrations despite its rapid elimination
Anabolic steroids			
Nandrolone decanoate	5–17 days (from injection)	Metabolism	Given as deep intramuscular injection (sustained release – see testosterone); the in vivo half-life is dependent on release from the depot injection, since the half-life for hydrolysis and the elimination of nandrolone from the circulation is only 4 hours
Stanozolol	Human data not available	Metabolism	Given orally; metabolised by conjugation and oxidation; half-life probably short since dosage is usually once daily
Antiandrogens			
Bicalutamide	7–10 days	Metabolism	Given orally; undergoes oxidation and conjugation, with the metabolites eliminated in urine and bile
Cyproterone acetate	2 days	Metabolism	Given orally; hydrolysed and conjugated with glucuronic acid and sulfate; metabolites eliminated in urine and bile
Finasteride	6 hours	Metabolism	Given orally; metabolised by hepatic oxidation
Flutamide	8 hours	Metabolism	Given orally; essentially complete oral bioavailability; rapid oxidation in the liver to an active hydroxy metabolite
Nilutamide (approved in USA not EU)	40–60 hours	Metabolism	Given orally; high oral bioavailability; five metabolites have been identified, one of which retains activity

47

Anaemia and haematopoietic colony stimulating factors

Anaemia

The definition of anaemia is rather arbitrary; in adults it equates to a blood concentration of haemoglobin below 135 g l^{-1} (normal $\simeq$ 154 g l^{-1}) in males or 115 g l^{-1} (normal $\simeq$ 135 g l^{-1}) in females. Lower concentrations can be normal in children. Anaemia causes symptoms such as shortness of breath and fatigue. Many individuals, however, have concentrations below these arbitrary values without apparent detriment. There are many causes of anaemia (Box 47.1).

Anaemias are classified by red cell size and haemoglobin content (Box 47.2).

Iron

Dietary iron is absorbed from the duodenum and upper jejunum. Absorption of iron occurs readily as haem, especially from meat sources; non-haem iron is inefficiently absorbed. Most dietary iron is in the ferric form although ferrous iron is more readily absorbed; conversion of ferric to ferrous iron is aided by reducing agents such as ascorbic acid and amino acids such as cysteine, while gastric acid increases the solubility of non-haem iron. Dietary vegetables contain ligands that make iron less soluble and reduce its absorption. Absorption of iron is substantially increased in iron deficiency.

Box 47.1

Causes of anaemia

Reduced red cell production
    Defective precursor proliferation, e.g. iron deficiency, anaemia of chronic disorders, marrow aplasia or infiltration
    Defective precursor maturation, e.g. vitamin B$_{12}$ or folate deficiency, myelodysplastic syndrome, toxins
Increased rate of red cell destruction
    Haemolysis
Loss of circulating red cells
    Bleeding

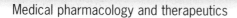

Box 47.2

Classification of anaemias by red cell characteristics

Hypochromic, microcytic (small size cells)
    Genetic, e.g. thalassaemia, sideroblastic anaemia
    Acquired, e.g. iron deficiency, sideroblastic anaemia
Normochromic, macrocytic (large size cells)
    With megaloblastic marrow: vitamin B_{12} or folate
       deficiency
    With normoblastic marrow: alcohol, myelodysplasia
Polychromatophilic, macrocytic
    Haemolysis
Normochromic, normocytic (normal size cells)
    Chronic disorders, e.g. infection, malignancy, autoimmune
       disease
    Renal failure
    Bone marrow failure

In the circulation, ferric iron is bound to the globulin transferrin and transported to the bone marrow and iron stores. Cellular iron uptake occurs via transferrin receptors. Intracellular iron is stored as a complex with the protein ferritin. Two-thirds of the iron in the body is present in circulating red cells. When ageing red cells are broken down by the reticuloendothelial system, the released iron is recycled.

Iron deficiency

The main cause of iron deficiency in the UK is abnormal loss of blood, particularly from the gut or exaggerated menstrual loss. Iron malabsorption can result from disease of the upper small intestine, for example coeliac disease, or following partial gastrectomy. Dietary deficiency is rarely a major cause in Western societies, but worldwide a vegetarian diet low in absorbable iron is the commonest contributory cause of iron deficiency.

Therapeutic iron preparations

Oral iron

Oral supplements are preferred and are given as ferrous salts, for example sulfate, fumarate or gluconate. Tablets are normally used but some patients find a syrup more acceptable. A daily dose of 200 mg of elemental iron produces the maximum rate of rise of haemoglobin; about one-third of this dose will be absorbed. Intolerance to oral iron is common, but unwanted effects can be minimised by taking iron supplements with food or by reducing the dose. Modified-release iron formulations have been developed to improve tolerance but much of the iron is released beyond the site where it is best absorbed. These formulations should only be used when other methods for improving iron tolerance are ineffective.

Unwanted effects

Unwanted effects include gastrointestinal intolerance, especially nausea and dyspepsia. The prevalence of these effects depends on both the dose of elemental iron and on psychological factors, rather than the iron salt used. There may also be diarrhoea or constipation; these are not dose-related. Patients should be warned that oral iron will turn their stools black.

Parenteral iron

Parenteral iron preparations are used for patients with intractable unwanted effects from oral preparations, those with severe uncorrectable malabsorption or with continuing heavy blood loss, and when compliance with oral treatment is poor. Parenteral iron does not raise the haemoglobin concentration any faster than oral iron.

Intramuscular: iron–sorbitol–citric acid

This complexed iron preparation is rapidly absorbed from a deep intramuscular injection site. Transferrin is saturated by high blood iron concentrations and about one-third of the iron is lost in urine, which may darken on standing. Approximately 30% is incorporated into red cells, the remainder of the retained iron being stored by macrophages in liver, bone marrow, spleen, etc. Between 10 and 20 injections are required over a 2–3 week period.

Unwanted effects

- Staining of the skin at the injection site
- Metallic taste
- Pain at the injection site
- Arthralgia.

Intravenous: iron–dextran

Iron–dextran is not bound to transferrin but accumulates in reticuloendothelial cells. It is usually given as a 'total dose' intravenous infusion, when the approximate total body deficit (haemoglobin and body stores) is estimated from the patient's size and haemoglobin concentration then replaced with a single slow iron infusion. Iron–dextran complex can be used intramuscularly but is very slowly absorbed from the injection site. Iron–dextran is only available by special supply on a 'named patient' basis in the UK.

Unwanted effects

Minor unwanted effects include flushing, headache, bronchospasm, diffuse pains and urticaria.

There may be anaphylactoid reactions including cardiovascular collapse. Facilities for resuscitation should always be available.

Therapeutic use of iron

The cause of iron deficiency should always be sought before resorting to symptomatic treatment with iron. If this is not done, serious disorders such as gastrointestinal malignancy can be overlooked. Oral iron supplements are adequate for most patients with mild or moderate iron deficiency anaemia, and, after an initial delay of a few days, should raise the haemoglobin concentration by about 1 g l^{-1} per day. After the haemoglobin concentration has been restored, oral iron supplements should be continued for 3 months to replenish tissue stores.

Failure to respond to oral iron can be caused by several factors:

- incorrect diagnosis, e.g. anaemia of chronic disorder, thalassaemia
- poor adherence to prescribed iron therapy
- inadequate iron dosage, e.g. in some modified-release formulations
- continuing excessive blood loss
- malabsorption
- concurrent deficiency of other haematinics.

Iron supplements are occasionally given for prophylaxis against iron deficiency at times of high demand for iron, e.g. pregnancy, or if the individual has menorrhagia, or if there is a poor diet. The reduced iron absorption after subtotal or total gastrectomy may also be overcome by long-term iron supplements.

Folic acid

Folic acid (pteroylglutamic acid) is ingested as conjugated polyglutamates or folates mainly in fresh leaf vegetables (in which it is heat labile) and in liver (where it is rather more heat stable). Folates are absorbed principally in the duodenum and jejunum. Before absorption, the polyglutamates are deconjugated to monoglutamate, then methylated and reduced to methyl tetrahydrofolate by dihydrofolate reductase. In tissues, folic acid is mainly in the more active polyglutamate form. Tetrahydrofolate is involved in synthesis of pyrimidines and purines and hence of DNA (see also Ch. 52).

Folate deficiency

The most obvious consequence of folate deficiency is a macrocytic anaemia with the presence of megaloblasts

---

Box 47.3

Causes of folate deficiency

- Poor diet: folate stores are adequate for a few weeks only. Lack of folate is uncommon in Western diets, but may be more common in the diet of elderly patients or in alcoholism.
- Increased requirements: e.g. pregnancy, malignancies, haemolytic anaemias, exfoliative dermatitis.
- Malabsorption: e.g. coeliac disease, tropical sprue.
- Drugs that interfere with folate metabolism: anticonvulsants (especially phenytoin, Ch. 23), methotrexate (Ch. 52), pyrimethamine (Ch. 51).

---

in the marrow, a feature it shares with vitamin B_{12} deficiency. Folate deficiency can arise for a number of reasons (Box 47.3).

Therapeutic use of folic acid

Folate deficiency almost always responds to oral folic acid supplements. Folic acid is converted by dihydrofolate reductase to tetrahydrofolic acid in target cells, then conjugated by polyglutamate synthetase. Treatment is usually given for 4 months to correct the anaemia and replace folate stores. For patients receiving drugs that inhibit the enzyme dihydrofolate reductase (e.g. methotrexate, Ch. 52; trimethoprim, Ch. 51) it is necessary to 'bypass' this enzyme blockade by giving the synthetic tetrahydrofolic acid, folinic acid (5-formyl tetrahydrofolic acid).

Folic acid is given prophylactically in pregnancy. It is given in higher doses if there is a history of neural tube defect in a previous pregnancy when it may protect against recurrence. Folic acid is also given during renal dialysis, to premature infants and in chronic haemolytic anaemia.

Treatment of combined vitamin B_{12} and folate deficiency with folic acid alone may correct the anaemia but neurological damage (see below) can be precipitated. Vitamin B_{12} deficiency must, therefore, be excluded before folic acid is used, or both administered if the deficiency is uncertain.

Vitamin B_{12}

The term vitamin B_{12} is usually used to cover all the cobalamin compounds that have biological activity. Bacteria are the only organisms that can synthesise cobalamin de novo. Humans obtain vitamin B_{12} from meat, and particularly liver, from animal products (milk, cheese, eggs, etc.) or from vegetables contaminated by bacteria. Absorption is by an unusual mechanism: dietary vitamin B$_{12}$ is complexed with a glycoprotein called intrinsic factor produced by gastric parietal cells. This complex is absorbed principally from the terminal ileum after binding to receptors on the luminal membranes of ileal cells.

In the blood, most vitamin B$_{12}$ is bound to a glycoprotein, transcobalamin I, from which it is rapidly taken up by the tissues, especially the liver, where about 50% of the body content of vitamin B$_{12}$ is stored. A second protein, transcobalamin II, is mainly responsible for enhancing vitamin B$_{12}$ uptake by the bone marrow via specific receptors. Vitamin B$_{12}$ is essential for isomerisation of methylmalonyl co-enzyme A to succinyl co-enzyme A, for isomerisation of α-leucine to β-leucine and also for methylation of homocysteine to methionine.

Vitamin B$_{12}$ deficiency

Impairment of vitamin B$_{12}$-dependent reactions affects DNA synthesis. The major organs affected by vitamin B$_{12}$ deficiency are those with a rapid cell turnover, i.e. bone marrow and the gastrointestinal tract.

Vitamin B$_{12}$ deficiency presents with a macrocytic anaemia and a megaloblastic bone marrow. The tongue becomes smooth and changes to the lining of the small bowel can lead to malabsorption. Damage to the posterior and lateral neuronal tracts in the spinal cord can also occur, leading to a condition known as subacute combined degeneration of the cord. The biochemical basis for the neurological damage is poorly understood: it may not be fully reversible after correction of vitamin B$_{12}$ deficiency.

Causes of vitamin B$_{12}$ deficiency include:

- diet: strict vegetarians (vegans) only
- intestinal malabsorption due to damage to the terminal ileum, for example Crohn's disease, lymphoma
- deficiency of intrinsic factor: pernicious anaemia (destruction of gastric parietal cells with achlorhydria and failure of intrinsic factor production), total and subtotal gastrectomy.

Therapeutic use of vitamin B$_{12}$

Most patients with vitamin B$_{12}$ deficiency have problems absorbing it from the gut, and treatment is usually by intramuscular injection of vitamin B$_{12}$ in aqueous solution. Hydroxocobalamin is the form of vitamin B$_{12}$ used for treating anaemia and has almost completely replaced cyanocobalamin since it is more highly bound to transcobalamins and less is excreted in the urine.

After initial injections on alternate days for 1–2 weeks to replenish stores, maintenance treatment, with injections every 2–3 months for life, is adequate. In the rare dietary causes of vitamin B$_{12}$ deficiency, oral cyanocobalamin supplements can be given, but otherwise oral treatment is never indicated.

Erythropoietin (epoetin)

Erythropoietin is a hormone released from the kidney which controls red cell production. Deficiency of erythropoietin in end-stage renal disease contributes to the anaemia that characterises this disorder. Human erythropoietin has been synthesised using recombinant DNA technology (epoetin).

Pharmacokinetics

Epoetin can be given intravenously or, more conveniently, subcutaneously. The red cell response is most rapid after intravenous use, but ultimately greater after subcutaneous injection. Doses are normally given two or three times weekly. Adequate iron stores are essential since erythropoiesis demands large amounts of iron.

Unwanted effects

- Flu-like symptoms early in treatment
- Hypertension, which is dose-dependent and can be severe, leading to encephalopathy with convulsions
- Thrombosis of synthetic arteriovenous shunts in patients receiving renal dialysis.

Therapeutic uses of epoetin

- Anaemia of end-stage renal disease. Other causes of anaemia should be excluded, and iron supplements may be needed to maximise the response. Anaemia can be corrected in more than 90% of patients and treatment improves quality of life. An improved, less atherogenic plasma lipid profile accompanies the treatment and may reduce the high cardiovascular mortality in renal failure.
- To increase red cell production prior to surgery. Autologous blood transfusion is becoming more popular to reduce the use of banked blood. Epoetin given twice weekly for 3 weeks before surgery can increase the number of units of blood that can be obtained.
- Anaemia associated with human immunodeficiency virus infection or AIDS.
- Anaemia associated with the chemotherapy of cancer by platinum-containing drugs (Ch. 52).

Drug treatment in other anaemias

Certain other anaemias require specific drug therapy.

Aplastic anaemia. Failure of haemopoietic stem cell production has many causes, including certain drugs (Box 47.4). Drugs do not have a major role in treatment. The anabolic steroid nandrolone (Ch. 46) is sometimes used, but its effectiveness is unpredictable. Antilymphocyte globulin is helpful in some patients with acquired aplastic anaemia, perhaps in combination with ciclosporin (Ch. 39).

Sideroblastic anaemia. This can also be caused by drugs (Box 47.5). It is characterised by accumulation of iron in erythroblasts, particularly in the mitochondria which lie in a ring around the nucleus. Staining for iron reveals the characteristic ring sideroblasts. Pyridoxine

supplements can increase the haemoglobin concentration in this disorder.

Autoimmune haemolytic anaemia. This can respond to immunosuppression with corticosteroids (Ch. 44).

β-Thalassaemia major. This is a genetic disorder of haemoglobin synthesis with a hyperplastic bone marrow and refractory anaemia. Blood transfusions or excessive iron supplements lead to iron overload with damage to the liver, heart and pancreas. Iron overload can be prevented with infusions of desferrioxamine (Ch. 53) together with vitamin C which enhances iron excretion. An oral iron chelator deferiprone is being evaluated in this condition, but it can cause neutropenia.

Sickle cell anaemia. This inherited disorder occurs when more than 80% of the haemoglobin is HbS; fetal haemoglobin (HbF) forms the remainder. Hydroxycarbamide (hydroxyurea) (Ch. 52) raises the HbF concentration. It also reduces the number of young red cells, which are those most likely to adhere to endothelium and occlude blood vessels. Hydroxycarbamide (hydroxyurea) may reduce the frequency and severity of sickle cell crises; long-term trials are in progress.

Box 47.4

Causes of aplastic anaemia

Drugs:
- cytotoxic agents
- chloramphenicol
- sulfonamides
- NSAIDs (especially phenylbutazone)
- gold salts
- carbimazole
- phenytoin
- carbamazepine
- phenothiazines
- chlorpropamide

Radiation
Infections, e.g. hepatitis, Epstein–Barr virus
Inherited, e.g. Fanconi anaemia
Malignant, e.g. myelodysplastic syndrome

Box 47.5

More common causes of sideroblastic anaemia

Congenital
Acquired
Myelodysplastic syndrome
Drugs:
- isoniazid
- chloramphenicol
- alcoholism
- lead poisoning

Drugs as a cause of anaemia

- Iron deficiency: especially drugs causing bleeding from the upper gut, e.g. NSAIDs.
- Aplastic anaemia (Box 47.4).
- Sideroblastic anaemia (Box 47.5).
- Haemolysis in glucose-6-phosphate dehydrogenase (G6PD) deficiency (Box 47.6). G6PD is involved in generating reduced glutathione, which protects red cells against oxidative stresses. Oxidant drugs produce haemolysis in deficient individuals, who are usually male (Ch. 53).

Box 47.6

Drugs causing haemolysis in glucose-6-phosphate dehydrogenase deficiency

Antimalarials
  Primaquine
  Pamaquine
Analgesics
  Acetylsalicylic acid (high dose)
Others
  Sulfonamides
  Nalidixic acid
  Dapsone

Neutropenia

Leucocytes are part of the first-line defence against pathogens. They include phagocytic cells (neutrophils, monocytes and eosinophils) and non-phagocytic cells (lymphocytes and basophils). In addition to their role in acute inflammation, all these cells participate in regulation of cellular and humoral immunity through production of cytokines (Ch. 39). A reduction in the number of circulating neutrophils (neutropenia) in particular increases the risk of serious infection. There are several causes of neutropenia (Box 47.7).

Drugs for neutropenia

Colony stimulating factors

Colony stimulating factors are molecules produced by many cells such as endothelial cells, monocytes and fibroblasts, which stimulate maturation of pluripotent stem cells in the bone marrow. Several of these factors have now been produced by recombinant DNA technology. They include: granulocyte-macrophage colony stimulating factor (GM-CSF) and granulocyte colony stimulating factor (G-CSF) which acts only on neutrophil cell lines.

- Filgrastim (unglycosylated recombinant human granulocyte-colony stimulating factor, rhG-CSF).
- Lenograstim (glycosylated recombinant human granulocyte-colony stimulating factor, rhG-CSF).
- Molgramostim (recombinant human granulocyte-macrophage colony stimulating factor, rhGM-CSF).

The molecules are glycosylated in their natural state, but this does not seem to be a pre-requisite for effectiveness.

Colony stimulating factors are given by prolonged intravenous infusion or subcutaneous injection to achieve sufficient stimulation of the bone marrow. A transient fall in circulating white cell numbers occurs within minutes of the injection, followed a few hours later by a substantial rise. After treatment with G-CSF, circulating neutrophils increase, while after GM-CSF there is also a smaller rise in monocyte and eosinophil counts.

Unwanted effects

- Bone pain
- Headache
- Fatigue
- Nausea
- Myeloproliferative disorders with long-term treatment
- Osteoporosis with long-term treatment.

> **Box 47.7**
>
> **Causes of neutropenia**
>
> Inherited
>   Congenital agranulocytosis
>   Cyclical neutropenia
> Acquired
>   Viral infection, e.g. hepatitis, influenza, rubella, infectious mononucleosis
>   Bacterial infection
>   Radiotherapy
>   Drugs, especially cytotoxic drugs, carbimazole
>   Autoimmune
>   Hypersplenism
>   Marrow infiltration

Therapeutic use of colony stimulating factors

The use of these drugs remains controversial in many indications.

Congenital neutropenia. There is concern over the risk of promoting myeloid malignancy with prolonged use in this condition.

Chemotherapy-induced neutropenia. The duration of neutropenia may be reduced, with a reduction in associated infection. However, there is no evidence that long-term survival of the patient is improved.

Mobilisation of progenitor cells into peripheral blood for harvesting prior to bone marrow transplantation. The white blood cell count rises 7–12 days after treatment, and the cells are obtained via a cell separation machine.

FURTHER READING

Anderlini P, Przepiorka D, Champlin R, Körbling M (1996) Biologic and clinical effects of granulocyte colony-stimulating factor in normal individuals. *Blood* 88, 2819–2825

Frewin R, Henson A, Provan D (1997) Iron deficiency anaemia. *Br Med J* 314, 360–363

Goodnough LT, Monk TG, Andriole GL (1997) Erythropoietin therapy. *N Engl J Med* 336, 933–939

Hoffbrand V, Provan D (1997) Macrocytic anaemias. *Br Med J* 314, 430–433

Muirhead N (1997) The clinical impact of recombinant human erythropoietin. *J Roy Coll Phys Lond* 31, 125–129

Self-assessment

In questions 1–4 the first statement, in italics, is true. Are the accompanying statements also true?

1. *Pernicious anaemia is caused by reduced vitamin B_{12} absorption due to autoimmunity that inhibits intrinsic factor release from the parietal cell.*

   a. Vitamin B_{12} is absorbed from the stomach.
   b. In vitamin B_{12} deficiency treatment is required for life.
   c. In a patient with pernicious anaemia the blood film shows macrocytosis.

2. *The most common causes of megaloblastic anaemias are vitamin B_{12} or folate deficiency.*

   a. Both vitamin B_{12} and folate are essential for DNA synthesis. A product of folate is necessary for purine and pyrimidine synthesis and vitamin B_{12} is also necessary for the formation of a cofactor in the synthesis of purines and pyrimidines.
   b. Folate deficiency can be associated with drug therapy, examples of which are methotrexate, trimethoprim and phenytoin.
   c. Folic acid cannot be given orally.

3. *Erythropoietin is a product of the kidney that stimulates progenitor cells to generate erythrocytes.*

   a. Chronic renal failure can result in a deficiency in erythropoietin.

4. *Colony stimulating factors (CSF) are formed from many cells and control the formation and survival of neutrophils, monocytes and eosinophils.*

   a. CSFs reduce the release of progenitor cells of neutrophils from bone marrow into the circulation.

5. Case history question

   A 40-year-old female complained to her general practitioner of fatigue and heavy menstrual periods lasting 7 days and occurring every 28 days. Her GP noted that she was pallid; her haemoglobin level was 67 g l^{-1} and mean cell volume was 61 fl. Other blood measurements of platelets and white cell counts were unremarkable.

   a. How would you interpret these data and what are the possible reasons?
   b. What biochemical tests could help the diagnosis?

   The tests confirmed iron deficiency anaemia.

   c. What pharmaceutical preparations should be given?

   Several iron formulations were tried as the patient felt unwell taking ferrous sulfate.

   d. What unwanted effects might the patient experience?
   e. Where is iron absorbed?
   f. In what dietary form is iron optimally absorbed?

   After 2 months of oral iron therapy the haemoglobin value was 80 g l^{-1}.

   g. Is this a sufficient response?

   The patient is intolerant of oral iron.

   h. What could be the reasons for the poor response?
   i. What alternative treatment could be administered?

   Her haemoglobin rose to 115 g l^{-1} over 2–3 weeks.

The answers are provided on pages 627.

Anaemia and haematopoietic colony stimulating factors

Drug	Half-life	Elimination	Comments
Iron			
Oral formulations			
Ferrous sulfate Ferrous fumarate Ferrous gluconate Ferrous glycine sulfate Polysaccharide–iron complex Sodium feredetate			Given orally; often given as co-formulations with folic acid; extent of absorption depends on form, the presence of food and iron status; water-soluble forms are the sulfate and gluconate, whereas the fumarate and glycine sulfate are only sparingly soluble
Parenteral formulations			
Iron sorbitol	–	Renal	Given by deep intramuscular injection; rapidly absorbed from injection site; about 30% is excreted in urine before the remainder enters normal iron pool
Iron dextran	–	–	Given by slow intravenous injection or intravenous infusion; extensive uptake by macrophage-rich spleen with effective release for erythrocyte formation
Drugs for megaloblastic anaemias			
Cyanocobalamin	Dose-dependent	Renal + metabolism	Given orally or by intramuscular injection; dose-dependent absorption and elimination; free cyanocobalamin is eliminated by glomerular filtration (and, like creatinine, can be used to determine GFR); the excretion increases with dose from 5% after 25 μg to 85% after 1000 μg; metabolism gives cobalamin
Folic acid	Dose-dependent	Renal	Given orally with 70–80% absorption; low doses are retained in cells and higher doses are eliminated in urine; folic acid per se does not occur naturally in the food
Hydroxocobalamin	Dose-dependent	Renal + metabolism	Given by intramuscular injection; elimination by glomerular filtration with 25% excreted at 500 μg and 29% at 1000 μg; excretion is complete by 24 hours after dosage
Drugs used in hypoplastic, haemolytic and renal anaemias			
Epoetin alfa and beta	4–6	Metabolism	Given by subcutaneous or intravenous injection; catabolised by target cells after internalisation
Treatment of iron overload			
Desferrioxamine mesilate (deferoxamine mesilate)	6	Metabolism + renal	Given by subcutaneous infusion; chelating agent used for iron overload (or aluminium in dialysis patients); eliminated unchanged in urine (15–65%) and by metabolism to inactive products

Lipoprotein metabolism

Lipid and lipoprotein metabolism is complex and the following account is a very brief summary, sufficient to establish the mechanism of action of drugs used to correct lipid abnormalities.

Cholesterol and triglycerides

Cholesterol is a ubiquitous building block in the body, and triglycerides are an important energy source. Cholesterol is a sterol that is mainly synthesised in the liver. Its synthesis involves several enzymes, but the rate-limiting step is catalysed by HMG-CoA (β-hydroxy-β-methylglutaryl-coenzyme A) reductase. It is then either transported into the circulation or secreted into the bile after incorporation into bile salt micelles (Fig. 48.1). A small amount of cholesterol is absorbed from the gut, either following dietary ingestion or by enterohepatic circulation of bile salts. Intracellular cholesterol in the liver acts by a negative feedback mechanism to reduce further hepatic cholesterol synthesis.

Triglycerides are the major dietary fat. They can also be synthesised in the liver from free fatty acids, or derived from excess carbohydrate in the diet. Triglycerides are stored in adipose tissue from which they can be mobilised as non-esterified free fatty acids to act as an energy substrate during periods of hepatic glycogen depletion.

Lipoproteins

Lipids (triglycerides and esters of cholesterol) circulate in plasma encased in a coat of polar phospholipids, cholesterol and apolipoproteins. The apolipoprotein–lipid complexes are termed lipoproteins. They are usually classified according to the density of the particles into very-low-density (VLDL), low-density (LDL) and high-density (HDL) lipoproteins. The least dense and largest diameter particles, known as chylomicrons, are exclusively concerned with the transport of dietary lipid to the liver. Their low density and large size reflect their high content of triglycerides (Table 48.1).

457

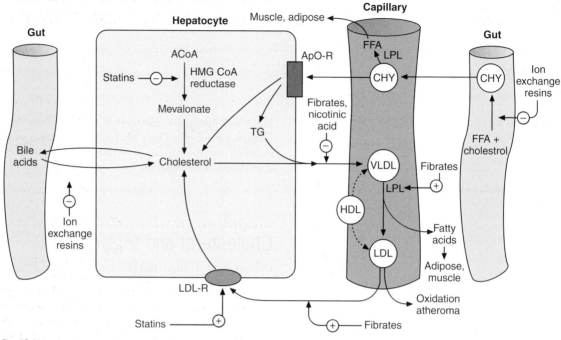

Fig. 48.1

The main steps in lipoprotein formation and metabolism. LDL-R, LDL receptor; ApO-R, apolipoprotein receptor; CHY, chylomicron; LPL, lipoprotein lipase; FFA, free fatty acid; TG, triglycerides; +, increases activity; −, decreases activity; −−→, transfer of cholesterol. Drug target sites are shown in red.

Table 48.1
The apoliprotein and lipid composition of the circulating lipoproteins

Lipoprotein	Major associated apolipoproteins	Cholesterol (%)	Triglyceride (%)
Chylomicrons	Apo A/apo C/apo B$_{48}$	3	90
VLDL	Apo C/apo B$_{100}$/apo E	20	50
LDL	Apo B$_{100}$	50	7
HDL	Apo A	40	6

Note: the balance of lipid content of the lipoprotein consists of phospholipids.

Important steps in lipoprotein metabolism

Processing of lipids absorbed from the gut (Fig. 48.1)

Triglycerides and cholesterol with associated apolipoproteins circulate in the plasma as chylomicrons after absorption and processing from the gastrointestinal tract. Hydrolysis of triglycerides is carried out by lipoprotein lipase (found in blood, liver and endothelial cells) and requires the chylomicron-associated apolipoprotein C as a cofactor (Table 48.1). The free fatty acid released by this hydrolysis can then be utilised by muscle and adipose tissue as an energy source. After removal of the triglycerides, the remaining lipoprotein

fragments bind to apolipoprotein receptors (ApO-R in Fig. 48.1) in the liver and are taken up into hepatocytes. After uptake into the liver, cholesterol can be processed in a variety of ways including:

- conversion to bile salts
- secretion in bile
- incorporation into VLDL.

Liver processing of lipids

Liver cholesterol (as esters) and triglycerides synthesised in the liver can be released from the liver into the circulation as VLDL complexes. Triglycerides are hydrolysed from VLDL by lipoprotein lipases that are present on the surface of endothelial cells in capillaries in muscle and adipose tissue (LPL in Fig. 48.1); the resulting free fatty acids are made available for uptake into muscle and adipose tissue. The resulting low-density lipoprotein (LDL) fragment contains a high concentration of cholesterol but a lower concentration of triglyceride compared to VLDL (Table 48.1). LDL is taken up into liver cells by specific uptake receptors (LDL-R in Fig. 48.1). However, if there is excess LDL or deficient receptor numbers, the circulating levels of LDL rise. Oxidation of LDL cholesterol and other reactions lead to formation of lipid-rich deposits in arterial walls as atheromatous plaques (see below).

Low-density lipoprotein

Several tissues that take up cholesterol have a genetically controlled cell-surface receptor for LDL. The receptor–LDL particle complex is internalised, the cholesterol released and the receptor returned to the cell surface. In the liver, as the cell content of cholesterol increases, there are two important feedback effects that limit cholesterol accumulation: (i) inhibition of HMG-CoA reductase activity, (ii) downregulation of LDL receptors. If the latter occurs in the presence of excess circulating cholesterol, then increased vessel wall uptake of cholesterol–LDL complex also occurs by non-receptor scavenger mechanisms and this enhances atherogenesis (see 'Hyperlipidaemias and Atheroma' section below).

High-density lipoprotein

HDL obtains most of its lipid content from chylomicrons and VLDL during lipolysis. It also takes up cholesterol esters from peripheral tissues and transfers it from HDL to VLDL and LDL and ultimately to the liver. HDL can also deliver cholesterol directly to the liver by a mechanism that does not utilise uptake of the whole lipoprotein (not shown in Fig. 48.1). Overall, the role of HDL is believed to be protective, reducing the risk of atherogenesis.

Hyperlipidaemias and atheroma

Abnormalities of plasma lipoprotein metabolism produce an excess of circulating cholesterol and/or triglyceride concentrations. Their clinical importance lies in their relationship to the production of atheroma (mainly cholesterol with a contribution from triglycerides) and pancreatitis (triglycerides).

Injury to endothelium encourages monocyte attachment and LDL oxidation. Oxidised LDL is taken up into macrophages, and macrophages migrate into the tissue. These modified macrophages (foam cells) form the fatty streaks of atherosclerosis. Further cytokine release and inflammatory processing leads to the formation of the fibrous cap surmounting the lipid-based plaque.

By contrast, the HDL concentration shows an inverse relationship to atheroma, presumably due to its involvement in reverse cholesterol transport to the liver. High plasma triglycerides are associated with low levels of HDL cholesterol and are usually associated with increased production of VLDL, the main carrier of triglycerides in plasma.

Variations in the pattern of lipoproteins can result from:

- Dietary factors.
- Primary (inherited) disorders of enzymes or receptors involved in lipid metabolism. Most inherited hyperlipidaemias are polygenic. However, an important inherited defect is familial hypercholesterolaemia, a single recessive gene disorder that affects 1 in 500 of the population who have reduced synthesis of LDL receptors.
- Secondary lipid disorders, when hyperlipidaemia results from diseases that affect lipid metabolism, for example liver disease, nephrotic syndrome, hypothyroidism.

The WHO has adopted a classification for the various patterns of hyperlipidaemia; this is shown in Table 48.2.

Table 48.2
The Fredrickson classification of dyslipidaemias

Type	Triglyceride	Total cholesterol	LDL cholesterol	Raised lipoprotein	Atheroma risk
I	+ + +	+	N	Chylomicrons	N
IIa	N	+ +	+ +	LDL	+++
IIb	+ +	+ +	+ +	LDL/VLDL	+++
III	+ +	+	N	VLDL and chylomicron remnants	++
IV	+ +	N/+	N	VLDL	++
V	+ + +	+	N	VLDL/chylomicrons	N

N = Normal; + = slightly raised; + + = moderately raised; + + + = extremely raised.

Drugs for hyperlipidaemia

HMG-CoA reductase inhibitors ('statins')

Examples: simvastatin, pravastatin

Mechanism of action and effects

HMG-CoA reductase inhibitors competitively inhibit the enzyme that catalyses the rate-limiting step in synthesis of cholesterol by the liver (Fig. 48.1). The fall in cholesterol available for bile acid synthesis produces a compensatory upregulation in the number of LDL receptors on the cell surface, with increased clearance of circulating LDL cholesterol. Statins also reduce the hepatic production of VLDL and therefore reduce circulating triglycerides, although the mechanism of this effect is unclear. A modest increase in HDL cholesterol is often seen. Statins also have several other actions, some of which may be distinct from their ability to reduce plasma lipids (Box 48.1). The contribution of these to the beneficial actions of statins is unknown.

Pharmacokinetics

The statins are well absorbed from the gut. Simvastatin is a prodrug (Ch. 2) which is activated by first-pass metabolism in the liver by cytochrome P450 (CYP3A). Further metabolism inactivates the drug and little active compound reaches the circulation. Pravastatin is a hydrophilic drug that undergoes little metabolism. Its half-life is short and elimination is mainly renal.

Unwanted effects

- Gastrointestinal upset
- CNS effects, for example dizziness, blurred vision, headache

---

Box 48.1

Non-lipid effects of statins

- Restored function to vascular endothelium that has been functionally damaged by hypercholesterolaemia. It is not known whether this is a direct effect or a consequence of reduction in plasma LDL cholesterol
- Stabilisation of atherosclerotic plaques by altered smooth muscle proliferation and migration (inhibited by simvastatin, unchanged by pravastatin)
- Changes in haemostasis: pravastatin decreases plasma fibrinogen and enhances fibrinolysis
- Reduction of inflammatory cell infiltration into atherosclerotic plaques

---

- Transient disturbance of liver function tests
- Myalgia or myositis, particularly when used in combination with fibrates or nicotinic acid.

Bile acid binding (anion-exchange) resins

Example: colestyramine

Mechanism of action

Bile acid binding resins are insoluble, non-absorbable compounds that bind bile salts in the gut and prevent enterohepatic circulation of bile acids. Bile acids are synthesised from cholesterol in the liver, a process that is initiated by the enzyme cholesterol 7α-hydroxylase. They are secreted into the duodenum to aid absorption of dietary fat, reabsorbed in the terminal ileum and returned to the liver in the portal circulation. When reabsorption is impaired, there is a compensatory increase in bile acid synthesis in the liver leading to further elimination of cholesterol. Intracellular cholesterol depletion in the liver results in upregulation of LDL receptors and as a result LDL cholesterol in blood is cleared more rapidly, with a fall in circulating levels. Stimulation of VLDL synthesis produces a small rise in plasma triglycerides. There is a small rise in HDL cholesterol, but the mechanism is unclear.

Unwanted effects

- Unpalatability: sachets containing several grams of powder have to be taken, usually mixed with food. The taste and texture limit patient acceptability, so that resins are no longer widely used.
- Diarrhoea.
- Interference with the absorption of certain drugs, for example digoxin (Ch. 7), warfarin (Ch. 11), thyroxine (Ch. 41). These drugs should be given at least 1 hour before or 4 hours after a resin.

Fibrates

Examples: bezafibrate, gemfibrozil, ciprofibrate

Mode of action

The main effect of these drugs is to activate gene transcription factors encoding for proteins that control lipoprotein metabolism. These factors are nuclear hormone receptors known as peroxisome proliferation activated receptors (PPARs). There are several consequences of PPAR activation:

- Increased lipoprotein lipase activity, which enhances the clearance of triglycerides from lipoproteins in the plasma (Fig. 48.1).
- Free fatty acid uptake by the liver is increased due to induction of a fatty acid transport protein in the cell membrane. In the liver, conversion to acyl-coenzyme A derivatives is enhanced as a result of increased acyl-CoA synthetase activity. The fatty acids are, therefore, less available for hepatic triglyceride synthesis.
- LDL cholesterol uptake by the liver is increased due to formation of less dense LDL particles which have greater affinity for hepatic LDL receptors.
- Plasma HDL is increased because of increased production in the liver.

Pharmacokinetics

Fibrates are well absorbed from the gut and highly protein bound in the plasma. Excretion is primarily by the kidney although some metabolism occurs in the liver. The half-lives of bezafibrate and gemfibrozil are short. Newer fibrates have long half-lives.

Unwanted effects

- Gastrointestinal upset.
- Increased lithogenicity of bile theoretically increases the risk of gallstones but this has not been a problem with the drugs mentioned here.
- Myalgia or myositis are uncommon.
- Drug interactions include inhibition of warfarin (Ch. 11).

Nicotinic acid and derivatives

Examples: nicotinic acid, acipimox

Mechanism of action

Nicotinic acid is a B vitamin which, when used in pharmacological doses, has effects on lipids. Reduced free fatty acid mobilisation from adipocytes leads to decreased VLDL synthesis in the liver. Circulating triglycerides are therefore substantially reduced and LDL cholesterol modestly reduced. HDL cholesterol is increased, possibly as a result of hepatic lipase inhibition.

Pharmacokinetics

Nicotinic acid is well absorbed from the gut. Hepatic metabolism occurs at low doses but is saturable, and large doses are excreted unchanged in the urine. It has a very short half-life. Acipimox is a synthetic derivative of nicotinic acid which is longer-acting, but is rather less effective for lowering LDL cholesterol.

Unwanted effects

- Nicotinic acid is often poorly tolerated but unwanted effects can be minimised by gradual dosage increases. Acipimox is better tolerated at currently recommended dosages.
- Cutaneous vasodilation (mediated by prostaglandins) is particularly troublesome and causes flushing and itching. A small dose of aspirin taken 30 minutes before nicotinic acid, or taking the drug with food will reduce this.
- Gastrointestinal upset and peptic ulceration.
- Glucose intolerance with high doses of nicotinic acid (not seen with acipimox).
- Exacerbation of gout.

Fish oils

Long-chain polyunsaturated omega-3 fatty acids, for example eicosapentaenoic acid (EPA) and docosahexanoic acid (DHA), are found in high quantities in oily fish such as mackerel and sardines. Since they are poor substrates for enzymes that synthesise triglycerides, they lead to production of triglyceride-poor LDL and reduce triglycerides in plasma, although cholesterol is increased. They also increase conversion of VLDL to LDL, and increase circulating LDL cholesterol. Other effects of fish oils may be important for reduction of coronary artery disease, for example reduction of plasma fibrinogen and impairment of platelet aggregation (Ch. 11). Large quantities are necessary.

Unwanted effects

- Gastrointestinal upset
- Prolonged bleeding time.

Management of hyperlipidaemia

The major risk associated with a raised LDL cholesterol is cardiovascular disease. The relationship is strongest with coronary atherosclerosis and peripheral vascular atherosclerosis. The relationship to cerebrovascular disease and atherothrombotic stroke is less strong. HDL cholesterol is protective against atherosclerosis; an HDL cholesterol of less than 1.0 mmol l^{-1} is associated with the highest risk of disease. The ratio of total cholesterol:HDL cholesterol provides a much more sensitive indicator of relative risk of cardiovascular disease than total cholesterol alone, improving the predictive values by about 15-fold.

While a high total cholesterol:HDL ratio predicts the relative risk of cardiovascular disease, the absolute risk (i.e. the numbers of individuals in the population under study who will develop disease in unit time) will be determined by the coexistence of other risk factors (see below).

Raised plasma triglycerides are an independent predictor of the risk of atherosclerosis, but less so than raised plasma cholesterol. Nevertheless, when raised triglycerides coexist with an atherogenic cholesterol profile, the overall risk is enhanced. A markedly raised plasma triglyceride concentration (>12 mmol l⁻¹) poses a progressively increasing risk of acute pancreatitis. Isolated hypertriglyceridaemia should be treated intensively for this reason alone.

Before embarking on management of the hyperlipidaemias, secondary causes such as diabetes, hypothyroidism or nephrotic syndrome should be excluded or treated.

Primary prevention of cardiovascular disease

Coronary atheroma has a multifactorial aetiology, and any strategy for primary prevention must consider all relevant treatable factors. Treatment of hyperlipidaemia with drugs for primary prevention should only be considered if there is a high absolute risk of disease, and should not be based on the lipid level alone. Important factors include:

Smoking. Smoking doubles the risk of coronary artery disease. Stopping smoking reduces risk to that of a non-smoker in 3–5 years (see Ch. 5).

Hypertension (see Ch. 6). Although more effective for prevention of stroke, treating hypertension also reduces the risk of myocardial infarction, especially in older people with hypertension.

Physical activity. A physically active life style reduces risk of myocardial infarction by up to 50%, compared to a sedentary life style.

Maintaining ideal body weight. Obesity (see Ch. 37) increases the risk of myocardial infarction by up to 50%.

Mild-to-moderate alcohol consumption. A modest alcohol intake (see Ch. 54) can reduce the risk of myocardial infarction by about one-third.

Postmenopausal hormone replacement therapy (Ch. 45).

Low-dose aspirin. This is less effective for primary prevention than for secondary prevention (Ch. 11) but is useful in selected high-risk individuals.

Control of diabetes. The evidence that close control of plasma glucose reduces subsequent vascular events is increasing. Since the risk of ischaemic heart disease in diabetes is at least twice that of non-diabetics, more intensive management of coexistent risk factors in diabetics should also be undertaken.

Cholesterol. This is a powerful predictor of future cardiovascular disease, especially in young people. Recent trials show that reducing plasma total cholesterol by 25–30% (with a reduction in LDL cholesterol of 30–35%) using a statin reduces the subsequent risk of myocardial infarction or vascular death by about 30%. Dietary management is the treatment of first choice, with a reduction in saturated fat intake and an increase in mono-unsaturated fats. Increasing antioxidants in the diet by eating more fresh fruit and vegetables reduces oxidation of LDL cholesterol and therefore makes it less atherogenic. The ability of cholesterol-lowering drugs (particularly statins) to prevent ischaemic heart disease has been demonstrated in many trials. The question exercising the minds of health economists is not whether treatment is effective, but when it becomes cost-effective. As part of a multiple risk factor intervention strategy, drug therapy has a role for those at highest absolute risk, usually because several other risk factors coexist or there is a history of premature coronary artery disease in a first-degree relative. To aid the identification of high-risk individuals, risk tables have been produced. The level of risk at which drug treatment is recommended varies; in the UK it is suggested that it should be targeted to those who have an annual risk of myocardial infarction or cardiovascular death of 3% or more. Once treatment is started the target plasma cholesterol should be less than 5 mmol l⁻¹ (LDL cholesterol less than 3 mmol l⁻¹).

Secondary prevention of cardiovascular disease

Once cardiovascular disease is clinically apparent, the subsequent risk of death from vascular events is high. Those at highest risk will already have experienced a myocardial infarction or an episode of unstable angina. At slightly lower absolute risk are those with stable angina pectoris or peripheral vascular disease. Several studies have confirmed that treatment of even modestly raised plasma cholesterol concentrations in such individuals reduces the subsequent risk of both fatal and non-fatal cardiovascular events. These patients are at much greater absolute risk than those without clinical coronary artery disease who have similar, or even higher plasma cholesterol concentrations. Current evidence supports the use of statins as first-line therapy; trials with fibrates have shown less marked benefit. The target cholesterol concentration is the same as for primary prevention. Lowering plasma cholesterol for secondary prevention of coronary artery disease should be only one aspect of a comprehensive strategy for improving prognosis. This is discussed more fully in Chapter 5.

Mechanisms of prevention of coronary events

There is a close relationship between the amount of LDL cholesterol reduction and the reduced risk of coronary events in most studies. Overall, there is a 2–3% reduction in risk for every 1% reduction in plasma total cholesterol concentration. Reducing plasma cholesterol probably stabilises existing atheromatous plaques by preventing lipid accumulation in their core and reducing the risk of plaque rupture. Statins prevent the growth of existing coronary artery plaques and reduce the formation of new plaques. Other actions of statins, such as reduction in thrombogenicity of blood and inhibition of smooth muscle proliferation in atheromatous plaques, may also contribute but their role remains speculative.

Management of hypertriglyceridaemia

When triglycerides are markedly raised, non-pharmacological methods of treatment are often useful. These include control of diabetes, weight loss and reduction of alcohol intake. If these are insufficient, then drug therapy may be necessary. Modest hypertriglyceridaemia in association with hypercholesterolaemia will usually respond to a statin.

Extremely high plasma triglyceride concentrations (often associated with 'type V' hyperlipoproteinaemia) usually respond well to a fibrate or to nicotinic acid. Combination therapy with a statin and a fibrate may be necessary in some high-risk individuals to achieve an acceptable lipid profile.

FURTHER READING

Crouse JR, Byington RP, Furberg CD (1998) HMG-CoA reductase inhibitor therapy and stroke risk reduction: an analysis of clinical trials data. *Atherosclerosis* 138, 11–24

Farmer JA, Gotto AM Jr (1996) Choosing the right lipid-regulating agent. *Drugs* 52, 649–661

Ginsberg HN (1998) Effects of statins on triglyceride metabolisms. *Am J Cardiol* 81(4A), 32B–35B

Grundy SM (1998) Consensus statement: role of therapy with 'statins' in patients with hypertriglyceridaemia. *Am J Cardiol* 81(4A), 1B–6B

Havel RJ, Rapaport E (1995) Management of primary hyperlipidaemia. *N Engl J Med* 332, 1491–1498

Maher V, Sinfuego J, Chas P, Parekh J (1997) Primary prevention of coronary heart disease. *Drugs* 54, 1–8

Pearson TA (1998) Lipid-lowering therapy in low-risk patients. *JAMA* 279, 1659–1661

Rosenson RS, Tangney CC (1998) Antiatherothrombotic properties of statins. *JAMA* 279, 1643–1650

Staels B, Dallongeville J, Auwerx J et al. (1998) Mechanism of action of fibrates on lipid and lipoprotein metabolism. *Circulation* 98, 2088–2093

Wood D (1998) European and American recommendations for coronary heart disease prevention. *Eur Heart J* 19 (suppl 1A), A12–A19

Self-assessment

In questions 1 and 2 the first statement, in italics, is true. Are the accompanying statements also true?

1. *Different drug classes available for treating hyperlipidaemia act at differing steps in the lipoprotein metabolic pathway.*

   a. In individuals with high HDL cholesterol there is a lowering in the risk of coronary disease if the HDL cholesterol levels are reduced.
   b. An important contributor to the development of hypercholesterolaemia is a genetic defect.
   c. Anion exchange resins act by enhancing the absorption of bile acids from the gut.

2. *Statins reduce cholesterol levels by inhibiting the rate-limiting enzymatic step (HMG-CoA reductase) in its synthesis.*

   a. Decreased hepatic cholesterol synthesis results in increased numbers of HDL receptors.
   b. Simvastatin lowers serum LDL cholesterol by 5%.
   c. Co-administration of bile acid binding resins and statins has no greater effect than giving each drug separately.

3. Case history question

   A 58-year-old man has recovered from an anterior myocardial infarction. His fasting plasma cholesterol is 7.8 mmol l^{-1}. You want to reduce his risk of a further myocardial infarction by lowering his cholesterol.

   a. What advice would you give him?
   b. What drug would you recommend and why?
   c. What reduction in plasma cholesterol would you expect, and when would you expect an adequate response?
   d. How do statins work?
   e. What target total cholesterol would you aim for?
   f. What unwanted effects would you warn him about?
   g. If the target cholesterol is not attained, how could you reduce cholesterol further?
   h. How do the additional drugs you have recommended work?

   The answers are provided on pages 627–628.

Drugs used to treat hyperlipidaemias (all drugs given orally unless otherwise stated)

Drug	Half-life (h)	Elimination	Comments
HMG-CoA reductase inhibitors			
Atorvastatin	32–36	Metabolism	Bioavailability is 14% (as drug) and 30% (as HMG-CoA reductase inhibition) because the first-pass metabolites are active; bioavailability is lower if taken with food or in the evening; oxidised by CYP3A4 to metabolites that are responsible for much of the activity
Cerivastatin	2–3	Metabolism	Good oral bioavailability; metabolised in the liver; metabolites retain activity but parent drug is largely responsible for cholesterol-lowering effect
Fluvastatin	1	Metabolism	Bioavailability is 30%; extensive hepatic uptake and oxidation; metabolites are conjugated and excreted in bile; parent drug is the active form
Pravastatin	1–2	Renal + metabolism	Low oral bioavailability (17%) which is decreased by food and is due to poor absorption plus first-pass metabolism; eliminated by renal tubular secretion plus oxidative metabolism; parent drug is the active form
Simvastatin	2 (activity)	Metabolism	A lactone prodrug which is converted to the active ring-opened acid analogue; oral bioavailability as the acid is low (about 5%); metabolised by hepatic CYP3A4 to active products
Bile acid binding resins			
Colestyramine	Not relevant	Not absorbed	Not absorbed
Colestipol	Not relevant	Not absorbed	Not absorbed
Fibrates (most fibrates are carboxylic acid derivatives that are eliminated unchanged and as acyl glucuronides formed largely in the kidneys)			
Bezafibrate	1–5	Renal + metabolism	Complete oral bioavailability; eliminated equally by renal excretion (unchanged) and by metabolism (conjugation and oxidation)
Ciprofibrate	27–28	Metabolism	Complete oral bioavailability; eliminated by glucuronidation, but very low clearance (about 40 ml per hour); contraindicated in severe renal dysfunction
Clofibrate	18–25 (CA)	Metabolism	Prodrug which has been discontinued in UK; given as ethyl ester of clofibric acid (CA); clofibric acid is excreted as the glucuronide
Fenofibrate	20–27 (FA)	Metabolism	Ester prodrug of fenofibric acid (FA); good oral bioavailability (60–90%) as fenofibric acid (negligible ester absorbed intact); fenofibric acid is eliminated mainly as the acyl glucuronide
Gemfibrozil	1–2	Renal + metabolism	Complete oral bioavailability; about one-half of the dose is excreted unchanged, with the remainder as hydroxylated metabolites and their conjugates
Nicotinic acid and derivatives			
Acipimox	1–2	Renal	Complete oral bioavailability; polar pyridine-*N*-oxide derivative which has a low volume of distribution; undergoes limited reduction to the pyridine analogue (<5%) and is eliminated by renal excretion
Nicotinic acid (niacin)	0.3–0.8	Metabolism + renal	Rapidly and completely absorbed; at therapeutic doses about one-third is excreted unchanged and the remainder is oxidised or conjugated with glycine

continued

Drug compendium

Drugs used to treat hyperlipidaemias (all drugs given orally unless otherwise stated) *(continued)*

Drug	Half-life (h)	Elimination	Comments
Other treatments			
Ispaghula	Not relevant	Not relevant	Soluble fibre which probably acts by reducing the reabsorption of bile acids in the bowel
Omega-3 marine triglycerides	Not relevant	Not relevant	Used for treating triglyceridaemias, but can aggravate hypercholesterolaemia

THE SKIN AND EYES

49

Skin disorders

Topical applications

Topical treatments for skin disorders usually have two components: a base and the active ingredient, for example corticosteroid, antifungal agent, tar. Four types of base are used:

- ointments are greases such as white or yellow soft paraffin.
- creams are emulsions of water in a grease or grease in water that are less greasy than ointments, they are absorbed more quickly into the skin and are often used as a vehicle for active ingredients.
- pastes are suspensions of powder in an ointment and will stay where they are put on the skin; their main use is to apply noxious chemicals that should be confined to one area of the skin
- lotions are any kind of liquid; they are used on wet surfaces and hairy areas and their main advantage is that they do not make a mess.

The choice between an ointment or cream depends on patient preference unless the skin is very dry, when an ointment is better.

Atopic and contact dermatitis

Dermatitis is a syndrome that has several possible causes.

Atopic dermatitis (eczema). This is often associated with asthma and hayfever and has a familial tendency. In common with atopic asthma (Ch. 12), T-lymphocytes proliferate, particularly T helper type 2 cells (Ch. 39). Affected skin is red, scaly and extremely dry. There may be vesicles and weeping and crusting over the skin surface. Scratching produces excoriation and thickening of the skin.

Contact dermatitis. An external agent gives rise to direct irritation or to sensitisation involving a delayed hypersensitivity response (Ch. 38). The latter can be a response to topical application of drugs. Once the skin has been sensitised, the potential for further reaction persists indefinitely.

Treatment of atopic dermatitis

- Emollients are helpful as hydrophobic agents that seal the surface of the skin and reduce water loss.

469

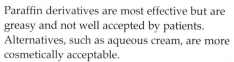

Paraffin derivatives are most effective but are greasy and not well accepted by patients. Alternatives, such as aqueous cream, are more cosmetically acceptable.

- Topical corticosteroid ointment (Ch. 44) is effective but, in general, the least potent corticosteroids should be used whenever possible to minimise unwanted effects. The anti-inflammatory effect of these drugs makes them the mainstay of treatment.
- Sedative antihistamines (Ch. 38) taken orally at night assist sleep although they have little direct effect on itching. Recently, a topical formulation of the tricyclic antidepressant doxepin (see Ch. 22) has been introduced to treat itch. It is uncertain whether its antihistamine activity is the major mode of action. For some patients, ciclosporin (Ch. 39), systemic corticosteroids (Ch. 44) or ultraviolet light therapy can reduce itch.
- Systemic antibiotics are given for secondary infection.
- Tar bandages on the limbs are messy but aid healing and prevent scratching.

Treatment of contact dermatitis

- Provision of a barrier to an irritant, for example wearing gloves, or removing an allergen may be sufficient.
- Dilute topical corticosteroid ointment (Ch. 44).
- Potassium permanganate soaks can help to dry up exudative lesions.

Psoriasis

Psoriatic skin lesions are produced by a very rapid proliferation of epidermal cells. Cell turnover is increased from about 28 days to 3–4 days, which prevents adequate maturation. Instead of producing a normal keratinous surface layer the skin thickens, forming a silvery scale with dilated upper dermal blood vessels. Inflammatory cells such as T-lymphocytes infiltrate into the dermis and epidermis. The process is driven by an immune reaction in the dermis, with cytokine production, which is initiated by an unknown antigen. The basic defect is genetically determined. Plaques usually affect elbows, knees, lower back, buttocks, scalp and nails. Various subtypes of the condition are recognised. An inflammatory arthritis also occurs in some patients. There are several treatments, both topical and systemic, but none produces long-term remission.

Topical therapy

Emollients (see atopic dermatitis above). These reduce scaling and itching and may be sufficient in mild psoriasis. They can also be used with a keratolytic.

Keratolytics. These break down keratin and soften skin, which improves penetration of other treatments. Salicylic acid ointment is most frequently used for more troublesome psoriasis.

Vitamin D analogues (e.g. calcipotriol). Vitamin D regulates epidermal proliferation and differentiation. It also has immunosuppressant properties. Vitamin D analogues are clean and simple to apply and particularly useful for chronic plaque psoriasis, although complete clearing of the plaques is unusual. Ointment has greater emollient effect than cream but is more messy. Calcipotriol should not usually be used for the face, where it often causes irritation; this is less troublesome elsewhere. Excessive use can lead to hypercalcaemia. The ease of use of these compounds makes them a popular choice if a keratolytic is insufficient.

Dithranol. This anthroquinone decreases cell division and is very effective in healing psoriatic plaques. In hospital it is applied in a stiff paste so that the dithranol does not come into contact with, and burn, normal skin. It is left in contact with the plaque for 24 h. At home, dithranol is used as a cream that is applied to the plaque for 30 min and then washed off. The oxidation products of dithranol stain the skin brown, leaving discoloration of healed areas for a few days. They also stain bedding and clothes a mauve colour that will not wash out. Since dithranol irritates normal skin, it should not be used in flexures.

Coal tar preparations. Crude coal tar is a mixture of a large number of hydrocarbons that have a cytostatic action. It enhances the healing effect of ultraviolet B radiation on psoriatic lesions. The main disadvantage is messiness and its efficacy when used alone is modest. More refined tar preparations have greater patient acceptability but are even less effective.

Phototherapy. Ultraviolet light produces improvement in most patients by inhibiting DNA synthesis and depleting intraepidermal T-lymphocytes. It should not be used on individuals who are very fair and who burn in the sun. Ultraviolet B ('sunburn' wavelength 290–320 nm) at least three times per week is very useful if patients have extensive small plaques of psoriasis. Pretreatment removal of scale is essential. Long wavelength ultraviolet A (320–400 nm) requires more specialised equipment and prior administration of an oral photosensitising drug such as psoralen (a process called photochemotherapy, PUVA). Psoralen probably locates between pyrimidine base pairs in the DNA helix and inhibits cell replication. PUVA is usually reserved for severe, resistant psoriasis and it is far more effective than treatment with ultraviolet B. Psoralen can produce nausea, and headache acutely. The long-term risks of PUVA include accelerated skin ageing and an increased incidence of skin cancer.

Topical corticosteroid preparations. These should be used sparingly on limited areas. Unwanted effects can be troublesome (Ch. 44). Withdrawal of high-potency corticosteroid can produce a rebound phenomenon and even generalised pustular psoriasis.

Topical retinoids, e.g. tazarotene. Retinoids are discussed more fully under systemic treatments. Tazarotene is available as a gel for treatment of plaque psoriasis and has minimal systemic absorption. Unlike other retinoids, tazarotene is selective for retinoic acid receptor (RAR) proteins with no affinity for retinoid X receptors (RXR). This may reduce its unwanted effects, which are mainly local irritation with pruritis. It should be avoided for 1 month before conception because of potential teratogenic actions.

Systemic treatments

Systemic treatment is reserved for the most severe forms of disease.

Methotrexate (Chs. 39 and 52). This is a very effective treatment at low dosages for resistant and widespread disease. Its main actions are cytostatic and immuno-suppressant. Oral or intramuscular dosing is commonly used once a week; bone marrow depression and hepato-toxicity with liver fibrosis are the main complications. Blood counts must be checked every 2–3 months and liver biopsies performed every 1–2 years to monitor treatment.

Retinoids. This term covers vitamin A (retinol) and therapeutically useful synthetic vitamin A derivatives such as etretinate and its active metabolite acitretin. Acitretin is now used in preference to etretinate. Given orally, they are anti-inflammatory and cytostatic. Vitamin A, and its metabolites retinaldehyde and retinoic acid, are involved in epithelial cell growth and differentiation. Retinoids enter cells by endocytosis and interact with two forms of retinoic acid nuclear receptor, RARs and RXRs (see above), which are related to steroid/thyroid hormone receptors. The retinoid receptor complex initiates gene transcription and may affect cell growth and differentiation by modulation of growth factors and their receptors. Response of psoriatic lesions is delayed by up to 2 months. The half-life of etretinate is very long (up to 6 months) because of sequestration in subcutaneous fat, while that of acitretin is about 2 days. Elimination of retinoids is by hepatic metabolism. Unwanted effects are almost universal and include dry lips and nasal mucosa, dryness of the skin with localised peeling over the digits and transient thin-ning of hair. These effects are dose dependent and reversible. Longer-term problems include ossification of ligaments, increased plasma triglycerides and, to a lesser extent, plasma cholesterol. There is a high risk of teratogenesis and women must use adequate contra-ception during treatment and stop treatment for 2 years before conception.

Ciclosporin or tacrolimus (Ch. 39). These immuno-suppressants are effective in psoriasis at lower doses than those required for prevention of allograft rejection. However, remissions induced by these drugs are usually short.

Future therapies

Drugs are under development that inhibit tumour necrosis factor activity or inhibit various functions of T-lymphocytes.

Acne

Acne most commonly arises in adolescence and often regresses in the late teens or early twenties. Acne affects areas of skin with large numbers of sebaceous glands: the face, back and chest. There is increased production of sebum, which distends the pilosebaceous duct producing a small closed papule (comedo) called a whitehead. Hyperkeratosis at the mouth of the hair follicle blocks the duct. If the duct then opens, compacted follicular cells at the tip give comedones the appearance of a blackhead. A resident anaerobic bacterium, *Propionibacterium acnes*, degrades triglycerides in sebum to free fatty acids and glycerol. It also produces chemotactic factors and inflammatory mediators. These, and the irritant free fatty acids, produce inflamed lesions of pustules, nodules or multilocular cysts if the lesions coalesce. The inflamma-tory lesions can scar with permanent disfigurement.

There is a genetic background to acne, which deter-mines the rate of sebum production, particularly in response to androgens. Androgens, which are produced at puberty, induce hypertrophy of sebaceous glands and the excess secretion rate in predisposed individuals triggers the acne.

Treatment of acne

There are several effective treatments for acne. The choice will depend on the nature of the lesions and their severity. Topical treatments do not influence the rate of production of sebum.

● Benzoyl peroxide has antibacterial and keratolytic actions that reduce the numbers of comedones. It produces scaling and skin irritation, which limit its use to short treatment periods.
● Topical antimicrobials, for example clindamycin, erythromycin, tetracycline (Ch. 51) are less effective than oral antimicrobials but have fewer unwanted effects. Their efficacy is similar to that of benzoyl peroxide with less skin irritation; tetracycline is least likely to cause bacterial resistance. They are used for mild to moderate acne and are particularly useful in pregnant women since there is no systemic absorption.
● Oral antimicrobials against *P. acnes* are used for inflammatory acne (papules/pustules). Penetration into sebaceous follicles is poor, but they produce some improvement after 2–3 months, requiring 4–6 months of treatment for maximal benefit. Treatment should be given for extended periods since relapse

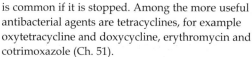

is common if it is stopped. Among the more useful antibacterial agents are tetracyclines, for example oxytetracycline and doxycycline, erythromycin and cotrimoxazole (Ch. 51).

- Azelaic acid is an aliphatic dicarboxylic acid that has an antibacterial action against propionibacteria and is effective against bacteria that have become resistant to erythromycin and tetracycline. It also inhibits the division of keratinocytes, which may reduce follicular plugging and prevent the development of comedones. It is applied topically; the most frequent unwanted effects are local burning, scaling or itching. Azelaic acid is most effective for mild to moderate acne, especially of the face.
- The antiandrogen cyproterone acetate (Ch. 46) is useful in women with moderate or severe acne and is usually given in combination with ethinylestradiol (Ch. 45). The combination reduces sebum flow by 40%. Alternatively, estrogen can be given with a non-androgenic progestogen such as norgestimate or desogestrel. Improvement can take 2–4 months.
- Isotretinoin is a vitamin A derivative that has a keratolytic action which unblocks the pilosebaceous follicles and allows flow of sebum to extrude the plug. The mechanism of action is similar to that of etretinate (see under psoriasis). It also reduces sebum production by up to 90% by decreasing sebocyte proliferation (this action is probably independent of effects on nuclear retinoid receptors). Topically it produces erythema and scaling, which can be minimised by starting with a low concentration. It is used orally in severe acne and gives an almost 100% chance of complete remission. High doses can produce prolonged remission. Unwanted effects include dry lips, nose and eyes, muscle and joint aches and increased plasma triglycerides. Teratogenesis is a major problem and, although the half-life of the metabolites is less than 2 days, conception should be avoided during and for 1 month after stopping treatment.

Choice of treatment for acne

Initially, management of non-inflammatory comedones is by topical treatment such as azelaic acid or retinoids. For early inflammatory lesions, a topical antimicrobial or benzoyl peroxide can be considered. More severe inflammatory acne usually requires topical or systemic antimicrobials with topical retinoid. Systemic treatment with isotretinoin is used for more severe and unresponsive patients. Estrogen and antiandrogen therapy are alternatives for women, and oral contraceptives can be of benefit.

Wound healing

Becalpermin

Mechanism of action and use

Becalpermin is a human recombinant platelet-derived growth factor (PDGF). Endogenous PDGF is synthesised by megakaryocytes, macrophages, fibroblasts, smooth muscle cells and endothelial cells. Platelets release PDGF after tissue injury. PDGF contributes to tissue healing by encouraging cell chemotaxis and activation of inflammatory cells and by increasing extracellular matrix deposition, cell mitogenesis and cell protein synthesis. This enhances granulation tissue in wounds. Becalpermin is used to enhance healing of chronic neuropathic diabetic foot ulcers.

Pharmacokinetics

Belcalpermin is applied topically as a gel. There is negligible systemic absorption.

Unwanted effects

A local erythematous rash can occur. Concern over the possibility of local carcinogenesis appears unfounded in short-term studies.

FURTHER READING

Brown SK, Shalita AR (1998) Acne vulgaris. *Lancet* 351, 1871–1876

Charman C (1999) Atopic eczema. *Br Med J* 318, 1600–1604

Friedmann PS (1998) Allergy and the skin. II: Contact and atopic eczema. *Br Med J* 316, 1226–1229

Greaves MW, Weinstein GD (1995) Treatment of psoriasis. *N Engl J Med* 332, 581–588

Leyden JJ (1997) Therapy for acne vulgaris. *N Engl J Med* 336, 1156–1162

Orfanos CE, Zouboulis CC, Almond-Roesler B et al. (1997) Current use and future potential role of retinoids in dermatology. *Drugs* 53, 358–388

Stern RS (1997) Psoriasis. *Lancet* 350, 349–353

Self-assessment

In questions 1–3, the first statement, in italics, is true. Are the following statements also true?

1. *Atopic dermatitis is the most common form of dermatitis and is an inflammatory condition with a familial tendency. It involves acute and chronic inflammation.*

   a. Topical corticosteroids should not be used in atopic dermatitis.
   b. Antihistamines given orally can reduce itching in atopic dermatitis.

2. *T-lymphocytes are important cells in psoriasis.*

   a. In severe resistant psoriasis, immunosuppressant drugs are contraindicated.
   b. Retinoids reduce cell growth and differentiation.

3. *Severe inflammatory acne should be treated with topical or systemic antimicrobials and a topical retinoid.*

   a. Suitable topical antimicrobials for inflammatory acne are erythromycin or clindamycin.
   b. Antibiotic resistance of *Propionibacterium acnes* does not occur.

4. Case history question

   > A 7-year-old girl with a history of asthma has developed a red, scaly and dry rash in her knee and elbow flexures and on her arms and cheeks. The rash is extremely itchy and she is scratching the affected areas causing excoriation and weeping. Her mother had atopic dermatitis when she was young.

   a. What is the possible diagnosis?
   b. What treatments should be tried initially?
   c. What other factors should be considered in the treatment of this young girl?

   The answers are provided on pages 628.

Drugs used in the treatment of skin disorders

Drug[a]	Half-life (h)[b]	Elimination	Comments
Corticosteroids			
Aclometasone dipropionate	–	–	No data available; topical pharmacokinetics probably similar to beclometasone
Beclometasone dipropionate	–	Metabolised and eliminated in faeces	Only about 2% is absorbed from the forearm but much higher absorption occurs from forehead (7%), scrotum (36%), the eyelids (40%) and from inflamed skin; hydration of the skin increases drug uptake and absorption
Betamethasone esters	–	Metabolism	Poor absorption with variations between different sites (see beclometasone)
Clobetasol propionate	–	Metabolism	Very poor absorption (see beclometasone); suppression of adrenocortical function is possible in patients with psoriasis
Clobetasone butyrate	–	Metabolism	Poorly absorbed (see beclometasone)
Desoximetasone	–	Metabolism (?)	Few data available; possible reduction in plasma cortisol in patients with psoriasis given long-term treatment suggests the possibility of significant absorption under such circumstances (a similar result was not obtained when intact skin was treated)
Diflucortolone valerate	–	Metabolism	Few data available; transdermal absorption is probably similar to beclometasone; only weak adrenocortical effects compared with clobetasol propionate
Fludroxycortide (flurandrenolone)	–	Metabolism	No published data have been identified; the route of elimination is predicted as no data are available
Fluocinolone acetonide	–	Metabolism	Poorly absorbed (see beclometasone); the route of elimination is predicted as no data are available
Fluocinonide	–	Metabolism	Poorly absorbed (see beclometasone); the route of elimination is predicted as no data are available
Fluocortolone	–	Metabolism	Few data available after topical dosing (not surprisingly it causes cortisol suppression after oral dosage but comparable topical data are not available)
Fluticasone propionate	2–5	Metabolism	Poorly absorbed transdermally (see beclometasone); half-life is following inhalation exposure
Halcinonide	–	Metabolism	Poorly absorbed (see beclometasone); higher risk of cortisol suppression than with betamethasone valerate (but better response) especially with occlusion; the route of elimination is predicted as no data are available.
Hydrocortisone (and butyrate)	1.5	Metabolism	Poorly absorbed transdermally (see beclometasone); half-life is for hydrocortisone
Mometasone furoate	–	Metabolism	Very poor absorption (see beclometasone); extensively metabolised with metabolites eliminated in urine and bile
Triamcinolone acetonide	2–5	Metabolism	Poorly absorbed from the skin (see beclometasone); rapidly eliminated from the blood by oxidation and then conjugation
Drugs for eczema and/or seborrheic dermatitis			
Gamolenic acid	–	Metabolism	Taken orally; metabolised to dihomogammalinolenic acid (DGLA), which is incorporated into cell membranes; scant evidence to support its value in atopic eczema
Ichthammol	–	–	A sulfonated shale oil that is used as an ointment or cream
Lithium succinate	–	–	Used as an ointment with zinc sulfate; high concentration used (8%) but absorption has not been defined
Drugs for psoriasis			
Coal tar	–	Metabolism	Also used for eczema and seborrheic dermatitis; coal tar contains polycyclic aromatic hydrocarbons which are oxidised (and activated) by CYP1A2; high transdermal absorption

continued

Drugs used in the treatment of skin disorders (continued)

Drug[a]	Half-life (h)[b]	Elimination	Comments
Drugs for psoriasis (continued)			
Psoralen (8-methoxypsoralen)	–	Metabolism	Unlicensed product given before ultraviolet A irradiation to increase effectiveness (PUVA treatment).
Calcipotriol (calcipotriene)	–	Metabolism	Vitamin D analogue; about 5% absorbed after topical application; few data available (very short plasma half-life in animal studies)
Tacalcitol	–	Metabolism	Vitamin D_3 analogue (1,24-dihydroxyvitamin D_3); negligible absorption after topical dosage
Tazarotene	18 (TA)	Metabolism	Retinoid; poorly absorbed across the skin; hydrolysed in skin to tazarotenic acid (TA), which is further metabolised; TA is responsible for binding to retinoid receptors
Acitretin	50	Metabolism	Given orally; retinoid; teratogenic risk; long half-life owing to low hepatic extraction and metabolism
Ciclosporin	27	Metabolism	Given orally; bioavailability is about 30%; oxidised by intestinal and hepatic CYP3A4
Dithranol (anthralin)	–	Metabolism	Poorly absorbed across the skin; metabolised within the skin
Methotrexate	8–10	Metabolism	Given orally; good oral absorption (20–95%); metabolised by the formation of polyglutamates (which are active and retained intracellularly) and by oxidation
Drugs for acne			
Azelaic acid	0.75	Renal	Low absorption (about 4%); eliminated unchanged in the urine (plus some limited β-oxidation); as for many (most?) topical drugs, absorption rate-limited kinetics result in a half-life after topical dosage (2 h) that is considerably longer than the elimination half-life
Benzoyl peroxide	–	Metabolism	Powerful oxidising agent that is reduced to benzoic acid; about 5% of the benzoic acid is absorbed
Adapalene	–	–	Retinoid-like drug; binds to nuclear but not cytosolic retinoid receptors; very low topical absorption; very few data available
Isotretinoin	10–20	Metabolism	Given topically; retinoid (13-*cis*-retinoic acid); isomerises to *all-trans*-retinoic acid; may be given orally but known to be a human teratogen; activity is largely owing to *all-trans*-retinoic acid
Tretinoin	1–2	Metabolism	Given topically; retinoid (*all-trans*-retinoic acid); metabolised by oxidation and formation of an acyl glucuronide; half-life is derived from studies following its formation from vitamin A

[a]The majority of treatments are given topically and show very slow and limited absorption. All drugs given topically unless otherwise stated.
[b]The systemic half-lives (when given) are not an indication of duration of action of topical formulations.

The eye

Vision depends upon the eye converting light input into an electrical signal to be carried to the brain through the optic nerve. The ciliary smooth muscles alter the shape of the lens, allowing the eye to accommodate to objects at different distances. The autonomic nervous system innervates these ciliary muscles. They also control the iris, which determines the size of the pupil and the amount of light entering the eye.

Accommodation. The ciliary muscle is a circular or constrictor muscle that is attached to the lens by suspensory ligaments. The ciliary muscle receives parasympathetic innervation. When the muscle is relaxed, tension on the suspensory ligaments stretches and flattens the lens inside its capsule, which adjusts visual acuity for distant vision. Paralysis of the ciliary muscle is known as cycloplegia. Stimulation of the parasympathetic innervation contracts the ciliary muscle, which relaxes the suspensory ligaments. The lens assumes a more globular shape, which accommodates the eye for near vision.

Pupil size. This is determined by the relative tone in the two muscles of the iris. The circular (constrictor) muscle is the more powerful and receives parasympathetic nervous innervation. The radial (dilator) muscle is sympathetically innervated. Constriction of the pupil is known as miosis, dilation is called mydriasis. The light reflex and accommodation for near vision both invoke a response in the parasympathetic nervous system producing pupillary constriction. Dilation of the pupil is caused by shortening of the iris muscle, which moves it towards the cornea and narrows the angle between the iris and the cornea.

Drainage of aqueous humour. The space between the cornea, at the front of the eye (Fig. 50.1) and the lens is filled with a clear liquid known as aqueous humour. Contraction of the ciliary muscle aids drainage of aqueous humour through the trabecular meshwork into the episcleral veins. If drainage of this fluid is impaired, the intraocular pressure rises, leading to **glaucoma** and progressive loss of vision. Dilation of the pupil also restricts drainage of aqueous humour through the trabecular meshwork. This predisposes to primary acute angle-closure glaucoma (Fig. 50.1). Conversely, constriction of the iris makes the pupil smaller and moves the pupil away from the trabecular meshwork of the canal of Schlemm, facilitating drainage.

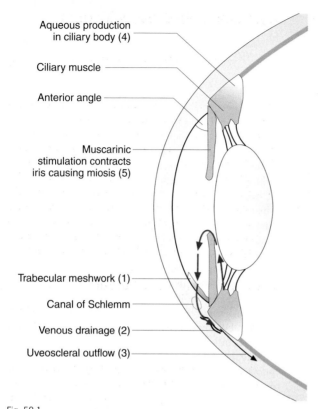

Cholinergic agonists, e.g. pilocarpine
(i) constrict iris (5)
   open anterior angle
(ii) constrict ciliary muscle
   enhance aqueous drainage (1,2)

Carbonic anhydrase inhibitors,
e.g. acetazolamide, decrease
aqueous production (4)

Beta blockers reduce aqueous
production (4), increase outflow (1)

Selective stimulants of α_2-adrenergic
receptors decrease aqueous
production (4) e.g. apraclonidine,
brimonidine

Prostaglandin $F_{2\alpha}$ analogues,
e.g. lanaprost, enhance uveoscleral
outflow (3)

→ Route of drainage of aqueous humor

Aqueous production
in ciliary body (4)

Ciliary muscle

Anterior angle

Muscarinic
stimulation contracts
iris causing miosis (5)

Trabecular meshwork (1)

Canal of Schlemm

Venous drainage (2)

Uveoscleral outflow (3)

Fig. 50.1
The route of drainage of aqueous humour from the eye and the sites and mechanisms of action of drugs used in the treatment of glaucoma.

Glaucoma

Glaucoma is a group of disorders, characterised by raised intraocular pressure, that lead to ischaemia of the optic nerve head and damage to retinal nerve fibres. Progressive visual defects occur, initially as scotomas (blind spots) in the peripheral visual field. These scotomas enlarge, coalesce and eventually lead to reduced visual acuity. Glaucoma is the second most common cause of blindness in the UK.

Glaucoma can result from a developmental defect or a degenerative process (primary glaucoma) or can be secondary to another disease process. Primary glaucoma is the most common type and can be either open-angle or closed-angle depending on the configuration of the drainage angle of the eye. Aqueous humour is constantly secreted by the ciliary body and is influenced by innervation from the autonomic nervous system; it flows round the iris and through the pupil to the anterior chamber (Fig. 50.1). **Open-angle glaucoma** is caused by obstruction in the trabecular meshwork that drains the anterior chamber of the eye to the episcleral veins through the canal of Schlemm. **Angle-closure glaucoma** is less common, usually acute in onset and results from the iris taking up close proximity against the trabecular meshwork and preventing drainage. This occurs often in an individual with a shallow anterior chamber, such as occurs in long-sighted individuals. Chronic angle-closure glaucoma is rare. α_2-Adrenoceptor stimulation in the ciliary body reduces the production of aqueous humour. β_1-Adrenoceptor stimulation, however, increases the production of aqueous humour.

Drugs used in the eye

Topical application

Drugs applied in solution to the anterior surface of the eye can penetrate to the anterior chamber and the ciliary muscle, principally via the cornea. The high water content of the cornea makes lipid solubility less important for adequate penetration than with transdermal drug delivery, but formulation of the carrier is important to avoid irritation of the conjunctivae. There is little diffusion to more posterior structures of the eye.

Systemic absorption of drug following topical application to the surface of the eye can occur either via conjuctival vessels or from the nasal mucosa after drainage of excess drug via the tear ducts. Topical administration of drugs to the eye may, therefore, produce systemic effects. Drainage can be reduced by shutting the eyes for at least 1 min after putting the drops in and by compressing the nasolacrimal duct at the medial corner of the eye with a finger. Both eye drops and ointments are usually administered into the pocket that can be formed by gently pulling the lower eyelid (the lower fornix).

Microbial contamination is a potential problem once eye preparations are opened. Multiple-application containers have preservative added to reduce the risk, but prolonged use of opened containers is not advisable.

Drugs for glaucoma

Sympathomimetics

Examples: brimonidine, apraclonidine, epinephrine, dipivefrine

Epinephrine (adrenaline) and its prodrug, dipivefrine, are mydriatic by stimulating α_1-adrenoceptors in the iris and should not be used in angle-closure glaucoma. They improve drainage through the trabecular meshwork and decrease aqueous production by α_2-adrenoceptor stimulation. Epinephrine is rarely used now. The prodrug dipivefrine is converted to epinephrine in the eye and has the advantage of greater penetration through the cornea. The α_2-adrenoceptor agonist drugs apraclonidine and brimonidine decrease ciliary body aqueous humour production and are not mydriatic. α_1-Adrenoceptor agonists should be used with care in patients with hypertension and heart disease.

Beta-adrenoceptor antagonists (β-blockers)

Examples: timolol, betaxolol

The β-blockers probably act by reducing the formation of aqueous humour. They have no effect on accommodation or pupil size, which makes them the treatment of first choice for glaucoma. However, systemic absorption can produce the typical unwanted effects associated with these compounds (Ch. 5) and the same contraindications apply as for oral use. Timolol is a non-selective β-blocker; betaxolol is 'cardioselective'.

Carbonic anhydrase inhibitors

Examples: acetazolamide, dorzolamide

The action of the carbonic anhydrase inhibitors is discussed in Chapter 14. The isoenzyme carbonic anhydrase is found primarily in red blood cells and the eye, where it plays a key role in controlling aqueous humour production. Carbonic anhydrase is responsible for about 70% of the Na^+ that enters the anterior chamber, which is followed by water to maintain isotonicity. Inhibition of the enzyme, therefore, reduces aqueous humour production.

Acetazolamide is taken orally; dorzolamide is a topical preparation for the eye with fewer systemic unwanted effects. They have a duration of action of 6–12 h.

Prostaglandin F$_{2\alpha}$ analogues

Example: latanoprost

Latanoprost is an analogue of prostaglandin F$_{2\alpha}$. This drug increases uveoscleral outflow of aqueous humour. The major disadvantage is an increase in brown pigmentation of the iris. It has a long duration of action, of 1–2 days.

Miotic drugs (muscarinic agonists)

Example: pilocarpine

Pilocarpine (see also Ch. 4) is usually given for angle-closure glaucoma to contract the pupillary muscle to produce miosis and open up the drainage channels in the anterior chamber of the eye. Ciliary muscle spasm is an undesirable consequence and produces blurred vision and an ache over the eye (especially in younger patients). The miosis effect lasts about 4 h, but prolonged miosis can be achieved by the use of Ocuserts®, a small plastic reservoir that releases drug in the lower fornix of the eye for up to a week. Ciliary muscle contraction may also improve uveoscleral outflow. Pilocarpine can be used together with other drugs in simple open-angle glaucoma.

Mydriatic and cycloplegic drugs

Examples: atropine, homatropine, cyclopentolate, tropicamide

The parasympathetic antagonists (see also Ch. 4) are both mydriatic (dilating pupil) and cycloplegic (paralysing ciliary muscle). Tropicamide is weak and short acting (about 3 h), which makes it useful to dilate the pupil for fundal examination. Cyclopentolate and homatropine both last for up to 24 h and are more powerful; the former has a more rapid onset of action. Atropine is long acting, the effect persisting for up to 7 days. The longer-acting compounds are used to prevent adhesions (posterior synechiae) in patients with anterior uveitis.

The degree of cycloplegia will depend on the dose of drug; small doses produce pupil dilation with insufficient diffusion to affect accommodation profoundly. Patients should not drive after receiving a cycloplegic and care must be taken using these drugs in patients predisposed to acute angle-closure glaucoma.

Other topical applications for the eye

Several other drugs are used topically in the eye for particular indications.

Antimicrobial agents. The antimicrobial drugs (Ch. 51) are given for local infection such as blepharitis, conjunctivitis or trachoma (caused by chlamydial infection). Aqueous solutions are rapidly diluted or flushed away by lachrimation; ointments are often given for longer action, for example at night. Examples of broad-spectrum agents are gentamicin, chloramphenicol, ciprofloxacin, fusidic acid, neomycin and chlortetracycline (the last for trachoma).

Antiviral agents. Antiviral drugs (Ch. 51) are mainly used for herpes simplex infection, which causes dendritic corneal ulcers. Aciclovir is most frequently used.

Corticosteroids. Local inflammatory conditions such as uveitis and scleritis are treated with corticosteroids, for example dexamethasone or prednisolone (Ch. 44). Care must be taken to exclude a viral dendritic ulcer and glaucoma before using them, since these conditions can be exacerbated by corticosteroids. Prolonged use of corticosteroids can lead to thinning of the sclera or cornea.

Antiallergic agents. Topical antihistamines such as antazoline (usually given in combination with the sympathomimetic xylometazoline) (Ch. 38) or sodium cromoglicate (Ch. 12) can be given for allergic conjuctivitis.

Local anaesthetics. Tetracaine (amethocaine) or lidocaine (lignocaine) eye drops provide surface anaesthesia (Ch. 18) for minor surgical procedures or tonometry (pressure measurements for the anterior chamber).

Artificial tears. A variety of compounds can be used for the dry eyes associated with Sjögren's syndrome, for example hypromellose or the mucolytic agent acetylcysteine.

Cocaine. Application of cocaine causes local anaesthesia but also pupillary dilatation. It is now rarely used. It brings about this effect as it prevents the re-uptake of noradrenaline released from sympathetic nerves, thus causing constriction of the radial muscles of the iris. Cocaine can be used in the eye to test for Horner's syndrome. A lesion of the sympathetic supply to the iris would result in pupil constriction that could not be reversed by cocaine.

Treatment of glaucoma

In open-angle glaucoma, reducing intraocular pressure can slow the rate of progression sufficiently to prevent significant visual impairment. A target pressure reduction of at least 30% below the presenting pressure is usually set.

Topical β-blockers remain the treatment of choice, when there are no contraindications, because of their lack of ocular unwanted effects. If a β-blocker cannot be used, the choice of a second-line drug lies between a muscarinic agonist (usually pilocarpine), a topical carbonic anhydrase inhibitor, a sympathomimetic agent or a prostaglandin analogue. Many ophthalmologists consider surgery if the first-line treatment fails. This is usually carried out by laser burns to the trabecular meshwork. The effect of this approach is often short lived, and drug treatment may still be required. Drainage surgery is an alternative approach. Combinations of drugs are sometimes used for patients with resistant disease, although their effects are less than additive.

Angle-closure glaucoma is treated by iridotomy to provide a channel for aqueous humour to flow through the iris. If drug therapy is required after surgery, then a topical β-blocker can be used.

FURTHER READING

Alward WLM (1998) Medical management of glaucoma. *N Engl J Med* 339, 1298–1307

Coleman AL (1999) Glaucoma. *Lancet* 354, 1803–1810

Self-assessment

In questions 1 and 2 the first statement, in italics, is true. Are the accompanying statements also true?

1. *The production of aqueous humour is not altered in glaucoma but drainage is reduced.*

   a. Epinephrine is the drug of choice in patients with narrow-angle glaucoma.
   b. Stimulation of α_2-adrenoceptors in the ciliary body reduces aqueous humour production.
   c. Tropicamide should be avoided in patients with glaucoma.

2. *Accommodation of the lens is controlled by the parasympathetic autonomic nervous supply to the ciliary muscle.*

   a. Cocaine is a local anaesthetic that does not alter pupil size when administered topically.
   b. Cyclopentolate is a longer-acting mydriatic drug than tropicamide.
   c. Pilocarpine causes accommodation for near vision.

3. Case history question

   During a routine eye examination, the optician noted a chronically raised intraocular pressure in a 56-year-old woman. Further tests revealed she had open-angle (simple) glaucoma.

   a. What is thought to be the main cause of open angle glaucoma?
   b. What drugs could be used for this condition?
   c. What precautions should be taken when using these drugs?

   The answers are provided on pages 628–629.

Drugs used in the eye[a]

Drug	Half-life (h)[b]	Elimination	Comments
Antibacterials			
Chloramphenicol	5 (2–12)	Metabolism	Eliminated mainly by glucuronidation
Chlortetracycline	5–6	Bile + renal	About 20% of absorbed drug will be eliminated in the urine with the remainder in the bile
Ciprofloxacin	3–4	Renal + metabolism	Eliminated by glomerular filtration, renal tubular secretion plus metabolism (15%)
Framycetin	–	–	No relevant kinetic data are available
Fusidic acid	9	Metabolism	Metabolised in liver and metabolites excreted in bile
Gentamicin	1–4	Renal	Eliminated by glomerular filtration
Lomefloxacin	8	Renal	Eliminated by renal excretion and the elimination rate is proportional to creatinine clearance; there is also significant 'non-renal' clearance (the difference between plasma clearance and renal clearance) but the nature of this is not known (metabolism, biliary excretion?)
Neomycin	2	Renal	Eliminated by glomerular filtration
Ofloxacin	6–7	Renal (+ metabolism)	Eliminated by kidneys plus limited metabolism (<5%)
Polymyxin B	–	–	No relevant kinetic data available
Propamidine isetionate	–	–	No relevant kinetic data available
Antivirals			
Aciclovir	3	Renal (+ metabolism)	Eliminated largely by renal tubular secretion + filtration; only about 10% is metabolised to inactive excretory products
Corticosteroids			
Betamethasone	35–55	Metabolism	Phosphate ester hydrolysed to betamethasone, which is inactivated by metabolism
Clobetasone butyrate	–	Metabolism	Only used topically; systemic disposition has not been defined
Dexamethasone	2–4	Metabolism	Metabolised in the liver by CYP3A4-mediated oxidation to the 6-hydroxy compound
Fluorometholone	–	Metabolism	Only used topically; metabolism probably occurs locally in the eye; systemic disposition has not been defined
Hydrocortisone acetate	1–2	Metabolism	Metabolised by oxidation to cortisone and reduction to dihydro- and tetrahydrocortisol
Prednisolone	2–4	Metabolism	Extensively metabolised but all pathways have not been defined
Rimexolone	1–2	Metabolism (+ bile)	The elimination half-life has been estimated by the fact that steady-state levels are achieved after 5–7 h; few other data available
Other anti-inflammatory preparations			
Antazoline	–	–	Histamine H_1 receptor antagonist; no relevant kinetic data are available
Azelastine	17	Metabolism	Histamine H_1 receptor antagonist; metabolised by hepatic P450 to active desmethyl metabolite
Emedastine	3–4	Metabolism	Histamine H_1 receptor antagonist; eliminated in urine largely as oxidised metabolites plus about 5% as the unchanged drug
Levocabastine	35–40	Renal (+ metabolism)	Histamine H_1 receptor antagonist; extensive absorption (30–60%) has been found following ocular administration; elimination is largely as the unchanged compound (plus the acyl glucuronide) in urine
Lodoxamide	8	Renal	Mast cell stabiliser; eliminated largely in the urine as the parent drug; few data available

continued

Drugs used in the eye[a] *(continued)*

Drug	Half-life (h)[b]	Elimination	Comments
Other anti-inflammatory preparations *(continued)*			
Nedocromil	2	Renal	Highly polar compound showing slow absorption across membranes; once in the blood it is eliminated rapidly by renal excretion (a slower late phase with a half-life of 14 h has been reported but this is probably of little clinical relevance)
Sodium cromoglicate	1–1.5	Renal	Highly polar drug that shows limited absorption across cell membranes; absorbed drug is eliminated largely in the urine
Mydriatics and cycloplegics			
Atropine	2–5	Metabolism + renal	Antimuscarinic; probably well absorbed; undergoes limited hydrolysis, plus oxidation and conjugation; about 30% of the dose is excreted unchanged in the urine
Cyclopentolate	2	?	Antimuscarinic; peak plasma concentrations occur about 30 min after giving eye drops; method of elimination has not been described
Homatropine	–	–	Antimuscarinic; probably well absorbed; no relevant kinetic data are available
Tropicamide	0.3 (or less)	?	Antimuscarinic; rapidly absorbed after ophthalmological dosage; peak plasma concentration occurs at 5 min, decreasing rapidly to undetectable levels by 2 h
Phenylephrine	2–3	Metabolism + renal	Sympathomimetic α_1-selective adrenoceptor agonist; eliminated in urine as glucuronic acid and sulfate conjugates and as parent compound (15–20% after intravenous dosage)
Local anaesthetics			
Lidocaine (lignocaine)	2	Metabolism	Metabolised by dealkylation, catalysed by CYP3A4, followed by hydrolysis
Oxybuprocaine	–	Metabolism	Few kinetic data available; about 90% recovered in urine as parent drug and metabolites within 9 h (therefore half-life is 3 h or less)
Proxymetacaine	–	–	No relevant kinetic data available.
Tetracaine (amethocaine)	Very short (?)	Metabolism	Any absorbed drug would be very rapidly hydrolysed by plasma pseudocholinesterase.
Treatment of glaucoma			
Miotics			
Carbachol	–	–	Muscarinic agonist; no relevant kinetic data are available
Pilocarpine	1	Metabolism	Few details available; oxidised to an acid analogue; ocular effects persist for 4–14 h
Sympathomimetics			
Epinephrine (adrenaline)	0.1	Metabolism	Any absorbed compound would be very rapidly cleared from the blood
Brimonidine	3	Metabolism	Agonist at α_2-adrenoceptors; metabolised by human liver preparations to oxidised products; relative importance of metabolism and other routes of elimination have not been defined
Dipivefrine	–	–	No relevant kinetic data available
Guanethidine	2 days	Renal	Very slow elimination; the true terminal half-life may be as long as 8 days (few data available)

continued

Drugs used in the eye[a] *(continued)*

Drug	Half-life (h)[b]	Elimination	Comments
Beta-blockers			
Betaxolol	13–24	Metabolism (+ some renal)	Selective for β_1-adrenoceptors; oxidised in liver and metabolites eliminated in urine
Carteolol	3–7	Renal + metabolism	Mostly eliminated in urine unchanged; the main metabolite (8-hydroxycarteolol) is a more potent β-adrenoceptor antagonist
Levobunolol	5–8	Metabolism + renal	Eliminated in urine as parent drug (about 15%), as a reduced metabolite and as conjugates of the parent drug and metabolite
Metipranolol	5	Metabolism	Various pathways of metabolism, including deacetylation giving a highly active metabolite (which is responsible for in vivo activity on cardiac β-adrenoceptors); the role of local metabolism in relation to ocular effect is not known
Timolol	2–5	Metabolism (+ some renal)	Non-selective β-blocker, eliminated by metabolism and renal excretion (20%)
Carbonic anhydrase inhibitors			
Acetazolamide	6–9	Renal	Eliminated in urine without detectable metabolism
Dorzolamide	Weeks	Renal (+ metabolism)	Blood concentrations are not detectable after ophthalmological use; an active de-ethylated metabolite has been reported; retained in red blood cells which gives rise to an elimination half-life on cessation of the treatment of weeks
Prostaglandin analogues			
Latanoprost	0.3 (acid)	Metabolism	Analogue of $PGF_{2\alpha}$; the parent compound can be measured in the plasma during the first hour after ophthalmological administration; metabolised to an active acid metabolite, which has a half-life of 0.3 h; the reduction of intraocular pressure occurs at about 8–12 h (so systemic disposition gives no indication of therapeutic effect)

[a]Drugs are usually given topically to reduce systemic side-effects.
[b]The half-life data in this table refer to the systemic fate following absorption into the general circulation.

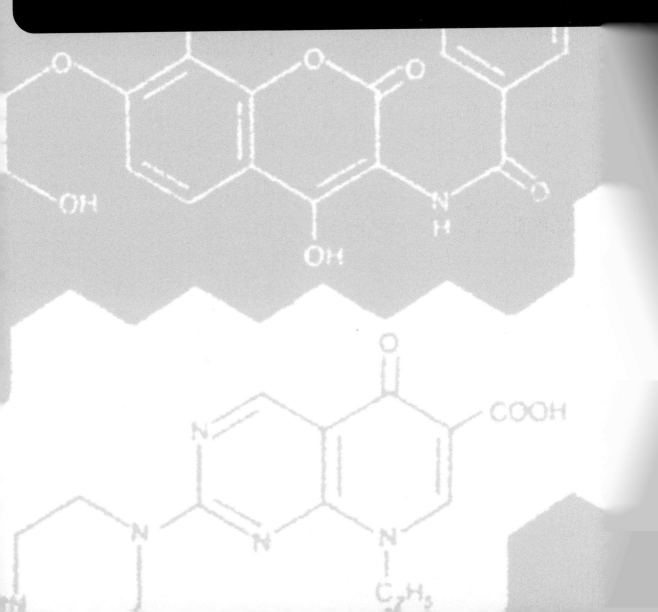

CHEMOTHERAPY

Chemotherapy of infections

Antimicrobial agents are natural or synthetic chemical substances that suppress the growth of, or destroy, microorganisms including bacteria, fungi and viruses. The term antibiotic is widely used but strictly should be reserved for antimicrobial agents derived from microorganisms; the terms antimicrobial or the more restrictive terms antibacterial, antifungal and antiviral are used in this chapter. In order to avoid unwanted effects, in man most antimicrobial agents are designed to have actions on processes that are unique to the pathogen. They must also be able to reach the site of infection. Microorganisms can acquire resistance to an antimicrobial and will then no longer be affected by the drug.

Bacterial infections

Classification of antibacterial agents

Antibacterial agents can be classified in several overlapping ways.

Firstly, they can be considered bacteriostatic or bactericidal. This categorisation depends largely on the concentration of drug that can be safely achieved in plasma without causing significant toxicity in the patient. Bacteriostatic antibacterials inhibit bacterial growth but do not destroy the cell at concentrations in plasma that are safe. The natural immune mechanisms of the body are used to eliminate the organism. Such drugs will be less effective in immunocompromised individuals or when organisms are dormant and not dividing. Bactericidal antibacterials kill microorganisms at safe plasma concentrations, but even so body immune mechanisms still play a role in elimination of the organism; Some bactericidal agents are more effective when cells are actively dividing; therefore, by preventing cell division, co-prescribed bacteriostatic agents may, in fact, make bactericidal antibacterials less effective.

Secondly, antibacterials can be grouped according to their various mechanisms of action (Fig. 51.1):

- agents that inhibit the synthesis of peptidoglycans of the bacterial cell wall or activate enzymes which disrupt the cell wall (e.g. β-lactams)

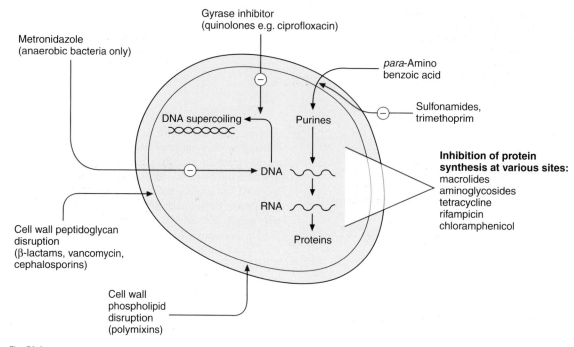

Fig. 51.1

A simplified scheme of the sites of action of the main classes of antibacterial drugs.

- agents that act directly on the cell phospholipid membrane and affect permeability, leading to leakage of intracellular contents (e.g. polymyxins)
- agents that alter the ribosomal function thereby causing a reversible inhibition of protein synthesis (e.g. aminoglycosides, macrolides); a high degree of selectivity for bacteria is possible because bacterial ribosomes differ structurally from those in humans
- agents that block metabolic pathways which are essential for the life of the bacteria (e.g. trimethoprim)
- agents that interfere with replication of DNA or RNA in the microorganism by interfering with DNA supercoiling (e.g. quinolones).

Thirdly, antibacterials may be classified according to whether their spectrum of activity against bacteria is limited (narrow spectrum) or extensive (broad spectrum).

Finally, they can be classified by chemical structure. In the following text the antibacterial agents are grouped according to their mechanism of action and then by their chemical structure. However, cross-referencing to other methods of classification is necessary. (The drug compendium is organised according to the BNF.)

Resistance

When an antimicrobial is ineffective against a microorganism in doses that can be safely used in humans, the organism is said to be resistant to the antimicrobial agent. There are four mechanisms by which a microorganism can protect itself against an antibacterial drug (Fig. 51.2).

- Modification of the organism such that it produces enzymes that inactivate the drug. For example, β-lactamase enzymes inactivate penicillin and acetylating enzymes can inactivate aminoglycosides.
- Modification of the organism such that penetration of the drug is reduced or it is pumped out faster than it can enter; for example, absence of the membrane protein D2 porin in resistant *Pseudomonas aeruginosa* prevents penetration of the β-lactam antibacterial imipenem.
- Structural change in the target molecule for the antibacterial drug. For example, low affinity of penicillin-binding proteins in resistant enterococci reduces binding of cephalosporins; mutation may prevent the binding of aminoglycosides to the previously sensitive 30S unit of ribosomes.
- Production of a bypass pathway to overcome the effect of the antibacterial drug. For example, resistant organisms have developed mutant dihydrofolate reductase resistant to trimethoprim inhibition.

Resistance to antibacterial agents can be inherent in the microorganism or can be acquired by modification of the genetic structure of the microorganism. The major mechanisms by which bacteria acquire resistance to antibacterial drugs are spontaneous mutation, conjugation, transduction and transformation.

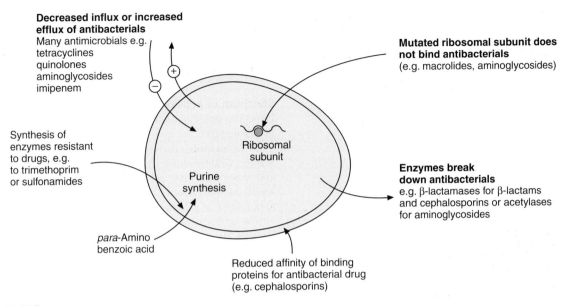

Decreased influx or increased efflux of antibacterials
Many antimicrobials e.g. tetracyclines quinolones aminoglycosides imipenem

Mutated ribosomal subunit does not bind antibacterials
(e.g. macrolides, aminoglycosides)

Synthesis of enzymes resistant to drugs, e.g. to trimethoprim or sulfonamides

Ribosomal subunit

Purine synthesis

Enzymes break down antibacterials
e.g. β-lactamases for β-lactams and cephalosporins or acetylases for aminoglycosides

para-Amino benzoic acid

Reduced affinity of binding proteins for antibacterial drug (e.g. cephalosporins)

Fig. 51.2
Mechanisms by which bacteria can resist antibacterial drugs.

Spontaneous mutation. In this process, a single-step genetic mutation in a bacterial population leads to selective growth of the resistant strain in the presence of an antibacterial drug.

Conjugation. Direct cell to cell contact is a way of exchanging genetic material that confers antibacterial resistance and usually involves transfer of self-replicating circular fragments of DNA called plasmids, which can contain multiple resistance genes. Plasmids can remain outside the genome of the microorganism or can be incorporated into it (a transposon).

Transduction. Bacteria are susceptible to infection by viruses known as bacteriophages. During replication of the bacteriophages, the host cell's DNA (containing resistance genes) may be replicated along with viral DNA and taken into the virus. The phage carrying the resistance genes can then infect other bacterial cells and spread resistance.

Transformation. Uptake of DNA from dead bacteria by live bacteria can spread resistance genes.

Resistance is also a major problem for infections with protozoa (e.g. malaria) and viruses (e.g. human immunodeficiency virus (HIV)) but is less significant in fungal infections (apart from in immunodeficient patients). Resistance in protozoa and viruses is discussed below in the individual sections.

Antibacterial agents

The antibacterial agents described are grouped by their mechanism of action and then by their chemical structure.

Agents affecting cell wall: β-lactam antibacterials

This group of drugs all have a β-lactam ring in common, which is responsible for their activity (Fig 51.3). The β-lactams include penicillins, cephalosporins and cephamycins, monobactams and carbapenems. Some are susceptible to enzymic attack by β-lactamases (penicillinases) but some are structurally modified to confer resistance to the β-lactamases.

Penicillins

Examples:
Penicillins: benzylpenicillin, phenoxymethylpenicillin
Aminopenicillins: ampicillin, flucloxacillin, amoxicillin
Ureidopenicillins: piperacillin
Amidinopenicillin: pivmecillinam
Carboxypenicillin: ticarcillin

Mechanism of action

Penicillins consist of a thiazolidine ring connected to a β-lactam ring to which is attached a side-chain (Fig. 51.3). The side-chain determines many of the antibacterial and pharmacological characteristics of a particular type of penicillin. The β-lactam antibacterials inhibit synthesis of the peptidoglycan layer of the cell wall, which surrounds

β-lactam ring

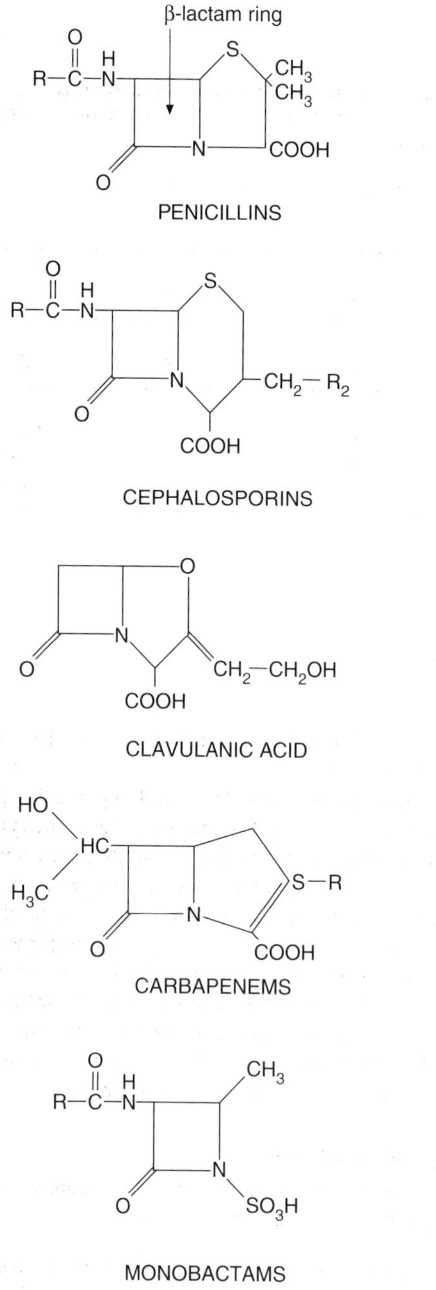

PENICILLINS

CEPHALOSPORINS

CLAVULANIC ACID

CARBAPENEMS

MONOBACTAMS

Fig. 51.3
The structural backbone of β-lactam antibacterial agents and the β-lactamase inhibitor clavulanic acid.

certain bacteria and is essential for their survival. Peptidoglycan synthesis occurs in three stages and the last stage of cross-linking is inhibited by penicillin, which binds to the transpeptidase involved in the cross-linking process. The β-lactam ring contains structural similarities to one of the constituents of the peptidoglycan layer. The antibacterial effect is confined to dividing cells, which become unable to maintain their transmembrane osmotic gradient; this leads to cell swelling, which is followed by

rupture and cell death. Some bacterial cells also contain enzymes that, if activated, lead to cell lysis. The β-lactam antibacterials bind to specific penicillin-binding proteins and reduce the action of the natural inhibitor of this lytic process, leading to lysis of the cell wall.

Spectrum of activity
Penicillins differ considerably in their spectrum of activity (Table 51.1).

Benzylpenicillin (penicillin G) is active against many aerobic Gram-positive bacteria, Gram-negative cocci and many anaerobic microorganisms. Gram-negative bacilli are not sensitive. Benzylpenicillin is susceptible to the action of β-lactamase (see below).

The addition of an acyl side-chain to the β-lactam nucleus produces derivatives such as flucloxacillin (floxacillin), which prevent the access of β-lactamase to the β-lactam ring. The downside is that flucloxacillin is generally less effective than benzylpenicillin against the bacteria that do not produce β-lactamase. Flucloxacillin is, therefore, usually reserved for treating β-lactamase producing staphylococci, which are particularly common in hospitals.

Ampicillin and amoxicillin are aminopenicillins that have an extended spectrum of activity to include activity against many Gram-negative bacteria. They are destroyed by β-lactamase and are somewhat less effective than benzylpenicillin against Gram-positive cocci.

Other extended-spectrum penicillins include ureidopenicillins (e.g. piperacillin), which are active against *Pseudomonas aeruginosa*, and amidinopenicillins (e.g. pivmecillinam), which are active mainly against Gram-negative bacteria. Carboxypenicillins (e.g. ticarcillin) are not widely used now, but have some activity against *Pseudomonas* species.

Clavulanic acid is a potent inhibitor of β-lactamase that is structurally related to the β-lactam antibiotics, although it has little intrinsic antibacterial activity (Fig. 51.3). When given in combination with penicillins that are destroyed by β-lactamase, such as amoxicillin and ticarcillin, they can be used to treat infections caused by β-lactamase-producing organisms that are otherwise insensitive to penicillins. Other β-lactamase inhibitors are also available.

Resistance
Resistance to penicillins is most often due to the production of β-lactamase which hydrolyses the β-lactam ring (Fig. 51.2). Some Gram-positive bacteria release extracellular β-lactamases particularly *Staphylococcus aureus*. In Gram-negative bacteria, the β-lactamases are located between the inner and outer cell membranes in the periplasmic space. The information for β-lactamase production is encoded in a plasmid and this may be transferred by transduction or conjugation to other bacteria.

Table 51.1
Example of penicillins and their properties

	β-Haemolytic streptococci	Staphylococcus aureus		Enterobacteriaceae (coliforms)	Pseudomonas aeruginosa	Bacteroides fragilis
		β-Lactamase negative	β-Lactamase positive			
Benzylpenicillin/ phenoxymethylpenicillin	++	+	0	0	0	++
Broader spectrum Amoxicillin/ampicillin	++	+	0[a]	++	0	0
β-Lactamase resistant Flucloxacillin	+	+	+[b]	0	0	0
Antipseudomonal Ticarcillin	++	+	0[a,c]	+	+	+/0
Azlocillin	++	+	0[a]	+	+	+/0
Piperacillin	++	+	0[a]	+	+	+/0

++, active; +, variable activity; 0, inactive.
[a] Can be used combined with a β-lactamase inhibitor.
[b] Resistance is developing.
[c] Ticarcillin only available with clavulanic acid.

Pharmacokinetics

Benzylpenicillin and phenoxymethylpenicillin. Only about one-third of an orally administered dose of benzylpenicillin is absorbed, the rest is destroyed in the stomach. Benzylpenicillin is, therefore, restricted to intramuscular or intravenous routes of administration. The phenoxymethyl derivative (penicillin V) is more stable in an acid environment and is better absorbed from the gut. Maximum concentrations in blood occur rapidly in 30–60 min. Penicillins are widely distributed throughout the body, although transport across the meninges is poor unless they are acutely inflamed (e.g. in meningitis), when penetration by the antibacterial is improved. The half-life of most penicillins is short (see drug compendium table) because they are very rapidly eliminated by the kidneys, mainly by active tubular secretion. Effective plasma concentrations of penicillins when given alone are usually maintained by frequent dosing or by intravenous infusion. The action of penicillin can be prolonged by combining it with a local anaesthetic such as procaine, and giving the formulation by intramuscular injection. Penicillin is then released slowly from the intramuscular depot, maintaining plasma concentrations for up to 24 h. A second method for prolonging effective plasma concentrations is to co-administer probenecid, which competitively inhibits the tubular secretion of penicillin (Ch. 2).

Flucloxacillin, ampicillin and amoxicillin. Flucloxacillin and amoxicillin are rapidly and almost completely absorbed from the gut but ampicillin is incompletely absorbed. These drugs have short half-lives. They can be administered parenterally if required

and are eliminated by the kidney in a similar way to benzylpenicillin.

Other penicillins. The amidinopenicillin pivmecillinam is a prodrug for oral use. The carboxypenicillin ticarcillin is only available in combination with clavulanic acid for parenteral use and as prodrug formulations that can be absorbed orally. These drugs are excreted renally. The ureidopenicillin piperacillin is given parenterally. Piperacillin is also available in combination with the β-lactamase inhibitor tazobactam. Biliary excretion eliminates about a quarter of piperacillin; therefore, at high doses, kinetics alter as a result of reduced renal and biliary clearances.

Unwanted effects

Penicillins are normally very safe antibacterials with a high therapeutic index.

- Hypersensitivity reactions. Manifestations of allergy to penicillins include rashes, fever, vasculitis, serum sickness, exfoliative dermatitis, Stevens–Johnson syndrome and anaphylactic shock. Cross-allergy occurs among various penicillins and to a lesser extent with cephalosporins. Penicillins and their breakdown products bind to proteins and act as haptens, stimulating the production of antibodies that mediate the allergic response (Ch. 39).
- Aminopenicillins (e.g. amoxicillin) frequently produce a non-allergic maculopapular rash in patients with glandular fever.
- Reversible neutropenia and eosinophilia can occur with prolonged high doses.

- Grand-mal seizures can occur with excessively high cerebrospinal fluid (CSF) concentrations of penicillin (a risk in patients with renal failure).
- Diarrhoea can occur as a result of disturbance of normal colonic flora, especially with broad-spectrum penicillins.

Cephalosporins

Examples:

First generation: cefadroxil, cefalexin, cefradine

Second generation: cefaclor, cefuroxime

Third generation: cefotaxime, cefixime, ceftazidime

Mechanism of action

Cephalosporins, like penicillins, have a β-lactam ring. To this ring is fused a dihydrothiazine ring, which makes them more resistant to hydrolysis by β-lactamases (Fig. 51.3). They inhibit bacterial cell wall synthesis in a manner similar to that of the penicillins.

Spectrum of activity

Cephalosporins are often classified by 'generations'. The members within each generation share similar antibacterial activity. However, the pharmacokinetics of individual drugs within each generation vary and there are examples within each generation of cephalosporins that can only be given parenterally. Succeeding generations tend to have increased activity against Gram-negative bacilli, usually at the expense of Gram-positive activity, and increased ability to cross the blood–brain barrier (Table 51.2).

The first-generation oral cephalosporins (e.g. cefadroxil or cefalexin) have activity against staphylococci and most streptococci except enterococci. They cross the blood–brain barrier only poorly. Second-generation oral cephalosporins such as cefuroxime are, in addition, active against some Gram-negative organisms such as *Haemophilus* species. Third-generation oral cephalosporins have improved β-lactamase stability and are able to penetrate the cerebrospinal fluid in useful quantities. Cefixime, which belongs to this group, improves on the Gram-negative activity of the other two generations and adds *Proteus* and *Klebsiella* species to its spectrum. However, it has no activity against staphylococci (Table 51.2).

Resistance

Some cephalosporins are sensitive to enzymatic hydrolysis of the β-lactam ring but susceptibility is considerably less with the later generations.

Pharmacokinetics

The pharmacokinetics of the cephalosporins vary greatly. First-generation oral cephalosporins are usually well absorbed. Several second- and third-generation drugs, for example cefuroxime and cefotaxime, are acid labile and must be given by a parenteral route. Cefuroxime has been formulated as a prodrug (cefuroxime axetil) for oral use, which has good absorption and is hydrolysed at first pass through the liver to cefuroxime. Most cephalosporins are primarily excreted by the kidney and have short half-lives. Cefixime is mainly eliminated by biliary excretion and has an intermediate half-life.

Unwanted effects

- Nausea and vomiting.
- Skin rashes.
- Cephalosporins can produce hypersensitivity reactions similar to those observed with the penicillins. Between 6 and 18% of patients who are allergic to penicillin show cross-allergy to cephalosporins. A history of a serious reaction to penicillin precludes the administration of cephalosporins.
- Diarrhoea can be caused by disturbance of normal bowel flora. This is more common with oral cephalosporins.

Monobactams

Example: aztreonam

Aztreonam is a β-lactam antibacterial related to the penicillins but with a single ring structure ('monocyclic β-lactam'). It has little cross-allergenicity with the penicillins and has been successfully administered to patients with proven penicillin allergy. Its spectrum of activity is limited to Gram-negative bacteria including *Ps. aeruginosa*, *Neisseria meningitidis* and *N. gonorrhoeae* and *Haemophilus influenzae* with none against Gram-positive bacteria or anaerobes. Aztreonam is given intramuscularly or intravenously and is β-lactamase resistant. It is excreted via renal tubular excretion and has a short half-life. Unwanted effects are similar to those of other β-lactam antibacterials.

Carbapenems

Examples: imipenem, meropenem

Imipenem is a β-lactam agent that has an extremely broad spectrum of bactericidal activity and is potent against

Table 51.2
Examples of cephalosporins and their spectra of activity

	Staphylococcus aureus	Haemophilus influenzae	Enterobacteriaceae (coliforms)	Pseudomonas aeruginosa	Bacteroides fragilis	Ability to cross blood-brain barrier	Resistance to β-lactamase
First generation							
Cefadroxil/cefradine (oral)	+	0	+	0	0	+/0	+
Cefradine (parenteral)	+	0	+	0	0	+/0	+
Second generation							
Cefuroxime axetil (oral)	++	++	++	0	+[a]	++	++
Cefuroxime (parenteral)	++	++	++	0	+	++	++
Third generation							
Cefixime (oral)	0	+++	++	0	0	++	++
Cefotaxime (parenteral)	+	+++	+++	0	+	++	++
Ceftazidime	0	0	+	++	0	+/0[b]	++

Staphylococcus aureus is a Gram-positive staining organism. Other illustrative bacteria are Gram negative staining.

+++, very active; ++, active; +, variable activity; 0 inactive.
[a]Cefoxitine (a cephamycin) is active.
[b] Some cephalosporins penetrate better into the CNS in the presence of inflamed meninges.

Gram-positive cocci, including some β-lactamase-producing pneumococci, Gram-negative bacilli, including *Ps. aeruginosa, Neisseria suppurans* and *Bacteroides* species, and also many anaerobic bacteria. It can penetrate the blood–brain barrier and is resistant to β-lactamases. Imipenem is rapidly metabolised by dihydropeptidases in the kidney and so is given in combination with cilastatin, a compound that inhibits dihydropeptidase-induced destruction. Meropenem is not inactivated by the renal enzyme and can be given alone. Both imipenem and meropenem are given intravenously; imipenem can also be given by deep intramuscular injection. They are mainly renally excreted and have short half-lives. Unwanted effects are similar to those of other β-lactam antibacterials.

Other agents affecting cell wall

Glycopeptides

Examples: vancomycin, teicoplanin

Mechanism of action

Vancomycin and teicoplanin are high-molecular-weight glycopeptide compounds that act by inhibiting bacterial cell wall synthesis specifically by inhibiting the growth of the essential peptidoglycan constituents (Fig. 51.1). They may also have effects on RNA synthesis. They are bactericidal.

Spectrum of activity

Vancomycin and teicoplanin are active only against Gram-positive bacteria, particularly staphylococci, as they do not penetrate the Gram-negative bacterial cell wall. They are usually reserved for serious staphylococcal infection or for bacterial endocarditis not responding to other treatments. Vancomycin is also effective against *Clostridium difficile*, which colonises the colon when normal flora are disturbed, causing antibiotic-associated colitis; metronidazole is preferred for this indication, but some strains are resistant to metronidazole.

Resistance

Acquired resistance is uncommon.

Pharmacokinetics

Both vancomycin and teicoplanin are very poorly absorbed orally and are, therefore, usually given by intravenous infusion, or in the case of teicoplanin by intramuscular injection. Oral administration of vanco-mycin is useful only for treating antibiotic-associated colitis. Both drugs are excreted by the kidneys; vancomycin has an intermediate half-life, teicoplanin a long half-life.

Unwanted effects

- Ototoxicity occurs with very high plasma levels but nephrotoxicity is less common. This toxicity may be enhanced if vancomycin or teicoplanin are used in combination with an aminoglycoside.
- Thrombophlebitis can occur at the site of infusion.
- Skin rashes: rapid intravenous injection of vancomycin produces generalised erythema, the 'red man' syndrome.
- Blood disorders, including leucopenia, thrombo-cytopenia.
- Gastrointestinal upset.

Polymyxins

Example: colistin

Mechanism of action

Polymyxins bind to bacterial membrane phospholipids and alter permeability to K^+ and Na^+. The cell's osmotic barrier is lost, and susceptible organisms are killed by lysis (Fig. 51.1).

Spectrum of activity

Polymyxins have bactericidal action against Gram-negative organisms including *Pseudomonas* species but are inactive against Gram-positive bacteria and most fungi.

Resistance

Acquired resistance is rare.

Pharmacokinetics

Colistin is very poorly absorbed from the gut and is usually given by inhalation or topically to the skin. Penetration into joint spaces or CSF is poor. It is excreted unchanged in the kidney, with an intermediate half-life. It is sometimes given by mouth for bowel sterilisation.

Unwanted effects

Substantial toxicity limits the use of polymyxins by systemic administration.

- Nephrotoxicity produces a dose-related but reversible renal impairment.
- Neurotoxicity produces dizziness, circumoral parasthaesiae and convulsions. Rarely, neuromuscular blockade can produce respiratory paralysis.

Agents affecting bacterial DNA

Quinolones (fluoroquinolones)

Examples: ciprofloxacin, norfloxacin, levofloxacin

Mechanism of action

Quinolones inhibit replication of bacterial DNA. They block the activity of DNA gyrase, the enzyme that forms DNA supercoils and is essential for DNA replication and repair (Fig. 51.1). The effect is bactericidal.

Spectrum of activity

Ciprofloxacin has a broad spectrum of activity and is active against many organisms resistant to penicillins, cephalosporins and aminoglycosides. Its spectrum includes most Gram-negative bacteria including *H. influenzae, Ps. aeruginosa, N. gonorrhoeae,* and *Enterobacteria, Campylobacter* and *Pseudomonas* species. It has only weak activity against streptococci and staphylococci. Ciprofloxacin has poor activity against anaerobic cocci and bacilli. Levofloxacin has greater activity against pneumococci than ciprofloxacin.

Resistance

Resistance to ciprofloxacin is relatively uncommon and may be produced by a mutation that results in a DNA gyrase that is less susceptible to the drug's action or by reduced drug penetration into the cell (Fig. 51.2). Plasmid-mediated resistance has not been found.

Pharmacokinetics

Oral absorption of ciprofloxacin is variable but adequate. It is widely distributed in body tissues and fluids; CSF penetration is poor unless there is meningeal inflammation. The majority of the drug is eliminated unchanged by the kidney, partly by tubular secretion, but about 20% is excreted in the bile and a similar amount is metabolised in the liver. An intravenous formulation is available. Ciprofloxacin has a short half-life. Levofloxacin has a longer half-life than ciprofloxacin and exhibits a 'post-antibiotic' effect. When levofloxacin has been administered, it continues to inhibit growth even if concentrations of drug have fallen to undetectable levels.

Unwanted effects

The incidence of unwanted effects is low:

- Gastrointestinal upset: nausea, vomiting, diarrhoea.
- Central nervous system (CNS) effects: dizziness, headache, tremors. Rarely, convulsions can occur.
- Photosensitive skin rashes.
- Pain and inflammation in tendons.

- Drug interaction: the plasma concentrations of theophylline (Ch. 12), warfarin (Ch. 11) and ciclosporin (Ch. 39) are increased by ciprofloxacin and norfloxacin through inhibition of hepatic metabolism; this can produce toxicity.

Metronidazole and tinidazole

Mechanism of action

Metronidazole is bactericidal only after it is degraded to an intermediate transient toxic metabolite, which inhibits bacterial DNA synthesis and breaks down existing DNA. Only some anaerobes and some protozoa contain the nitroreductase that converts metronidazole to the antibacterial derivative. The intermediate metabolite is not produced in human cells, or in aerobic bacteria. It is bactericidal. It is equally active against dividing and non-dividing cells.

Spectrum of activity

Metronidazole and tinidazole are mainly active against anaerobic bacteria and protozoa, including *Bacteroides* and *Clostridium* species, *Trichomonas vaginalis, Giardia lamblia.* It is also an amoebicidal drug active against *Entamoeba histolytica.* It is an important drug for treating antibiotic-induced colitis (pseudomembranous colitis) caused by *C. difficile.* It can be used prophylactically prior to surgery. Metronidazole and tinidazole are important constituents of the triple or quadruple therapy utilised for the elimination of *Helicobacter pylori* (Ch. 33).

Resistance

Acquired resistance is not high but is developing. For example, in some countries a significant percentage of strains of *H. pylori* are resistant to metronidazole and some outbreaks of *C. difficile*-induced colitis are resistant. In some patients, this resistance results from bacteria lacking nitroreductase.

Pharmacokinetics

Metronidazole is well absorbed orally and can also be given intravenously, as vaginal pessaries or rectal suppositories. Rectal absorption is high, and this route is often preferable to intravenous administration if the drug cannot be taken by mouth. Metronidazole penetrates well into body fluids including vaginal, pleural and cerebrospinal fluids and can cross the placenta. It is mainly metabolised by the liver and has an intermediate half-life. Tinidazole is similar but has a longer duration of action.

Unwanted effects

- Mild gastrointestinal symptoms often occur and patients complain of a metallic taste.
- Intolerance to alcohol may occur by a mechanism that is similar to the disulfiram reaction (Ch. 54).
- Skin rashes.

Nitrofurantoin

Mechanism of action

Nitrofurantoin is probably activated by reduction to unstable metabolites inside bacteria, which produces DNA disruption. It is bactericidal, especially to organisms in acid urine.

Spectrum of activity

Nitrofurantoin is active against most Gram-positive cocci and *Escherichia coli* and its use is confined to infection of the urinary tract; *Pseudomonas* species are naturally resistant, as are many *Proteus* species.

Resistance

Chromosomal resistance occurs but is not common.

Pharmacokinetics

Nitrofurantoin is well absorbed from the gut. The half-life is short in the plasma, and therapeutic concentrations are not achieved. It is excreted unchanged in the urine by both glomerular filtration and tubular secretion but also appears in the bile. Urinary concentrations are high enough to treat lower urinary tract infections, but the low tissue concentrations are often inadequate for acute pyelonephritis.

Unwanted effects

- Gastrointestinal upset is common including anorexia, nausea and vomiting.
- Pulmonary toxicity with long-term use produces acute allergic pneumonitis or chronic interstitial fibrosis.

Agents affecting bacterial protein synthesis

Macrolides

> Examples: erythromycin, azithromycin, clarithromycin

Mechanism of action

Macrolides interfere with bacterial protein synthesis by binding reversibly to the 50S subunit of the bacterial ribosome. The action is primarily bacteriostatic (Fig. 51.1).

Spectrum of activity

Erythromycin has a similar spectrum of activity to broad-spectrum penicillins. It is effective against Gram-positive organisms and gut anaerobes but has poor activity against *H. influenzae*. It is also used for infections by *Legionella*, *Mycoplasma*, *Chlamydia*, *Mycobacteria* and *Campylobacter* species and for pertussis infections (*Bordetella pertussis*). Although erythromycin is primarily bacteriostatic, it is bactericidal at high concentrations for some Gram-positive species, such as group A streptococci and pneumococci. Azithromycin has a similar spectrum of activity to erythromycin but enhanced activity again *H. influenzae*. Clarithromycin has slightly greater activity than erythromycin and is also used as part of the multidrug treatment of *H. pylori* (Ch. 33).

Resistance

Bacteria become resistant by a mutation that modifies the target sites on the ribosome.

Pharmacokinetics

Erythromycin is adequately absorbed from the gut. It is destroyed at acid pH and is, therefore, given as an enteric-coated tablet or as an ester prodrug (erythromycin ethyl succinate), which is acid stable. It can also be administered intravenously. Azithromycin and clarithromycin are acid stable and well absorbed from the gut.

Erythromycin and clarithromycin are metabolised in the liver and have short half-lives. Care should be taken in hepatic impairment. Azithromycin is released slowly from the tissues and has a long half-life.

Unwanted effects

- Epigastric discomfort, nausea, vomiting and diarrhoea are common with the oral preparation of erythromycin. Azithromycin and clarithromycin are better tolerated.
- Skin rashes.
- Cholestatic jaundice can occur with erythromycin, usually if treatment is continued for more than 2 weeks.
- Prolongation of the Q–T interval on the electrocardiograph, with a predisposition to ventricular arrhythmias (Ch. 8).
- Erythromycin and clarithromycin inhibit P450 drug-metabolising enzymes and can elevate levels of drugs requiring these enzymes for metabolism. Examples include carbamazepine (Ch. 23) and ciclosporin (Ch. 39).

Aminoglycosides

> Examples: gentamicin, netilmicin, streptomycin, tobramycin, amikacin

Mechanism of action

The aminoglycosides are similar in their properties but some differences may be exploited in particular clinical circumstances as illustrated below. Aminoglycosides inhibit protein synthesis in bacteria by binding irreversibly to the 30S ribosomal subunit (Fig. 51.1). This inhibits translation from mRNA to protein and also increases the frequency of misreading of the genetic code. Aminoglycosides are bactericidal.

Spectrum of activity

Aminoglycosides are active against many Gram-negative bacteria (including *Pseudomonas* species) and some Gram-positive organisms but are inactive against anaerobes; these bacterial species are unable to take up the aminoglycosides into their cells. Aminoglycosides are particularly useful for serious Gram-negative infections, when they have a complementary and synergistic action with agents that disrupt cell wall synthesis (e.g. penicillins). Gentamicin is the most widely used aminoglycoside. Streptomycin is mainly used as part of the drug regimen to treat *Mycobacterium tuberculosis* (see below).

Resistance

Resistance is increasingly a problem with the aminoglycosides and can occur by several mechanisms. It is transferred by plasmids and is principally caused by production of degradative enzymes that acetylate, phosphorylate or adenylate aminoglycosides in the bacterial periplasmic space. Bacterial uptake of the modified drug is poor (Fig. 51.2). Amikacin is less susceptible to these enzymes. Changes in the ribosomal proteins in resistant bacteria can also reduce drug binding and antibacterial effectiveness. Netilmicin remains effective against many gentamicin-resistant bacteria. Resistance resulting from reduced penetration of the drug can be overcome by co-administration of antibacterials that disrupt cell wall synthesis.

Pharmacokinetics

Aminoglycosides are poorly absorbed from the gut and are, therefore, given parenterally. They have short half-lives and are rapidly and entirely excreted by the kidney. They do not cross the blood–brain barrier; however they cross the placenta and can damage the VIIIth cranial nerve in the fetus (see below). Blood concentrations should always be measured to guide dosing. Peak concentrations and trough concentrations are important, both to ensure bactericidal efficacy and to minimise the risk of toxic effects. Once-daily dosage regimens for aminoglycosides are becoming more popular and are no more toxic than multiple daily dosages.

Tobramycin is also available as a preservative-free solution for administration by nebuliser for the management of patients with cystic fibrosis whose respiratory tracts are colonised by *Ps. aeruginosa*.

Unwanted effects

Most unwanted effects of aminoglycosides are dose related and many are reversible; they are probably related to high trough concentrations of the drug.

- Ototoxicity can lead both to vestibular and auditory dysfunction. Prolonged treatment or high plasma drug concentrations lead to accumulation of aminoglycoside in the inner ear, resulting in often irreversible disturbances of balance or deafness. Ototoxicity can be enhanced by loop diuretics; (Ch. 14). Netilmicin appears to cause less ototoxicity than the other aminoglycosides.
- Renal damage occurs through retention of aminoglycosides in the proximal tubular cells of the kidney. It is usually reversible and is manifest initially by a defect in the concentrating ability of the kidney, with mild proteinuria followed by a reduction in the glomerular filtration rate.
- Acute neuromuscular blockade can occur, usually if the aminoglycoside is used in association with anaesthesia (Ch. 17) or administration of other neuromuscular-blocking agents (Ch. 27). It is caused by inhibition of prejunctional acetylcholine release in association with reduced postsynaptic sensitivity, and it is reversed by intravenous Ca^{2+} salts.

Tetracyclines

Examples: tetracycline, oxytetracycline, doxycycline, minocycline

Mechanism of action

Tetracyclines enter bacteria mainly by an active uptake mechanism not found in human cells. They are bacteriostatic and inhibit bacterial protein synthesis by binding reversibly to the 30S subunit of ribosomes.

Spectrum of activity

Tetracyclines have a broad spectrum of activity against many Gram-positive and Gram-negative bacteria and in infections caused by rickettsiae, amoebae, *Chlamydia psittici*, *Trachomatis coxiella*, *Vibrio cholerae*, and *Mycoplasma*, *Legionella* and *Brucella* species. They are useful in acne (Ch. 49). Minocycline is active against *N. meningitidis*, unlike other tetracyclines.

Resistance

Resistance to the tetracyclines develops slowly, but in the UK is now widespread among most Gram-positive and several Gram-negative organisms, limiting the drugs' usefulness. Microorganisms that have developed resistance to one tetracycline frequently display resistance to the others. In most, resistance is carried by plasmids and results from decreased uptake of the drug into bacteria (Fig. 51.2). In other cases, the binding of tetracyclines to bacterial ribosomes is decreased.

Pharmacokinetics

Tetracyclines are incompletely absorbed from the gut, particularly if taken with food. Absorption of tetracycline and oxytetracycline is further impaired by milk, aluminium, calcium or magnesium salts (antacids; Ch. 33), iron and increased intestinal pH; tetracyclines bind to divalent and trivalent cations forming inactive chelates (Ch. 56).

The tetracyclines diffuse reasonably well into sputum, urine and peritoneal and pleural fluid and cross the placenta. They have poor penetration into CSF. All of the tetracyclines have intermediate or long half-lives, with doxycycline and minocycline having the longest. Tetracyclines are concentrated in the liver and some drug is excreted via the bile into the small intestine, from where it is partially reabsorbed. Drug concentrations in the bile may be three to five times higher than in the plasma.

Tetracyclines are mainly eliminated unchanged in the urine, with the exception of doxycycline, which is largely eliminated in the bile.

Unwanted effects

- Nausea, vomiting and epigastric discomfort commonly occur after oral administration.
- Tetracyclines in children produce permanent yellow-brown discoloration of the growing teeth by chelating with Ca^{2+} and, in some, cause enamel hypoplasia. They should be avoided during the latter half of pregnancy and in children in the first 12 years of life.
- Anti-anabolic effects can occur in human cells from inhibition of protein synthesis (not seen with doxycycline or minocycline). In patients with impaired renal function, this can lead to uraemia.
- Benign intracranial hypertension causes headache and visual disturbances.

Chloramphenicol

Mechanism of action

Chloramphenicol inhibits protein synthesis in bacteria by binding reversibly to the 50S subunit of bacterial ribosomes (Fig. 51.1). It inhibits peptide bond formation by impairing the reading of mRNA. The effect is mainly bacteriostatic but can be bactericidal in some organisms.

Spectrum of activity

Chloramphenicol is a broad-spectrum antimicrobial, active against many Gram-positive cocci (both aerobic and anaerobic) and Gram-negative organisms. The sensitivities of all bacteria are variable but it has a bactericidal effect on *E. coli*, *Streptococcus pneumoniae*, *H. influenzae*, *N. meningitidis*, *B. pertussis*, salmonellae, shigellae, *V. cholerae* and *Salmonella*, *Shigella* and *Bacteroides* species. Some streptococci and staphylococci are inhibited.

Because of its toxicity, chloramphenicol is reserved for life-threatening infections, particularly with *H. influenzae* or typhoid fever. It is used topically for conjunctivitis (Ch. 50).

Resistance

Resistance is caused by the production of an enzyme that inactivates the drug by acetylation. This enzyme is plasmid mediated. It is produced by many Gram-negative bacteria but can also be induced in Gram-positive bacteria. Resistant strains may also show reduced uptake of the drug.

Pharmacokinetics

Chloramphenicol is well absorbed orally but an ester prodrug is used to disguise its bitter taste when it is given as a syrup. Intramuscular injection leads to inadequate plasma concentrations and so the intravenous route is preferred for parenteral administration. Chloramphenicol is widely distributed into many tissues including CSF and the biliary tree. It crosses the placenta and is present in breast milk. Chloramphenicol is almost completely metabolised in the liver and has a short half-life.

Unwanted effects

- The most important unwanted effect is bone marrow toxicity. Reversible anaemia, thrombocytopenia or neutropenia can occur particularly in patients receiving high or prolonged dosing. Aplastic anaemia is rare, but usually fatal.
- Premature infants and babies of less than 2 weeks of age have immature hepatic enzymes, particularly glucuronyl transferase, and reduced renal drug elimination. Chloramphenicol can accumulate in these children, causing the 'grey baby syndrome'. Initial symptoms include vomiting and cyanosis followed by hypothermia, vasomotor collapse and an ashen grey discoloration of the skin. There is a high mortality.

Lincosamides

Example: clindamycin

Mechanism of action

Clindamycin inhibits bacterial protein synthesis in a similar manner to the macrolide antibacterials. The mechanism of action and the ways that resistance develop are similar to those of erythromycin.

Pharmacokinetics

It is well absorbed orally and is used for staphylococcal bone infection such as osteomyelitis and as prophylaxis for endocarditis in individuals who cannot take penicillins. It is also effective against Gram-positive cocci.

Unwanted effects

- Gastrointestinal irritation
- Pseudomembranous colitis
- Skin rashes and hepatic dysfunction have also been reported.

Fusidic acid

Mechanism of action

Fusidic acid is a steroid that inhibits bacterial protein synthesis by preventing binding of transfer RNA to the ribosome.

Spectrum of activity

Fusidic acid is a narrow-spectrum antibacterial, mainly active against Gram-positive organisms. It is commonly used for treatment of penicillin-resistant *S. aureus*. It is bactericidal.

Resistance

Resistance is fairly frequent when fusidic acid is used alone; consequently, it is usually given in combination with another drug. Resistance occurs either by mutation or by plasmid conjugation.

Pharmacokinetics

Oral absorption is complete, but an intravenous formulation is available. Penetration into synovial fluid and soft tissues is good. Fusidic acid is extensively metabolised in the liver and has an intermediate half-life.

Unwanted effects

- Thrombophlebitis with intravenous infusions.
- Cholestatic jaundice.
- Gastrointestinal intolerance.

Streptogramins

Examples: quinupristin with dalfopristin

Mechanisms of action and use

Streptogramins are isolated from *Streptomyces pristinae spiralis*. A mixture of quinupristin with dalfopristin binds to the 50S subunit of the bacterial ribosome and inhibits the late phase of protein synthesis. The combination acts synergistically and should be reserved for serious infections not treatable with other antimicrobials.

Spectrum of activity

Streptogramins are used for serious aerobic Gram-positive infections including methicillin-resistant *Staphylococcus aureus* (MRSA) and vancomycin-resistant *Enterococcus faecium*.

Pharmacokinetics

The streptogramins are administered intravenously; their metabolism is complex and several active metabolites are formed by cytochrome P450 enzymes. The main route of elimination is faecal. The half-lives of both quinupristin and dalfopristin are very short at about 45 min.

Unwanted effects

- Nausea and vomiting.
- Injection site reactions.
- Hepatitis.

Oxazolidinones

Example: linezolid

Mechanisms of action

The oxazolidinones are a new group of drugs active against non-replicating bacteria through binding to the ribosomal 30S subunit, mRNA and formylmethionine.

Spectrum of activity

Linezolid is active against a range of Gram-positive organisms including MRSA and also vancomycin-resistant *E. faecium*.

Pharmacokinetics

Linezolid is well absorbed orally with a half-life of 5 hours.

Unwanted effects

- Headache.
- Nausea and vomiting.
- Diarrhoea.

Agents affecting bacterial metabolism

Sulfonamides

Examples: sulfadiazine, sulfamethoxazole

The therapeutic importance of the sulfonamides has diminished because of the spread of resistance, and there are now few (nonetheless important) indicated first-choice uses, generally in combination with trimethoprim (see below).

Mechanism of action

Unlike humans, bacteria cannot utilise external folic acid, a nutrient that is essential for cell growth and is used to manufacture purines for incorporation into DNA. Bacteria must synthesise it from *para*-aminobenzoic acid (PABA). Sulfonamides are structurally similar to PABA and inhibit the enzyme dihydrofolate synthetase in the synthetic pathway for folic acid. High concentrations of PABA can overcome the effectiveness of sulfonamides (Fig. 51.4).

Spectrum of activity

Sulfonamides have a bacteriostatic action against a wide range of Gram-positive and Gram-negative organisms and are also active against *Toxoplasma*, *Chlamydia* and *Nocardia* species. Because of the frequency of resistance, sulfonamides are given as sole therapy only for the treatment of nocardiosis or toxoplasmosis.

Resistance

Resistance is common and occurs through production of a mutated dihydrofolate synthetase that has reduced affinity for binding of sulfonamides (Fig. 51.2); resistance is transmitted in Gram-negative bacteria by plasmids. Resistance in *S. aureus* occurs as a result of excessive synthesis of PABA. Some resistant bacteria have reduced uptake of sulfonamides.

Pharmacokinetics

Sulfonamides are well absorbed orally. A parenteral preparation of sulfadiazine is available. They are widely distributed in the body and cross the blood–brain barrier and placenta.

Sulfonamides are metabolised in the liver, initially by acetylation, which shows genetic polymorphism (Ch. 2). The acetylated product has no antibacterial action but retains toxic potential. Substantial amounts of parent drug and *N*-acetyl metabolite are excreted by the kidney. Most sulfonamides have intermediate half-lives.

Unwanted effects

- Nausea and vomiting.
- Hypersensitivity reactions include rashes, vasculitis, and Stevens–Johnson syndrome.
- Sulfonamides can precipitate haemolysis in patients with glucose 6-phosphate dehydrogenase deficiency (Chs 47, 53).
- Crystalluria has been a potential problem with older sulfonamides in overdose or if the urine is acidic, but is unusual with newer sulfonamides, which are more soluble than earlier compounds.
- Sulfonamides should not be used in the last trimester of pregnancy or in neonates because the drug competes for bilirubin-binding sites on albumin. This can raise the concentration of unconjugated bilirubin and increases the risk of kernicterus.

Trimethoprim

Trimethoprim can be combined with sulfamethoxazole as co-trimoxazole.

Mechanism of action

Trimethoprim inhibits dihydrofolate reductase, which converts dihydrofolate to tetrahydrofolate (Fig. 51.4). The bacterial enzyme is inhibited at much lower concentrations than its mammalian counterpart. The combination of trimethoprim with the sulfonamide sulfamethoxazole (co-trimoxazole) acts synergistically to prevent folate synthesis by bacteria. However, resistance to the sulfamethoxazole component, and the incidence of unwanted effects limit the value of this combination.

Spectrum of activity

Trimethoprim has wide-spectrum bacteriostatic activity against Gram-positive and Gram-negative bacteria. The combination with sulfamethoxazole is also effective against the protozoan *P. carinii*, which causes pneumonia in patients with acquired immunodeficiency syndrome (AIDS) and this is now its major indication (see below). In many urinary and respiratory tract infections, trimethoprim alone gives results similar to the combination with sulfamethoxazole.

Resistance

Resistance to trimethoprim occurs in similar ways to that seen with sulfonamides.

Pharmacokinetics

Trimethoprim is well absorbed from the gut. Most is excreted unchanged by the kidney and it has an intermediate half-life. Both trimethoprim and co-trimoxazole are available for intravenous use.

The folic acid pathway:

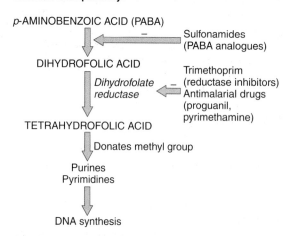

Fig. 51.4
Mechanism of action of the sulfonamides, trimethoprim and antimalarial drugs in the folic acid pathway.

Unwanted effects

- Nausea, vomiting and diarrhoea, which are usually mild.
- Skin rashes.
- Folate deficiency, leading to megaloblastic changes in the marrow, is rare except in patients with depleted folate stores.
- Marrow depression with agranulocytosis.

Agents used for tuberculosis

Tuberculosis is usually treated with a multidrug regimen because of resistance. The drugs used are described here and the treatment regimen is described on page 506.

Rifamycins

Examples: rifampicin, rifabutin

Mechanism of action and spectrum of activity

Rifamycins act by inhibition of DNA-dependent RNA polymerase and have a bactericidal action. Rifampicin (rifampin) has a broad spectrum of activity and is used in the treatment of mycobacterial infections (*M. tuberculosis* and *M. leprae*), brucellosis, legionella infections and serious staphylococcal infections. In tuberculosis, it is considered an essential drug in the UK. Rifabutin is also used for prophylaxis against *Mycobacterium avium intracellulare* infection in patients with infections with human immunodeficiency virus.

Resistance

Resistance develops rapidly, which limits the wider use of rifampicin as an antibacterial agent apart from the treatment of tuberculosis. It is acquired by a one-step genetic mutation of the DNA-dependent RNA polymerase.

Pharmacokinetics

Oral absorption is good, and an intravenous formulation of rifampicin is also available. Rifampicin is metabolised in the liver and has a short half-life, although undergoing some enterohepatic recycling. Rifabutin has a long half-life and can be given once daily.

Unwanted effects

- Nausea and anorexia.
- Pseudomembranous colitis with rifampicin.
- Hepatotoxicity, usually only producing a transient rise in plasma transaminases. Regular monitoring is recommended.
- Orange coloration of tears, sweat, urine.
- Induction of drug-metabolising enzymes in the liver (Ch. 2). Important interactions include reducing the levels of plasma estrogen in those taking oral contraceptives (Ch. 45), and reducing levels of phenytoin (Ch. 23), warfarin (Ch. 11) and sulfonylureas (Ch. 40).
- Various 'toxicity syndromes' occur, commonly with intermittent use, owing to sensitisation. They include renal failure, a shock-like syndrome and acute haemolytic anaemia.

Isoniazid

Mechanism of action

Isoniazid is an important and specific drug for the treatment of *M. tuberculosis*. Isoniazid inhibits production of long-chain mycolic acids, which are unique to the cell wall of *Mycobacteria* species. It is bactericidal against dividing organisms, but bacteriostatic on resting organisms.

Resistance

Resistance occurs through mutation. It is uncommon in developed countries but can be troublesome in developing countries and develops rapidly if isoniazid is used alone.

Pharmacokinetics

Oral absorption is good but reduced by food. Isoniazid is metabolised by acetylation in the liver, which is subject to genetic polymorphism (Ch. 2). Rapid acetylators show extensive first-pass metabolism and in slow acetylators isoniazid blood concentrations are twice those in rapid acetylators. The half-life is short but varies according to acetylator status.

Unwanted effects

- Nausea and vomiting.
- Peripheral neuropathy with high doses. This can be prevented by prophylactic use of oral pyridoxine supplements in high-risk patients, for example those with diabetes, alcoholism, chronic renal failure or malnutrition. Neuropathy is more common in slow acetylators.
- Hepatotoxicity. Regular monitoring with liver function tests is recommended.
- Systemic lupus erythematosus-like syndrome. Positive antinuclear antibodies are found in 20% of patients during long-term treatment, but fewer develop symptoms.

Pyrazinamide

Mechanism of action

Pyrazinamide may act through metabolites formed by the enzyme pyrazinamidase, which is found in *M. tuberculosis*. The product pyrazinoic acid produces an acid intracellular pH to destroy the cell. It is bactericidal to semi-dormant cells.

Resistance

Resistance develops rapidly if pyrazinamide is used as a sole treatment for tuberculosis.

Pharmacokinetics

Oral absorption is good and metabolism occurs in the liver. Pyrazinamide has a long half-life.

Unwanted effects

- Hepatotoxicity: a rise in plasma bilirubin usually requires cessation of treatment. Regular monitoring is recommended.
- Nausea and vomiting.
- Gout can occur through inhibition of uric acid excretion by the kidney.

Ethambutol

Mechanism of action

It is uncertain how ethambutol acts, but it probably impairs synthesis of the cell wall of mycobacteria. Ethambutol is primarily bacteriostatic. It is effective against *M. tuberculosis* and several other mycobacteria including *M. avium*, which can cause lung infections.

Resistance

Resistance develops slowly but is common during prolonged treatment of tuberculosis if ethambutol is used alone.

Pharmacokinetics

Oral absorption is good. Only a small amount is metabolised and most is eliminated unchanged by the kidney. The half-life is long.

Unwanted effects

- Headache, dizziness.
- Optic neuritis produces initial red/green colour blindness, then reduced visual acuity. It is dose related but usually reversible.

Streptomycin

Streptomycin was discussed above (see aminoglycosides). It is not used in the UK as first-line treatment for tuberculosis because of its toxicity and the need for parenteral administration.

Thiacetazone (not available in UK)

Mechanism of action

Thiacetazone is a bacteriostatic compound that is believed to form copper complexes within mycobacteria thus interfering with copper-dependent enzymes in the microorganism.

Resistance

Resistance develops in about 30% of mycobacteria if thiacetazone is used alone.

Pharmacokinetics

Oral absorption is slow and most thiacetazone is metabolised in the liver. The half-life is usually long but shows wide interindividual variation.

Unwanted effects

- Gastrointestinal upset including nausea, vomiting, anorexia, abdominal pain and diarrhoea are common.
- Blurred vision, giddiness.
- Hypersensitivity reactions with severe cutaneous reactions and hepatitis.

Other drugs used in the treatment of tuberculosis

Other drugs can be used as second-line treatments in multidrug-resistant tuberculosis. These include cycloserine, capreomycin, amikacin, ciprofloxacin, ethionamide and *para*-aminosalicylic acid.

Agents used for leprosy

The drugs recommended for treatment of leprosy, which is caused by *M. leprae*, are rifampicin (see above), dapsone and clofazimine.

Dapsone

Mechanism of action and spectrum of activity

Dapsone is similar to the sulfonamides and acts by inhibition of folate synthesis. It is the most active drug against *M. leprae*.

Resistance

Resistance can develop as for sulfonamides (see above).

Pharmacokinetics

Dapsone is orally active, is metabolised in the liver and undergoes enterohepatic recycling. It has a long half-life.

Unwanted effects

- Blood disorders: haemolysis, methaemoglobinaemia.
- Neuropathy.

Clofazamine

Clofazamine is a dye that interferes with DNA and is used as a second-line drug in the event of dapsone intolerance in those with leprosy. It is a long-acting drug that tends to accumulate. Unwanted effects include gastrointestinal upset, brownish-black discoloration of the skin and acne.

Principles of antibacterial therapy

The following guidelines outline the principles that should be considered in the choice of a safe and effective therapy.

Presumptive treatment. Most antibacterial therapy is started 'blind' without prior identification of the organism and its antibacterial drug sensitivities. Such treatment should be guided by the clinical diagnosis and a knowledge of the most common pathogenic organisms in the current situation. Local information about patterns of antibacterial resistance should be considered.

Drug spectrum. A drug with a narrow spectrum of activity should be used in preference to a broad-spectrum drug whenever possible. Unnecessary use of broad-spectrum drugs encourages the development of resistant organisms; this can present problems for the individual patient by the selection of resistant pathogens or overgrowth of resistant commensal organisms. For the community, the selection of resistant pathogens can create problems by rendering standard antibacterial therapy less reliable. Broad-spectrum antibacterial cover is sometimes appropriate, for example in a seriously ill patient when the infecting bacterium is unknown and a variety of bacteria can cause the condition being treated.

Combination therapy. Treatment with more than one antibacterial agent should not be used routinely. It may, however, be valuable to provide broad-spectrum cover in serious illness when the organism is unknown, for example the combination of cefotaxime and metronidazole to cover aerobic and anaerobic organisms in suspected Gram-negative septicaemia. When resistance is likely to develop readily to the first choice drug during protracted treatment, the use of combination therapy can minimise that risk, for example in the treatment of infective endocarditis or tuberculosis.

Bactericidal versus bacteriostatic drugs. In some situations bactericidal drugs are preferred to bacteriostatic agents, for example for the treatment of infective endocarditis or when the patient is immunocompromised. In most other situations the choice is probably not important.

Site of infection. This may determine the choice of drug, for example some antibacterials only achieve low concentrations in the biliary tree, urine, bone or CSF.

Mode of administration. Oral therapy is usually preferred to parenteral treatment. Exceptions include the treatment of serious infections when reliable blood concentrations are essential, if the drug is only available in parenteral formulation, or if gastrointestinal absorption may be unreliable, for example after abdominal surgery.

Duration of therapy. This should be as short as is compatible with adequate treatment of the infection. The decision is often arbitrary, for example 7–10 days in many infections. Some infections can be effectively treated over much shorter periods, for example courses of 1–3 days are usually adequate for lower urinary tract infections. For a few infections, long periods of treatment may be necessary to eliminate semidormant organisms or those in 'privileged sites' to which antibacterial penetration is poor. Examples include infective endocarditis, osteomyelitis and tuberculosis.

Chemoprophylaxis. The use of chemoprophylaxis to prevent infection is important in many situations. Common examples include prevention of meningococcal meningitis in close contacts of an infected patient, prevention of infective endocarditis in patients with diseased or artificial heart valves undergoing surgery or dental treatment, and preoperative prophylaxis before gut, biliary, thoracic or orthopaedic surgery.

Treatment of individual infections

This section is not intended to be comprehensive. It will outline the approach to antibacterial therapy in several common bacterial infections. The choice of antibacterial agent for these infections will depend on factors such as local patterns of bacterial resistance, which make universal recommendations impossible.

Upper respiratory tract infections

Most upper respiratory tract infections are caused by viruses, producing symptoms of the common cold. Symptomatic treatment is all that should be offered, with an antihistamine (e.g. chlorpheniramine; Ch. 38) or an anticholinergic spray (e.g. ipratropium; Ch. 12) to reduce rhinorrhoea and sneezing. An α-adrenoceptor agonist given orally or nasally (e.g. xylometazoline; Ch. 4) can reduce nasal congestion but prolonged use can provoke a rebound effect (rhinitis medicamentosa). A non-steroidal anti-inflammatory drug (NSAID; Ch. 29) can be used to reduce associated headache and malaise. Antibacterial drugs are widely prescribed for upper respiratory tract symptoms but have no benefit.

Sinusitis and otitis media

Sinusitis and otitis media accompany catarrhal conditions in childhood and frequently follow an upper respiratory tract infection. Sinusitis produces headache, facial pain, fever and purulent rhinorrhoea. A nasal decongestant such as an α-adrenoceptor agonist can be helpful, in conjunction with an analgesic. An antimicrobial may be beneficial in acute sinusitis. The most common infecting organisms are *H. influenzae* (which often produces β-lactamase) and *S. pneumoniae*. Suitable antibacterial drugs include co-amoxiclav, cefuroxime axetil or erythromycin. Chronic sinusitis usually requires correction of an anatomical obstruction in the nose.

Otitis media is very common in childhood and is often associated with enlargement of the adenoids. Increased pressure in the middle ear causes pain and perforation of the ear drum. The organisms responsible are similar to those causing acute sinusitis. In more than 80% of children, the condition is self-limiting over 2–3 days without treatment. An antibacterial should be used for protracted episodes of otitis media.

Lower respiratory tract infection

Acute bronchitis is usually a viral infection, which often takes 7–10 days to resolve without treatment and does not require antibacterial treatment unless there is an underlying risk factor for bacterial infection, such as chronic obstructive airways disease. In such cases, *S. pneumoniae* (pneumococcus), *H. influenzae* or *Moraxella catarrhalis* are common pathogens. Acute bacterial bronchitis can be treated with amoxicillin, co-amoxiclav or erythromycin. Quinolones such as ciprofloxacin are poorly active against pneumococci and are not drugs of first choice in this situation.

Primary community-acquired pneumonia is most commonly caused by *S. pneumoniae*, followed by *H. influenzae* and staphylococci. Atypical pneumonias are most often caused by *Legionella* or *Mycoplasma* species or by *Chlamydia pneumoniae*. Appropriate antibacterial treatment will be dictated by the most likely organisms. If pneumococcus is suspected, benzylpenicillin is the treatment of choice. However, resistance in pneumococci to benzylpenicillin is increasing, and in some areas a third-generation cephalosporin such as cefotaxime may be more appropriate. Alternatively, broad-spectrum therapy with erythromycin will cover most organisms, including atypical bacterial pneumonias. For severe community-acquired pneumonia, either an intravenous cephalosporin, such as cefuroxime, or amoxicillin combined with erythromycin is often used. Adjunctive treatment of pneumonia may include supplemental oxygen via a facemask, pain relief for pleurisy and ensuring adequate hydration.

Secondary pneumonias occur in patients with other concurrent diseases, often during a stay in hospital (nosocomial infection: hospital acquired). A wide range of pathogens may be involved and parenteral drug treatment is usually necessary. A cephalosporin, such as cefuroxime, or a macrolide, such as erythromycin, is the treatment of choice. For more severely ill patients, the addition of a second drug such as an aminoglycoside (e.g. gentamicin), a quinolone (e.g. ciprofloxacin) or an antipseudomonal penicillin (e.g. azlocillin) may be necessary. Alternatively a broader-spectrum third-generation cephalosporin such as ceftazidime could be given as monotherapy.

Pneumocystis carinii pneumonia

Pneumonia caused by *P. carinii* in patients with AIDS is treated with high doses of trimethoprim and sulfamethoxazole (co-trimoxazole) as the first-line treatment (see above). Some patients show adverse reactions to co-trimoxazole, or it is ineffective. Second-line drugs that can be given include pentamidine, atovaquone and trimetrexate.

Pentamidine. This drug interferes with nucleotide incorporation into DNA and RNA and may antagonise folate. It is also effective against trypanosomiasis and leishmaniasis. It is poorly absorbed orally and is given by inhalation or parenterally.

Atovaquone. This is orally active against *P. carinii* and also against *T. gondii* and *Plasmodia* and *Entamoeba* species (see also p. 519).

Trimetrexate. This can be used for treatment of *P. carinii* (see p. 520).

Urinary tract infections

Urinary tract infections are more common in women than men because of their shorter urethra. Infections can occur in structurally normal urinary tracts or in association with a structural genitourinary abnormality that impairs drainage of urine or acts as a focus for infection, such as a stone in the urinary tract. An indwelling urinary catheter is often associated with bacterial colonisation of the urine that is almost impossible to eradicate.

The most frequent bacterial cause of urinary tract infection is *E. coli*. Hospital-acquired infections are often caused by *Klebsiella*, *Enterobacter* and *Serratia* species or by *Ps. aeruginosa*, because these organisms can be selected as resistant bacteria following antibacterial usage. *Proteus mirabilis* is often found if there are stones in the urinary tract. Less commonly, staphylococci, especially *Staphylococcus saprophyticus*, are responsible.

Uncomplicated urinary tract infection is confined to the bladder (cystitis) and can be treated by short courses (1–3 days) of an aminopenicillin such as amoxicillin or co-amoxiclav, the choice depending on local resistance patterns. Alternative agents include a first-generation cephalosporin, such as cefalexin, trimethoprim or nitrofurantoin. A quinolone such as ciprofloxacin can be useful for *Ps. aeruginosa* infections.

Complicated urinary tract infections also involve the kidney (pyelonephritis) or the prostate in males and require longer courses of treatment. For pyelonephritis, initial intravenous therapy is usually initiated with broad-spectrum agents such as aztreonam, ciprofloxacin or cefuroxime; treatment is usually continued for 7–14 days. In patients who have developed prostatitis, oral treatment with trimethoprim, erythromycin or ciprofloxacin is recommended for at least 4 weeks.

If infection occurs in patients with an indwelling urinary catheter, then treatment is only recommended if the patient develops systemic symptoms of infection, for example fever or rigors.

Long-term antibacterial prophylaxis against urinary tract infections may be necessary to prevent recurrent infection in patients with underlying urinary tract abnormalities. Suitable agents, usually given at low dosage, include trimethoprim, nitrofurantoin or cefalexin.

Gastrointestinal infection

Gastroenteritis (a syndrome that includes nausea, vomiting, diarrhoea and abdominal discomfort) can result from ingestion of bacterial pathogens. Severe disease of the large intestine can cause dysentery, an inflammatory disorder often associated with fever, abdominal pain and blood and pus in the faeces.

'Food poisoning' of bacterial origin can occur from ingestion of a pre-formed bacterial toxin (e.g. from *Clostridium botulinum* or *S. aureus*), with onset of symptoms usually within hours, or it can be caused by ingested bacteria in the bowel (e.g. *Campylobacter* or *Salmonella* species).

The most common cause of bacterial diarrhoea (especially in children in developing countries) is *E. coli*, which produces powerful enterotoxins. In other circumstances, *Salmonella* species, *Campylobacter* species, *Vibrio cholerae*, *Shigella* species or various other organisms are responsible. However, in the UK, diarrhoea is usually caused by viruses and is self-limiting.

If diarrhoea is severe, fluid replacement is often necessary. Antimicrobial treatment is not usually recommended even if bacterial infection is suspected unless there are systemic symptoms such as fever, rigors and hypotension. In such cases, erythromycin or ciprofloxacin can be useful for *Campylobacter* enteritis. Salmonella infections or shigellosis can be treated with ciprofloxacin or trimethoprim unless *Salmonella typhi* is suspected, when ciprofloxacin or chloramphenicol are used.

Antibacterial agents can themselves cause diarrhoea, which usually resolves rapidly when the drug is withdrawn. However, if it is complicated by pseudomembranous colitis, then oral metronidazole or oral vancomycin can be used.

Biliary tract infection

Acute cholecystitis or cholangitis are often caused by *E. coli* and most often occur if there is biliary obstruction. Supportive treatment with fluid and electrolytic replacement is usually required. Antibacterial therapy with a cephalosporin, aminopenicillin or gentamicin is usually effective. Combination therapy with the addition of gentamicin to one of the other agents is recommended if the infection is severe, or alternatively a ureidopenicillin such as piperacillin can be given alone. Treatment is usually given for 7–10 days.

Osteomyelitis

Infection of bone produces necrotic tissue and generates an avascular privileged site for bacteria that antibacterial drugs only penetrate to a limited extent. Organisms involved include *S. aureus*, which adheres readily to bone matrix, various streptococci, *Serratia* species, *Ps. aeruginosa* and enteric Gram-negative rods.

Early antibacterial treatment is essential, with intravenous therapy for 6 weeks to achieve a cure. Surgical intervention may be necessary to remove necrotic tissue. The choice of drug depends on the suspected organisms. First-line treatment is often with clindamycin or flucloxacillin combined with fusidic acid. If *H. influenzae* is identified, then amoxicillin or cefuroxime are usually used. If long-term therapy is necessary for chronic refractory osteomyelitis, then an oral quinolone such as ciprofloxacin can be substituted.

Septicaemia

Septicaemia is a bacterial infection involving the blood stream and can present with fever, or, if more severe, can result in circulatory collapse, hypotension and shock. This is a medical emergency requiring intensive fluid replacement, plasma volume expansion and electrolyte correction. If the source of infection is not clinically apparent, then empirical therapy is given to cover as wide a range of potential infecting organisms as possible. Suitable treatment would be with an aminoglycoside such as gentamicin combined with a broad-spectrum penicillin (e.g. amoxicillin) or a broad-spectrum cephalosporin (e.g. cefotaxime or ceftazidime). Alternatively, a carbapenem such as meropenem can be used alone. If anaerobic infection is suspected then metronidazole is added.

Immunocompromised patients are at particularly high risk from septicaemia. A combination of gentamicin with a broad-spectrum penicillin or cephalosporin could be given in this situation. Other authorities recommend gentamicin combined with either piperacillin and the β-lactamase inhibitor tazobactam or with meropenem. If anaerobic infection is suspected, then metronidazole is usually added; flucloxacillin or vancomycin are added if Gram-positive infection is suspected. Patients who fail to respond to such triple therapy may have a fungal infection, for which amphotericin can be added (see below).

Infective endocarditis

The majority of cases of infective endocarditis are caused by bacterial pathogens, most commonly oral streptococci, followed by enterococci, *S. aureus* and coagulase-negative staphylococci. Endocarditis usually arises on the endothelial surface of a pre-existing heart defect (e.g. valvular heart defect, ventricular septal defect) or on a prosthetic heart valve. It arises when organisms enter the blood stream and become established on the endocardium, where they may adhere to pre-existing fibrin–platelet vegetations. Bacteria enter the blood during dental procedures, vigorous teeth cleaning or during some surgical procedures.

Untreated infection can destroy the infected heart valve or produce severe haemodynamic disturbance. Systemic complications can also arise from embolisation of vegetation from the valve, from bacteraemia or through immune complexes that form in response to the infection.

When suspected, treatment should be started after blood cultures have been obtained. If the organism is not known, then treatment is usually started with intravenous benzylpenicillin combined with low-dose gentamicin. If the organism is sensitive to penicillin, then the benzylpenicillin is continued for 4 weeks and the gentamicin stopped after 2 weeks. In penicillin-allergic patients, vancomycin is substituted for benzylpenicillin. For staphylococcal endocarditis, flucloxacillin is given in combination with either gentamicin or fusidic acid; for penicillin-allergic patients, vancomycin is used alone.

Antibacterial prophylaxis prior to dental treatment or certain surgical or other procedures is extremely important for individuals with a cardiac lesion that places them at risk of endocarditis. A single large dose of amoxicillin should be given immediately before the procedure, or clindamycin if the individual is allergic to penicillin or has taken penicillin in the previous month. For high-risk individuals (e.g. with a prosthetic valve or previous endocarditis), amoxicillin is combined with gentamicin, and a second dose of amoxicillin is given after the procedure.

Meningitis

Bacterial meningitis is a medical emergency. The most likely organism depends on the age of the patient (Table 51.3).

Empirical selection of therapy is usually necessary, and treatment should be started at the first suspicion of meningitis. A single dose of benzylpenicillin can be given if the patient is outside hospital, but cefotaxime is the preferred treatment in hospital. If the meningitis was caused by meningococci or *H. influenzae*, rifampicin is given for 2–4 days before hospital discharge. Close contacts of patients with meningococcal or *H. influenzae* meningitis are usually given rifampicin as prophylaxis against infection.

Tuberculosis

M. tuberculosis readily develops resistance to single drug therapy. Three or four drugs are used for the first 2 months until bacterial sensitivities are known, when treatment is continued with two drugs for a further 6 months to achieve a cure. In some cases, more prolonged treatment may be necessary, especially for tuberculous meningitis or for resistant organisms. A standard regimen in the UK includes rifampicin and isoniazid for 6 months. In addition, pyrazinamide is usually given for the first 2 months. Ethambutol is added if there is an increased risk of resistance to isoniazid (e.g. after previous treatment for tuberculosis, immunosuppression, contact with drug-resistant organisms). Ethambutol is not used for treatment of young children because of difficulty in monitoring for eye toxicity. Streptomycin is used in some countries in the initial phase of treatment. In countries that cannot afford rifampicin, thiacetazone is often used with isoniazid and initially streptomycin. Compliance can be a major problem in the treatment of tuberculosis, and combination tablets are often used to maximise this. In developed countries directly observed treatment (DOT) has been instituted to improve compliance. This can result in major improvements in eradication rates.

Table 51.3
Organisms causing bacterial meningitis

Age	Organism
<1 month	Group B streptococci
1 month to 4 years	*Haemophilus influenzae*
>4 years to young adult	*Neisseria meningitidis* (meningococcus)
Older adults	*Streptococcus pneumoniae* (pneumococcus)

Fungal infections

Fungi usually infect skin or superficial mucous membranes but also, more rarely, internal organs. Most fungal infections occur because of an underlying defect in host resistance. Fungi grow readily in immuno-suppressed individuals or following the suppression of normal flora with antibiotics. Treatment with general measures such as good hygiene and avoidance of sources of infection is an important complement to the use of antifungal agents.

Compared with antibacterial drugs, only a few agents have been developed that have activity against fungi, and many of these are toxic to humans. A simplified outline of the ways in which antifungal drugs work is shown in Figure 51.5. The following account does not give details of the management of individual fungal infections.

Antifungal agents

Polyene antifungal agents

Examples: nystatin, amphotericin

Mechanism of action
Polyenes bind to ergosterol in the cell wall of fungi and promote leakage of intracellular ions and disruption of membrane active transport mechanisms. They can be fungistatic or fungicidal.

Spectrum of activity
Nystatin is particularly effective against infections with *Candida* species. Amphotericin is active against all common fungi that cause systemic infection (*Candida, Aspergillus, Mucor* and *Cryptococcus* species).

Resistance
Acquired resistance is rare but can occur in immuno-suppressed patients with AIDS. Moulds and yeasts develop a mutation that permits synthesis of the cell membrane without using ergosterol.

Pharmacokinetics
Nystatin is too toxic for systemic use and is not absorbed from the gastrointestinal tract. It is therefore used topically, for example as cream or vaginal pessaries for superficial infections, or orally for buccal and bowel infections.

Amphotericin is poorly absorbed from the gut and is administered intravenously, or given topically for buccal and bowel infections. It can also be given intrathecally for fungal meningitis. Amphotericin is eliminated slowly via the biliary tract and kidney and has a very long half-life of up to 2 weeks. New delivery

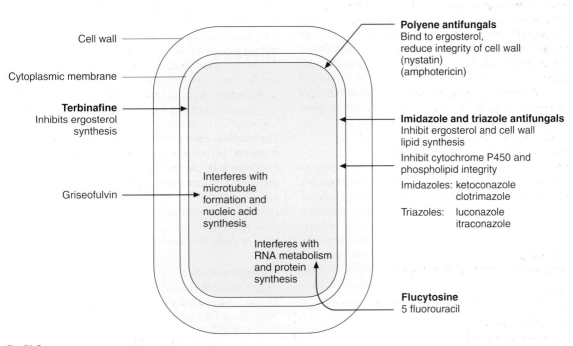

Fig. 51.5
Sites at which antifungal drugs exert their actions on fungi.

Cell wall

Cytoplasmic membrane

Terbinafine
Inhibits ergosterol synthesis

Griseofulvin

Interferes with microtubule formation and nucleic acid synthesis

Interferes with RNA metabolism and protein synthesis

Polyene antifungals
Bind to ergosterol, reduce integrity of cell wall (nystatin) (amphotericin)

Imidazole and triazole antifungals
Inhibit ergosterol and cell wall lipid synthesis

Inhibit cytochrome P450 and phospholipid integrity

Imidazoles: ketoconazole clotrimazole

Triazoles: luconazole itraconazole

Flucytosine
5 fluorouracil

vehicles for amphotericin have been developed to reduce its nephrotoxicity. These formulations deliver the drug in a lipid environment that helps to concentrate it at the site of infection. Formulations include liposomes in which the drug is dissolved (phospholipid membrane vesicles), lipid complexes in which the lipid exists in ribbons interspersed with amphotericin, or a colloidal dispersion of lipid discs that incorporate the drug.

Unwanted effects

Nystatin is virtually free of both toxic and allergic unwanted effects when used topically. Intravenous infusion of amphotericin is commonly associated with:

- fever and rigors during the first week of therapy
- anorexia, nausea and vomiting
- nephrotoxicity, which is the major limiting factor in treatment: it is dose related, reduces glomerular filtration rate and produces hypokalaemia through tubular leakage of K⁺; lipid and liposomal formulations substantially reduce the risk of nephrotoxicity and are particularly useful to treat patients with pre-existing renal impairment.

Imidazoles

Examples: ketoconazole, clotrimazole, miconazole

Mechanism of action

The imidazoles alter the cell membrane fluidity of fungi by inhibiting 14α-demethylase, which is responsible for conversion of lanosterol to ergosterol. This alters cell membrane synthesis, reduces the activity of membrane-associated enzymes and increases cell wall permeability. The result is inhibition of cell growth and replication. The enzyme inhibited belongs to the cytochrome P450 system; similar inhibition of cytochrome P450 enzymes can occur in human tissue.

Spectrum of activity

The imidazoles are active against a wide variety of filamentous fungi and yeasts, including *Candida* species. Clotrimazole and miconazole are used for vaginal candidiasis and for dermatophyte infections (e.g. ringworm (tinea); causative species varies geographically but generally are *Trichophyton*, *Microsporon*, or *Epidermophyton* species). Ketoconazole can be used for systemic mycoses, resistant mucocutaneous candidiasis, resistant vaginal candidiasis or dermatophyte infections; hepatotoxicity limits its clinical value.

Resistance

The development of resistance is rare, except during long-term use in patients with AIDS. The mechanism may involve a mutation in the target enzyme, or development of an active pump that removes drug from the cell.

Pharmacokinetics

Absorption of imidazoles from the gastrointestinal tract is incomplete, but adequate blood concentrations of ketoconazole can be achieved. Many compounds (e.g. clotrimazole) are only used in topical formulations for superficial infections, for example skin and vagina. The imidazoles are metabolised in the liver and have intermediate or long half-lives.

Unwanted effects

These are unusual with topical formulations. Systemic ketoconazole causes:

- gastrointestinal upset: nausea, vomiting, abdominal pain
- itching.
- hepatitis: asymptomatic elevation of liver enzymes is common; more severe hepatic reactions are unusual but can be fatal: liver function tests must be monitored during systemic use of ketoconazole
- high doses of ketoconazole suppress androgen production in males and can cause oligospermia or gynaecomastia; this is an effect mediated by inhibition of cytochrome P450 enzyme systems.
- drug interactions: ketoconazole can inhibit metabolism of drugs that are eliminated by cytochrome P450; if co-prescribed with terfenadine (Ch. 38) this can lead to arrhythmias detected as prolongation of the Q–T interval on the ECG (Ch. 8).

Triazoles

Examples: fluconazole, itraconazole

The triazoles have a similar mechanism of action and spectrum of activity to the imidazoles (see above). Fluconazole is used for candidiasis or for cryptococcal infection. Itraconazole is used for mucocutaneous candidiasis and for dermatophyte infections such as pityriasis versicolor (caused by an organism known as *Malassezia furfur* or *Pityriasis orbiculare*) and tinea corporis or pedis (ringworms).

Pharmacokinetics

Oral absorption is good. Intravenous (fluconazole) and topical (itraconazole) formulations are also available. The triazoles are metabolised in the liver and have very long half-lives of about 36 h. Fluconazole penetrates well into CSF, which is useful for treatment of fungal meningitis.

Unwanted effects

- Gastrointestinal upset can occur, including abdominal pain, nausea and diarrhoea.
- Abnormalities of liver function and occasionally hepatitis or cholestasis occur, more commonly during prolonged treatment with itraconazole. Monitoring of liver function tests during systemic treatment is essential.
- Skin rashes occur, including Stevens–Johnson syndrome.

Flucytosine

Mechanism of action

Flucytosine is converted to 5-fluorouracil selectively in fungal cells. This acts as an antimetabolite that competes with uracil for incorporation into fungal RNA. If some 20–40% of uracil is replaced by 5-fluorouracil, protein synthesis is inhibited. DNA synthesis can also be inhibited.

Spectrum of activity

Flucytosine is only active against yeasts such as *Candida* and *Cryptococcus* species. It is used for systemic infections, often in combination with amphotericin.

Resistance

Resistance occurs readily and occurs through a mutation that produces a deficiency of the enzyme which metabolises flucytosine or through excessive synthesis of uracil, which competes with the antimetabolite.

Pharmacokinetics

Flucytosine is well absorbed from the gut and is also available for intravenous use. It is mainly eliminated unchanged in the urine and has a short half-life.

Unwanted effects

- Gastrointestinal intolerance: nausea, abdominal pain and diarrhoea.
- High concentrations produce reversible bone marrow depression.

Griseofulvin

Mechanism of action

Griseofulvin inhibits dermatophyte mitosis by impairing the polymerisation of microtubule protein.

Spectrum of activity

Griseofulvin is active against dermatophytes such as *Microsporum*, *Epidermophyton* and *Trichophyton* species.

Resistance

Resistance has not been shown.

Pharmacokinetics

Griseofulvin is well absorbed from the gut and is selectively concentrated in skin and nail beds; only low concentrations are found in plasma. Elimination is by metabolism in the liver and the half-life is long.

Unwanted effects

- Gastrointestinal upset: nausea and diarrhoea.
- Headache, dizziness, fatigue.
- Skin rashes, including photosensitivity.

Terbinafine

Mechanism of action

Terbinafine is an allylamine that inhibits squalene epoxidase, an enzyme that converts squalene to ergosterol in the cell wall; consequently, cell wall synthesis is impaired. The intracellular accumulation of squalene is probably cytotoxic.

Mechanism of resistance

Resistance is similar to that for imidazole antifungals.

Pharmacokinetics

Terbinafine penetrates well into the stratum corneum and hair follicles after topical use. After oral administration it is metabolised in the liver and has a long half-life.

Unwanted effects

Unwanted effects are unlikely with topical use of the drug.

- Gastrointestinal upset can include nausea, taste disturbance, abdominal discomfort and diarrhoea.
- Skin rashes occur, which are occasionally severe.

Viral infections

Viruses are small infective particles consisting of DNA or RNA (DNA viruses or RNA viruses), inside a protein coating (capsule), which in some viruses may be further surrounded by a lipoprotein coating. The proteins can have antigenic properties. Viruses lack any inherent metabolic machinery and must parasitically attach to and enter host cells in order to survive and replicate. To do this, some viruses produce enzymes to facilitate their own replication. In this procedure they can acquire phospholipids of host cell origin. Viruses access host cells after binding to recognition sites that are endogenous receptors for many other cellular constituents, for example adrenoceptors, cytokine receptors, etc.

The host will normally eliminate the virus after infection of the cell by actually killing the infected cell. Cytotoxic T-lymphocytes recognise the viral surface

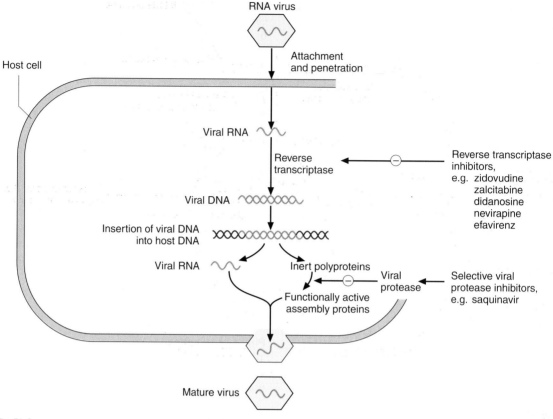

Fig. 51.6
Principles of RNA virus replication and sites of action of antiviral drugs. For details see text.

proteins that are expressed by infected cells. The host can also produce antibodies that bind to and inactivate virus particles extracellularly. Vaccination is designed to mimic this approach.

Viruses, therefore, share many of the host's metabolic processes, which make it difficult to damage the virus without damaging the host. Importantly, antiviral drugs are only effective while the virus is replicating, so the earlier they are given in the course of the infection the more likely they are to work. An outline of the replication of RNA and DNA viruses is shown in Figure 51.6 and 51.7. Since the replicative mechanisms involved may be distinctive to one type of virus, some antiviral drugs are specific for one or another class of virus.

New antiviral drugs are being introduced into clinical practice at an increasing rate. Currently, drugs are available to treat infection by herpes viruses, human immunodeficiency virus (HIV), cytomegalovirus (CMV), hepatitis B virus and influenza virus.

Resistance to antiviral drugs occurs readily. This relates to the high rate of natural occurrence of mutations in the viral genome and production of quasi-species of the virus. Viral polymerases have a high inherent error rate (especially RNA viruses) and viruses tolerate a large number of nucleoside mutations without

losing their infectivity. Normally the large variety of viral quasispecies will be dominated by the variant most selected for survival. However, use of an antiviral drug will select for growth of resistant variants.

Antiviral agents

Viral RNA reverse transcriptase inhibitors

Nucleoside analogue reverse transcriptase inhibitors

Examples: zidovudine, didanosine, zalcitabine

The reverse transcriptase inhibitors are active against RNA viruses, preventing viral RNA being transcribed as viral DNA in the host cell.

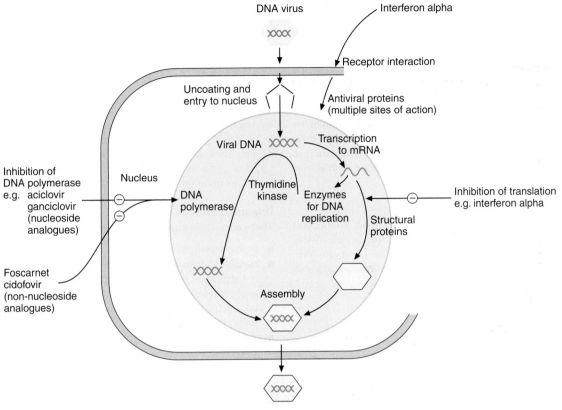

Fig. 51.7
Principles of DNA virus replication and sites of actions of antiviral drugs. For details see text.

Mechanism of action

The reverse transcriptase inhibitor drugs (Fig. 51.6) are activated by intraviral phosphorylation to the 5'-triphosphate form. Zidovudine is an analogue of the pyrimidine base thymidine, one of the constituents of the base pairs in DNA (Fig. 51.6). Didanosine is similar to zidovudine but is a purine analogue. Zalcitabine is a pyrimidine analogue that is phosphorylated via a different pathway from zidovudine.

These drugs inhibit RNA viral replication by an action on the viral enzyme reverse transcriptase, which generates viral DNA for insertion into the host DNA sequence. The inhibition is achieved by competitive binding of the activated drug to the enzyme–template–primer complex in place of the natural 5' deoxynucleoside triphosphates, thus terminating further chain elongation.

Mechanisms of resistance

Resistant strains emerge rapidly within weeks or months through mutation of the drug-binding site on the transcriptase enzyme that increases the affinity for natural substrate compared with the drug. Because of rapid development of resistance, multiple drug therapy is used for treatment.

Spectrum of activity

Reverse transcriptase inhibitors are used in the management of HIV infection and in AIDS.

Pharmacokinetics

Zidovudine is almost completely absorbed from the gut, and about a third undergoes first-pass metabolism in the liver. Elimination is by hepatic metabolism and the half-life is short. The pharmacokinetics of didanosine and zalcitabine are similar.

Unwanted effects

There are a number of unwanted effects that can lead to termination of therapy:

- neutropenia and anaemia are the most frequent unwanted effects (usually occurring in patients with advanced AIDS)
- gastrointestinal upset
- headache, nausea, insomnia
- myalgia or myositis, especially with high doses
- lactic acidosis with severe hepatomegaly
- peripheral neuropathy and pancreatitis are particular problems with zalcitabine and didanosine.

Non-nucleoside reverse transcriptase inhibitors

Examples: nevirapine, efavirenz

Mechanisms of action and resistance

This group of drugs have a similar mode of action to the nucleoside reverse transcriptase inhibitors but have greater antiviral activity. Resistance still emerges rapidly unless they are used in combination with at least two other antiretroviral drugs.

Pharmacokinetics

Oral absorption of nevirapine is very good. Elimination is via metabolism by hepatic cytochrome P450. Nevirapine has a very long half-life of about 30 h. Efavirenz is metabolised in a similar manner and also has a very long half-life.

Unwanted effects

The unwanted effects include:

- skin rash (severe in 10% patients)
- nausea
- headache, drowsiness, fatigue
- drug interactions with agents that affect hepatic cytochrome P450.

Viral RNA protease inhibitors

Examples: saquinavir, ritonavir, indinavir, nelfinavir

Mechanism of action

In HIV infection, there are some steps in viral replication that differ from the processes in host cells. RNA is converted into inactive polyproteins rather than the functional proteins that are the products in host cells. Proteases that are found only in viruses then cleave the polyproteins to the functionally active proteins required by the viruses for their continued existence (Fig. 51.6). Protease enzyme inhibitors are specific for the enzymes found in HIV. They block the infectivity of the viruses but do not affect virus activity in host cells that are already infected.

Mechanism of resistance

Resistance occurs by mutation in the amino acid sequence of the HIV protein that forms the target for the enzyme. Multiple mutations are required for high level resistance; over one-third of the amino acid residues in HIV protein can be changed without altering viral func-

tion. High plasma drug concentrations delay the onset of resistance, as does the combination of a protease inhibitor with two reverse transcriptase inhibitors. Sequential use of more than one protease inhibitor encourages high level resistance.

Pharmacokinetics

Oral absorption is high, but bioavailability varies among the drugs, being very low with saquinavir owing to high first-pass metabolism, and high with the other agents. They are all metabolised by the P450 enzyme CYP3A4 in the liver and have short half-lives. They are inhibitors of human cytochrome P450 enzymes.

Unwanted effects

There are a large number of unwanted effects:

- gastrointestinal disturbances
- metabolic disturbance, e.g. hyperlipidaemia, fat redistribution (buffalo hump), glucose intolerance
- nephrolithiasis is dose limiting with indinavir because of its low water solubility
- paraesthesiae with ritonavir
- drug interactions (Ch. 56): inhibition of the P450 enzyme CYP3A4 (Ch. 2) can enhance the unwanted effects of protease inhibitors; the concurrent use of inducers of CYP3A4 can lower plasma concentrations of the protease inhibitor and encourage viral resistance.

Viral DNA polymerase inhibitors

Nucleoside analogue DNA polymerase inhibitors

Examples: aciclovir, valaciclovir, ganciclovir

Mechanism of action

Aciclovir and the other drugs in this class are guanosine analogues that inhibit the synthesis of viral DNA (Fig. 51.7). They all require phosphorylation by viral enzymes that are not present in uninfected host cells before they exert their antiviral activity. They are phosphorylated by phosphorylation enzymes that have a variable presence in different viruses.

Aciclovir is activated by conversion to a monophosphate following phosphorylation of the drug by herpesvirus thymidine kinase. The monophosphate is then converted to a triphosphate derivative by other intracellular enzymes. The triphosphate derivatives are potent inhibitors of viral DNA polymerase. This terminates viral DNA synthesis and thus inhibits viral replication (Fig. 51.7).

CMV is relatively resistant to aciclovir. It does not possess thymidine kinase and phosphorylates the drugs via a different protein kinase, for which ganciclovir is a good substrate but aciclovir is not. Ganciclovir also has some differences from aciclovir in its mechanisms of action; it does suppress viral DNA replication but unlike aciclovir it does not act as a DNA chain terminator. Uninfected human cells cannot phosphorylate these drugs, which prevents cytotoxic effects in human tissue.

Spectrum of activity

Aciclovir is most active against herpes viruses (both simplex and zoster). It is only active against CMV at high doses. Treatment of herpes infections is only successful if it is given at the start of the illness. Valaciclovir has a similar spectrum of action to aciclovir but is a prodrug. Ganciclovir has much greater activity against CMV.

Mechanisms of resistance

Phosphorylation of this group of drugs by viral enzymes is essential for their activity. Viral mutants are selected that are unable to phosphorylate the drugs. Thymidine kinase-deficient mutants of herpes virus usually develop in immunocompromised individuals, for example those with AIDS or after bone marrow transplantation, when resistance rates average 5–10%.

Pharmacokinetics

Aciclovir can be given topically to the skin or eye, orally or intravenously. Absorption from the gut is poor. The drug is widely distributed, but concentrations in the CSF are low compared with those in plasma. Most elimination is via the kidney, and the half-life is short. Valaciclovir is an ester of aciclovir with higher oral bioavailability. Ganciclovir is given intravenously for acute infections since it is poorly absorbed from the gut; oral dosage forms for maintenance therapy are available; it penetrates into the CSF moderately well. It is eliminated by the kidney and has a short half-life. Ganciclovir undergoes little or no metabolism.

Unwanted effects

Most unwanted effects occur with intravenous use.

- Severe local phlebitis at an infusion site.
- Gastrointestinal disturbances.
- Skin rashes.
- Encephalopathy occurs in 1% of patients
- Nephrotoxicity is caused by crystallisation of the drug in the kidney; it can be limited by a high fluid intake.
- With ganciclovir, the commonest unwanted effect is bone marrow suppression, with neutropenia occurring in up to 40% of patients, and thrombocytopenia less frequently. The neutropenia can be prevented by the use of granulocyte or granulocyte–macrophage colony-stimulating factor (Ch. 47).

- Ganciclovir causes azoospermia by direct inhibition of sperm production.

Non-nucleoside analogue DNA polymerase inhibitors

Examples: foscarnet, cidofovir

Mechanisms of action

Foscarnet is an inorganic pyrophosphate compound that binds to the pyrophosphate binding sites of viral DNA polymerase, preventing DNA chain elongation. Affinity for the viral DNA polymerase is a hundred times greater than for the host cell DNA polymerase. These drugs are reversible inhibitors of CMV and herpes simplex replication. Cidofovir is similar in structure to aciclovir but contains a phosphate moiety. Its action is similar to that of foscarnet. Neither foscarnet nor cidofovir relies on intracellular activation for its antiviral activity (Fig. 51.7).

Pharmacokinetics

Both foscarnet and cidofovir are only available for intravenous use. They are eliminated by the kidney and have intermediate half-lives. Cidofovir is given with probenecid to inhibit its renal tubular secretion and minimise nephrotoxicity.

Unwanted effects

- Foscarnet causes gastrointestinal upset and mood disturbances.
- Both agents are highly nephrotoxic, causing a rise in plasma creatinine. Good hydration reduces kidney damage.

Other antiviral drugs

Tribavirin

Tribavirin (ribavirin) is used in the treatment of infections with hepatitis C virus and respiratory syncitial virus (RSV). It is discussed in Chapter 36.

Idoxuridine

The phosphorylated metabolite of idoxuridine is incorporated into viral DNA and impairs transcription. It is now little used. Idoxuridine has been used topically to treat superficial eye and skin infections caused by herpes simplex. For use on the skin, penetration is enhanced by dissolving it in dimethylsulfoxide (DMSO).

Amantadine

Amantadine is discussed in Chapter 13. It acts by inhibiting viral DNA replication at the stage of uncoating after entry into the cell. The clinically useful activity of amantadine is limited to the treatment of influenza A. It reduces the incidence of influenza A infection when used prophylactically and will shorten the symptoms and duration of the established illness if given early enough. Its use is only recommended for high-risk individuals for whom immunisation is contraindicated, or if immunisation was given less than 2 weeks before an outbreak.

Influenza virus neuraminidase inhibitor

Example: zanamivir

Mechanism of action

Influenza virus neuraminidase is a surface glycoprotein that cleaves sialic acid from a sugar residue. This promotes the spread of the virus by increasing penetration into respiratory epithelial cells, releasing virions from infected cells, promotes viral activation and induces cellular apoptosis. Zanamivir binds and inhibits only the neuraminidases of influenza A and B and is effective against isolates resistant to amantidine.

Pharmacokinetics

Zanamivir is administered by inhalation, where systemic absorption is only 4–17%. Absorbed drug is excreted unchanged and the half-life is short.

Unwanted effects

- Gastrointestinal disturbance.
- Bronchospasm.

Immunomodulators

Interferon alfa

Interferons are glycoproteins produced as part of the natural host defences in response to virus infections. There are three types: α, β and γ. Interferons α and β are produced by most cells in response to viral infection but production of interferon γ is limited to T-lymphocytes in response to antigens of viral and non-viral origin. Administration of the drug interferon alfa can prevent, but not cure, certain viral infections. The interferons have several actions, although the exact ways that they exert their benefit is unclear. These actions include binding to receptors on both RNA and DNA viruses and enhancing synthesis of intracellular enzymes that inhibit mRNA translation into viral proteins. This reduces the replication of viruses (Fig. 51.7). Interferon alfa is antiproliferative and immunomodulatory and alters cytokine induction.

Interferons have additional effects on human malignant cells (Ch. 52), reducing their rate of multiplication, possibly by reimposing normal control mechanisms. Macrophage and natural killer cell activity is also enhanced (Ch. 39).

Pharmacokinetics

Interferon alfa is not absorbed orally and must be given intramuscularly or subcutaneously. It is inactivated in renal tubular cells and also in target tissue cells. The half-life is short.

Unwanted effects

- An influenza-like illness that includes fever, chills, headache and myalgia.
- Bone marrow suppression is common.
- Neurological effects include confusion and seizures.

Clinical uses of interferon alfa

Clinical uses of interferon alfa include the treatment of:

- chronic hepatitis
- condylomata acuminata
- AIDS-related Kaposi's sarcoma
- hairy cell leukaemia
- recurrent or metastatic renal cell carcinoma (Ch. 52).

Palivizumab

Mechanism of action and use

Palivizumab is a humanised monoclonal antibody with human and murine antibody sequences produced by recombinant DNA technology. It has potent neutralising and fusion-inhibiting activity against RSV. It reduces the ability of RSV to replicate and infect cells by binding to an antigenic site on the surface of RSV. RSV is a common cause of mild respiratory illness in infants but can produce more severe illness in premature infants or those with congenital heart disease or bronchopulmonary dysplasia. It is given to at-risk children under the age of 2 years prior to commencement of the RSV season (October to April in the northern hemisphere) and monthly thereafter.

Pharmacokinetics

Palivizumab is given intramuscularly into the anterolateral aspect of the thigh. It has a long half-life of 20 days. The routes of metabolism and elimination are unknown.

Unwanted effects

- Fever.
- Injection site reactions.

Treatment of specific viral infections

HIV infection

There are several principles of antiviral therapy for HIV (retroviral) infection, which are now widely adopted. The most frequently used treatment regimens include a protease inhibitor combined with two nucleoside analogue reverse transcriptase inhibitors (e.g. saquinavir with zidovudine and zalcitabine). Such combinations are referred to as highly active antiretroviral therapy (HAART) and involve complex regimens that require compliance by the patient and careful assessment of the progress of viral suppression. Key principles include:

- Combination drug treatment should be started before substantial immunodeficiency is present. The goal is to suppress the virus before resistant mutants emerge or irreversible immune damage occurs. The current recommendation is to start treatment at the onset of an acute HIV syndrome, or within 6 months of seroconversion. Failing these, treatment is given if symptoms occur as a result of HIV infection.
- When resistance occurs, changes in drug therapy should involve the addition or change of at least two drugs. However, if toxicity limits the tolerability of one drug, a single substitution of a similar agent is a reasonable option.
- Optimal treatment should reduce the viral load to below detectable limits. This may take 6 months of adequate therapy to achieve.
- Failure to achieve full suppression of viral load should prompt a change in therapy if compliance is believed to be good. Poor compliance with therapy is likely to encourage the development of drug resistance (see above) and thus treatment failure. Drug therapy is ideally guided by patterns of resistance in the virus.

Prophylaxis after accidental exposure to the virus is now recommended. The regimen depends on the level of risk: two drugs are often used for moderate risk, or three drugs if the risk is high.

Varicella–zoster virus infections

Varicella–zoster virus (VZV) is a herpes virus responsible for both chickenpox and shingles (zoster). Shingles arises from reactivation of the virus, which lies dormant in a dorsal root ganglion after the primary chickenpox infection. Chickenpox is rarely treated with antiviral therapy, although the use of oral aciclovir reduces lesion formation and results in quicker healing.

Zoster is most commonly found in the elderly and the immunosuppressed. The rash is often preceded by pain for 1–4 days. Oral antiviral drug therapy reduces pain and accelerates healing but must be given while the virus is still replicating. Oral aciclovir is often used and is particularly indicated for those older than 55 years (who are at greater risk of complications), for ophthalmic infections or in immunosuppressed patients. Complications occur in 15–20% of those with zoster and include meningoencephalitis, motor nerve paralysis, ocular complications and postherpetic neuralgia. The use of aciclovir has little effect on the risk of developing postherpetic neuralgia but does reduce the risk of motor nerve damage. Corticosteroids have no value as an adjunctive treatment to aciclovir. Valaciclovir may be more effective for resolving symptoms than aciclovir. Analgesics are often required in the early phases of zoster, and postherpetic neuralgia may require specific therapy (Ch. 19).

Herpes simplex virus infections

Herpes simplex virus exists in two forms: type 1 produces either oral or genital ulceration and type 2 produces genital ulceration. Oral herpes infection will respond to early topical application of aciclovir. Primary genital herpes produces multiple painful lesions and responds to oral aciclovir given for 5 days. Recurrent lesions occur from reactivation of latent virus in the dorsal root ganglia, producing symptoms that are usually less severe than with primary episodes. After initial therapy with aciclovir, continuous prophylactic therapy can be given to prevent further relapses.

Cytomegalovirus infection

CMV infection is common and usually produces mild symptoms. However, it can be devastating in immunosuppressed patients. Troublesome complications in this group include retinitis (which can threaten sight), gastrointestinal manifestations (including oesophagitis, gastritis, cholecystitis or colitis), pneumonia and CNS involvement.

Intravenous ganciclovir is the treatment of choice for severe manifestation of CMV infection. For retinitis, oral ganciclovir is used to prevent relapse. Oral ganciclovir may be of particular value for the prevention of CMV infection, particularly in bone marrow transplant recipients in whom CMV pneumonia is a major potential complication. Combined therapy with ganciclovir and CMV immunoglobulin may be more effective than ganciclovir alone for treatment of pneumonia in this group.

Protozoal infections

Malaria

Four species of the protozoan *Plasmodium* produce malaria in humans: *P. vivax, P. ovale, P. malariae* and *P. falciparum*. Sporozoites are formed by repeated division of oocysts in the body of the mosquito and are transferred into host blood in the anopheles mosquito saliva during a blood meal. The parasite is sequestered in the liver and divides to form tissue schizonts (Fig. 51.8). When the pre-erythrocytic (liver) sexual cycle is complete, the liver cells rupture and 20 000–40 000 merozoites escape into the blood and invade erythrocytes. They then undergo the erythrocytic cycle, multiplying asexually in the erythrocytes. The red cells then rupture and release merozoites to invade other red cells. Merozoites in the plasma at this stage are termed gametocytes. A mosquito biting an infected individual ingests gametocytes that then go through a development cycle in the mosquito to form sporozoites.

At the pre-erythrocytic stage in the liver, some schizonts from *P. vivax* and *P. ovale* rather than being released as merozoites remain in the liver, forming hypnozoites. These form a reservoir of parasites that are difficult to eradicate and can emerge to give relapses months or years after the initial infection. Release of merozoites in the human every 2 or 3 days causes repeated bouts of tertian or quartan fever. The duration of the infection varies with the parasite. Because *P. vivax* and *P. ovale* continue to multiply in the liver as hypnozoites, drugs that treat only the erythrocytic phase will not produce a radical cure (elimination of all parasites) in these patients and relapsing infection can occur.

P. falciparum and *P. malariae* only multiply in erythrocytes, but disease can recrudesce if parasites are not completely eliminated from the blood.

Clinical symptoms include chills as merozoites enter blood from ruptured erythrocytes. Nausea, vomiting and headache are common. A fever follows and the attack concludes with sweating. *P. falciparum* produces the most severe symptoms because it causes agglutination of red cells, which produces capillary thrombosis, especially in the brain leading to cerebral malaria.

Antimalarial drugs

Chloroquine

Mechanism of action

Erythrocytes infected by malaria parasites concentrate chloroquine more than 100-fold since it binds to a break-

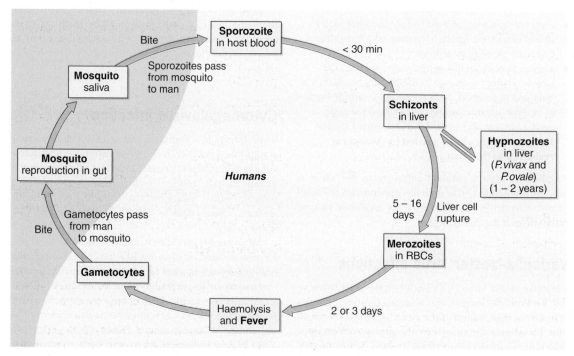

Fig. 51.8
Life-cycle of malarial parasite.

down product of haemoglobin induced by the parasite. Three mechanisms of action have been proposed but are unproven:

- Chloroquine is digested by the erythrocyte-resident parasite, and this raises lysosomal pH, which will reduce the ability of the parasite to digest haemoglobin and inhibit its growth.
- Chloroquine interacts with ferriprotoporphyrin IX, which is formed during digestion of haemoglobin, an action that prevents further degradation of haemoglobin by the parasite.
- A third possibility is inclusion of chloroquine among the nucleic acids in the parasite's DNA, inhibiting gene expression.

Chloroquine (and its close relative hydroxychloroquine) also possesses slow-onset anti-inflammatory activity, which is useful in the treatment of rheumatoid arthritis (Ch. 30).

Pharmacokinetics
Chloroquine is a 4-aminoquinoline that is completely absorbed from the gut, or it can be given intravenously. It has a very high volume of distribution because of selective concentration in melanin-containing tissues, for example the retina of the eye, and in the liver, spleen and kidney. Approximately half is converted in the liver to active metabolites, the rest is excreted unchanged by the kidney. The half-life is very long during chronic dosing; an initial half-life of up to 6 days is followed by a second slow phase of tissue elimination with a half-life greater than 1 month.

Unwanted effects

- Nausea, vomiting, diarrhoea, abdominal pain can occur, which may be caused by anticholinesterase activity (Chs. 27 and 28).
- Cardiovascular depression occurs after intravenous use, with hypotension and heart block; these are quinidine-like effects (Ch. 8).
- Retinopathy can occur with cumulative doses, producing retinal pigmentation and visual field defects. Visual function should be monitored.
- Skin rashes and itching.

Mefloquine

Mechanism of action
Mefloquine is similar to chloroquine, although binding to DNA does not occur.

Pharmacokinetics
Mefloquine is an amino alcohol that is well absorbed from the gut and has a high affinity for lung, liver and lymphoid tissue. Extensive metabolism occurs in the liver but the elimination half-life is very long, in excess of 20 days.

Unwanted effects

- CNS effects: dizziness, vertigo, headache. Less commonly, severe psychiatric disturbance can occur and mefloquine should not be given to individuals with a previous history of psychiatric disorder.
- Gastrointestinal effects occur that are similar to those seen with chloroquine.

Primaquine
Primaquine is an unlicensed drug in the UK and only available for individual 'named' patients.

Mechanism of action
Unlike structurally related drugs, primaquine only affects the exoerythrocytic parasite. It enters the parasite in the liver and may inhibit mitochondrial respiration. The active metabolites also bind to parasitic DNA (cf. chloroquine).

Pharmacokinetics
Primaquine is an 8-aminoquinolone that is completely absorbed from the gut and rapidly metabolised in the liver, producing active compounds. The half-life is intermediate.

Unwanted effects

- Intravascular haemolysis can occur in patients with glucose 6-phosphate dehydrogenase deficiency (Ch. 47).
- Gastrointestinal effects are similar to those seen with chloroquine.

Quinine

Mechanism of action
Quinine is similar to chloroquine in its action but does not bind to DNA.

Pharmacokinetics
Quinine is well absorbed from the gut but can also be given by intravenous infusion. Metabolism in the liver is extensive and the half-life is intermediate in healthy subjects, becoming long in severe malaria.

Unwanted effects

- Cinchonism: tinnitus, headache, nausea, visual disturbances with vertigo and hearing loss if severe.
- Stimulation of insulin secretion producing hypoglycaemia.
- Quinidine-like effects on the heart (Ch. 8) with bradycardias, heart block or ventricular tachycardia. Most often this occurs with intravenous loading doses.

Pyrimethamine

Mechanism of action

Selective inhibition of dihydrofolate reductase in the parasite reduces folic acid synthesis (Fig. 51.4). Pyrimethamine should only be given in combination with a sulfonamide derivative, either sulfadoxine or dapsone.

Pharmacokinetics

Pyrimethamine is well absorbed from the gut and undergoes extensive hepatic metabolism. The half-life is very long, approximately 2–6 days.

Unwanted effects

Pyrimethamine is usually well tolerated; occasional effects are:

- photosensitive rashes
- megaloblastic anaemia due to inhibition of human folate metabolism (with chronic therapy).

Proguanil

Mechanism of action

Proguanil inhibits plasmodial dihydrofolate reductase (Fig. 51.4), mainly through its active metabolite. This inhibits folate production in both pre-erythrocytic and erythrocytic parasites. It is usually used for malaria prophylaxis, in combination with chloroquine.

Pharmacokinetics

Absorption of proguanil from the gut is good, and extensive metabolism occurs in the liver to cycloguanil, a potent active derivative. The half-life of proguanil is long; that of cycloguanil is short.

Unwanted effects

- Mouth ulcers.
- Epigastric discomfort.

Treatment of malaria

Chemotherapy of malaria falls into three categories:

- rapid-acting *blood* schizonticides (to kill schizonts in *acute* malaria): chloroquine, quinine, mefloquine
- slow-acting *blood* schizonticides (to *prevent* blood infections): pyrimethamine, proguanil
- tissue schizonticides (to eliminate *liver* parasites): primaquine.

The recommended drug to use within each category depends on the type of parasite and the pattern of resistance where the infection was acquired. If the infecting organism is unknown, it is assumed to be *P. falciparum*, which carries the greatest risk. Latest recommendations should be obtained from tropical disease advisory centres.

Examples are given for current recommended treatments for acute attacks of high and low-risk malaria.

For *P. falciparum*, chloroquine resistance is common. Oral quinine or mefloquine are given initially (intravenous quinine is used for serious infections). This is followed by pyrimethamine with sulfadoxine for 7 days or by doxycycline (see Antibacterials above) if the plasmodia are resistant to sulfadoxine.

For benign malaria, chloroquine is given initially. For *P. vivax* and *P. ovale*, primaquine is then given to destroy hepatic parasites.

Prophylaxis against malaria

The recommendations for prophylaxis depend on patterns of resistance in the area to be visited. Where resistance is low, chloroquine or proguanil are often recommended. For many areas a combination of both drugs is desirable. Mefloquine is recommended in some areas when there is a high risk of chloroquine-resistant malaria. In some parts of southeast Asia, doxycycline can be used for prophylaxis. Prophylaxis must also take into account the unwanted effects of the drugs and other factors such as pregnancy and renal or hepatic impairment. Prophylaxis must be continued for 1 month after leaving a malarious area to protect against infection acquired immediately prior to departure.

Other protozoal infections

Details of the natural history of other protozoal infections are not given in this book. Important drugs available in the UK for these conditions are discussed below. An outline of therapeutic uses is given in Table 51.4.

Pentamidine

Indications

Pentamidine is used in *Pneumocystis carinii* pneumonia, leishmaniasis and trypanosomiasis.

Mechanism of action and uses

Pentamidine undergoes active uptake into the cell where it probably inhibits DNA synthesis and ribosomal synthesis of protein and phospholipid. It is cytotoxic to *P. carinii* in the non-replicating state. Because of its toxicity, pentamidine is usually reserved for patients who are intolerant of co-trimoxazole, which is the drug of first choice for pneumocystis pneumonia (see Antibacterials above).

Pharmacokinetics

Pentamidine is given intravenously or inhaled as an aerosol for pneumocystis pneumonia. It can be given by deep intramuscular injection for leishmaniasis or trypanosomiasis. Inhalation is particularly useful for

Table 51.4
Selected protozoan infections and antiprotozoal drugs

Protozoa	Disease	Drug examples
Plasmodium	Malaria	Chloroquine, halofantine, mefloquine, primaquine, quinine, proguanil, pyrimethamine
Entamoeba histolytica	Amoebic dysentery	Metronidazole, tinidazole, diloxanide
Trichomonas vaginalis	Vaginitis	Metronidazole, tinidazole
Giardia lamblia	Gastrointestinal dysfunction	Metronidazole, tinidazole, mepacrine
Leishmania	Cutaneous or visceral (kala-azar) leishmaniasis	Stibogluconate, pentamidine
Trypanosomes	Trypanosomiasis, Chagas' disease, sleeping sickness	Suramin, nifurtimax, benznidazole, eflornithine, pentamidine, melarsoprol
Toxoplasma gondii	Encephalomyelitis, toxoplasmosis	Pyrimethamine plus sulfadiazine, trimetrexate
Pneumocystis carinii	Pneumocystis pneumonia	Co-trimoxazole, pentamidine, atovaquone, trimetrexate

pneumocystis pneumonia (which affects immunocompromised patients, especially those with AIDS), since lung concentrations are low after intravenous administration. Pentamidine is metabolised in the liver and has a long half-life.

Unwanted effects

- Inhaled pentamidine produces bronchial irritation with cough and bronchospasm.
- Intravenous pentamidine is nephrotoxic, can produce irreversible hypoglycaemia and life-threatening arrhythmias such as ventricular tachycardia.

Sodium stibogluconate

Indication
Visceral leishmaniasis.

Mechanism of action
Sodium stibogluconate is an organic pentavalent antimony derivative that may act by binding to thiol groups in the parasite.

Pharmacokinetics
Sodium stibogluconate must be given parenterally, either by intramuscular injection or slow intravenous infusion. It has a short half-life and is eliminated by the kidney.

Unwanted effects

- Anorexia and vomiting.
- Cough and substernal pain during intravenous infusion.

Diloxanide furoate

Indication
Chronic amoebiasis.

Mechanism of action
Unknown.

Pharmacokinetics
Hydrolysis in the gut liberates diloxanide and furoic acid; 90% of the diloxanide is then absorbed and rapidly conjugated in the liver. Diloxanide has a short half-life. The unabsorbed fraction of diloxanide may contribute to the drug's effectiveness in amoebic dysentery.

Unwanted effects
Gastrointestinal effects include flatulence, anorexia, nausea and diarrhoea.

Atovaquone

Indications
Infections with *P. carinii* and *Toxoplasma gondii*.

Mechanisms of action
Atovaquone is used as a second line agent in patients with *P. carinii* infections and is used for treating patients with *T. gondii* infection (see above). In *P. carinii*, atovaquone does not inhibit folate but interferes in DNA synthesis by inhibiting pyrimidine synthesis. It is selective for protozoa, which cannot utilise preformed pyrimidines. It is able to kill *Pneumocystis* organisms rather than just delaying growth. It is also active against *Plasmodium* species and *Entamoeba histolytica* and *Trichomonas vaginalis*.

Pharmacokinetics
Oral absorption of atovaquone is poor but is improved with food. There is limited metabolism and it has a long half-life.

Unwanted effects

- Gastrointestinal effects: diarrhoea, nausea.
- Rash.
- Neutropenia.

Trimetrexate

Indications

P. carinii infection where standard treatment is not tolerated (see above) and *T. gondii* infection.

Mechanisms of action

Trimetrexate is a dihydrofolate reductase inhibitor (Fig. 51.4). Calcium folinate must be given to avoid bone marrow depression, gastrointestinal ulceration and renal and hepatic dysfunction.

Pharmacokinetics

Trimetrexate is administered parenterally and does not cross the blood–brain barrier. It is metabolised in the liver and has an intermediate half-life.

Unwanted effects

- Blood disorders: thrombocytopenia, anaemia.
- Gastrointestinal effects: diarrhoea, ulcers.
- Plasma electrolyte disturbances.
- Renal and hepatic dysfunction.

Helminth infections

Details of the natural history of helminth infections are not given here, but an outline of the more commonly encountered conditions is given in Table 51.5. Drugs specifically for helminth infections are discussed below.

Antihelminthic agents

Ivermectin

Indications

Filiariasis (especially onchocerciasis), hookworm, strongyloides.

Mechanism of action

Ivermectin is a macrocyclic lactone. It produces an influx of Cl⁻ via an action on cell membrane ion channels, producing hyperpolarisation of the filariae and muscle paralysis. In the UK, it is an unlicensed drug, available on a 'named' patient basis only.

Pharmacokinetics

Ivermectin is well absorbed from the gut and is excreted mainly in the faeces. It undergoes some hepatic metabolism and has a long half-life. Treatment with a single dose reduces microfilarial levels for several months, and it can be repeated every 6–12 months if necessary.

Unwanted effects

- Itching.
- Skin rash.

Diethylcarbamazine

Indication

Filariasis.

Mechanism of action

The mechanism of action of diethylcarbamazine is not well understood. It may inhibit arachidonic acid metabolism in the filariae. It also triggers exposure of antigens on the surface coat, leading to antibody-mediated destruction.

Pharmacokinetics

Oral absorption is good, and approximately half the drug is metabolised in the liver; the rest is excreted unchanged in the kidney. The half-life is intermediate. Treatment is usually required for 2–3 weeks to eliminate the microfilariae.

Unwanted effects

Most problems are caused by release of antigens from dying filariae. The onset is about 2 h after dosing and is almost diagnostic of the disease. The reaction is occasionally severe and life threatening. The reaction includes:

- fever

Table 51.5
Helminth infections

Helminth	Common name	Drug examples
Enterobius vermicularis	Threadworm	Mebendazole, piperazine
Ascaris lumbricoides	Roundworm	Mebendazole, piperazone, levamisole
Toxocara canis	Dog roundworm	Tiabendazole, diethylcarbamazine
Taenia species	Tapeworm	Niclosamide, praziquantel
Ancylostoma species, *Necator* species	Hookworm	Mebendazole, ivermectin, albendazole
Microfilariae (e.g. *Loa loa*, *Wuchereria bancrofti*, *Brugia malayi*)		Diethylcarbamazine, ivermectin
Strongyloides stercoralis		Tiabendazole, albendazole, ivermectin
Echinococcus granulosa	Hydatid disease	Albendazole

- headache
- nausea
- muscle and joint pains
- itching
- postural hypotension.

Benzimidazoles

Examples: tiabendazole, mebendazole, albendazole

Indications

Tiabendazole: threadworm, mixed worm infestations (but not filariasis)
Mebendazole: threadworm, roundworm, whipworm, hookworm
Albendazole: hydatid cysts, strongyloides.

Mechanism of action

The benzimidazoles bind to tubulin, preventing its polymerisation into the cytoskeletal microtubules. The effect is selective for parasitic tubulin and the drugs are active against the adults, larvae and eggs.

Pharmacokinetics

Oral absorption of tiabendazole is almost complete and metabolism in the liver is extensive. The half-life is short. Oral absorption of mebendazole and albendazole is very poor; the little drug that is absorbed is metabolised in the liver. These drugs act principally from within the gut.

Unwanted effects

- Gastrointestinal effects are common with tiabendazole and include anorexia, nausea, vomiting and diarrhoea. They are less severe with the other agents.
- Dizziness, drowsiness can occur with tiabendazole.

Piperazine

Indications

Threadworm and roundworm.

Mechanism of action

Piperazine competitively inhibits the effect of acetylcholine on the smooth muscle of the worm, producing a reversible flaccid paralysis.

Pharmacokinetics

Absorption of piperazine is rapid from the gut, but little is known about its handling after absorption.

Unwanted effect

Gastrointestinal upset can occur.

Niclosamide

Indication

Tapeworm infection.

Mechanism of action

Niclosamide inhibits generation of ATP by preventing phosphorylation of ADP in mitochondria. It is ineffective against larval worms. Purgatives are usually given after niclosamide to remove viable ova from the gut.

Pharmacokinetics

Some oral absorption (up to 20%) occurs, with subsequent liver metabolism.

Unwanted effects

- Gastrointestinal upset: nausea, abdominal pain.
- Lightheadedness.
- Pruritis.

Praziquantel

Indications

Tapeworm infection and schistosomiasis.

Mechanism of action

It is not well understood how praziquantel acts; it is known to interfere with Ca^{2+} homeostasis in the parasite, causing muscular paralysis and increasing cell membrane permeability. Praziquantel is unlicensed in the UK and is available only on a 'named' patient basis.

Pharmacokinetics

Praziquantel is well absorbed from the gut and penetrates well into most tissues; it has a short plasma half-life and is extensively metabolised by the liver.

Unwanted effects

- Dizziness, headache, lassitude.
- Gastrointestinal upset.

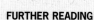

FURTHER READING

Antibacterial agents

Brown PD, Lerner SA (1998) Community-acquired pneumonia. *Lancet* 352, 1295–1302

Gold HS, Moellering RC (1996) Antimicrobial-drug resistance. *N Engl J Med* 335, 1445–1453

Gaya H (1998) Empirical therapy of infections in neutropenic patients. *Br J Haematol* 101 (suppl 1), 5–9

Goldenberg DL (1998) Septic arthritis. *Lancet* 351, 197–202

Hancock REW (1997) Peptide antibiotics. *Lancet* 349, 418–422

Hawkey RM (1998) The origins and molecular basis of antibiotic resistance. *Br Med J* 317, 657–660

Lew DP, Waldvogel FA (1997) Osteomyelitis. *N Engl J Med* 336, 999–1007

Nicolle LE (1997) A practical guide to the management of complicated urinary tract infection. *Drugs* 53, 583–592

Stamboulian D, Carbone E (1997) Recognition, management and prophylaxis of endocarditis. *Drugs* 54, 730–744

Vogel F (1995) A guide to the treatment of lower respiratory tract infections. *Drugs* 50, 62–72

Westphal J-F, Brogard J-M (1999) Biliary tract infections. *Drugs* 57, 81–91

Antifungal agents

Alexander BD, Perfect JR (1997) Antifungal resistance trends towards the year 2000. *Drugs* 54, 657–678

Allen TA (1998) Liposomal drug formulations. *Drugs* 56, 747–756

Gupta AK, Einarson TR, Summerbell RC et al. (1998) An overview of topical antifungal therapy in dermatomycoses. *Drugs* 55, 645–674

Kauffman CA, Carver PL (1997) Antifungal agents in the 1990s. *Drugs* 53, 539–549

Quagliarello VJ, Scheld WM (1997) Treatment of bacterial meningitis. *N Engl J Med* 336, 708–716

Antiviral agents

Balfour HH (1999) Antiviral drugs. *N Engl J Med* 340, 1255–1268

Barry M, Mulcahy F, Back DJ (1998) Antiretroviral therapy for patients with HIV disease. *Br J Clin Pharmacol* 45, 221–228

British HIV Association Co-ordinating Committee (1997) British HIV Association guidelines for antiretroviral treatment of HIV seropositive individuals. *Lancet* 349, 1086–1092

Cox NJ, Subbarao K (1999) Influenza. *Lancet* 354, 1277–1282

Flexner C (1998) HIV-protease inhibitors. *N Engl J Med* 338, 1281–1292

Gubareva LV, Kaiser L, Hayden FG (2000) Influenza virus neuraminidase inhibitors. *Lancet* 355, 827–835

Panel on Clinical Practices for Treatment of HIV Infection (1998) Guidelines for the use of antiretroviral agents in HIV-infected adults and adolescents. *Ann Intern Med* 128, 1079–1100

Pillay D, Zambon M (1998) Antiviral drug resistance. *Br Med J* 317, 660–662

Snoeck R, Andrei G, de Clercq E (1999) Current pharmacological approaches to the therapy of varicella zoster virus infections. *Drugs* 57, 187–206

Vandamme A-M, Laethem KV, de Clercq E (1999) Managing resistance to anti-HIV drugs. *Drugs* 57, 337–361

Antiprotozoal agents

Herwaldt BL (1999) Leishmaniasis. *Lancet* 354, 1191–1199

White NJ (1996) The treatment of malaria. *N Engl J Med* 335, 800–806

Antihelminthic agents

de Silva N, Guyatt H, Bundy D (1997) Antihelminthics. *Drugs* 53, 769–788

Liu LX, Weller PF (1996) Antiparasitic drugs. *N Engl J Med* 334, 1178–1184

Self-assessment

In questions 1–7, the first statement, in italics, is true. Are the accompanying statements also true?

1. *Resistance to antibacterials can be generated by organisms increasing efflux or decreasing uptake of drugs, producing enzymes that metabolise drugs, replacing essential microbial enzymes that could be inhibited by antibacterials with mutant enzymes that are no longer inhibited, or developing mutated ribosomal subunits that do not bind antibacterials.*

   a. Benzylpenicillin has a short half-life as it is rapidly excreted by the kidneys.
   b. Broad-spectrum penicillins do not result in disturbances in normal colonic flora.
   c. The antipseudomonal penicillin azlocillin is β-lactamase resistant.
   d. Penicillins are bactericidal by binding to bacterial ribosomal-binding sites.

2. *A number of cephalosporins exist that show a range of activities against Gram-positive and Gram-negative bacteria and high central nervous system penetration.*

   a. Cefotaxime is a third-generation cephalosporin. It crosses the blood–brain barrier and is not broken down by β-lactamases.
   b. Patients that are allergic to penicillins cannot be given cephalosporins.

3. *The carbapem imipenem is a broad-spectrum β-lactamase effective against many Gram-positive and Gram-negative organisms.*

   a. Imipenem is rapidly metabolised.
   b. Imipenem is a bacteriostatic antibacterial.

4. *The quinolone ciprofloxacin is active against many Gram-negative and Gram-positive organisms but has weak activity against streptococci and staphylococci. It has a relatively low incidence of unwanted effects.*

   a. Ciprofloxacin can be used for *Pseudomonas aeruginosa* infections in cystic fibrosis.
   b. Ciprofloxacin can safely be given together with theophylline in asthmatics.

5. *Macrolide antibiotics (e.g. erythromycin, clarithromycin) can be used as part of the regimen to eliminate* Helicobacter pylori *and* Legionella *infection.*

   a. Erythromycin commonly causes gastrointestinal disturbances.
   b. Gentamicin has relatively low incidence of unwanted effects.
   c. Gentamicin is not active when given orally.

6. *Metronidazole can be used as part of the regimen for eradicating* Helicobacter pylori *and for treatment of pseudomembranous colitis resulting from overgrowths with* Clostridium difficile.

   a. Antibacterials do not reduce the development of serious illness for patients with sore throat.
   b. Tetracyclines should be avoided in pregnancy and young children.
   c. Vancomycin is active against β-lactamase-producing Gram-positive bacteria.

7. *Because of problems with resistance,* Mycobacterium tuberculosis *is always treated with at least two drugs acting at different sites.*

   a. Rifampicin is an important drug for the treatment of tuberculosis and also serious Legionnaire's disease and leprosy.
   b. Isoniazid is active against a wide range of bacteria.
   c. Co-trimoxazole is the drug of choice for hospital-acquired acute urinary tract infection.
   d. Trimethoprim administration can result in folate deficiency.

8. Case history 1

   > Mr JW, age 40 years, living at home was previously healthy but saw his GP in August, 5 days after returning from a conference abroad where he had stayed in a large hotel and indulged his passion for frequent whirlpool baths. He had characteristic symptoms of pneumonia, including pleuritic chest pain and sudden development of fever and cough, producing yellow sputum. Physical examinations and chest radiograph corroborated the diagnosis.

   a. Before the results of the microbiological test were available, what treatment would you commence and what route of administration would you use?
   b. How do the drugs you are proposing to give work?

9. Case history 2

   > Mr RH, age 80 years, has influenza and is admitted to hospital when he develops symptoms similar to Mr JW and becomes seriously ill. A chest radiograph also shows multiple abscesses.

   a. What treatment would you commence before microbiological results are available?
   b. What antibacterial can be used if the organism is not treatable by β-lactamase-resistant penicillins?

10. Case history 3

A 31-year-old homosexual male was admitted with shortness of breath, cough and generalised chest discomfort. Chest radiograph revealed diffuse bilateral opacities and a blood gas analysis demonstrated an arterial partial oxygen pressure (Pa_{O_2}) of 8.0 kPa (normal range 11.0–14.0). Gram sputum culture was non-contributory. A bronchoalveolar lavage was performed and transbronchial biopsies taken.

a. What is the likely clinical diagnosis?
b. What microscopic investigation could be useful and what could they show?
c. How should the patient be managed and what factors need to be considered?
d. What drug treatment could expose a patient to the increased risk of opportunistic infection similar to that occurring in this instance?
e. What needs to be considered after initial treatment?

11. Case history 4

Twenty-four hours after attending a convention, a patient became ill with a temperature, abdominal pain, vomiting and diarrhoea. Faeces were collected and inoculated onto culture plates with several different types of culture medium. Pale coloured colonies that were non-lactose fermenting were identified.

a. What organisms could be causing this infection?
b. How should this patient be managed?
c. What food is most likely to cause this infection?

The answers are provided on pages 629–531.

Drug compendium

Drugs used for infections

Drug	Half-life (h)	Elimination	Comments
Antibacterial drugs			
Penicillins			
Amoxicillin	1	Renal (+ metabolism)	Broad-spectrum penicillin; given orally, by i.m. injection or by i.v. injection or infusion; good oral bioavailability (90%) not influenced by food; rapid renal excretion
Ampicillin	1–2	Renal (+ metabolism)	Broad-spectrum penicillin; given orally, by i.m. injection or by i.v. injection or infusion; low oral bioavailability which is reduced if taken with food; eliminated largely by renal clearance
Benzylpenicillin (penicillin G)	0.5–1	Renal (+ metabolism)	Given by i.m. injection, slow i.v. injection or i.v. infusion; unreliable oral absorption owing to hydrolysis by gastric acid; rapidly eliminated by renal excretion; depot formulation (procaine benzyl penicillin) is available as i.m. injection
Flucloxacillin (floxacillin)	0.8–1.2	Renal (+ metabolism)	β-Lactamase resistant; given orally, by i.m. injection or by i.v. injection or infusion; high oral bioavailability (80%), absorption delayed by food; cleared largely by the kidneys
Phenoxymethylpenicillin (penicillin V)	0.5	Renal + metabolism	Given orally; rapidly but incompletely (60%) absorbed from the gut; eliminated equally by renal excretion unchanged and as the penicilloic acid metabolite
Piperacillin	0.7–1.3	Renal (+ bile)	Antipseudomonal; given by deep i.m. injection or by i.v. injection (over 3–5 min) or infusion; poorly absorbed from the gut, therefore not given orally; not metabolised
Pivmecillinam	–	Hydrolysis	Antipseudomonal; given orally; rapidly and extensively hydrolysed prodrug for mecillinam; mecillinam has a half-life of 1–2 h
Ticarcillin	1	Renal	Antipseudomonal; given by i.v. infusion in combination with clavulanic acid; excreted mostly in the urine unchanged
Cephalosporins and other β-lactams			
Aztreonam	1.7	Renal	Given by deep i.m. injection or by i.v. injection (over 3–5 min) or infusion; not given orally as very poor absorption (<1%); rapidly eliminated by renal clearance without metabolism
Cefaclor	0.5–1	Renal (+ metabolism)	Given orally; rapidly and extensively absorbed; eliminated largely by the kidneys plus limited metabolism (15%)
Cefadroxil	1–2	Renal	Given orally; rapidly and completely absorbed (not affected by food); eliminated unchanged (>90%)
Cefalexin	1	Renal	Given orally; rapidly and completely absorbed; eliminated unchanged.
Cefamandole	0.5–1.5	Renal	Given by deep i.m. injection or by i.v. injection (over 3–5 min) or infusion; rapidly eliminated in urine unchanged
Cefazolin	1.6–2.2	Renal	Given by deep i.m. injection or by i.v. injection (over 3–5 min) or infusion; eliminated unchanged in urine but with little renal tubular secretion
Cefixime	2.5–3.8	Renal + bile	Given orally; absorbed slowly and incompletely (50%); excreted more slowly than other cephalosporins (not eliminated by renal tubular secretion)
Cefotaxime	0.9–1.3	Renal + metabolism	Given by deep i.m. injection or by i.v. injection (over 3–5 min) or infusion; renal excretion (with some tubular secretion) is major route of elimination but metabolism accounts for 20% of dose

continued

Drugs used for infections *(continued)*

Drug	Half-life (h)	Elimination	Comments
Cephalosporins and other β-lactams (continued)			
Cefoxitin	1	Renal	Given by deep i.m. injection or by i.v. injection (over 3–5 min) or infusion; eliminated by glomerular filtration plus extensive tubular secretion
Cefpirome	1.4–2.3	Renal	Given by i.v. injection or infusion; eliminated by glomerular filtration with negligible secretion
Cefpodoxine	1.9–3.2	Renal	Given orally as the proxetil derivative prodrug, which is absorbed rapidly and quantitatively hydrolysed to cefpodoxine; only about 50% of the dose is absorbed and the fraction absorbed is increased by low gastric pH; cefpodoxine is eliminated by glomerular filtration and secretion
Cefprozil	1.0–1.4	Renal + metabolism	Given orally; rapidly and completely absorbed; eliminated by glomerular filtration (main route) and renal tubular secretion plus metabolism
Cefradine	?	Renaal	Given orally, by deep i.m. injection or by i.v. injection (over 3–5 min) or infusion; completely absorbed but rate affected by food; eliminated unchanged in urine
Ceftazidime	1.8–2.2	Renal	Given by deep i.m. injection or by i.v. injection (over 3–5 min) or infusion; eliminated unchanged by glomerular filtration
Ceftriaxone	6–9	Renal + bile	Given by deep i.m. injection or by i.v. injection (over 3–5 min) or infusion; eliminated unchanged; long half-life is probably a result of extensive plasma protein binding (95%)
Cefuroxime	1.2	Renal	Given orally, by deep i.m. injection or by i.v. injection (over 3–5 min) or infusion; the oral formulation is the axetil derivative prodrug, which is quantitatively hydrolysed to cefuroxime and absorbed better if taken after food; cefuroxime is eliminated equally by renal filtration and secretion
Imipenem (with cilastatin)	1	Renal + metabolism	Given by deep i.m. injection or i.v. infusion; eliminated unchanged in urine and also hydrolysed by a renal enzyme; always given with cilastatin, which inhibits the renal enzyme (although this does not have a major impact on half-life or clearance)
Meropenem	1	Renal + metabolism	Given by i.v. injection (over 5 min) or i.v. infusion; eliminated by kidneys (80%) and hepatic metabolism (20%)
Quinolones			
Cinoxacin	1.5	Renal + metabolism	Given orally; complete absorption but the rate is reduced by food; eliminated by kidneys (60%) and metabolism to inactive products (40%)
Ciprofloxacin	3–4	Renal + metabolism	Given orally or as i.v. infusion; good bioavailability (50–80%); eliminated by glomerular filtration, renal tubular secretion plus metabolism (15%); the relatively long half-life results from a high apparent volume of distribution (3 l kg^{-1}) not low clearance
Levofloxacin	6–8	Renal (+ metabolism)	Given orally or as i.v. infusion; complete bioavailability (unaffected by food); eliminated largely unchanged by the kidneys
Nalidixic acid	1.5	Metabolism	Given orally; essentially complete bioavailability; eliminated by hepatic metabolism (oxidation + conjugation)
Norfloxacin	3	Renal + metabolism	Given orally; bioavailability has not been defined, but absorption is reduced by 30% if taken with food; eliminated by kidneys (filtration + secretion) plus metabolism (about 10%)

continued

Drugs used for infections (continued)

Drug	Half-life (h)	Elimination	Comments
Quinolones (continued)			
Ofloxacin	6–7	Renal (+ metabolism)	Given orally or as i.v. infusion; rapid and complete oral absorption; eliminated by kidneys plus limited metabolism (<5%)
Macrolides			
Azithromycin	40–60	Bile	Given orally; bioavailability is 37% (owing to poor absorption) and is reduced by food; eliminated largely by biliary excretion of the parent drug (mol. wt. 785 Da); does not induce P450 isoenzymes
Clarithromycin	3	Metabolism + renal	Given orally or by i.v. infusion; bioavailability is 55% (owing to first-pass metabolism); eliminated by metabolism and renal excretion; half-life increased to 9 h at high doses; induces CYP3A4
Erythromycin	1–1.5	Metabolism (+ bile + urine)	Given orally or by i.v. infusion; oral formulations are as ester prodrugs; eliminated largely by CYP3A4 in the liver (plus gut wall after oral dosage?); inhibits CYP3A4
Aminoglycosides			
Amikacin	2	Renal	Given by i.m. injection, slow i.v. injection or i.v. infusion; eliminated by glomerular filtration
Gentamicin	1–4	Renal	Given by i.m. injection, slow i.v. injection, i.v. infusion or by intrathecal injection; eliminated by glomerular filtration
Kanamycin	3	Renal	Given by i.m. injection or i.v. infusion; eliminated by glomerular filtration
Neomycin	2	Renal	Given orally; very poor absorption (<5%); eliminated by glomerular filtration
Netilmicin	2.5	Renal	Given by i.m. injection, slow i.v. injection or i.v. infusion; eliminated by glomerular filtration
Tobramycin	2–3	Renal	Given by i.m. injection, slow i.v. injection or i.v. infusion; eliminated by glomerular filtration
Tetracyclines			All given orally; no parenteral formulations are available
Demeclocycline	10–15	Renal + bile	Oral bioavailability is 66% (owing to poor absorption); equal amounts excreted unchanged in urine and bile
Doxycycline	18–22	Bile + urine	High oral bioavailability (>90%); eliminated in bile (20–40%) and urine (20–26%)
Lymecycline	10	?	Few kinetic data available
Minocycline	12–16	Bile + urine + metabolism	Oral bioavailability (>90%); bile is major route of elimination; only 30% has been recovered in excreta (possibly chemical decomposition in vivo rather than metabolism?)
Oxytetracycline	9	Urine + bile	Variable absorption (up to 60%); renal excretion is major route of elimination
Tetracycline	9	Bile + urine	Irregular and incomplete absorption; eliminated in bile and urine, with some metabolism
Sulfonamides			
Sulfadiazine	7–12	Metabolism + renal	Given orally or by i.v. infusion (silver sulfadiazine cream is available for topical use); completely absorbed from the gut, but first-pass metabolism reduces the bioavailability to 60–90%; metabolised by acetylation, and parent drug and acetyl metabolite eliminated by kidney

continued

Drugs used for infections *(continued)*

Drug	Half-life (h)	Elimination	Comments
Sulfonamides (continued)			
Sulfamethoxazole	9 (6–20)	Metabolism + renal	Given orally or by i.v. infusion; given in combination with trimethoprim (see below); eliminated mainly by acetylation
Trimethoprim	9–17	Renal + metabolism	Essentially complete absorption and bioavailability; eliminated largely by the kidneys (filtration + secretion) with some oxidative metabolism (20%)
Other antibiotics			
Chloramphenicol	5 (2–12)	Metabolism	Given orally or by i.v. injection or infusion; high oral bioavailability (80–90%); eliminated mainly by glucuronidation
Clindamycin	2.5	Metabolism (+ renal)	Given orally, by deep i.m. injection or by i.v. infusion; rapidly and extensively absorbed after oral dosage; mostly eliminated by hepatic metabolism with two of the metabolites being active; elimination in saliva may give a bitter taste
Colistin	4–8	Renal	Given orally (for bowel sterilisation), by i.m. injection, i.v. injection or infusion, or by inhalation (nebuliser); not absorbed orally; eliminated by renal excretion
Fusidic acid (sodium fusidate)	9	Metabolism	Given orally or by i.v. infusion; essentially completely bioavailable after oral dosage; metabolised in liver and metabolites excreted in bile
Linezolid	5	Metabolism + renal	Given orally or by i.v. infusion; eliminated by oxidative metabolism (not P450) to inactive carboxylic acid metabolites; about 30% is excreted unchanged in urine
Methenamine	?	Metabolism	Given orally for urinary tract infections; broken down in acid stomach contents so given as enteric-coated formulation; gives rise to urinary excretion of formaldehyde; half-life is 6 h (or less) because 90% is eliminated in 24 h
Metronidazole	6–9	Metabolism + renal	Given orally, rectally or by i.v. infusion; complete oral bioavailability; metabolites are eliminated slowly, primarily in the urine
Nitrofurantoin	0.3–1	Renal + metabolism	Given orally for urinary tract infections; complete oral bioavailability; over 40% is excreted rapidly unchanged by filtration and renal tubular secretion; about 20% metabolised by nitroreduction
Quinupristin plus dalupristin	0.5–1.0	Metabolism	Given by i.v. infusion; treatment reserved for MRSA or patients who cannot be treated with other regimens; both drugs are rapidly cleared from the blood and converted into active metabolites which are eliminated in the bile
Teicoplanin	32–176	Renal	Given by i.m. injection, i.v. injection or infusion; slowly eliminated in urine without metabolism; slower elimination than vancomycin because its higher lipid solubility gives a higher volume of distribution, and because renal excretion is limited by extensive reabsorption and high plasma protein binding (90%)
Tinidazole	12–14	Metabolism + renal	Given orally; complete oral bioavailability; about 25% excreted unchanged and the remainder metabolised and eliminated via urine and bile
Vancomycin	5–11	Renal	Given orally (for colitis) or by i.v. infusion; negligible absorption from the gut; eliminated by glomerular filtration
Antituberculous drugs			
Capreomycin	?	Renal + ?	Used in combination with other drugs when resistance to first-line drugs occurs; given by deep i.m. injection; about 50% is eliminated by renal excretion; old drug with few data available

continued

Drugs used for infections *(continued)*

Drug	Half-life (h)	Elimination	Comments
Antituberculous drugs *(continued)*			
Cycloserine	4–30	Renal + metabolism	Used in combination with other drugs when resistance to first-line drugs occurs; given orally; high oral bioavailability (> 90%); 60–70% excreted in urine and the remainder is metabolised
Ethambutol	10–15	Renal + metabolism	First-line drug (initial phase only); given orally; good oral bioavailability (80%); cleared by glomerular filtration + renal tubular secretion, plus < 10% metabolism
Isoniazid	0.5–2 (RA), 2–6.5 (SA)	Metabolism	First-line drug; given orally or by i.m. or i.v. injection; high oral bioavailability; eliminated largely by acetylation with slow acetylators (SA) having higher blood concentrations than rapid acetylators (RA); other minor metabolites may be linked to hepatotoxicity
Pyrazinamide	10–24	Metabolism + renal	First-line drug (initial phase only); given orally; high oral bioavailability; metabolised in liver to the active compound pyrazinoic acid, which is eliminated in urine
Rifabutin	35–40	Metabolism (+ renal)	New drug that is an analogue of and alternative to rifampicin (see below); given orally; bioavailability is 20% decreasing to 12% (owing to autoinduction); eliminated largely by CYP3A, which it induces during chronic treatment; only about 5% is excreted unchanged
Rifampicin (rifampin)	1–6	Metabolism + renal + bile	Given orally or by i.v. infusion; high oral bioavailability (percentage not defined); eliminated by a number of routes; induces CYP3A4
Streptomycin	2–9	Renal	Use is mainly restricted to resistant organisms; given by deep i.m. injection; poor and variable oral bioavailability (0–40%); eliminated by kidney (50–60%) but the fate of the remainder not known (metabolites?)
Drugs used in leprosy			
Clofazimine	10 days	Bile	Given orally; bioavailability is variable (20–85%) dependent on formulation and food (which enhances absorption); slowly eliminated unchanged in bile; urinary excretion is negligible (but enough to make urine red)
Dapsone	27	Metabolism + renal	Given orally; bioavailability is > 90%; undergoes polymorphic acetylation and N-glucuronidation (a rare reaction); metabolites undergo enterohepatic circulation; about 10% eliminated in urine unchanged.
Rifampicin	See above		
Antifungal agents			
Amphotericin	24–48	Renal	Given orally (for intestinal candidiasis) or by i.v. infusion; negligible oral absorption; slow renal excretion
Fluconazole	30	Renal + some metabolism	Given orally or by i.v. infusion; high oral bioavailability (90%); renal excretion accounts for 80% of clearance, with oxidation and conjugation a further 11%; weak inhibitor of CYP3A4
Flucytosine	3	Renal	Given by i.v. infusion; eliminated by glomerular filtration; about 1% is deaminated to 5-fluorouracil (which may explain the bone marrow toxicity)
Griseofulvin	10–21	Metabolism	Given orally; variable absorption, which is increased by ingestion with fatty foods (bioavailability not defined); eliminated by glucuronidation
Itraconazole	20	Metabolism	Given orally; oral bioavailability is 55%; eliminated by hepatic metabolism followed by biliary excretion; metabolised by and is a competitive inhibitor of CYP3A4

continued

Drugs used for infections (continued)

Drug	Half-life (h)	Elimination	Comments
Antifungal agents (continued)			
Ketoconazole	6–10	Metabolism + bile	Given orally; incomplete bioavailability owing to first-pass metabolism (absolute bioavailability has not been reported); metabolised by CYP3A4 and inhibits CYP3A4 metabolism of other drugs
Miconazole	24	Metabolism	Given orally; used for oral and intestinal infections; poorly absorbed from the gut; data indicate that up to 50% is absorbed from the gut but blood levels are too low to give a therapeutic effect
Nystatin	–	–	Given orally or topically (for vaginal and skin infections); not absorbed from the gastrointestinal tract or from intact skin
Terbinafine	11–17	Metabolism	Given orally; good oral bioavailability (80%); numerous pathways of metabolism; does not inhibit P450 isoenzymes
Antiviral agents			
Reverse transcriptase inhibitors			
Abacavir	1.5	Metabolism	Given orally; good oral bioavailability (80%); metabolised by alcohol dehydrogenase and glucuronidation; does not inhibit P450 isoenzymes
Didanosine	0.6–1.4	Renal + metabolism	Given orally; absorption is approximately 20–40% but affected by gastric acidity and food; about one-half of the absorbed fraction is excreted unchanged in the urine and the remainder metabolised (pathways not known)
Efavirenz	40–70	Metabolism	Non-nucleoside drug; given orally; variable and incomplete absorption; metabolised by CYP3A4 and CYP2B6, which it induces; half-life is shorter after regular dosage (40–55 h) compared with the first dose (50–75 h) (because of autoinduction)
Lamivudine	5–7	Renal (+ some metabolism)	Given orally; rapid and nearly complete absorption as parent drug (90%); eliminated largely in the urine unchanged; the intracellular half-life of the active trisphosphate metabolite (11–16 h) is longer than that of the parent drug in the plasma
Nevirapine	25–45	Metabolism	Non-nucleoside drug; given orally, high oral bioavailability (> 90%); metabolised by CYP3A4 which it induces; half-life is shorter after regular dosage (25–30 h) compared with a single dose (45 h) (because of autoinduction)
Stavudine	1–1.6	Renal + metabolism	Given orally; high oral bioavailability (> 80%); approximately equal amounts eliminated unchanged and by metabolism through normal pathways of pyrimidine biochemistry
Zalcitabine	1–2	Renal + metabolism	Given orally; high oral bioavailability (80–90%); about 75% is eliminated unchanged; metabolism is by normal pathways for pyrimidines (including phosphorylation)
Zidovudine	1	Metabolism + renal	Given orally or by i.v. infusion; oral bioavailability is about 65% owing to first-pass metabolism; most of the dose is metabolised by glucuronidation with limited excretion unchanged (about 20%); intracellular phosphorylation may be saturable, which may explain the apparent non-linear dose–response relationship

continued

Drugs used for infections *(continued)*

Drug	Half-life (h)	Elimination	Comments
Protease inhibitors			All given by oral route only
Indinavir	2	Metabolism (+ renal)	Oral bioavailability is only 18–20% owing to metabolism by CYP3A4 in gut wall and liver, and by efflux from enterocytes back into the gut lumen by the P-glycoprotein transporter (saturation of which results in increased absorption at high doses); eliminated solely by CYP3A4 metabolism; metabolites eliminated via the faeces
Nelfinavir	3.5–5	Metabolism + bile	Oral bioavailability in humans is not known; metabolised in liver by CYP3A4 with a major metabolite as active as the parent drug; metabolites plus parent drug (about 20%) are eliminated via the faeces
Ritonavir	3–5	Metabolism	Oral bioavailability in humans is not known; metabolised by CYP3A4 and is an inhibitor of the enzyme (more potent than other protease inhibitors); one of the metabolites is as active as the parent drug; metabolites eliminated in the faeces
Saquinavir	5–7	Metabolism	Oral bioavailability is low and variable (1–30%) (see indinavir for reasons) and is considerably influenced by food; metabolised by CYP3A4 and metabolites are eliminated in the faeces (different papers have reported average half-lives of between 1 and 7 h after oral dosage and 10–15 h after i.v. dosage, which suggests this inconsistency is an artefact of analytical sensitivity)
Viral DNA polymerase inhibitors			
Aciclovir (acyclovir)	3	Renal (+ metabolism)	Given orally, topically or by i.v. infusion; slowly and poorly absorbed from the gut (bioavailability = 10–20%); eliminated largely by renal tubular secretion + filtration; only about 10% is metabolised to inactive excretory products
Cidofovir	3	Renal	Given by i.v. infusion; phosphorylated analogue of aciclovir; undergoes further intracellular phosphorylation to mono-, di- and triphosphates, which have longer half-lives; eliminated by renal tubular secretion + filtration
Famciclovir (prodrug for penciclovir)	2 (penciclovir)	Metabolism (famciclovir), renal (penciclovir)	Given orally; inactive prodrug for penciclovir; negligible oral absorption intact but extensive conversion to penciclovir (77%); penciclovir is eliminated largely by renal excretion; triphosphate formed intracellularly has a longer half-life
Foscarnet	3–7	Renal	Given by i.v. infusion; highly polar compound; eliminated by glomerular filtration and renal tubular secretion + filtration.
Ganciclovir	4	Renal	Given orally or by i.v. infusion; very low oral bioavailability (3–7%), which is enhanced by food; eliminated largely by glomerular filtration.
Valaciclovir	3 (aciclovir)	Metabolism (valaciclovir), renal (aciclovir)	Given orally; rapidly and well absorbed (bioavailability 55%); rapidly and extensively metabolised to aciclovir; aciclovir is eliminated by the kidneys
Other antivirals			
Amantidine	10–15	Renal	Given orally; slowly but completely absorbed from the gut; eliminated by active renal tubular secretion plus filtration
Inosine pranobex	?	?	Given orally; very few data available; complex that probably decomposes to *p*-acetamidobenzoic acid, *N,N*-dimethylamino-2-propanol and inosine
Palivizumab	?	?	Given by i.m. injection; humanised monoclonal antibody; very few published data available

continued

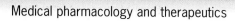

Drugs used for infections (*continued*)

Drug	Half-life (h)	Elimination	Comments
Other antivirals (*continued*)			
Tribavirin (ribavirin)	7–21 days	Metabolism + renal	Given orally or by inhalation; oral bioavailability is 50%; metabolised by hydrolysis of ribosyl group from triazole moiety, which is then excreted in urine; very slowly cleared from erythrocytes and tissue compartments (shorter half-lives are reported after single doses)
Zanamivir	2–5	Renal	Given by inhalation for influenza; very low absorption (< 20%); eliminated in urine

Antiprotozoal drugs

Antimalarials

Drug	Half-life (h)	Elimination	Comments
Atovaquone	3 days	Faeces + urine	Given orally with proguanil; poor and variable absorption influenced by food; most eliminated in faeces (but poor absorption)
Chloroquine	30–60 days	Renal + metabolism	Given orally or by i.v. infusion; complete oral bioavailability; limited metabolism (about 20%) but metabolite retains activity; mostly eliminated by filtration in the kidney; the very long half-life results from the very high volume of distribution (200 l kg^{-1}) and low renal clearance.
Halofantine	1–4 days	Metabolism	Given orally; poor and variable absorption, which is increased markedly if taken with food; the absorbed fraction is eliminated by cytochrome P450 oxidation
Mefloquine	15–33 days	Metabolism + renal	Given orally; good bioavailability (80%); metabolised by hydrolysis and metabolites eliminated in urine and bile; renal clearance accounts for about 10% of total
Primaquine	4–10	Metabolism (+ renal)	Given orally; rapidly absorbed with almost complete bioavailability; metabolised to carboxyprimaquine, which retains antimalarial activity and is implicated in haemolysis
Proguanil (prodrug for cycloguanil)	12–24	Metabolism	Given orally (alone or with atovaquone); high oral bioavailability; it is a prodrug for cycloguanil (which accounts for 19% of an oral dose) and which has a short half-life (2 h), so that plasma concentrations of the active metabolite are usually less than the parent drug
Pyrimethamine	2–6 days	Metabolism	Given orally (alone or with sulfadoxine or dapsone); well absorbed (human bioavailability is not known); numerous metabolites eliminated mainly in the faeces
Quinine	6–47	Metabolism (+ renal)	Given orally or by i.v. infusion; high oral bioavailability (80–90%); eliminated largely by metabolism by CYP3A4; also binds to and inhibits CYP2D6; may also be metabolised by CYP1A2 because smoking (which does not induce CYP3A4) increases its clearance

Other antiprotozoals

Drug	Half-life (h)	Elimination	Comments
Diloxanide furoate	–	Metabolism	Given orally (for amoebiasis); completely hydrolysed in the gut lumen and mucosa to diloxanide, which is incompletely absorbed; absorbed diloxanide is conjugated with glucuronic acid
Metronidazole	6–9	Metabolism + renal	Given orally; complete oral bioavailability; metabolites are eliminated slowly in urine.
Pentamidine	13 days	Metabolism + renal	Given by inhalation (nebuliser), by deep i.m. injection or i.v. infusion; metabolised by oxidation, and conjugation with sulfate and glucuronic acid

continued

Drugs used for infections (continued)

Drug	Half-life (h)	Elimination	Comments
Other antiprotozoals (continued)			
Stibogluconate	6	As pentavalent antimony	Given by i.v. injection (over at least 5 min); pentavalent antimony compound; pentavalent antimony eliminated in urine; very slow minor late elimination phase reported (half-life of 76 h) but chemical form of pentavalent antimony not defined
Tinidazole	12–14	Metabolism + renal	Given orally; complete oral bioavailability; about 25% excreted unchanged and the remainder metabolised and eliminated via urine and bile
Trimetrexate	14	Metabolism + renal	Given by i.v. injection (over 5–10 min) or i.v. infusion; action is similar to trimethoprim but 1000 times more potent; metabolised in liver and excreted unchanged in urine (about 10%)
Anthelminthic drugs			
Albendazole	8–12	Metabolism	Given orally; low oral bioavailability (parent drug not usually detectable); metabolised by *S*-oxidation; the parent compound and sulfoxide (SO) are active, while the sulfone C (SO)$_2$ is inactive
Diethylcarbamazine	?	?	No data available
Ivermectin	12	Metabolism	Named patient basis only; given orally; bioavailability is not defined; eliminated as metabolites in faeces
Levamisole	4–6	Metabolism	Named patient basis only; given orally; bioavailability 60–70%; oxidised in liver and conjugated with glucuronic acid
Mebendazole	3–9	Metabolism	Given orally; low bioavailability (20% for solutions, 2% for tablets); metabolites excreted in urine
Niclosamide	?	?	Given orally; few data available
Piperazine	?	Renal	Given orally; 5–30% of an oral dose is excreted in urine unchanged within 24 h; few data available
Praziquantel	2	Metabolism	Named patient basis only; given orally; probably extensive first-pass metabolism; rapidly metabolised and excreted
Tiabendazole	1.2	Metabolism	Given orally; rapidly and extensively absorbed; metabolised by oxidation and conjugation

i.m., intramuscular, i.v., intravenous; MRSA, methacillin-resistant *Staphylococcus aureus*.

52

Chemotherapy of malignancy

Approximately 20–25% of people in the western world die from cancer. Surgery and radiotherapy are valuable for treating localised cancers but are less effective in prolonging the patient's life once the tumour has spread to produce metastases. The successful treatment of cancer frequently involves a multidisciplinary approach, which also includes necessary psychological and social support. The introduction of cytotoxic chemotherapy to kill rapidly proliferating neoplastic cells has had a major impact on the successful treatment of malignant disease, especially diffuse tumours.

A wide range of different chemicals, with a variety of mechanisms and sites of action within the cell, has been introduced into clinical practice since the 1970s. Although the agents may differ in their specific cellular targets they nearly all rely on the rapid rate of growth and division of cancer cells to provide a degree of selectivity between normal and malignant tissue. The drugs share a number of generic properties and characteristics, both beneficial and adverse, which will be discussed first. Information on the major classes of drug will then be given with information on mechanisms of action and general toxic effects. There is an extensive drug compendium table, which also gives details of the clinical uses and adverse effects of specific drugs.

The rate of introduction of new anticancer drugs has decreased in recent years, largely because effective agents are already available. A placebo-controlled clinical trial of a new antineoplastic drug given as sole treatment is now unethical, and the efficacy of any new agent usually has to be assessed by its addition to the best available current therapy. Therefore, a successful new agent would have to show a clinically significant effect above that of current treatment. There are a number of in vivo animal tests for detecting antineoplastic activity, but these frequently overpredict the likely effectiveness of a compound in clinical use, because the animal tumours used as models have a much higher growth fraction (see below). For all these reasons, many recent advances in cancer chemotherapy have arisen from the more effective use of existing agents, by optimising drug combinations and regimens, and by minimising toxicity, rather than the introduction of novel compounds. The ability of molecular biological approaches to define the mechanisms of cell–cell communication, apoptosis etc., will undoubtedly prove a major stimulus for the production of new drugs with greater selectivity for cancer cells.

Molecular origins of cancer

Cancer probably arises from a combination of genetic mutations in a cell. These lead to activation of oncogenes, cell factors that cause cells to divide, and deletion of tumour suppressor genes. This leads to unregulated cell proliferation and also delays in programmed cell death (apoptosis). With many cancers, sequential gene defects result in progressive changes in the cell leading to metaplastic and dysplastic phases, and to invasive and ultimately metastatic cancer.

External regulators of cell growth and death include various growth factors, cytokines and hormones, which activate or suppress the genes controlling these functions. Gene mutations activating oncogenes may lead to expression of proteins that allow cell growth in the absence of stimulation by an external regulator. Abnormal regulation of tumour suppressor genes leads to the excessive production of proteins that inhibit cell death. It will also produce cells that are resistant to chemotherapy.

Growth factors secreted by cancer cells promote angiogenesis and increase blood supply to the tumour. Other secreted factors can impede the host's immune response to the cancer cells.

Proto-oncogenes are normal gene sequences that control cell proliferation and differentiation; they are capable of being activated to oncogenes, the expression of which leads to tumour development. Considerable attention is currently being given to the products of proto-oncogene activation, since these are often linked to cell growth factors and may provide useful targets for future drug development. Identification of the protein sequence and tertiary structure of the growth factors may allow new drug molecules to be designed to interact specifically with the growth factor (analogous to recent developments in the field of receptor pharmacology). However, whether this will increase the selectivity of drugs for neoplastic cells is unknown because selectivity may still be based on rates of growth and division. Other possible future approaches for therapy are to increase the effectiveness of tumour suppressor genes.

Clinical use of antineoplastic agents

Different forms of cancer differ in their sensitivity to chemotherapy. The most responsive include lymphomas, leukaemias, choriocarcinoma and testicular carcinoma, while solid tumours such as colorectal, adrenocortical and squamous cell bronchial carcinomas generally show a poor response. An intermediate response is shown by other cancers, for example those of the bladder, head and neck, oat cell bronchogenic tumours and sex-related cancers (breast, ovary, endometrium and prostate). The sensitivity within a patient may change during treatment with antineoplastic agents because of the development of resistance (see below).

Mechanisms of action

The majority of antineoplastic agents act on the process of DNA synthesis within the cancer cell, as summarised in Figure 52.1. Therefore, selectivity for cancer cells compared with normal tissues is determined by the rate of cell division and DNA synthesis. Resting cells, that is those in the G_0 phase (Fig. 52.2), are resistant to many antineoplastic drugs. Some antineoplastic drugs, such as the antimetabolites, work effectively only when the cells are in the appropriate phase of the cell cycle at the time of treatment with the drug; these are termed cell-cycle-specific agents (Fig. 52.2). Some drugs, such as the alkylating agents, nitrosoureas and cisplatin, have a 'hit and run' action on the DNA, and it is not critical when the cell is exposed because the drug effect becomes apparent later, when the cells attempt to undergo division.

The sensitivity of a cancer to treatment depends, therefore, on the growth fraction – that is the fraction of cells undergoing mitosis at any time. For example, in Burkitt's lymphoma, almost 100% of neoplastic cells are undergoing division, and the tumour is very sensitive and shows a dramatic response to a single dose of cyclophosphamide. In contrast, the growth fraction represents less than 5% of cells in a carcinoma of the colon, resulting in its resistance to chemotherapy. However, metastases from colonic carcinoma deposited in the liver and elsewhere initially have a high growth fraction and are sensitive to chemotherapy, which is frequently given following surgical removal of the primary tumour.

Studies using in vitro cancer cell lines have shown that:

- antineoplastic drugs produce a proportional cell kill, for example 99% of the cells present; in consequence, multiple treatments may be necessary to eradicate the cancer, with each treatment producing an exponential decrease in the number of viable cells remaining
- essentially complete eradication of tumour cells is necessary to prevent regrowth
- increased efficacy is obtained if treatment with cell cycle-specific drugs is timed to coincide with the appropriate phase of cell division within the cell population.

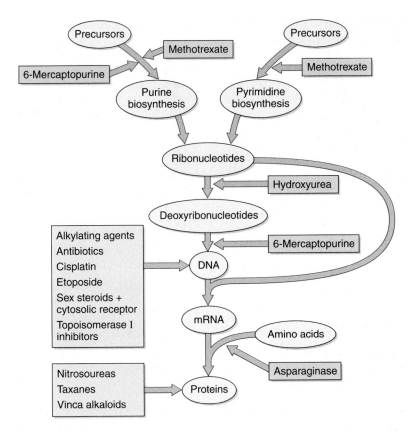

Fig. 52.1
Sites of action for the main groups of anticancer drugs.

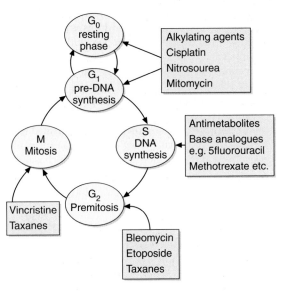

Fig. 52.2
Sites of action for the main groups of cell cycle-specific anticancer drugs.

Although these concepts apply to in vivo therapy of patients, the situation is complicated because there are risk–benefit considerations to be taken into account, and these may change with successive treatments. In addition, the immune system probably contributes to the final removal of residual malignant cells and yet most antineoplastic drugs compromise immunoresponsiveness, which will reduce this removal process. Finally, the periodicity of doses is less critical in vivo because cancer cell cycles are not synchronised within the target cell population between treatments.

Resistance

Resistance to chemotherapeutic agents may develop in a number of ways:

- reduced drug uptake into cancer cells, e.g. downregulation of the high-affinity reduced folate (tetrahydrofolic acid, THF) transport system limits the uptake of methotrexate
- use of alternative metabolic pathways and salvage mechanisms to circumvent a blocked biochemical process; such mechanisms are usually drug specific, e.g. induction of asparagine synthesis in cells exposed to crisantaspase (asparaginase).

- alteration of intracellular drug targets, e.g. production of topoisomerase II with reduced sensitivity to the inhibitory effects of anthracyclines
- increased inactivation of the compound within the cancer cell, e.g. high intracellular levels of glutathione-S-transferase inactivate cisplatin and alkylating agents
- reduced activation of prodrugs, e.g. low intracellular levels of deoxycytidine kinase reduces activation of cytarabine
- increased removal of the drug from the cancer cell; this involves increased transcription of the gene for P-glycoprotein ('P' for permeability), which acts as a carrier for the elimination from the cell of a number of cytotoxic compounds. The increased production of the P-glycoprotein carrier confers multidrug resistance to a number of structurally unrelated natural compounds, or their derivatives, including vinca alkaloids, etoposide, taxanes, anthracyclines, dactinomycin (actinomycin D), mitomycin C and mitozantrone. The carrier can be blocked by Ca^{2+} channel antagonists, such as nifedipine or verapamil, ciclosporin and tamoxifen, and these drugs may be added to cytotoxic drug regimens to minimise resistance.

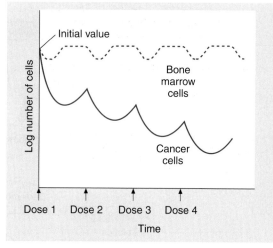

Fig. 52.3
Hypothetical dosing schedule to allow recovery of normal tissues. The malignant cells show a greater proportional kill because a greater fraction are in division at any time. Theoretically, the response of the malignant cells to dose 2 would be greater than for dose 1 if cell cycles became synchronised and dose 2 was given during the correct phase of the growth cycle. A typical dose interval would be 3–4 weeks. A minimum of 10^9 tumour cells are usually present when tumours are first detectable.

Adverse effects

Cytotoxic antineoplastic drugs are among the most toxic compounds given to humans. Many have a therapeutic index of approximately 1, that is the toxic dose usually is the therapeutic dose. Because drug selectivity is for tissues with a high growth fraction, it is not surprising that a number of normal non-malignant tissues are also affected. In addition to effects that occur in all rapidly dividing tissues, many chemotherapeutic drugs also have specific toxic effects on other tissues. Dosage regimens are usually designed so that normal tissues, especially bone marrow and gut, can recover between doses (Fig. 52.3).

Gastrointestinal tract. Mucosal cells have a rapid turnover. Toxicity can produce anorexia, mucosal ulceration or diarrhoea. Nausea and vomiting are common, especially with alkylating agents and cisplatin, and this may limit the patient's ability to tolerate an optimal dosage regimen.

Bone marrow. Myelosuppression is a serious consequence of treatment and can lead to severe leucopenia, thrombocytopenia and sometimes anaemia. These haematological consequences may limit the drug dosage that the patient is able to tolerate. There is a high risk of both infection and haemorrhage following cytotoxic chemotherapy (see the drug compendium table).

Hair follicle cells. Partial or complete alopecia may occur, but this is usually temporary.

Reproductive organs. Both sexes are affected and sterility can result, particularly after therapy with cyclophosphamide or cytarabine; women frequently have dysmenorrhoea or amenorrhoea. Because of the mechanisms of action of cytotoxic drugs, most would be expected to exhibit teratogenic activity. Pregnant women should not be exposed to cytotoxic drugs as patients or as members of the health-care team. Drugs that mimic or affect the activity of sex hormones are frequently used for the treatment of breast or prostate cancer, and these produce adverse effects on sexual function.

Growing tissues in children. Of particular concern in children is the possibility that intensive cytotoxic chemotherapy can impair growth. Children treated with cytotoxic drugs for malignancy also have an increased risk of a second malignancy (about 10%), which is often leukaemia.

Drug combinations

It is common practice to treat many cancers with a mixture of different antineoplastic drugs simultaneously, and there are numerous permutations used clinically. Criteria for selecting ideal combinations are:

- each drug should be an active antineoplastic drug in its own right (e.g. a second drug would not be given simply to increase the formation of an active metabolite of the first)

- each drug should have a different mechanism of action and target site within the cancer cell: this will increase efficacy while reducing the likelihood of resistance
- each drug should have a different site for any organ-specific toxicity (obviously all agents will affect tissues with a high growth factor).

Specific antineoplastic agents

The drug compendium table gives the uses of individual drugs and notes any unusual or limiting toxicity.

Agents affecting nucleic acid function

Alkylating agents

> Examples: cyclophosphamide, melphalan, busulfan, chlorambucil

The nitrogen mustards were developed from the sulfur mustard gases used in the trenches in World War I. These chemical warfare gases caused bone marrow suppression in addition to the respiratory toxicity for which they were developed. Replacement of the sulfur atom by nitrogen allowed the introduction of complex side-chains, which resulted in a range of more stable non-volatile agents that could be given therapeutically under controlled conditions. Alkylating agents contain reactive sites that bind to DNA or proteins, usually following an activation step that involves loss of part of the molecule (the leaving group).

Mechanism of action

The reactive alkylating group(s) in the molecule may be:

- *nitrogen mustard* $N-CH_2CH_2Cl$ (Cl is the leaving group), e.g. carmustine, chlorambucil, chlormethine (mustine), cyclophosphamide, estramustine, ifosfamide, lomustine, melphalan
- *sulfonate ester* $-CH_2OSO_2CH_3$ (SO_2CH_3 is the leaving group), e.g. bulsulfan, treosulfan
- *nitrosourea* $-N-N=O$, e.g. carmustine, lomustine
- *cyclic nitrogen derivative* (a three-membered ring with CH_2, CH_2 and N as the three components, e.g. thiotepa which has three of these rings attached to a central $P{\rightarrow}S$ group).

The mechanism of action is by covalent binding to DNA (nitrogen mustards, sulfonate esters and cyclic nitrogen compounds), which prevents DNA and RNA synthesis, and by binding to proteins (nitrosoureas), which blocks DNA repair. Because of the covalent nature of the product, these effects are not cell cycle specific.

The leaving groups in alkylating agents are highly reactive and produce a chemical species that binds covalently to sites within DNA, such as N-7 of guanine. The alkylated guanine in DNA may either be repaired or it may interfere with DNA replication by

- being misread
- undergoing further metabolism via ring opening
- cross-linking to another guanine via the remaining leaving group.

Many alkylating agents are bifunctional (have two leaving groups), which leads to cross-linking of the DNA chains.

Pharmacokinetics

The pharmacokinetic characteristics of the alkylating agents depend on the nature of the group(s) linked to the leaving group. The original and simplest drug is chlormethine (mustine), which is a nitrogen mustard with a simple methyl group; it is very unstable, and solutions have to be injected soon after preparation because decomposition occurs in minutes. Care is necessary when handling the toxic dosing solutions and mustine is now used much less commonly. A major advance in the use of nitrogen mustards was achieved with the introduction of cyclophosphamide, which is a chemically stable solid chemical that can be given orally. It is a prodrug that undergoes metabolic activation to produce two toxic metabolites: acrolein ($CH_2{=}CHCHO$) and phosphoramide mustard, which contains the $N-(CH_2CH_2Cl)_2$ group. Toxic metabolites of cyclophosphamide and ifosfamide are excreted in the urine. Melphalan and chlorambucil, which have an aromatic substituent, have short or very short half-lives and a substantial amount is excreted in the urine unchanged.

Unwanted effects

- Generalised cytotoxicity is common.
- Cyclophosphamide and ifosfamide cause bladder toxicity, with haemorrhagic cystitis; this may be prevented by prior treatment with mercaptoethane sulfonic acid (mesna) (Ch. 53). Bladder cancer may develop years after cyclophosphamide therapy.
- Fertility is reduced through impaired gametogenesis.
- A particular problem with the long-term use of alkylating agents, especially if combined with radiotherapy, is the development of acute myeloid leukaemia.

Platinum compounds

Examples: cisplatin, carboplatin

Mechanism of action

The platinum drugs enter cells and, after dissociation of the Cl⁻, generate a reactive complex that cross-links between guanine units in DNA. The result is similar to that of alkylating agents that break the DNA chain. They are particularly useful for ovarian and testicular tumours.

Pharmacokinetics

These drugs are poorly absorbed from the gut and are given by intravenous infusion. They are mainly excreted by the kidney as platinum compounds and have a long half-life mainly owing to extensive protein binding.

Unwanted effects

The unwanted effects of cisplatin are all more marked than those of carboplatin:

- severe nausea and vomiting
- nephrotoxicity with irreversible renal impairment; hydration is important to minimise the risk
- ototoxicity with hearing loss and tinnitus
- peripheral neuropathy.

Topoisomerase I inhibitors

Examples: irinotecan, topotecan

These are semi-synthetic derivatives of a cytotoxic alkaloid isolated from the Chinese tree *Camptotheca acuminata* that act as inhibitors of topoisomerase I.

Mechanism of action

The drugs inhibit topoisomerase I, which is important in DNA transcription and translation. The enzyme produces single-strand breaks that relieve the torsional strain in DNA; under normal cell conditions the strands are then religated. The drugs bind to the DNA–topoisomerase I complex and prevent religation. Although this binding is readily reversible, the consequences are irreversible, because cell death occurs when a double-strand break is produced at the DNA replication fork during S phase. Inhibition of DNA repair increases the sensitivity of the cell to ionising radiation. They are given as second-line treatments for metastatic cancer (see the drug compendium table).

Pharmacokinetics

They are large complex molecules that are given by intravenous infusion and are eliminated largely by hepatic metabolism.

Unwanted effects

General cytotoxicity, with dose-limiting myelosuppression.

Cytotoxic antibiotics

Examples: doxorubicin, epirubicin, mitozantrone, bleomycin

The cytotoxic antibiotics represent a diverse range of chemical structures:

- the 'rubicin' drugs are all quinone-containing four-ringed structures (planar anthraquinones) that contain an amino sugar group
- mitoxantrone (mitozantrone) has a three-ringed planar quinone structure with amino-containing side-chains and mitomycin is a non-planar tricyclic quinone.
- bleomycin and dactinomycin are complex peptide or glycopeptide derivatives.

Mechanisms of action

Although these antibiotics affect normal nucleic acid function, they also have a number of other mechanisms of action.

- Intercalation. This is shown particularly by the rubicins, with the planar ring system intercalating between DNA bases, and the amino sugar part binding to the deoxyribose phosphate groups. Intercalation blocks reading of the DNA template and also stimulates topoisomerase II-dependent DNA double-strand breaks.
- Free radical attack. The metabolism of the drugs gives rise to superoxide and hydroxyl radicals and hydrogen peroxide, which cause DNA damage and cytotoxicity.
- Membrane effects. Interference with membrane function can occur either directly or via oxidative damage.

In general the mechanisms of action are not cell cycle specific, although some members of the class are reported to show greatest activity at certain phases of the cycle, for example S phase (doxorubicin, mitoxantrone (mitozantrone)), G_1 and early S phase (mitomycin), and G_2 phase and mitosis (bleomycin).

Pharmacokinetics

The cytotoxic antibiotics are poorly absorbed from the gut and are given intravenously. They have very long half-lives, 1–2 days, and are eliminated by metabolism.

Unwanted effects

- General cytotoxicity can occur.
- Doxorubicin produces dose-related irreversible myocardial damage through free radical release and oxidative stress.
- Dilated cardiomyopathy and heart failure can result.

....

Antimetabolites

Antimetabolites interfere with normal metabolic pathways. They can be divided into folate antagonists and analogues of purine or pyrimidine bases.

Folic acid antagonists

Example: methotrexate

An astute clinical observation, that the administration of folic acid to children with leukaemia exacerbated their condition, led to the development of a folate antagonist methotrexate. This represented an important landmark in cancer chemotherapy.

Mechanism of action and uses

Folic acid in its reduced form (tetrahydrofolic acid; THF) is an important biochemical intermediate. It is essential for synthetic reactions that involve the addition of a single carbon atom during a biochemical reaction, such as the introduction of the methyl group into thymidylate and the synthesis of the purine ring system. During such reactions, THF is oxidised to dihydrofolic acid (DHF), which has to be reduced by dihydrofolate reductase back to THF before it can accept a further 1-carbon group. Methotrexate has a very high affinity for and inhibits the active site of mammalian dihydrofolate reductase. This blocks purine and thymidylate synthesis and inhibits the synthesis of DNA, RNA and protein. Methotrexate blocks dihydrofolate reductase and the 1-carbon cycle. It may show selectivity for cancer cells because these rely more on de novo synthesis of purines and pyrimidines, whereas normal tissues use salvage pathways (for preformed purines and pyrimidines) to a greater extent. Methotrexate is specific for S phase and slows G_1 to S phase.

Mechanisms of resistance of cancer cells to methotrexate include altered or increased cellular levels of dihydrofolate reductase, increased salvage of preformed thymidine and impaired uptake of methotrexate.

Folinic acid (leucovorin) is frequently administered shortly after high-dose methotrexate to rescue normal tissues and enhance selectivity for tumour cells.

Methotrexate is given for acute lymphoblastic leukaemia, non-Hodgkin's lymphomas and various other malignancies. It is also used in non-malignant conditions such as inflammatory joint diseases and psoriasis (Chs. 30 and 49).

Pharmacokinetics

Methotrexate is well absorbed from the gut but can also be given intravenously or intrathecally. It is eliminated by renal excretion, but a small amount may be retained for longer periods both strongly bound to the dihydrofolate reductase and intracellularly as polyglutamate conjugates.

Unwanted effects

- Methotrexate is toxic to normal tissues (especially the bone marrow).
- Hepatotoxicity can follow chronic therapy (as in psoriasis).
- Toxicity is increased in the presence of reduced renal excretion, and methotrexate should be avoided if there is significant renal impairment.

Base analogues

Examples: 5-fluorouracil (5-FU), cytarabine (cytosine arabinoside), 6-mercaptopurine

A number of useful chemotherapeutic agents have been produced by simple modifications to the structures of normal purine and pyrimidine bases (Fig. 52.4). These act in a number of ways to interfere with DNA synthesis (Table 52.1).

Pharmacokinetics

Base analogues tend to be absorbed and metabolised by the pathways involved with the corresponding normal (unmodified) base. Oral absorption is often erratic, and most are given intravenously. The urine is a minor route of elimination (up to 1% of the parent drug) and half-lives are short to intermediate.

Unwanted effects

- Typical cytotoxic effects are common.
- Allopurinol (Ch. 31) interferes with the metabolism of 6-mercaptopurine, and the dose should be reduced if these drugs are used concurrently.

....

Agents affecting microtubule function

Vinca alkaloids and etoposide

Examples: vincristine, vinblastine, etoposide

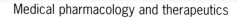

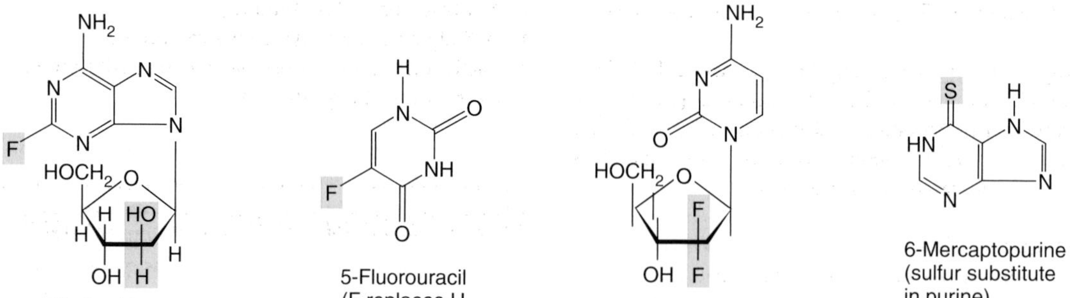

Fludarabine
(F replaces H
of adenosine)

5-Fluorouracil
(F replaces H
of uracil)

Gemcitabine
(F replaces H and
OH on arabinose ring)

6-Mercaptopurine
(sulfur substitute
in purine)

Fig. 52.4
The structure of some antimetabolites illustrating their similarity to normal bases and nucleotides (structural changes are highlighted).

Table 52.1
Mechanisms of action of base analogues

Analogue	Metabolism	Action	Cell cycle effect
Cladribine	Phosphorylated intracellularly by deoxycytidine kinase	The main action is by incorporation of the triphosphate into DNA and blocking DNA polymerase and DNA ligase	Not specific
Cytarabine	Phosphorylated intracellularly by deoxycytidine kinase	The main action is by incorporation of the triphosphate into DNA and blocking DNA polymerase and DNA ligase	Specific: mostly active in S phase
Fludarabine	Phosphorylated intracellularly by deoxycytidine kinase	The main action is by incorporation of the triphosphate into DNA and blocking DNA polymerase and DNA ligase	Specific: mostly active in S phase
5-Fluorouracil	Phosphorylated intracellularly to fluorouridine monophosphate (FUMP) and the deoxy analogue (FdUMP)	FdUMP inhibits thymidylate synthase, is converted to the triphosphate and is incorporated into DNA FUMP is converted to the triphosphate and is incorporated into RNA	Some selectivity for G_2 and S phases
Gemcitabine	Converted to a triphosphate	Triphosphate is incorporated into DNA and blocks elongation and promotes apoptosis	Specific for S phase
6-Mercaptopurine	Phosphorylated to mono- and triphosphate	Monophosphate inhibits de novo purine synthesis Triphosphates are incorporated into DNA and/or RNA giving cytotoxicity	Specific for S phase
Ralitrexed	–	Inhibits thymidylate synthase	
Tioguanine	Converted to intracellular nucleotides	Main action arises from incorporation of triphosphates into DNA and RNA The nucleotides causes 'pseudo' feedback inhibition of the synthesis of other purines and inhibits purine nucleotide interconvensions	Active in G_1 and S phases

The vinca alkaloids are complex natural chemicals isolated from the periwinkle plant (*Vinca rosea*). Etoposide
is a synthetic derivative of a compound that is extracted
from the mandrake root (*Podophyllum peltatum*) and is
sometimes called a 'podophyllotoxin'.

Mechanism of action and uses

Vinca alkaloids bind to tubulin and cause depolymerisation of microtubules, thus producing metaphase
arrest. They are therefore cycle specific. The vinca
alkaloids are used for various lymphomas and for

acute leukaemia. They are also effective in some solid tumours.

Etoposide is active during the G_2 phase and binds to the complex of DNA and topoisomerase II (an enzyme involved in the uncoiling and coiling of DNA during repair). The etoposide-bound complex prevents DNA replication and causes strand breaks.

Pharmacokinetics
The absorption of oral doses of vinca alkaloids is unpredictable and they are usually given intravenously. Etoposide can be given orally. Elimination is largely by metabolism with little renal excretion. They have long half-lives.

Unwanted effects
General cytotoxicity occurs, although the spectrum of adverse effects differs between different drugs, despite their close structural similarities (see drug compendium table).

Taxanes

Examples: paclitaxel, doxetaxel

The clinically used drugs are produced from taxane, which is a diterpenoid extracted from the bark of the Pacific Yew tree (*Taxus bretifolia*).

Mechanism of action
Taxanes promote the assembly of microtubules and inhibit their depolymerisation, leading to the formation of stable and non-functional microtubular bundles in the cell. They bind to a different site to that used by vinca alkaloids. The cell is inhibited during G_2 and M phases of the cell cycle. Microtubules are essential for numerous cellular functions, including maintenance of cell shape, motility, transport between organelles and cell division.

Taxanes are also radiosensitisers, since cells in the G_2 and M phases are more sensitive to radiation. The drugs are used for ovarian and breast cancer.

Pharmacokinetics
These drugs are given intravenously because of poor oral absorption. They are extensively metabolised in the liver and have short half-lives.

Unwanted effects
- General cytotoxicity.
- Severe hypersensitivity reactions can occur with hypotension, angioedema and bronchospasm; routine premedication with histamine (H_1 and H_2) receptor antagonists (Chs 33, 38) combined with a corticosteroid (Ch. 44) is recommended.

- Neutropenia is dose limiting.
- Arthalgia/myalgia syndrome can occur.
- Paclitaxel causes sensory neuropathy, with motor neuropathy at high dosages.

Miscellaneous anticancer drugs

Examples: altretamine, amsacrine, cristantaspase (asparaginase), dacarbazine, hydroxyurea (hydroxycarbamide), pentostatin, procarbazine, razoxane (dexrazoxane), temozolomide and tretinoin

These drugs represent a mixture of compounds with a variety of mechanisms of action. Further details are given in the drug compendium table.

Mechanisms of action
Most potential biochemical sites within the process of cell division have been investigated as targets for anticancer drugs. Actions of different drugs include:

- chelation of metal ions (razoxane)
- removal of asparagine for protein synthesis (cristantaspase)
- inhibition of incorporation of thymidine and adenine into DNA (procarbazine)
- inhibition of adenosine deaminase, which causes a build up of dATP, which inhibits the formation of other deoxyribonucleotide triphosphates (pentostatin)
- inhibition of reduction of ribonucleotides to deoxyribonucleotides (hydroxyurea)
- intercalation between DNA base pairs (amsacrine)
- covalent binding to macromolecules (altretamine)
- alkylating action, especially on thiol groups, to inhibit DNA repair (dacarbazine and temozolomide)
- increased cell differentiation by action on retinoid receptors (RAR and RXR) (tretinoin) (Ch. 49).

Pharmacokinetics
The drugs show a diverse array of pharmacokinetic characteristics (see the drug compendium table).

Unwanted effects
See the drug compendium table.

Antidotes (chemoprotectants)

Examples: folinic acid, mesna

The antidotes are chemical or class specific and may be given before, during or after chemotherapy to reduce adverse effects (see the drug compendium table). In addition, some anticancer drugs may modulate the biological effects of other active drugs; for example, razoxane chelates iron and reduces the cardiomyopathy of the cytotoxic anthracycline antibiotics.

Other drugs used for the treatment of cancer

Other drugs used in cancer therapy act to suppress cell division; for example drugs such as corticosteroids, antibiotics, cytokines or drugs acting to control the division of cells sensitive to sex hormones. Cancers that arise from cell lines possessing steroid receptors that promote their growth and cell division are frequently susceptible to inhibitory steroids.

Glucocorticoids. The glucocorticoids (Ch. 44) suppress lymphocyte mitosis and are used in leukaemia and lymphoma; they are also helpful in reducing oedema around a tumour.

Oestrogens. The estrogens (Ch. 45) suppress prostate cancer cells both locally and metastases and provide symptomatic improvement; gynaecomastia is a common unwanted effect.

Progestogens. The progestogens (Ch. 45) suppress endometrial cancer cells and kidney cancer metastases.

Estrogen antagonists. Cells in breast cancer can be suppressed by oestrogen antagonists (e.g. tamoxifen). Tamoxifen is active orally and binds competitively to oestrogen receptors. It shows both oestrogenic effects (on bone) and anti-oestrogenic effects (on breast tissue). Tamoxifen inhibits oestrogen-regulated genes and reduces the secretion of growth factors by tumour cells. Tumour cells are affected mainly in the G_2 phase of the cell cycle. Tamoxifen is extensively metabolised in the liver and has active metabolites with long half-lives; therefore, several weeks of treatment are necessary to achieve steady-state concentrations. Unwanted effects include hot flushes and amenorrhoea in premenopausal women and vaginal bleeding in postmenopausal women. Tamoxifen inhibits CYP3A4 and, therefore, reduces the metabolism of other substrates, such as warfarin.

Androgen antagonists. These drugs (e.g. flutamide; Ch. 46) suppress prostate cancer cells.

Gonadorelin analogues. These drugs (e.g. buserelin; Ch 43) suppress prostate cancer cells.

Aromatase inhibitors. Aromatase is the enzyme that converts androgens to oestrogens. Inhibitors of aromatase (e.g. formestane) reduce oestrogen production in postmenopausal women, who produce oestrogen mainly from androstenedione and testosterone in many tissues such as adipose tissue, skin, muscle and liver.

Aromatase is also present in the cells of two-thirds of breast carcinomas, and many breast cancers are oestrogen dependent.

Interferon. Interferon alfa has proved to be a disappointing agent despite the vast resources committed to its isolation in sufficient amounts for early clinical trials. It is used for certain lymphomas and solid tumours but is not the 'natural, side-effect free' agent that was hoped for when it was first isolated.

Aldesleukin (interleukin 2). Interleukin 2 is a lymphokine produced by T-lymphocytes that activates cytotoxic killer cells. Aldesleukin, made by recombinant DNA technology, has been given by intravenous infusion for the treatment of patients with metastatic renal carcinoma. Its efficacy has yet to be established but toxic effects include hypotension and oedema owing to capillary leakage, influenza-like symptoms, nausea, vomiting, diarrhoea, anaemia and thrombocytopenia.

Monoclonal antibodies. Some monoclonal antibodies (e.g. rituximab) can have highly specific effects, for example, the lysis of B-lymphocytes. Unwanted effects are common, especially during the first infusion.

Anticancer drug therapy for specific malignancies

The following discussion selects certain important cancers and outlines the role of chemotherapeutic drugs in their management. Trials produce a continued flow of improved therapeutic options, and this is a field of medicine that changes rapidly.

Gastric cancer

Surgery can be curative for early disease, but about 90% of patients present with advanced diseases. For these patients, chemotherapy with a combination of epirubicin, cisplatin and long-term intravenous infusion of 5-fluorouracil can reduce tumour bulk before surgical resection. Chemotherapy can be palliative in advanced disease, using 5-fluorouracil combined with cisplatin or methotrexate and doxorubicin. Radiotherapy is used for palliation of bone metastases.

Pancreatic cancer

Most pancreatic cancers present late and 5-year survival is rare because of liver metastases. Surgical resection is the treatment of choice. Chemotherapy with 5-fluorouracil and radiotherapy may shrink larger tumours and make surgery possible. Adjuvant chemotherapy combined with radiotherapy after resection in patients with resection margins free of tumour only produces a marginal improvement in survival. For patients with liver metastases, chemotherapy with gemcitabine may offer greater palliation than 5-fluorouracil.

Colorectal cancer

Surgery is the treatment of choice for patients with colorectal cancer without metastatic disease, and palliative surgery is often used even if spread has occurred. About 50% of colorectal tumours are cured by surgery; recurrence of rectal tumour is higher than colonic tumour. Adjuvant chemotherapy is often given, with 5-fluorouracil modulated by the use of folinic acid. This regimen has improved survival by 10–15% for locally invasive tumours. The major benefit is reduction of metastatic spread rather than of local recurrence. Perioperative intraportal chemotherapy with 5-fluorouracil is also under investigation. Once a patient has survived for 5 years, life expectancy is similar to that in the general population.

In advanced colorectal cancer, prolonged intravenous infusion of 5-fluorouracil doubles survival and improves quality of life. In rectal cancer, this treatment can be combined with radiotherapy. Irinotecan and other new cytotoxic agents are being investigated for patients who are resistant to 5-fluorouracil.

Lung cancer

There are four principal types of lung cancer. Non-small cell cancers (adenocarcinoma, squamous cell cancer and large cell cancer) account for about three-quarters of cases, with small cell cancer responsible for the remainder.

Surgical resection can be curative in the early stages for non-small-cell lung cancer. Radiotherapy is used after surgery when the tumour is not fully resectable, or for palliation of metastases. Chemotherapy has a limited place for advanced or recurrent disease but is mainly palliative. However, regimens including agents such as cisplatin and etoposide produce little or no survival advantage. Current interest is focusing on chemoradiotherapy, a combination of cyclical multidrug chemotherapy followed by radiotherapy. In these studies, cisplatin is often combined with one or more additional drugs. Small cell lung cancer is more sensitive to chemotherapy.

Melanoma

Survival in melanoma is related to tumour thickness, falling from >95% 5-year survival with superficial tumours to less than 50% survival if the depth is greater than 4 mm. Wide surgical excision is the treatment of choice. Postsurgical adjuvant chemotherapy does not improve survival or disease-free outcome. Immunotherapy with Bacillus Calvette Guérin (BCG) may produce a benefit for patients who had a negative tuberculin skin test before therapy. The use of granulo-cyte–macrophage colony-stimulating factor (GM-CSF) has shown promising preliminary results. Currently, interferon-alfa is the only agent shown to increase disease-free survival. For metastatic disease, current therapy rests mainly on single-agent chemotherapy with dacarbazine or the vinca alkaloids (vincristine or vinblastine), which produce responses in 10–20% of patients. Combination chemotherapy increases toxicity with no improvement in response. Immunotherapy with interferon-alfa has produce similar response rates to chemotherapy, and a combination of interferon-alfa and dacarbazine may have additive or synergistic effects.

Kidney cancer

Nephrectomy is the treatment of choice for early-stage kidney cancer. However, up to one-third of patients have metastases at the time of diagnosis. Options for chemotherapy include:

- chemotherapy with a combination of the antimetabolites fluorouracil and gemcitabine; the response is generally low, with fewer than 15% patients showing a partial or complete response
- progestogens produce a response in about 10% of patients
- immunotherapy with interferon-alfa produces a response rate of about 10%; aldesleukin (interleukin 2) has a slightly higher success rate of about 15%; combination therapy with low doses of both agents may be more effective than either alone.

Bladder cancer

Superficial bladder tumours are removed surgically, but recurrence rates are high. Adjuvant chemotherapy with intravesical cytostatic drugs such as thiotepa, doxorubicin, mitomycin C or epirubicin have been used, but long-term survival is not altered. Intravesical immunotherapy with BCG looks more promising. Invasive tumours are usually treated by surgery and radiotherapy. Chemotherapy is sometimes given before surgery (neoadjuvant chemotherapy) or after surgery or radiotherapy (adjuvant chemotherapy). Currently, no survival advantage has been shown for either approach.

Prostate cancer

Treatment is largely determined by the extent of spread of the cancer. There are several options.

- 'Watchful waiting' for localised disease confined to the prostate. This is usually used for individuals with a life expectancy under 10 years, since many tumours do not progress in this time.
- Radiotherapy for localised disease or locally advanced disease. Impotence follows therapy in 40–70%.

- Radical prostatectomy for localised disease. Impotence is a common sequel, occurring in 30–70%.
- Hormonal therapy for lymph node or distant metastases. Testosterone reduction can be achieved by bilateral orchidectomy or the use of gonadotrophin-releasing hormone (GnRH) analogues such as goserelin (Ch. 43). Antiandrogen therapy (e.g. with flutamide or cyproterone acetate; Ch. 46) can be added to block adrenal androgen activity, although the advantages of such therapy are unproven.
- Hormone-refractory diseases can be treated by combination chemotherapy with drugs such as doxorubicin with fluorouracil or estramustine with vinblastine. Response rates of about 50% can be achieved. Painful metastatic deposits can be treated with radiotherapy or with strontium-89, which is taken up by sclerotic metastases.

Testicular cancer

Testicular tumours are either seminomas or non-seminomatous germ cell tumours, depending on the tissue of origin.

For seminoma, treatment choice includes:

- radiotherapy for localised disease, which gives cure rates up to 95%
- For more advanced disease, chemotherapy with carboplatin is usually used.

For non-seminomatous germ cell tumours, treatment includes:

- orchidectomy for localised disease, which has a 95% cure rate.
- chemotherapy for more advanced or recurrent disease (occurs in 20% of patients). Combination chemotherapy often includes cisplatin, etoposide and bleomycin, which produces a 70–80% complete remission rate.

Ovarian cancer

Initial surgery for ovarian cancer is followed by chemotherapy for all disease that is not localised to the ovary (which occurs in 80% of cases). About 70% of these patients respond to chemotherapy, with complete remission in 10–20%. Options include:

- carboplatin or cisplatin alone: this is the most widely used first-line treatment
- for patients refractory to standard chemotherapy, the addition of paclitaxel achieves palliation in 25–35% of cases.

The role of intraperitoneal drug delivery and more intensive combination chemotherapy is the subject of several current studies.

Endometrial cancer

Surgery is the usual initial treatment for endometrial cancer. Subsequent irradiation is used for extrauterine metastases. Disseminated disease can be treated by hormone therapy with progestogens, but responses are low (less than one-third of patients) and may depend on the presence of progesterone receptors on the tumour cells. Adjuvant chemotherapy is currently being studied.

Breast cancer

Limited surgery is the treatment of choice for very early disease and oestrogen receptor-positive tumours; it is usually followed by local radiotherapy. The risk of invasive recurrence is low and is treated by mastectomy followed by chemotherapy. Chemotherapy or hormonal therapy is used for larger locally invasive tumours or distant spread, with treatment started before surgery. Determination of the hormone receptor status of the tumour is an important guide to chemotherapy. Options for hormonal therapy for oestrogen receptor-positive tumours include:

- anti-oestrogen therapy, e.g. with tamoxifen
- ovarian ablation for premenopausal women as an alternative approach
- aromatase inhibitors, e.g. formestane for postmenopausal women
- progestogens (Ch. 45)
- gonadotrophin-releasing hormone (GnRH) analogues such as goserelin (Ch. 43).

Treatment is usually given for 5 years. The 10–20% of patients who become unresponsive to one hormonal treatment may still benefit from use of an alternative class of drug. For oestrogen receptor-negative tumours, or hormonally unresponsive disease, chemotherapy is used. Examples of current regimens include doxorubicin or paclitaxel alone or combined, which produces response rates of up to 40%.

Acute myeloid leukaemias

The acute myeloid leukaemias are a heterogenous group of disorders (Box 52.1) that are differentiated on morphological grounds. Acute myeloid leukaemia is responsible for up to 15% of childhood leukaemias and is the commonest leukaemia of adult life. Complications result from bone marrow failure, and management of serious infection or bleeding are important issues in supportive care. The risk of infection is amplified by chemotherapy. The initial aim of chemotherapy is to reduce 'blast' cells in the marrow to below 5% of the total cell population (remission) with induction therapy and then to eradicate the leukaemic cells with consolidation therapy.

In the induction phase, cyclical intravenous chemotherapy with three or more drugs is used to reduce the development of resistance, usually giving four courses with 3–5 weeks between courses. A typical regimen consists of daunorubicin, cytarabine and either tioguanine or etoposide in younger patients (under 60 years of age). Consolidation is achieved with further courses of similar therapy. Bone marrow transplantation may be considered after remission is achieved. In children, treatment for the central nervous system is also given with intrathecal methotrexate. For acute promyelocytic leukaemia, the best initial response is obtained with tretinoin, a vitamin A derivative (see Ch. 49) and consolidation achieved by the addition of daunorubicin.

Acute lymphoblastic leukaemia

Acute lymphoblastic leukaemia is most common in children under 10 years of age, with a few cases occurring after age 40 years. Supportive therapy is similar to that for acute myeloid leukaemia.

Remission is achieved with vincristine, crisantaspase, prednisolone and often doxorubicin or daunorubicin. Consolidation therapy is initially with at least two multidrug intensification modules using a combination of cytarabine, tioguanine, daunorubicin, vincristine, prednisolone and etoposide. Continuation therapy is continued after the first 5 months with vincristine and prednisolone for at least 2 years. Eradication of cranial disease is important, using intrathecal methotrexate or cranial irradiation.

The results of treatment in childhood are excellent, with about 70% 5-year survival; this falls to 30% if the disease occurs in adult life.

Chronic myeloid leukaemia

Chronic myeloid leukaemia occurs in all age groups but is rare in children. Most patients have an initial chronic course, lasting 3–4 years, followed by transformation to an accelerated phase, when survival is just 3–6 months. In younger patients, allogenic bone transplantation is the treatment of choice after high-dose chemotherapy.

For older patients, hydroxyurea is usually given to reduce the white cell count. Once symptoms are relieved, treatment with interferon alfa is substituted and can achieve remission in up to 80% of patients. Survival is prolonged by up to 20 months with this regimen. Busulfan is an alternative chemotherapeutic agent for patients who cannot tolerate hydroxyurea.

For advanced disease, combination chemotherapy can be considered, such as the regimen used for acute myeloid leukaemia.

Chronic lymphocytic leukaemia

Chronic lymphocytic leukaemia is predominantly a disease of the elderly. Cure is unusual and median survival is 5–8 years. Treatment may not be necessary if the disease is causing few problems; oral chlorambucil, often combined with prednisolone, can be given for up to 6 months to regress the disease. Transformation of the disease to a more aggressive form can occur after several years, when combination chemotherapy should be considered.

Fludarabine is the second-line treatment of choice. It is used intravenously for relapse after treatment with chlorambucil. Response rates of about 50% have been reported, with remissions lasting, on average, 8 months.

Malignant lymphomas

The malignant lymphomas are a diverse group of disorders comprising Hodgkin's disease and a variety of non-Hodgkin's lymphomas, which are classified by histopathological and cytochemical techniques. Low-grade non-Hodgkin's lymphomas are managed in a similar way to chronic lymphatic leukaemia and have a similar prognosis. Non-Hodgkin's lymphomas of intermediate grade are curable in about 40% of patients using courses of combination chemotherapy with cyclophosphamide, doxorubicin, vincristine and prednisolone on six occasions. Radiotherapy is sometimes also used as adjunctive treatment. More intensive therapy is required for high-grade non-Hodgkin's lymphomas.

For Hodgkin's disease, radiotherapy is curative if the tumour is located. For more extensive disease, combination chemotherapy is the usual approach.

Multiple myeloma

Multiple myeloma is mainly a disorder of the elderly. Treatment is aimed at suppression of the monoclonal protein in the blood. Supportive therapy is often required to treat hypercalcaemia, renal impairment and infection. Rehydration and analgesia for bone pain are often required.

Chemotherapy is usually with oral melphalan and prednisolone in pulses for 4–6 weeks. This reduces the myeloma protein in blood by more than 50% in half of the patients. Median survival with this treatment is 3 years.

High doses of intravenous melphalan or combination therapy with vincristine, doxorubicin and dexamethasone produces up to 70% response rate and may be justifiable in younger patients who tolerate the associated toxicity better. Autologous bone marrow transplant is used as salvage therapy after intensive chemotherapy and can produce 30–50% complete remission.

FURTHER READING

Drugs and drug action

Ambudkar SV, Dey S, Hrycyna CA, Ramachandra M, Pastan I, Gottesman MM (1999) Biochemical, cellular, and pharmacological aspects of the multidrug transporter. *Annu Rev Pharmacol Toxicol* 39, 361–398

Bailly C (2000) Topoisomerase I poisons and suppressors as anticancer drugs. *Curr Med Chem* 7, 39–58

Burden DA, Osheroff N (1998) Mechanism of action of eukaryotic topoisomerase II and drugs targeted to the enzyme. *Biochim Biophys Acta* 1400, 139–154

Dubowchik, GM, Walker MA (1999) Receptor-mediated and enzyme-dependent targeting of cytotoxic anticancer drugs. *Pharmacol Ther* 83, 67–123

Garrett MD, Workman P (1999) Discovering novel chemotherapeutic drugs for the third millennium. *Eur J Cancer* 35, 2010–2030

Jordan MA, Wilson L (1998) Microtubules and actin filaments: dynamic targets for cancer chemotherapy. *Curr Opin Cell Biol* 10, 123–130

Links M, Lewis C (1999) Chemoprotectants: a review of their clinical pharmacology and therapeutic efficacy. *Drugs* 57, 293–308

Njar VC, Brodie AM (1999) Comprehensive pharmacology and clinical efficacy of aromatase inhibitors. *Drugs* 58, 233–255

Nooter K, Stoter G (1996) Molecular mechanisms of multidrug resistance in cancer chemotherapy. *Pathol Res Pract* 192, 768–780

Pommier Y, Pourquier P, Fan Y, Strumberg D (1998) Mechanism of action of eukaryotic DNA topoisomerase I and drugs targeted to the enzyme. *Biochim Biophys Acta* 1400, 83–105

Stein WD (1997) Kinetics of the multidrug transporter (P-glycoprotein) and its reversal. *Physiol Rev* 77, 545–590

Young A, Rea D (2000) Treatment of advanced disease. *Br Med J* 321, 1278–1281

Urogenital cancer

Bosl G-J, Motzer RJ (1997) Testicular germ-cell cancer. *N Engl J Med* 337, 242–253

Frydenburg M, Stricker PD, Kaye KW (1997) Prostate cancer diagnosis and management. *Lancet* 349, 1681–1687

Horwick A, Huddart R, Dearnaley D (1998) Markers and management of germ-cell tumours of the testes. *Lancet* 352, 1535–1538.

Rose PG (1996) Endometrial carcinoma. *N Engl J Med* 335, 6400–6409

Van der Meijden AP (1998) Bladder cancer. *Br Med J* 317, 1366–1369

Vogelzang NJ, Stadler WM (1998) Kidney cancer. *Lancet* 352, 1691–1696

Breast cancer

Hortobaggyi GN (1998) Treatment of breast cancer. *N Engl J Med* 339, 974–984

Howell A, Dowsett M (1997) Recent advances in endocrine therapy of breast cancer. *Br Med J* 315, 863–866

Osborne CK (1998) Tamoxifen in the treatment of breast cancer. *N Engl J Med* 339, 1609–1618

Other cancers

Bastin KT, Curley R (1995) Non-small-cell lung carcinoma. *Drugs* 49, 362–375

Cohen GL, Falkson CI (1998) Current treatment options for malignant melanoma. *Drugs* 55, 791–799.

Hendliz A, Bleiberg H (1995) Diagnosis and treatment of gastric cancer. *Drugs* 49, 711–720

Midgley R, Kerr D (1999) Colorectal cancer. *Lancet* 353, 391–399

Sporn JR (1999) Practical recommendations for the management of adenocarcinoma of the pancreas. *Drugs* 57, 69–79

Acute leukaemias

Burnett AK, Eden OB (1997) The treatment of acute leukaemia. *Lancet* 349, 270–275

Pui C-H, Evans WE (1998) Acute lymphoblastic leukemia. *N Engl J Med* 339, 605–615

Chronic leukaemias

Goldman J (1997) Chronic myeloid leukaemia. *Br Med J* 314, 657–660

Mead, GM (1997) Malignant lymphomas and chronic lymphocytic leukaemia. *Br Med J* 314, 1103–1105

Multiple myeloma

Bataille R, Harousseau J-L (1997) Multiple myeloma. *N Engl J Med* 336, 1657–1664

Self-assessment

1. What are the criteria for combination chemotherapy of cancer? How well do the following treatment regimens meet the criteria?

   a. Acute lymphoblastic leukaemia (ALL; initial phase for induction of remission): intravenous vincristine (1.5 mg m²), subcutaneous crisantaspase (6000 units m²), prednisolone (40 mg m²).
   b. Hodgkin's lymphoma (MOPP regimen): intravenous mustine (6 mg m²), intravenous vincristine (oncovine) (1.5 mg m²), oral procarbazine (100 mg m²) and oral prednisolone (40 mg m²).
   c. Testicular teratoma (in an adult): intravenous etoposide (120 mg m²), intravenous bleomycin (30 mg) and intravenous cisplatin (20 mg m²).

2. Why are the doses of anticancer drugs corrected to surface area rather than simply body weight (e.g. mg/kg body weight)? Does the use of surface area correction result in higher or lower doses for children compared with simple body weight correction (Table 52.2)?

Table 52.2
Examples of surface area calculation

Age (years)	Body weight (kg)	Height (cm)	Body surface area (m²)
0.5	7.4	65.8	0.350
1.0	9.9	74.7	0.434
3	14.5	96.0	0.613
6	21.5	116.8	0.835
Adult			
Male	72.1	175.3	1.874
Female	60.3	167.6	1.681

Surface area is calculated using a nomogram or the equation:

$$A = 71.84\ W^{0.425}\ H^{0.725}$$

where A is surface area (in cm²), W is weight (in kg) and H is height (in cm).

The answers are provided on pages 631.

Drugs used in the treatment of cancer

Drug	Half-life (h)	Elimination	Comments	Unusual or limiting toxicity[a]
Alkylating agents				
Busulfan	2–3	Metabolism	Given orally; 'metabolism' is largely by interaction with thiol groups, such as cysteine, the products of which are further metabolised and eliminated; mainly used for effects on the bone marrow (e.g. chronic myeloid leukaemia)	Myelosuppression and irreversible bone marrow aplasia; rare pulmonary fibrosis
Carmustine (BCNU)	0.4–0.5	Metabolism	Given i.v.; unstable reactive molecule that cross-links DNA and the nitroso function inactivates DNA repair; crosses blood–brain barrier; metabolites eliminated in urine; used for myeloma, lymphoma and brain tumours	Renal damage; delayed pulmonary fibrosis
Chlorambucil	1–2	Metabolism	Given orally usually after fasting; 'metabolised' at alkylating groups owing to reactivity and in the liver by β-oxidation of the carboxylic acid side-chain; used mainly in lymphocytic leukaemia, Hodgkin's and ovarian cancer	Vomiting
Chlormethine (mustine)	–	Metabolism	Given i.v. as a freshly prepared solution by a fast-running infusion; extremely unstable and reactive; volatility poses occupational risk; much less commonly used (it is the M in the MOPP (MVPP) regimen)	
Cyclophosphamide	4–10	Metabolism	Given orally or by i.v. injection; good penetration of blood–brain barrier; metabolic oxidation by cytochrome P450 (CYP2B1 and CYP3A4) leads to bioactivation; wide interpatient variability; widely used	Haemorrhagic cystitis (see mesna, antidote)
Estramustine	20–24	Metabolism	Given orally (an oestrogen molecule linked to a nitrogen mustard group); acts as an alkylating agent especially on microtubule proteins, and increases circulating oestrogen levels; the phosphate ester, which is given orally, is dephosphorylated to the active drug, which is oxidised in the steroid ring; used for prostate cancer	
Ifosfamide	4–15	Metabolism	Given by i.v. injection; metabolic fate is similar to cyclophosphamide	Cystitis (see mesna, antidote)
Lomustine (CCNU)	1–5 (4-OH)	Metabolism	Given orally; bifunctional drug similar to carmustine; oxidised to 4-hydroxy compound (4-OH) completely in the gut wall and liver during first-pass metabolism; mainly used for Hodgkin's disease and some solid tumours	Permanent bone marrow damage
Melphalan	1.5	Metabolism	Given orally or by i.v. injection; oral absorption is incomplete and variable; does not cross blood–brain barrier in useful amounts; pathways of metabolism are not well defined; used mainly for myeloma	
Thiotepa	1–3 (thiotepa), 10–21 (TEPA)	Metabolism	Given by intravesicular injection; extensively absorbed from bladder lumen; bioactivated by cytochrome P450 (CYP2B and CYP2C) to TEPA (the active form), in which sulfur is replaced by oxygen; used for bladder cancer	
Treosulfan	1–2		Given orally or by i.v. injection; high oral bioavailability; metabolised by loss of reactive groups through non-enzymatic reactions; leaving groups are eliminated as methylsulfonic acid; used mainly for ovarian cancer	Allergic alveolitis; pulmonary fibrosis

continued

Drugs used in the treatment of cancer *(continued)*

Drug	Half-life (h)	Elimination	Comments	Unusual or limiting toxicity[a]
Cytotoxic antibiotics				
Aclarubicin	1–9 (10–20 as active metabolite M1)	Metabolism	Given i.v.; rapidly taken up by cells; crosses blood–brain barrier in useful amounts; metabolised to active (M1) and inactive metabolites; activity linked to parent drug and M1; used for non-lymphocytic leukaemia in relapsed/resistant patients	Bone marrow suppression
Bleomycin	2–4	Metabolism + renal	Given i.v. or i.m.; slow uptake by tissues; hydrolysed by enzyme 'bleomycin hydrolase', which largely inactivates the drug; low levels of the hydrolase correlate with cytotoxicity; used for testicular cancer, lymphomas and squamous cell carcinoma	Dermatological effects; progressive pulmonary fibrosis
Dactinomycin (actinomycin D)	36	Renal + bile	Given i.v.; negligible metabolism; mainly used for paediatric solid tumours	Bone marrow toxicity; gastrointestinal toxicity
Daunorubicin	24–48 (5 as liposomes)	Metabolism + bile	Given i.v.; undergoes metabolic reduction and redox cycling, giving toxic superoxide radicals and H_2O_2; long half-life owing to slow release from tissues; metabolite retains activity; used for acute leukaemias and AIDS-related Kaposi's sarcoma (as a liposome preparation)	Bone marrow toxicity
Doxorubicin	2–10	Metabolism	Given i.v.; reduced in liver to doxorubicinol which is further metabolised and excreted, largely in the bile; does not cross blood–brain barrier; widely used for leukaemias, lymphomas and a variety of solid tumours	Myelosuppression; cardiotoxicity
Epirubicin	11–69	Metabolism (+ renal)	Given i.v.; reduced to epirubicinol and also conjugated in amino sugar ring; very wide interpatient variability in kinetics; does not cross blood–brain barrier; uses are similar to doxorubicin	Myelosuppression; cardiotoxicity (less than doxorubicin)
Idarubicin	12–35 (50–70 idarubicinol)	Metabolism	Given orally or i.v.; oral bioavailability is low and variable (4–50%); metabolised by reduction to idarubicinol (which has a longer half-life and retains activity) and by hydrolysis of the amino sugar moiety; used mainly for acute leukaemias and advanced breast cancer (non-responsive to first-line treatments)	Myelosuppression
Mitomycin	0.5–1.5	Metabolism	Given i.v.; reduced to a hydroquinone, which gives rise to a highly unstable alkylating species that cross-links DNA; metabolism gives toxic superoxide and hydroxyl radicals; mainly used for upper gastrointestinal and breast cancers and by bladder instillation for superficial bladder tumours	Myelosuppression; nephrotoxicity; lung fibrosis
Mitoxantrone (mitozantrone)	4–220	Renal + metabolism	Given by i.v. infusion; metabolised in the liver by side-chain oxidation to inactive metabolites; extremely wide interpatient variability in half-life; long half-life may result from high tissue uptake and affinity; used to treat breast cancer	Myelosuppression; cardiotoxicity
Antimetabolites				
Cladribine	7	Metabolism	Given by i.v. infusion; chlorine-substituted purine; purine; undergoes intracellular phosphorylation to the active triphosphate form; used for hairy cell leukaemia	Myelosuppression; neurotoxicity

continued

Drugs used in the treatment of cancer _(continued)_

Drug	Half-life (h)	Elimination	Comments	Unusual or limiting toxicity[a]
Antimetabolites (continued)				
Cytarabine (cytosine arabinoside)	1–3	Metabolism	Given i.v., s.c. or intrathecally; undergoes intracellular phosphorylation to the active triphosphate form; metabolism to uracil arabinoside gives inactivation; used for acute leukaemias	Myelosuppression
Fludarabine phosphate	7–20	Renal + metabolism	Given i.v.; fluorine-substituted purine riboside; phosphate is rapidly hydrolysed to give fludarabine, which enters the cell and is phosphorylated to a triphosphate; used for B-cell chronic lymphocytic leukaemia	Myelosuppression
Fluorouracil	0.25	Metabolism	Given orally, topically or i.v. (normal route); fluorine-substituted uracil; converted to fluorouracil monophosphate intracellularly and then to di- and triphosphates; catabolised in the liver by dihydropyrimidine dehydrogenase; used for cancers of the gastrointestinal tract and malignant and premalignant skin lesions	Relatively low toxicity (not usually the limiting drug given)
Gemcitabine	0.2–0.5	Metabolism	Given i.v.; deoxycytidine analogue with two fluorine atoms in the deoxyribose moiety; bioactivated by intracellular conversion to the active triphosphate; inactivated by deamination to difluorodeoxyuridine; used for palliative treatment of patients with non-small cell lung and pancreatic cancer	Limited toxicity
5-Mercaptopurine	1–1.5	Metabolism	Given orally; sulfur-substituted purine; poor oral bioavailability owing to first-pass metabolism (about 20%); bioactivated by intracellular phosphorylation; inactivated by xanthine oxidase (interaction with allopurinol); used almost exclusively for maintenance therapy for acute leukaemias	Limited toxicity
Methotrexate	8–10	Renal + metabolism	Given orally, i.v., i.m. or intrathecally; folate analogue; taken up into cells by the reduced folate carrier and undergoes polyglutamate formation (like folate); the polyglutamates are retained for months (the half-life refers to the non-glutamate form); eliminated mainly by the kidneys with some as a hydroxy metabolite; contraindicated in renal impairment; used for maintenance therapy for childhood acute lymphoblastic leukaemia, choriocarcinoma, non-Hodgkin's lymphoma and some solid tumours	Myelosuppression (folinic acid is an 'antidote'– see below)
Raltitrexed	10–12 days	Renal + some metabolism	Given i.v.; prolonged retention within cells gives prolonged inhibition of thymidylate synthase and 3-weekly dosage intervals; forms polyglutamates intracellularly; used for palliation of metastatic colon cancer	Myelosuppression
Tioguanine (6-thioguanine)	3–6	Metabolism + renal	Given orally; bioavailability is 25–50%; rapidly taken up by cells; converted to corresponding nucleotide intracellularly; which is retained within cells; methylation of the 6-thio group is the major route of metabolism; used for acute leukaemias	Myelosuppression

continued

Drugs used in the treatment of cancer (continued)

Drug	Half-life (h)	Elimination	Comments	Unusual or limiting toxicity[a]
Vinca alkaloids and etoposide				
Etoposide	4–8	Metabolism	Given orally or i.v.; oral absorption is 25–75%; eliminated in urine and bile mainly as metabolites; used for small cell carcinoma of the bronchus, lymphomas and testicular cancer	Myelosuppression; alopecia
Vinblastine	20–80	Metabolism	Given i.v.; metabolised by hepatic CYP3A4 and metabolites eliminated in bile and urine; used for acute leukaemias, lymphomas and non-solid tumours (e.g. breast and lung)	Myelosuppression
Vincristine	85	Metabolism	Given i.v.; metabolised in liver; metabolites eliminated mainly in the bile; uses as for vinblastine	Neurotoxicity (peripheral and autonomic neuropathy) (recovery is slow but complete)
Vindesine	25	Metabolism + renal	Given i.v.; metabolised by CYP3A4 and metabolites are eliminated in bile and urine; up to 10% excreted unchanged in urine; uses are similar to vinblastine	Myelosuppression
Vinorelbine	28–44	Metabolism	Given i.v.; semisynthetic vinca alkaloid made from vinblastine; metabolised by CYP3A4 and metabolites are eliminated in bile and urine; used for advanced breast and non-small cell lung cancer	Myelosuppression
Platinum compounds				
Carboplatin	1.5	Renal	Given i.v.; active form produced by interaction with water; eliminated by glomerular filtration; good correlation between AUC in blood (see Ch. 2), creatinine clearance and myelosuppression; the excretion of total platinum (Pt) (equivalent to 'metabolites') is much slower than that of the parent compound; used for ovarian cancer and some other solid tumours	Myelosuppression (plus some nausea and vomiting – less than cisplatin)
Cisplatin	24–60	Renal	Given i.v.; active form produced by interaction with water; eliminated by kidney; some sources give the half-life as up to 60 h, and these values relate to total Pt not cisplatin per se; used for solid tumours such as ovarian cancer and testicular teratoma	Nausea and vomiting; nephrotoxicity; myelosuppression; ototoxicity
Oxaliplatin	27	Renal	Given i.v.; has a 1,2-diaminocyclohexane ligand (which increases the formation of DNA adducts) and an oxalate ligand on the Pt atom; half-life relates to free Pt because the parent drug undergoes rapid hydration and ligand-exchange reactions; used for metastatic colorectal cancer	Neurotoxicity
Taxanes				
Docetaxel	11	Metabolism (+ renal)	Given by i.v. infusion; metabolised by CYP3A4-mediated oxidation; metabolites eliminated in the bile; a small amount (<10%) excreted changed in urine; used for advanced or metastatic anthracycline-resistant breast cancer	Hypersensitivity reactions; myelosuppression; peripheral neuropathy; fluid retention

continued

Drugs used in the treatment of cancer *(continued)*

Drug	Half-life (h)	Elimination	Comments	Unusual or limiting toxicity[a]
Taxanes (continued)				
Paclitaxel	19	Metabolism	Given by i.v. infusion; metabolised by CYP2C8 and CYP3A4 to different metabolites, which are eliminated in bile; used for advanced ovarian cancer and as secondary treatment for breast and non-small cell lung cancer	Hypersensitivity reactions; myelosuppression; periperal neuropathy
Topoisomerase I inhibitors				
Irinotecan	6	Metabolism + renal	Given by i.v. infusion; metabolised by esterase to a highly active metabolite and by CYP3A4 to largely inactive metabolite; activity resides in parent drug and esterase product; some renal excretion (10–20%); used for metastatic colorectal cancer	Myelosuppression; gastrointestinal effects
Topotecan	2–3	Renal + hydrolysis	Given by i.v. infusion; undergoes pH-dependent hydrolysis of the lactone ring, which results in inactivation; enzymatic metabolism is only a minor route of elimination; used for metastatic ovarian cancer when first-line treatment has failed	Myelosuppression; gastrointestinal effects
Miscellaneous anticancer drugs				
Altretamine	5–10	Metabolism	Given orally; metabolites are cytotoxic and bind to tissue macromolecules; used for advanced ovarian cancer where other treatments have failed	Peripheral and central neurotoxicity; nausea and vomiting
Amsacrine	4–7	Metabolism	Given as i.v. infusion; metabolites formed in the liver and eliminated as bile; used for acute myeloid leukaemia	Myelosuppression (fatal arrhythmias when there is hypokalaemia)
Crisantaspase (asparaginase)	7–13	Metabolism	Given by intramuscular or s.c. injection; enzyme isolated from *Erwinia chrysanthemi*; taken up by reticuloendothelial system and degraded; used for acute lymphoblastic leukaemia	Anaphylaxis; nausea; CNS depression; hyperglycaemia
Dacarbazine	5	Renal + metabolism	Given i.v.; activated by P450-mediated metabolism to a cytotoxic and alkylating metabolite; about 50% is excreted in the urine unchanged; used for metastatic melanoma and soft tissue sarcomas	Myelosuppression; intense nausea and vomiting
Hydroxyurea (hydroxycarbamide)	2–6	Urine	Given orally; eliminated by glomerular filtration; used for chronic myeloid leukaemia	Myelosuppression
Pentostatin	3–15	Renal	Given i.v.; eliminated by kidneys with negligible metabolism; clearance correlates with creatinine clearance; used for hairy cell leukaemia	Myelosuppression; immunosuppression
Procarbazine	?	Metabolism (+ renal)	Given orally; eliminated by hepatic metabolism via CYP1A2, which gives rise to methyl radicals; limited renal excretion (5% of dose); crosses blood–brain barrier; ingestion with alcohol may give a disulfiram-like effect; used in Hodgkin's disease	Nausea; myelosuppression; rash

continued

Drugs used in the treatment of cancer *(continued)*

Drug	Half-life (h)	Elimination	Comments	Unusual or limiting toxicity[a]
Miscellaneous anticancer drugs (continued)				
Razoxane (dexrazoxane)	2–4	Metabolism	Given orally; metabolised in the liver; limited value for leukaemias; dextroisomer is approved by FDA to prevent cardiac complications associated with cases of chemotherapy (by chelating iron and preventing redox cycling with, for example, doxorubicin)	
Temozolomide	2	Metabolism	Given orally; structural analogue of dacarbazine (see above) and converted to the same active compound non-enzymatically; eliminated as metabolites; used as a second-line treatment for malignant glioma	Myelosuppression
Tretinoin (all-*trans*-retinoic acid)	1–2	Metabolism	Given orally; eliminated by oxidation, conjugation with glucuronic acid, and isomerisation to the less active *cis*-isomer; used for remission of acute promyelocytic leukaemia	Numerous symptoms (highly teratogenic)
Antidotes (chemoprotectants)				
Folinate (leucovorin) and levofolinate	0.75	Metabolism	Given orally or by i.m. or i.v. injection; given 24 h after methotrexate to speed recovery from myelosuppression; formyl group is used for thymidate synthesis and folate enters body pool	
Amifostine	<0.2	Metabolism	Given by i.v. infusion; rapidly cleared by uptake into normal tissues where it is hydrolysed; used prior to cytotoxic treatment to reduce the risk of neutropenia-related infection in patients treated with cisplatin or cyclophosphamide, and to reduce cisplatin nephrotoxicity	Hypotension
Mesna	1	Renal + metabolism	Given orally or by i.v. injection; highly polar molecule that contains a sulfhydryl (SH) group; eliminated in the urine; some dimerisation of SH group to a disulfide, which is eliminated in the urine and reduced back to mesna; given either before (oral) or with (i.v.) cyclophosphamide or ifosfamide treatment to prevent urothelial toxicity	
Other drugs used for the treatment of cancer			These are drugs that affect the cancer per se; other drugs used in the management of patients with cancer (e.g. anti-emetics) are described in the appropriate chapter	
Aldesleukin (interleukin 2)	0.5–6	Metabolism	Given by s.c. injection; recombinant interleukin 2; taken up and degraded by the kidneys; the half-life is that seen after i.v. dosage; s.c. dosage gives prolonged low plasma levels with a half-life of 3–12 h; use restricted to metastatic renal cell carcinoma	Severe toxicity; pulmonary oedema; hypotension; plus bone marrow, hepatic, renal, thyroid and CNS toxicity
Diethylstilbestrol	2–3 days	Metabolism	Given orally; eliminated by conjugation with glucuronic acid; undergoes enterohepatic recycling; used rarely for prostate cancer, and occasionally for breast cancer	Nausea; fluid retention; thrombosis; impotence and gynaecomastia in men; hypercalcaemia and bone pain in women

continued

Drugs used in the treatment of cancer (*continued*)

Drug	Half-life (h)	Elimination	Comments	Unusual or limiting toxicity[a]

Other drugs used for the treatment of cancer (*continued*)

Drug	Half-life (h)	Elimination	Comments	Unusual or limiting toxicity[a]
Ethinylestradiol	8–24	Metabolism	Given orally; may be used for breast cancer (see contraceptive hormones)	See contraceptive hormones (Ch. 45)
Fosfestrol	2–3 days (DES)	Metabolism	Given orally or by slow i.v. injection; phosphate ester of diethylstilbestrol (DES), which is hydrolysed by phosphatases; used for prostate cancer	See diethylstilbestrol (above)
Interferon alfa	3–4	Metabolism	Given by s.c. or i.v. injection; catabolised by kidney; slow absorption from s.c. dosage with peak concentrations at 4–8 h; used for certain lymphomas and solid tumours	Nausea; lethargy; ocular effects; depression; myelosuppression; cerebrovascular, liver and kidney problems
Prednisolone	2–4	Metabolism	Given orally, topically and by i.m. injection; injectable form is the acetate ester as an aqueous suspension; high oral bioavailability (70–80%); extensively metabolised but all pathways have not been defined; has a marked antitumour effect in acute lymphoblastic leukaemia, Hodgkin's disease and non-Hodgkin's lymphoma (also used in palliative care)	See corticosteroids (Ch. 44)
Rituximab	60	Metabolism	Given by i.v. infusion; monoclonal chimaeric mouse/human antibody that causes lysis of B-lymphocytes; the elimination of the peptide has a shorter half-life for the first infusion compared with subsequent dosage; used for chemotherapy-resistant advanced follicular lymphoma	Fever; chills; nausea; allergic reactions
Gestonorone caproate	–	Metabolism	Progestogen; given by i.m. injection; few kinetic data available; probably undergoes hydrolysis of the caproate ester group to liberate the steroid; used to treat endometrial cancer and benign prostatic hypertrophy	Usually mild effects only
Medroxy-progesterone acetate	30	Metabolism	Progestogen; given orally or by deep i.m. injection; complete oral bioavailability; eliminated as conjugated metabolites; used for endometrial, prostate and renal cancer	Glucocorticoid effect at high doses
Megestrol acetate	15–20	Metabolism	Progestogen; given orally; complete oral bioavailability; metabolised largely by oxidation followed by conjugation; used for breast and endometrial cancer	Usually mild
Norethisterone (norethindrone)	5–12	Metabolism	Progestogen; given orally; complete oral bioavailability; metabolised by reduction of the ketone group to an alcohol, which is conjugated; used for breast cancer	

Drugs for breast cancer

Drug	Half-life (h)	Elimination	Comments	Unusual or limiting toxicity[a]
Tamoxifen	7 days	Metabolism	Non-steroidal anti-oestrogen; given orally; high bioavailability; oxidised by CYP2C and CYP3A isoenzymes; used for oestrogen receptor-positive breast cancer	Exacerbation of pain from bone metastases

continued

Drugs used in the treatment of cancer *(continued)*

Drug	Half-life (h)	Elimination	Comments	Unusual or limiting toxicity[a]
Drugs for breast cancer (continued)				
Aminoglutethimide	12	Renal + metabolism	Aromatase inhibitor; eliminated in urine unchanged (50%) and as *N*-acetyl and other metabolites; largely replaced by selective aromatase inhibitors but still sometimes used for treatment of prostate cancer	Drug fever; drowsiness; adrenal hypofunction
Anastrozole	40–50	Metabolism (+ renal)	Selective aromatase inhibitor; given orally; metabolised by oxidation and formation of an *N*-glucuronide (rare reaction); a small amount is excreted unchanged; used for advanced breast cancer in postmenopausal women	Hot flushes; vaginal dryness and bleeding; gastrointestinal effects
Formestane	5–10 days	Metabolism	Aromatase inhibitor; given by deep i.m. injection; metabolised in liver mostly by conjugation with glucuronic acid; used for postmenopausal breast cancer	Numerous effects
Letrozole	2 days	Metabolism	Selective non-steroidal aromatase inhibitor; given orally; high oral bioavailability; oxidised in the liver by CYP3A4 to an inactive metabolite; used for advanced breast cancer in postmenopausal women that is not responsive to other anti-oestrogens	Hot flushes; nausea; gastrointestinal effects
Toremifene	5 days	Metabolism	Non-steroidal oestrogen receptor antagonist; given orally; metabolised by CYP3A4-mediated demethylation; metabolite retains weak activity; undergoes enterohepatic circulation; used for hormone-dependent metastatic breast cancer in postmenopausal women	Hot flushes; vaginal bleeding and discharge plus numerous other effects
Drugs for prostate cancer				
Bicalutamide	7–10 days	Metabolism	Anti-androgen; given orally; undergoes oxidation and conjugation; metabolites excreted in urine and bile; used for advanced prostate cancer; used to cover the 'flare' associated with administration of gonadorelin analogues	Hot flushes; pruritus; gynaecomastia plus rare serious hepatic and cardiovascular effects
Buserelin	3–6 min	Metabolism + renal	Gonadorelin analogue; given by s.c. injection for 7 days and then nasally; peptide hormone; metabolism plus some excreted in urine; used for advanced prostate cancer	May cause tumour 'flare' leading to spinal cord compression; ureteric obstruction and bone pain
Goserelin	4	Metabolism	Gonadorelin analogue; potent LHRH agonist; given by s.c. implant into the anterior abdominal wall; metabolised by peptidase-mediated hydrolysis; used for prostate cancer and advanced breast cancer	(See buserelin)
Leuprorelin acetate (leuprolide)	3–4	Metabolism	Gonadorelin analogue; given by s.c. or i.m. injection; metabolised by proteases; used for advanced prostate cancer	See buserelin; plus muscle weakness; hypertension; palpitations
Triptorelin	3	Metabolism	Gonadorelin analogue; given by i.m. injection; metabolised by proteases; used for advanced prostate cancer (and endometriosis)	(See buserelin)
Cyproterone acetate	2 days	Metabolism	Anti-androgen; given orally; hydrolysed and conjugated with glucuronic acid and sulfate; metabolites eliminated in urine and bile; used for prostate cancer and to cover 'flare' of gonadorelin analogues	(See bicalutamide)

continued

Drugs used in the treatment of cancer (continued)

Drug	Half-life (h)	Elimination	Comments	Unusual or limiting toxicity[a]
Drugs for prostate cancer (continued)				
Flutamide	8	Metabolism	Anti-androgen; given orally; complete bioavailability; rapid oxidation in the liver to an active hydroxy metabolite; used for advanced prostate cancer and to cover the 'flare' of gonadorelin analogues	(See bicalutamide)

AIDS, acquired immunodeficiency syndrome; AUC, area und the curve for plasma concentration versus time; FDA, US Food and Drug Administration; LHRH, luteinising hormone releasing hormone; i.m., intramuscular; i.v., intravenous; s.c., subcutaneous

[a]The toxicity that is typical for a class of drug is described in the general text for that class; toxicity given in this table represents 'non-class' effects and/or severe dose-limiting toxicity.

GENERAL FEATURES:
TOXICITY AND PRESCRIBING

53

Drug toxicity and overdose

Most therapeutic drugs are developed for their ability to interfere with human homeostatic mechanisms in order to produce a beneficial response; only antimicrobial agents and parasiticides have the theoretical possibility of a therapeutic response without some direct action on human metabolic or physiological processes. Several therapeutic agents, for example atropine (belladonna), tubocurarine (curare), ergot alkaloids (causing St Anthony's fire), digoxin (digitalis) and dicoumarol (causing haemorrhagic disease in cattle) have actions that were first recognised as a result of either accidental or intentional poisonings. It is hardly surprising, therefore, that all drugs are capable of producing adverse effects.

The relationship between a drug and a poison was recognised five centuries ago when Paracelsus stated: 'all things are toxic and it is only the dose which makes a thing a poison'. Many of the medicines prescribed today were first used as plant extracts, for example digitalis glycosides and opium extracts. It was the identification and isolation of the active chemical entities in such plant extracts that allowed the dose and purity of the active ingredient to be controlled sufficiently to optimise the ratio between risk and benefit. The current vogue for 'natural, herbal remedies' may be considered to represent a backward step as far as the control of safety and efficacy of drugs is concerned.

Drug toxicity can develop during the normal therapeutic use of a drug or as a result of an acute overdose. In some cases, toxicity occurs in most treated patients because of the nature of the drug, for example cytotoxic agents used for cancer chemotherapy. Significant toxicity is rare with the majority of widely prescribed drugs when used at recommended dosages. There is considerable interpatient variability in the development of adverse reactions, and toxicity may be reduced by taking into account variables that are known to increase vulnerability prior to drug administration, such as age, concurrent disease or body weight, when selecting both the drug and the dosage. Usually a reduction in dosage or a change of drug during chronic treatment will reduce the severity of adverse effects (but see immunological mechanisms discussed below).

Toxicity following an acute overdose usually produces predictable adverse reactions, which may be life threatening and/or prejudice long-term health. Rapid treatment is then required and this may be aimed at preventing further drug absorption, increasing drug elimination/inactivation and managing the adverse effects produced.

This chapter is, therefore, divided into two main sections: drug toxicity, which discusses mechanisms for adverse effects produced both during normal drug therapy and after an overdose and drug overdose, which is concerned with the management of drug overdose.

Drug toxicity

This section provides a framework for classifying adverse effects, rather than an exhaustive catalogue of drugs and their toxicities. The toxic effects of drugs are more numerous than their beneficial properties. Prescribers should be alert to both predicted and un-expected reactions to medicines and should consider the risk–benefit ratio for the particular patient and the suitability of alternative drugs and/or treatments. Patients should also be informed of the risk–benefit balance inherent in their treatment. Prescription information leaflets included with the dispensed medicine represent a useful way of providing such advice.

It should be appreciated that all drugs are associated with some risk of toxicity, although both the severity and incidence differ widely between drugs. The acceptability of a risk of toxicity is inversely related to the severity of the disease being treated; for example, serious idiosyncratic reactions with incidences of 1 in 10 000 have led to the withdrawal of some non-steroidal anti-inflammatory drugs (NSAIDs), whereas cancer chemotherapeutic agents may result in serious toxicity in nearly all patients. In addition 'one man's cure is another man's poison' because the beneficial effects of a drug in one situation (e.g. the antidiarrhoeal effect of opioids) may be an adverse effect in other circumstances (e.g. constipation, when used for pain relief). Therefore, even classification of the nature of effect into beneficial or adverse may depend on the condition being treated.

A useful indication of the safety margin available to the physician (and patient) is given by the therapeutic index (TI):

$$\text{Therapeutic index} = \frac{\text{Dose resulting in toxicity}}{\text{Dose giving therapeutic response}}$$

Drugs such as diazepam have a TI of about 50 and it is difficult for even the most inept doctor to poison patients with diazepam. In contrast, digoxin has a TI of only about 2 and for such drugs, toxicity may be precipitated by relatively small changes in dosage regimen, bioavailability or the clearance of the drug from the body. The TI relates to serious adverse effects and does not indicate the potential for minor unwanted effects, which can inconvenience the patient enough for them to stop treatment.

Types of drug toxicity

Toxicity is frequently divided into two main types:

type A: these effects are dose related and largely predictable

type B: these effects are not dose related but are idiosyncratic and unpredictable.

Our understanding of the mechanisms involved in toxicity has increased greatly in recent years, and this provides a useful framework for students to integrate future knowledge:

- pharmacological: type A
- biochemical: type A and some type B
- immunological: type B
- unknown: mostly type B?

Pharmacological toxicity

The toxic reaction is an extension of the known pharmacological properties of the drug at its site(s) of action (Table 53.1). There are numerous examples in this book where the adverse effects listed are a direct consequence of excessive therapeutic action (response 1 in Fig. 53.1). The change in response with increase in dose from subtherapeutic to therapeutic to toxic has given rise to the concept of a 'therapeutic window' within which most patients should show a beneficial response with minimal risk of adverse effects (response 1 in Fig. 53.1).

Table 53.1
Drugs with adverse effects that are related to their primary therapeutic properties

Drug	Adverse effect
Warfarin	Haemorrhage
Insulin	Hypoglycaemia
β-Adrenoceptor antagonists (β-blockers)	Heart block when used as an antiarrhythmic
Loop diuretics	Hypokalaemia
General anaesthetics	Medullary depression
Acetylcholinesterase inhibitors	Muscle weakness

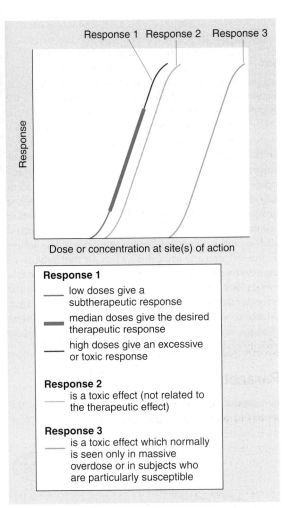

Response 1
___ low doses give a
subtherapeutic response

___ median doses give the desired
therapeutic response

___ high doses give an excessive
or toxic response

Response 2
___ is a toxic effect (not related to
the therapeutic effect)

Response 3
___ is a toxic effect which normally
is seen only in massive
overdose or in subjects who
are particularly susceptible

Fig. 53.1
Dose–response relationships in relation to toxicity.

This concept is particularly valuable in the interpretation of measurements of drug concentrations in plasma to monitor compliance and to assess likely response (Table 53.2).

In many other cases, the toxic reaction may be unrelated to the primary therapeutic effect (Table 53.3) and may be caused by a secondary or alternative effect that is not the primary aim of the treatment given (response 2 in Fig. 53.1). This toxicity would usually be present to a limited extent in patients receiving therapeutic doses (e.g. response 2 in Fig. 53.1).

The separation of therapeutic and toxic dose–response curves is a measure of the TI. If these are very close (e.g. response 2 in Fig. 53.1) then there is little safety margin and most patients will exhibit some degree of toxicity, for example myelosuppression with cytotoxic anticancer drugs.

A high TI (response 3 in Fig. 53.1) results from a form of toxicity that would not be seen with normal therapeutic doses, for example heart failure caused by myocardial depression in patients with normal left ventricular function taking β-blockers. However, some patients may be uniquely sensitive to the toxic effect because of their genetics or their physical condition, for example β-blockers may precipitate heart failure in patients with pre-existing impaired left ventricular function.

Pharmacological toxicity is the most common cause of adverse effects. Such toxicity can be minimised by an assessment of the risk–benefit balance for the individual patient. This should take into account factors that may influence both pharmacokinetics and sensitivity, including age, physiological status (e.g. renal function), concurrent medication, disease processes, environmental aspects (e.g. smoking), etc.

Table 53.2
Therapeutic windows based on plasma concentrations

Drug	Therapeutic concentration range[a]		Toxic response
	Minimum	Maximum[b]	
Aspirin (analgesia) (μg ml^{-1})	20	300	Tinnitus, metabolic acidosis
Carbamazepine (μg ml^{-1})	4	10	Drowsiness, visual disturbances
Digitoxin (ng ml^{-1})	15	30	Bradycardia, nausea
Digoxin (ng ml^{-1})	0.8	3	Bradycardia, nausea
Gentamicin (μg ml^{-1})	2	12	Ototoxicity, renal toxicity
Kanamycin (μg ml^{-1})	10	40	Ototoxicity, renal toxicity
Phenytoin (μg ml^{-1})	10	20	Nystagmus, lethargy
Theophylline (μg ml^{-1})	10	20	Tremor, nervousness

[a]The values given represent average values only, patients will vary in their inherent sensitivity and response to particular concentrations. The concept of a therapeutic window also applies to situations where the response can be measured directly (e.g. blood clotting control with warfarin and hypoglycaemia with oral hypoglycaemics).
[b]The maximum concentration may be based on toxicity related to the primary therapeutic response (e.g. carbamazepine) or an unrelated effect (e.g. gentamicin).

Table 53.3
Drugs with adverse effects unrelated to their primary therapeutic use

Drug	Adverse effect
Opioid analgesic	Respiratory depression when used for analgesia
β-Blocker	Reduction in heart rate when used for hypertension
Anticonvulsant	Sedation, when used for epilepsy

Because of the predictable nature of pharmacological toxicity, it is possible to co-prescribe drugs that will minimise toxic effects. Examples include anti-emetics given with cancer chemotherapy, vitamin B_6 given with isoniazid, and leucovorin (folinic acid) given after methotrexate.

Biochemical toxicity

This toxicity or tissue damage is caused by an interaction of the drug, or an active metabolite, with cell components, especially macromolecules. A generalised scheme is given in Figure 53.2. For most approved drugs, this form of toxicity is characterised during both preclinical studies in animals and early clinical trials (Ch. 3), for example by monitoring changes in serum enzyme levels.

In some situations, an understanding of the mechanism of toxicity has allowed the development of appropriate treatments. An example is the key observation that the thiol (-SH) group of the tripeptide glutathione provides a cytoprotective mechanism for preventing cell damage caused by highly reactive chemical species, such as certain drug metabolites (see below). The nature of the cell damage caused depends on the stability of the reactive chemical (metabolite); extremely unstable metabolites may bind covalently to and inactivate the enzyme that forms them; more stable species may diffuse to a distant site, for example DNA and initiate changes, such as cancer. Some examples of biochemical toxicity and their treatment are given below.

Paracetamol

Paracetamol-induced hepatotoxicity represents the results of an imbalance between inactivation of para-

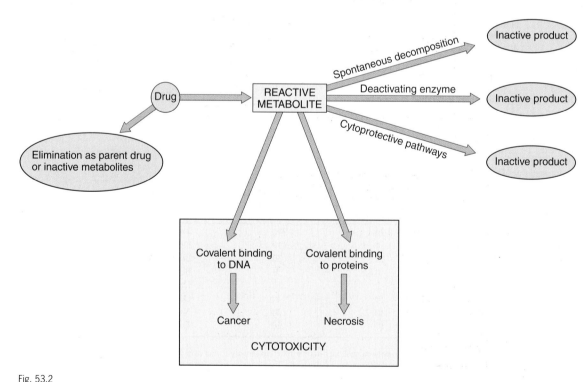

Fig. 53.2
Metabolism and cytotoxicity. The extent of cytotoxicity depends on (i) the balance between the activation process and alternative pathways of elimination of the parent drug, and (ii) the balance between inactivation of the reactive metabolite and the production of biochemically adverse effects. Therapeutic interventions are aimed at either increasing elimination of the parent drug or enhancing cytoprotective pathways.

cetamol via conjugation with glucuronic acid and sulfate and activation via oxidation by cytochrome P450 to an unstable metabolite that binds covalently to proteins and causes cell necrosis. Low doses are safe because they are eliminated by conjugation with little oxidation. However, in overdose the conjugation reactions are saturated and there is increased cytochrome P450-mediated oxidation to an unstable quinone-imine metabolite (Fig. 53.3). Early after an overdose, much of the toxic metabolite is inactivated by a cytoprotective pathway involving glutathione, but as the available glutathione becomes depleted there is increased covalent binding and cell death. This mechanism explains the site of toxicity (centrilobular necrosis in the liver because of the large amounts of cytochrome P450 present) and the increased toxicity seen in patients

treated with inducers of cytochrome P450 (especially alcohol-related induction of CYP2E1). An understanding of the mechanism of toxicity of paracetamol led to the development of treatment with N-acetylcysteine, which enhances the cytoprotective processes by providing an additional source of thiol groups for conjugation of the active metabolite and protection of thiol groups in proteins (see below).

The sulfur-containing amino acid methionine can also prevent paracetamol-induced hepatotoxicity and a combination of paracetamol plus methionine (comethiamol) is available. Such a formulation may prove to be of particular value to high-risk groups such as children (because of the greater risk of accidental overdose) and alcoholics (because of the possibility of induction of CYP2E1 and depressed glutathione levels).

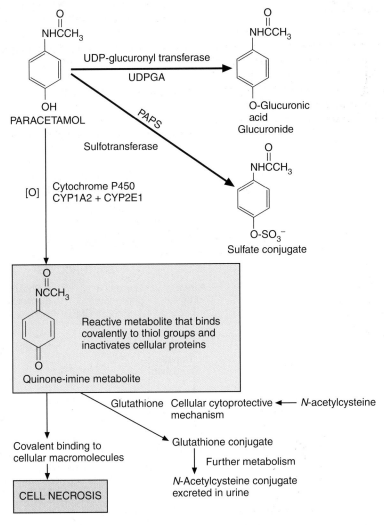

Fig. 53.3
Pathways of paracetamol metabolism. In overdose the concentrations of 3′-phosphoadenosine 5′-phosphosulfate (PAPS) (for sulfation) and glutathione (for cytoprotection) are depleted and extensive macromolecular binding leads to hepatocellular necrosis. UDPGA, uridine diphosphate glucuronic acid.

Cyclophosphamide

Cyclophosphamide is an anticancer drug that is converted to highly toxic metabolites which are eliminated in the urine and cause haemorrhagic cystitis (Ch. 52). This can be prevented by prior treatment with mesna (mercaptoethane sulfonic acid), which possesses both a thiol group for cytoprotection and a highly polar sulfonic acid group, which results in high renal excretion and delivery of this cytoprotective molecule to the bladder epithelium. Because of its polarity, mesna is absorbed from the gut slowly and incompletely but is eliminated rapidly. It is, therefore, given intravenously prior to cyclophosphamide and to cover the period of maximum excretion of toxic metabolites. It is not yet known if mesna will also protect the urinary bladder from the delayed consequence of cyclophosphamide, that is from bladder cancer that arises about 10–20 years after initial treatment.

Isoniazid

Isoniazid, which is used for the treatment of tuberculosis (Ch. 51), causes hepatitis in about 0.5% of patients. This is believed to occur through increased formation of a reactive metabolite, N-acetylhydrazine, which is formed by acetylation followed by oxidative metabolism. Fast acetylators (see Ch. 2) form more N-acetylhydrazine than do slow acetylators but, unexpectedly, they are not more sensitive to isoniazid toxicity. The biochemical basis for the susceptibility of some patients to the hepatotoxic metabolite is not known; it is possibly related to the balance between further activation of N-acetylhydrazine (by cytochrome P450-mediated oxidation) and detoxication of N-acetylhydrazine, which is by further acetylation. Consequently, fast acetylators may produce more active metabolite and also inactive it more rapidly.

Chloroform

Chloroform is no longer used clinically because of hepatotoxicity, which is mediated by the generation of reactive free radicals during its metabolism.

Spironolactone

Spironolactone (Ch. 14) is oxidised by cytochrome P450. The metabolite formed in the testes binds to and destroys testicular cytochrome P450 and this causes a decrease in the metabolism of progesterone to testosterone (which is also catalysed by a cytochrome P450). This effect, combined with an antiandrogenic action at receptor sites, results in gynaecomastia and decreased libido.

Aromatic amines and nitrites

Aromatic amines, such as the antileprosy drug dapsone and some antimalarials, may cause both haemolysis and methaemoglobinaemia through the generation of toxic metabolites. The active metabolite is formed in the liver and released into the circulation. In the presence of oxygen, the active metabolite oxidises haemoglobin (Fe^{2+}) to methaemoglobin (Fe^{3+}) and is oxidised itself (Fig. 53.4). Because of the large amounts of haemoglobin in the blood, compared with the amount of drug given,

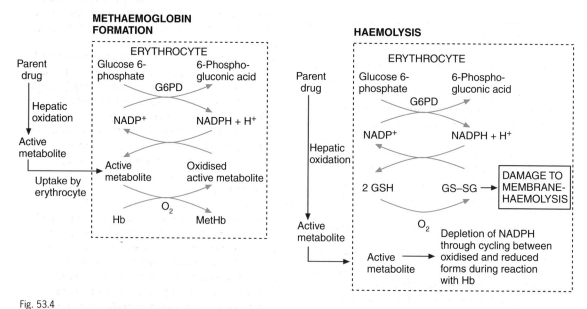

Fig. 53.4
Mechanisms of methaemoglobinaemia and haemolysis. Hb, Haemoglobin; G6PD, glucose 6-phosphate dehydrogenase; GS–SG, glutathione dimer (oxidised form); GSH, glutathione (reduced form), NADP, nicotinamide adenine dinucleotide phosphate. High concentrations of reduced glutathione are necessary for maintaining cell membrane integrity; a build-up of oxidised glutathione is associated with haemolysis. The active metabolite may also react with glutathione directly to lower GSH concentrations.

this would be inconsequential, except that the oxidised active metabolite can be recycled back to the active metabolite by reduction with NADPH (reduced nicotinamide adenine dinucleotide phosphate) in the erythrocyte. Consequently, one molecule of the metabolite is able to oxidise many molecules of haemoglobin. The recycling depends on the presence of NADPH, which is formed during the metabolism of glucose 6-phosphate via glucose 6-phosphate dehydrogenase (G6PD) (Fig. 53.4). Haemolysis arises from accumulation of oxidised glutathione (GS–SG in Fig. 53.4) in the erythrocyte; oxidised glutathione accumulates because recycling of the drug metabolite linked to the formation of methaemoglobin causes depletion of NADPH, which is the cofactor essential for the reduction of oxidised glutathione.

The amounts of G6PD, and hence of NADPH, are determined genetically and the incidence of G6PD deficiency is high in Blacks and very high in Mediterranean races, such as the Kurds. Such subjects have limited NADPH reserves and, therefore, have a decreased ability to reduce either the oxidised drug metabolite or the oxidised glutathione (Fig. 53.4). Because they have insufficient NADPH to drive the interconversion of the oxidised active metabolite and the active metabolite, they are less susceptible to drug-induced methaemoglobinaemia. However, the deficiency in NADPH means that this can be depleted rapidly and the oxidised glutathione cannot be reduced; therefore they are very susceptible to haemolysis. Given the geographical distribution of G6PD deficiency, it is ironic that the amino groups associated with this form of toxicity are found in drugs used to treat tropical infections.

....

Immunological toxicity

Immunological toxicity is frequently referred to as 'drug allergy' and is the form of toxicity with which patients may be most familiar, for example penicillin allergy. Immunological mechanisms are implicated in a number of common adverse effects, such as rashes and fever, but may also be involved in organ-directed toxicity. Although the term allergy may not be strictly correct for all forms of immunologically mediated toxicity, it is probably better than hypersensitivity, which has also been used to describe an elevated sensitivity to any mechanism or effect.

Low-molecular-weight compounds (<1100 Da) are not able to elicit an allergic response unless the compound, or a metabolite, forms a stable or covalent bond with a macromolecule. The process has been recognised for many years and is summarised in Figure 53.5.

Immunologically mediated toxicity shows a wide range of characteristics:

- toxicity is unrelated to pharmacological toxicity but has been implicated in some forms of biochemical toxicity following the formation of a reactive, covalently binding metabolite
- toxicity is unrelated to dose: once the antibody has been produced even very small amounts of antigen can trigger a reaction
- there is normally a lag of at least 3 days between initial exposure and the development of symptoms; however, the first dose of a subsequent treatment may give an immediate reaction
- cross-reactivity is possible between compounds that share the same antigen-determinant or antibody-recognition moiety, such as the penicilloyl group of penicillins
- the incidence varies between different drugs, for example from about 1 in 10 000 for phenylbutazone-induced agranulocytosis to 1 in 20 for ampicillin-related skin rashes
- the response is idiosyncratic but genetically controlled; individual responsiveness cannot be predicted, but individuals who have a history of atopic disease are more likely to develop a drug allergy.

The effects produced may be subdivided into the classical four types of allergic reaction (see also Ch. 38).

- Type I: immediate or anaphylactic reactions. These are mediated via IgE antibodies attached to the surface of basophils and mast cells; the release of numerous mediators, for example histamine, 5-hydroxytryptamine (5HT) and leukotrienes, produces effects that include urticaria, bronchial constriction, hypotension, oedema and shock. A skin-prick challenge test usually produces an acute inflammatory response. Examples of drugs having this type of effect are penicillins and peptide drugs such as crisantaspase.
- Type II: cytotoxic reactions. The antigen is formed by the drug binding to a cell membrane; subsequent interaction of this antigen with circulating IgG, IgM or IgA antibodies activates complement and initiates cell lysis. Loss of the carrier cell can result in thrombocytopenia (e.g. digitoxin, cephalosporins, quinine), neutropenia (e.g. phenylbutazone, metronidazole), and haemolytic anaemia (e.g. penicillins, rifampicin (rifampin) and possibly methyldopa).
- Type III: immune-complex reactions. The antigen–antibody interaction occurs in serum and the complex formed is deposited on endothelial cells, basement membranes, etc. to initiate a more localised inflammatory reaction, for example arteritis and nephritis. Examples include serum sickness (urticaria, angio-oedema, fever) with penicillins, lupus erythematosus-like syndrome with hydralazine and procainamide (especially in slow acetylators) and possibly NSAID-related nephropathy.

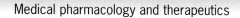

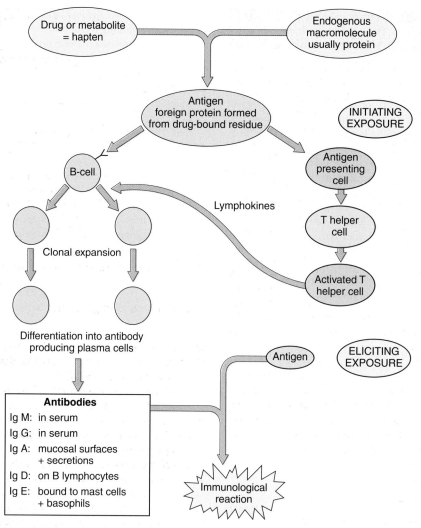

Fig. 53.5
Mechanisms of drug allergy. The initial exposure produces an antigen, which results in the production of antibodies via B-cell clonal expansion and differentiations; this is stimulated by activated T helper cells. The eliciting exposure occurs later (usually at least 3 days later, during which time therapy may or may not be continuing); antigen–antibody interaction exposes a complement-binding site, which triggers the reaction. The nature of the immunological reaction depends on the nature of the antibody and/or localisation of the antigen. Immunosuppressant drugs such as cyclophosphamide, methotrexate and azathioprine act primarily to block the clonal expansion stage; ciclosporin is highly selective and prevents helper T-cell activation without myelosuppression.

- Type IV: cell-mediated reactions. Reaction to the eliciting exposure is delayed. The reactions occur mostly in skin through the formation of an antigen between the drug (hapten) and skin proteins. This is followed by an infiltration of sensitised T-lymphocytes, which recognise the antigen and release lymphokines to produce local inflammation, oedema and irritation, for example contact dermatitis.

In addition to true immunologically mediated toxicity, as described above, there are examples of so-called 'allergic' reactions, such as aspirin hypersensitivity, which show many of the characteristics given above (e.g. rashes, induction of asthma in susceptible patients,

cross-reactivity with other aromatic acids such as benzoates) but for which a true immunological basis has not been demonstrated.

It has been estimated that 'drug allergy' accounts for about 10% of adverse drug reactions but that severe reactions are very rare. For example, only about 5 patients in 10 000 develop an anaphylactic reaction to penicillins, but about one-half of these are sufficiently serious to warrant hospital treatment, which is aimed at blocking the effects on the airways and heart and preventing further mediator release (see Ch. 38). However, given the large numbers of patients receiving drugs such as penicillins, 'drug allergy' is an important source of iatrogenic morbidity.

Drug overdose

Self-poisoning can be either accidental or deliberate. Approximately a quarter of a million episodes are believed to occur each year, although less than 40% of these reach hospital. Deaths from self-poisoning still average about 2000 each year in England and Wales. Accidental poisoning is common in children under 5 years of age, at which age it often involves household products as well as medicines. A second peak of self-poisoning occurs in the teens and early twenties, when it is more frequent in girls. The incidence then progressively falls with increasing age. Most deliberate self-poisoning represents 'parasuicide' or attention-seeking behaviour. True suicide attempts comprise a minority of events, occurring most frequently in patients over 45 years. However, it is important to recognise that the severity of poisoning bears little relationship to suicidal intent. About 30% of the deaths from deliberate overdose are in patients over 65 years of age: self-poisoning at this age occurs most often in response to depression or specific life events such as bereavement.

The drugs most frequently used for self-poisoning are benzodiazepines, analgesics and antidepressants. Alcohol is often taken together with these drugs. It is important to attempt to identify the cause of the poisoning since it may influence treatment. However, it should be remembered that information from the patient about which drug was taken, how much and the time of overdosing is frequently unreliable.

Management principles

The management of drug overdose has a number of principal aims (Fig. 53.6).

....
Managing adverse effects

Immediate measures

There are clear immediate measures required when a patient presents with a possible drug overdose:

- obtain a clear history if possible
- preserve any evidence, for example bottles, written notes, etc.
- remove patient from contact with poison if appropriate, for example gases, corrosives
- assess vital signs: pulse, respiration and pupil size; inspect the patient for injury
- ensure a clear airway; patients who are breathing but unconscious should be placed in the coma position.

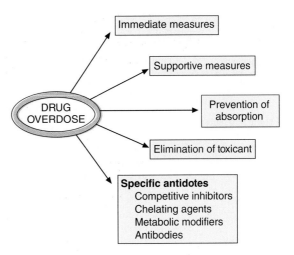

Fig. 53.6
Principles underlying the management of drug overdose.

Supportive measures

Examples of drugs producing specific unwanted effects in overdose are shown in Table 53.4. There are a number of effects produced by drug overdose that will require supportive measures (Fig. 53.7).

Cardiac or respiratory arrest. These may result from a toxic effect of the drug on the heart, depression of the respiratory centre or from metabolic disturbance. In some circumstances, recovery is possible even after prolonged resuscitation.

Cardiovascular complications, including hypotension and arrhythmias. A low blood pressure should be treated if it is accompanied by poor tissue perfusion or low urine output. Arterial dilation and peripheral venous pooling can result from depression of the vasomotor centre and produce a low central venous pressure. This should be raised to 10–15 cmH$_2$O (measured from the midaxillary line) by intravenous infusion of a colloid solution, for example dextran polymers. If blood pressure is low with a normal or raised central venous pressure, this suggests myocardial depression. Inotropic drugs such as dobutamine (Ch. 7) should then be used.

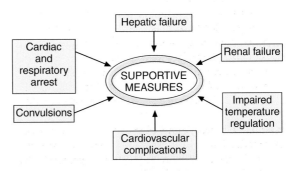

Fig. 53.7
Main effects of overdose requiring supportive measures.

Table 53.4
Complications of acute poisonings

Complications	Cause	Examples of poisons
Cardiac arrest	Direct cardiotoxicity	Many
	Hypoxia	Many
	Electrolyte/metabolic disturbance	Many
Central nervous system depression		Many
Convulsions	Direct neurotoxicity	Tricyclic antidepressants, theophylline
	Hypoxia	Many
Hypotension	Myocardial depression	β-Blockers, tricyclic antidepressants, dextropropoxyphene
	Peripheral vasodilation	Many
Arrhythmia	Direct cardiotoxicity	β-Blockers, tricyclic antidepressants, verapamil, digoxin
	Hypoxia	Many
	Electrolyte/metabolic disturbance	Many
Renal failure	Hypotension	Many
	Rhabdomyolysis	Narcotic drugs, hypnotics, ethanol, carbon monoxide
	Direct nephrotoxicity	Paracetamol, heavy metals
Hepatic failure	Direct hepatotoxicity	Paracetamol, carbon tetrachloride
Respiratory depression	Direct neurotoxicity	Sedatives, hypnotics, narcotics

Disturbances of cardiac rhythm should only be treated if they are severe; however, it is essential to correct metabolic disturbances that predispose to arrhythmias, for example hypothermia, hypoxia, hypercapnia, hypo- or hyperkalaemia and acidosis.

Convulsions. These may be caused by a treatable underlying change such as hypoxia, hypoglycaemia or hypocalcaemia, or they may be a direct toxic effect of the drug on neuronal function. Diazepam, intravenously or rectally (Ch. 20), is the treatment of choice. Artificial ventilation with neuromuscular blockade (Ch. 27) is used if the fits cannot be controlled.

Renal failure. Kidney damage is usually a consequence of prolonged hypotension. Other causes include a direct nephrotoxic effect of the drug and renal damage produced by the products of toxic muscle necrosis (rhabdomyolysis).

Hepatic failure. This usually results from the direct toxic effects of specific agents, such as paracetamol.

Impaired temperature regulation. Hypothermia is common, caused by depression of metabolic rate with reduced heat production and by increased heat loss from cutaneous vasodilatation. Rewarming reduces the risk of serious ventricular arrhythmias. By contrast, aspirin can produce hyperthermia by uncoupling cellular oxidative phosphorylation.

Reducing toxicity

The amount of poison that is available to cause the adverse effects can be reduced by:

- minimising further absorption
- maximising elimination
- negating effects with antidotes, etc.

Prevention of absorption of poisons

There are three principal methods of preventing further absorption of the drug:

Emesis. Vomiting can be induced in a conscious patient who has not ingested a corrosive agent. Stimulation of the pharynx can be tried in children but is often ineffective. Ipecacuanha is sometimes advocated to induce vomiting. It is a plant extract, containing emetine and cephaeline, that irritates the stomach and stimulates the medullary vomiting centre. Most patients vomit within 30 min and prolonged vomiting can occur. There are doubts as to its effectiveness in removing drug from the stomach and the unwanted effects of ipecacuanha (nausea, drowsiness and lethargy) may mask symptoms of the overdose; in consequence the routine use of emetics is no longer recommended.

Gastric aspiration and lavage. This should not be considered in unconscious patients without protection of the airway by an endotracheal tube to prevent aspiration of gastric contents. A large-bore orogastric tube is used to aspirate gastric contents initially and then to lavage with doses of water at body temperature. Its effectiveness is unproven. Gastric lavage is recommended normally for up to 2 h after ingestion of a significant amount of drug. There may be benefit for up to 4 h after aspirin and/or in unconscious patients and for up to 4–6 h after a life-threatening overdose of tricyclic antidepressants.

Activated charcoal. This formulation has a large adsorbent area and is given as a suspension in water. Activated charcoal adsorbs, or binds, the drug and

Table 53.5
Drug adsorption onto activated charcoal

Drug/compounds not adsorbed	Drugs/compounds adsorbed
Acids	Aspirin
Alkalis	Carbamazepine
Cyanide	Dapsone
DDT (insecticide)	Digoxin
Ethanol	Ecstacy
Ethyleneglycol (antifreeze)	Paraquat (herbicide)
Ferrous salts	Phenobarbital
Lead	Quinine
Lithium	Sustained-release preparations
Mercury	Theophylline
Methanol	Tricyclic antidepressants
Organic solvents	

retains it in the gastrointestinal lumen; not all drugs are adsorbed onto charcoal (Table 53.5). About 10 g of charcoal is required to every 1 g of poison, which makes it impractical for poisons that are usually ingested in large quantities, for example paracetamol. An initial dose of charcoal can prevent drug absorption if given within 4 h of drug ingestion. Repeated administration over 24–36 h achieves further adsorption of drug in the small intestine. Drug is continuously being transferred in both directions across the gut wall, with the concentration gradient normally favouring net absorption. If drug in the bowel is adsorbed onto the charcoal, this lowers the free concentration and can result in net transfer into the gut and enhanced elimination of the compound from the body. Constipation is the major unwanted effect of charcoal; charcoal should not be given in the absence of bowel sounds because of the risk of obstruction.

Elimination of poisons

There are three principal methods of enhancing elimination of the drug: activated charcoal (see above), renal elimination and haemodialysis/haemoperfusion.

Renal elimination. Forced diuresis with intravenous infusion of large quantities of fluid has been advocated in the past for drugs that are mostly eliminated unchanged by the kidney or if renally excreted metabolites are toxic. A major potential disadvantage of forced diuresis is serious disturbance of fluid or electrolyte balance and it is not now used. Altering urine pH can be effective in increasing the renal elimination of drugs that are weak electrolytes. This is achieved by increasing the ionisation of the drug, which reduces reabsorption from the renal tubule by lowering its lipid solubility (Ch. 2). Only a modest increase in urinary flow rate is required. Weak acids are more readily excreted in alkaline urine (alkaline diuresis) while the converse is true for weak bases (acid diuresis). Alkalinisation of the urine can be achieved with sodium bicarbonate and acidification with ammonium chloride.

Haemodialysis or haemoperfusion. These are reserved for the most severely poisoned patients, and large amounts of drug must be retained in the plasma (a low apparent volume of distribution; see Ch. 2) for the techniques to be successful. Haemodialysis relies on diffusion of the drug across a semipermeable membrane from blood to the dialysis fluid. Haemoperfusion involves adsorption of drug from blood as it passes down a column containing activated charcoal or a resin.

Specific antidotes

Antidotes are only available for a minority of drugs commonly involved in poisonings. Some important examples are given below.

Competitive inhibitors

- Atropine acts at muscarinic receptors to block the parasympathetic effects of organophosphorus insecticides.
- Naloxone acts at opioid receptors to reverse the effects of narcotic analgesics.
- Flumazenil is an antagonist at benzodiazepine receptors. It is rarely needed for the treatment of intentional overdose, because fatalities are uncommon with this class of drug. It is of value in reversing the effects of benzodiazepines when toxicity occurs in patients with chronic liver disease.

Chelating agents

Chelating agents act by forming a complex with the drug or chemical, which reduces the free concentration:

- desferrioxamine for ferrous ions
- dicobalt edetate for cyanide
- dimercaprol for gold, lead, mercury and arsenic
- penicillamine for copper and lead
- sodium calcium edetate for lead.

Compounds that affect drug metabolism

Ethanol is used in the treatment of methanol poisoning, because it acts as a competitive substrate for alcohol dehydrogenase, preventing formation of the toxic metabolites formaldehyde and formic acid.

N-Acetylcysteine provides a substrate for conjugation of the cytotoxic metabolite of paracetamol when the natural conjugating ligand, glutathione, is depleted.

Antibodies

Digoxin can be neutralised in severe poisoning by specific antibody fragments. The antibodies are raised in sheep and cleaved to remove the antigenic crystalline (Fc) portion of the molecule while retaining the specific antigen-binding fragment (Fab).

Some specific common poisonings

Paracetamol

Paracetamol overdose can be fatal, with about 200 deaths occurring each year in England and Wales. Metabolism of paracetamol takes place in the liver, mainly producing non-toxic conjugates (Fig. 53.3). A small amount is oxidised by the cytochrome P450 system to an active metabolite that is inactivated by conjugation with the thiol group on glutathione. When hepatic glutathione is depleted (which occurs readily in overdose), the metabolite denatures protein to produce hepatic necrosis. Similar processes in the kidney can cause renal tubular necrosis.

Gastric aspiration and lavage is recommended within 4 h of a potentially serious paracetamol overdosage. In the first 24 h, there are few symptoms apart from nausea, vomiting, abdominal pain and sweating. Liver damage begins within 24 h after a large overdose, producing right upper quadrant pain and tenderness. The patient usually becomes jaundiced by 36–48 h and can progress to severe or even fatal liver failure. The most sensitive measures of liver damage are the prothrombin time, or the international normalised ratio (INR), and the plasma unconjugated bilirubin. Renal failure is seen in about a quarter of patients with severe liver damage.

Since antidotes are most effective when given early, blood should be analysed for paracetamol if there is any suspicion of poisoning. Antidotes used in paracetamol poisoning replace glutathione as a thiol donor in the liver; glutathione cannot enter liver cells from the blood and so a substitute is given. Methionine can be given orally as an initial measure but not to patients who have already been given activated charcoal because large amounts are needed and methionine would displace bound paracetamol. Patients admitted 4 h or more post-overdose are treated with intravenous N-acetylcysteine prior to the analysis of plasma paracetamol concentrations. This is currently the preferred treatment, although there is some evidence that N-acetylcysteine is more effective after oral administration, possibly because higher concentrations reach the liver. Treatment used to be confined to the first 15 h after overdose, but recent evidence suggests that liver damage can be reduced even when the antidote is delayed for up to 20–30 h. It may be useful even later after ingestion to reduce the severity of established liver damage. A graph is available (Fig. 53.8) to indicate the risk of liver damage for a given plasma paracetamol concentration related to the time of ingestion. The plasma concentration before 4 h is unreliable because absorption and distribution are still occurring. High plasma concentrations after 15 h must be inferred by extrapolation of the graph. Treatment is only necessary if potentially toxic paracetamol concentrations are detected. It is important to realise that toxicity can occur at much lower plasma paracetamol concentrations under certain circumstances:

- patients who have been using drugs such as alcohol or phenytoin that induce liver cytochrome P450 (Ch. 2) and hence increase the formation of the reactive metabolite
- patients with pre-existing liver disease
- malnourished/anorexic patients
- patients infected with human immunodeficiency virus.

All such patients should be treated if plasma paracetamol concentrations are only one-half of those given in Figure 53.8.

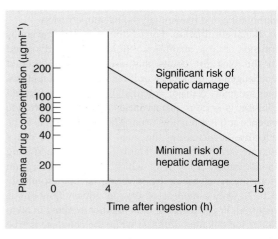

Fig. 53.8
Relationship between plasma paracetamol concentration and the risk of liver damage.

Salicylates

Although salicylate poisoning is becoming less common, there are still about 150 deaths each year in England and Wales. Aspirin is hydrolysed rapidly to salicylic acid after absorption but further metabolism, by conjugation, is rate limited. Symptoms of toxicity are nausea, vomiting, abdominal pain, tinnitus, hyperventilation and sweating. Agitation frequently occurs in adults, but children become comatose. The chain of metabolic events produced by aspirin is shown in Figure 53.9.

Gastric aspiration for up to 4 h after the overdose is widely practised since aspirin tends to remain in the stomach; however, activated charcoal may be better for reducing absorption and enhancing elimination. Correction of fluid, electrolyte and acid–base balance is fundamental to successful management; a fluid deficit of 3–4 l is not unusual in severe poisoning. Forced alkaline diuresis is no longer advocated to enhance salicylate elimination; simple alkalinisation of the urine to raise the pH above 7.5 is effective and safer. In severe poisoning, haemodialysis is the treatment of choice.

Tricyclic antidepressants

Approximately 400 deaths per year occur in England and Wales from overdose with tricyclic antidepressants.

Symptoms are caused by antimuscarinic effects and actions on the heart. The antimuscarinic effects delay gastric emptying and, therefore, gastric lavage or oral activated charcoal is used routinely for up to 4 h after the overdose and can be useful for up to 6 h. Induction of emesis is not used because of the risk of central nervous system (CNS) depression or convulsions with tricyclic antidepressants. Repeated doses of activated charcoal may be useful for large tricyclic antidepressant overdoses or when a sustained-release formulation has been taken, but they have little effect on the elimination of the drug. Other approaches are ineffective, and supportive measures are of greatest importance. Drowsiness and confusion are followed by coma in more severely poisoned patients. Cardiac depression can produce hypotension, and serious arrhythmias such as ventricular tachycardia can occur. Electrocardiographic monitoring is recommended for at least 24 h. Arrhythmias frequently respond to correction of acidosis. If this is not successful, phenytoin or direct current shock can be used. Drugs that depress cardiac contractility should be avoided.

Opioid analgesics

The triad of signs characteristic of opioid overdose are respiratory depression, pinpoint pupils and impaired consciousness (Ch. 19). They can be reversed rapidly by naloxone, which is a competitive antagonist at opioid μ-receptors. After the response to an initial intravenous bolus dose of naloxone, it is often necessary to give repeated boluses or a continuous infusion because the half-life of naloxone is very short compared with those of most opioids. The effect of naloxone in poisoning produced by buprenorphine is often incomplete, and nonspecific respiratory stimulants (Ch. 13) may also be needed. Acute poisoning with organophosphorus insecticides can produce signs that are similar to those with opioids, but naloxone will have no effect.

Ecstasy

Ecstasy (methylenedioxymethamphetamine; MDMA), toxicity is characterised by tachycardia, hyper-reflexia, hyperpyrexia and initial hypertension leading to hypotension. In severe cases, delirium, convulsions, coma and cardiac dysrhythmias may occur. MDMA is metabolised by CYP2D6 (Ch. 2) and genetic differences in this enzyme may result in wide interindividual differences in susceptibility to the toxic effects of MDMA. Some patients may present with hyponatraemia, possibly as a result of drinking excessive water as a precaution to prevent dehydration. Treatments include activated charcoal, but only for up to 2 h postingestion since MDMA is absorbed rapidly, plus diazepam, β-blockers and dantrolene as appropriate.

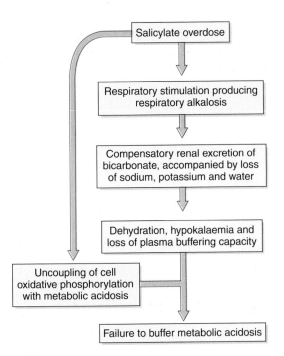

Fig. 53.9
The metabolic consequences of salicylate overdose.

FURTHER READING

Bateman DN (1994) NSAIDs: Time to re-evaluate gut toxicity. *Lancet* 343, 1051–1052

Buckley NA, Dawson AH, Whyte IM, Henry DA (1994) Greater toxicity in overdose of dothiepin than of other tricyclic antidepressants. *Lancet* 343, 159–162

Buckley NA, Dawson AH, Whyte IM, O'Connell DL (1995) Relative toxicity of benzodiazepines in overdose. *Br Med J* 310, 219–221

Edwards JG (1995) Suicide and antidepressants. Controversies on prevention, provocation, and self poisoning continue. *Br Med J* 310, 205–206

Hawton K, Ware C, Mistry H et al. (1995) Why patients choose paracetamol for self poisoning and their knowledge of its dangers. *Br Med J* 310, 164

Henry JA, Alexander CA, Sener EK (1995) Relative mortality from overdose of antidepressants. *Br Med J* 310, 221–224

Jick SS, Dean AD, Jick H (1995) Antidepressants and suicide. *Br Med J* 310, 215–218

Lee WM (1995) Drug-induced hepatotoxicity. *N Engl J Med* 333, 1118–1127

Park BK, Kitteringham NR, Pirmohamed M, Tucker GT (1996) Relevance of induction of human drug-metabolising enzymes: pharmacological and toxicological implications. *Br J Clin Pharmacol* 41, 477–491

Roujeau JC, Stern RS (1994) Severe adverse cutaneous reactions to drugs. *N Engl J Med* 331, 1272–1285

Vale JA, Proudfoot AT (1995) Paracetamol (acetaminophen) poisoning. *Lancet* 346, 547–552

Waring RH, Emery P (1995) The genetic origin of responses to drugs. *Br Med Bull* 51, 449–461

Self-assessment

1. Case history question

> A 70-year-old man with a history of depressive illness and alcohol abuse was prescribed a compound analgesic containing 500 mg paracetamol and 30 mg codeine phosphate. Eight hours after collecting his prescription he was seen as an emergency by his GP, who considered he had taken an overdose and he was admitted to hospital.

   a. What features might be seen soon after the overdosage and during the subsequent 24–48 h?
   b. Outline what suitable pharmacological treatments should be undertaken
   c. Would co-dydramol have been a safer alternative to prescribe?

   The answers are provided on pages 632.

54

Drugs of abuse

Drug abuse and dependence

A number of therapeutic drugs may be used as drugs of abuse because of their effects on the nervous system. Abuse is defined as any drug used in a manner that differs from the approved use in that culture. Examples include hypnotics and anxiolytics (Ch. 20) and opioid analgesics (Ch. 19), and these are discussed in the relevant chapters. This chapter covers other drugs that are encountered in clinical practice primarily because of their abuse potential. The effects of these agents are often complicated by the impurity and multiple constituents of samples of the abused drug.

Most drugs with potential for abuse also produce dependence. This is a syndrome that exists when an individual continues to take a drug because of the pleasurable effect it produces, despite adverse social consequences or medical harm that it might produce. Dependence produces varying degrees of need for the drug, from mild desire to a craving.

Dependence may be psychological, caused by the unpleasant psychological reaction or dysphoria that occurs on drug withdrawal, or physical, when there are abnormalities of behaviour and autonomic symptoms on withdrawal. Physical dependence causes symptoms on drug withdrawal that can be provoked by the use of a specific antagonist to the drug.

The biological basis of dependence is believed to be related to dopaminergic and serotoninergic activity arising in the ventral tegmental area, and relaying via the nucleus accumbens to the prefrontal cortex. The globus pallidus, amygdala, locus ceruleus and raphe nuclei are also involved in addiction. Most drugs of abuse release dopamine in these regions of the brain, and withdrawal leads to reduced dopaminergic function in the same areas. Dopamine D_2 receptors are primarily involved in drug-seeking behaviour by facilitating stimuli that release dopamine in the nucleus accumbens. Dopamine D_1 receptors may enhance this response. The nucleus accumbens is also involved in the motivational effects of food and sex. Other neurotransmitters including noradrenaline, 5-hydroxytryptamine (5HT, serotonin) and glutamate may also be involved in the genesis of dependence, but their role is less well understood.

Drugs of abuse

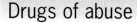

Central nervous system stimulants

Several drugs that have central stimulant properties are abused and produce dependence. Those more commonly encountered are considered here.

Cocaine

Cocaine is also known as 'coke', 'Charlie', 'crack' or 'snow'.

Mechanism of action and effects

Many of the psychic effects of cocaine may relate to inhibition of catecholamine reuptake into nerve terminals. This in turn may activate opioid systems in the brain, with upregulation of μ-receptors (Ch. 19). Cocaine binds strongly to the catecholamine reuptake transporters, particularly that for dopamine. Effects in the mesocorticolimbic dopaminergic pathways, possibly via dopamine D_2 receptors, appear to be important for reinforcing the use of the drug. Increased activity in serotonergic pathways may contribute to wakefulness. Changes in various pituitary neuroendocrine functions occur with more prolonged use; in particular, release of corticotrophin and luteinising hormone (LH) is enhanced. Tolerance to the psychic effects of cocaine is limited. One of the metabolites of cocaine, norcocaine, has direct vasoconstrictor activity.

Effects of cocaine include:

- intense euphoria
- alertness and wakefulness
- increased confidence and strength
- heightened sexual feelings
- indifference to concerns and cares
- severe emotional, but not physical, dependence through the reinforcing effect of the rapid onset, yet brief duration of action; this develops particularly rapidly with 'crack' cocaine
- despondency and despair rapidly follow withdrawal; after chronic use, withdrawal can produce a dysphoric mood with fatigue, vivid dreams, insomnia or excessive sleeping, increased appetite and either psychomotor retardation or agitation
- toxic psychosis, with delusions and sensations of great stamina, occurs with chronic use
- in overdose, excessive catecholamine concentrations produce fear, convulsions, hypertension, cardiac rhythm disturbances and hyperthermia; if severe, death can occur from respiratory depression and circulatory collapse (the cardiovascular toxicity can be treated with combined α- and β-adrenoceptor blockade, and seizures by intravenous diazepam)
- cocaine snuff produces necrosis of the nasal septum through its vasoconstrictor action.

Pharmacokinetics

Cocaine can be used orally, intranasally or by intravenous injection; the last gives a rapid onset of effect and avoids inactivation by first-pass metabolism. In the free base form it is smoked, often as 'crack' cocaine (mixed with sodium bicarbonate), which produces an intense psychic reaction. Cocaine is metabolised by plasma esterases and its half-life is very short.

Management of cocaine dependence

There are no recognised drug treatments for cocaine dependency. Behavioural treatments remain the main approach. Tricyclic antidepressants are sometimes advocated for severe depression on withdrawal.

Amphetamine and derivatives

Amphetamine, methamphetamine ('speed', 'uppers') and 3,4-methylenedioxymethamphetamine (MDMA, 'Ecstasy') are all drugs of abuse.

Mechanism of action and effects

The amphetamine drugs have indirect sympathomimetic effects (Ch. 4) and also inhibit neuronal reuptake of several monoamines, which produces central nervous system (CNS) stimulation. This is most marked in the reticular formation but occurs in many other areas of the brain. The D-isomer (dexamphetamine) is twice as potent as the L-isomer of amphetamine in its central stimulant activity. Effects include:

- euphoria, similar to that experienced with cocaine
- psychotic behaviour with prolonged use
- acute intoxication with amphetamine produces tremor, confusion, irritability, hallucinations and paranoid behaviour
- actions on the heart and circulation can lead to hypertension, cardiac arrhythmias, convulsions and death
- tolerance develops to some of the central effects of amphetamine, such as euphoria and anorexia, presumably through central monoamine depletion
- withdrawal leads to depression, anxiety and craving, soon followed by fatigue, sleep disturbance and increased appetite.

MDMA (Ecstasy) produces euphoria similar to that of amphetamine but with less stimulant effect. Disturbance of thermoregulatory homeostasis occurs, leading to a syndrome resembling heat stroke with hyperthermia and dehydration, usually after exertion in hot environments. The toxic effects of MDMA include cardiac arrhythmias, convulsions and severe metabolic acidosis, which may be fatal. The long-term toxicity is unknown.

Pharmacokinetics

Although amphetamine is sometimes used intravenously, absorption from the gut is rapid and complete. About half is then excreted unchanged in the urine, and the rest is metabolised in the liver. The half-life of amphetamine varies according to urine pH; if the urine is acid then greater ionisation increases excretion (Ch. 2) to produce a short half-life. By contrast, if urine pH is high, then the half-life is longer because of reduced ionisation which leads to greater tubule reabsorption of amphetamine. Metabolites of amphetamine are believed to contribute to the psychotic effects seen with long-term use.

Cannabis

Cannabis is also referred to as 'dope', 'pot' or 'hash'. Cannabis can be smoked as marijuana, which consists of dried leaves or flowers of the cannabis plant, or as resin scraped from the leaves of the plant and then dried, known as hashish. Solvent extraction of the resin produces cannabis oil, which can be added to tobacco.

Mechanism of action and effects

The mechanism of action of cannabis is unknown, although cannabinoids interact with specific receptors in the brain for which there is a natural ligand called anandamide. The receptor is found in greatest density in areas of the brain involved in cognition, memory reward, pain recognition and motor coordination. Some of the effects of cannabis may be mediated by changes in neuronal prostanoid synthesis.

- The psychic effects result largely from the derivative tetrahydrocannabinol (THC), which produces euphoria, heightened intensity of sensations, relaxation and sleepiness. This may be accompanied by panic reactions, hallucinations, paranoid feelings and depersonalisation. Psychotic reactions can occur in predisposed individuals. Recent memory is markedly impaired and complex mental tests are less well executed. Driving ability may be impaired.
- Effects on the cardiovascular system include tachycardia and increased systolic blood pressure with a postural fall.
- The tars inhaled during chronic use predispose to heart disease, chronic bronchitis and lung cancer.
- THC has an anti-emetic action, which has been used to prevent the nausea and vomiting (Ch. 32) associated with cancer chemotherapy (Ch. 52).
- Tolerance to the psychic effects of cannabis occurs with regular use.

Pharmacokinetics

Metabolism of THC is extensive, with some active metabolites being produced. The high lipid solubility of THC means that absorption from the lung or gut is high, with a large volume of distribution and a correspondingly long half-life. The psychic effects, however, only last 2–3 h after inhalation.

Hallucinogenic agents

Hallucinogens include lysergic acid diethylamide (LSD; 'acid') and psilocybin ('magic mushrooms').

Mechanism of action and effects

The actions of hallucinogens on the brain are probably related to presynaptic $5HT_{1A}$ receptor blockade in the dorsal raphe neurons. Presynaptic receptor blockade inhibits neuronal firing and decreases neuronal activity in the forebrain. However, LSD also acts as an agonist at postsynaptic $5HT_2$ receptors in the locus ceruleus. Tolerance occurs rapidly and appears to be related to downregulation of these receptors. The actions of LSD and psilocybin are similar.

- Psychic effects predominate at low doses.
- Visual hallucinations are frequent and auditory acuity is accentuated. Time appears to pass rapidly and emotions are altered with either elation or depression. The overall experience can produce a 'good' or a 'bad' trip. Serious psychotic reactions can occasionally occur.
- Excessive sympathetic nervous system stimulation with large doses produces nausea, dizziness, mydriasis, tremor, tachycardia and hypertension.
- Visual hallucinations occur with highest doses. There may be an overlap of sensory impressions so that music is 'seen' or colours 'heard', which can produce severe anxiety.
- Emotional dependence is frequent but physical dependence is not.

Pharmacokinetics

Oral absorption is good and the half-lives are short.

Nicotine

Mechanism of action

Addiction to smoking involves several factors, both pharmacological and non-pharmacological. Over 300 chemical compounds are present in tobacco smoke. The actions of nicotine are believed to be of major importance but are not solely responsible for the effects of smoking. Nicotine produces dose-related responses. At low doses, stimulation of aortic and carotid chemoreceptors enhances sympathetic nervous system activity (Ch. 4). At higher doses, there is direct stimulation of the nicotinic N_1 receptors on autonomic ganglia (Ch. 4). At even higher doses, nicotine acts as a ganglion-blocking agent. Initial stimulation of autonomic nervous tissue is

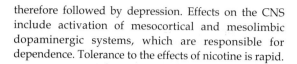

therefore followed by depression. Effects on the CNS include activation of mesocortical and mesolimbic dopaminergic systems, which are responsible for dependence. Tolerance to the effects of nicotine is rapid.

Pharmacokinetics of nicotine

Nicotine is absorbed from the mouth in its unionised form, which is found in the alkaline environment of cigar and pipe tobacco smoke. Acid cigarette smoke ionises nicotine, which can then only be absorbed in adequate amounts from the larger surface area of the lung. Nicotine can also be absorbed transdermally. It is metabolised in the liver and has a short half-life.

Effects of nicotine and tobacco

Tobacco components including nicotine have effects on a number of organ systems.

Respiratory effects. The lungs are the first area to be in contact with the chemical components and are also exposed to particles and gases.

- Reduction of activity of cilia in bronchi decreases clearance of lung secretions.
- An increase in carboxyhaemoglobin concentration in blood reduces oxygen carrying capacity. This may be important in patients with ischaemic heart disease, increasing the chance of provoking angina.
- Increased mucus secretion leads to chronic bronchitis and chronic obstructive lung disease. Progressive destruction of the supporting tissue in the bronchioles produces emphysema and airway obstruction.
- The risk of lung cancer is increased to about 20 times that of a non-smoker. Inhalation of tobacco smoke is a major contributory factor and explains the greater risk in cigarette smokers. Giving up smoking reduces the risk progressively over about 10 years of abstinence. The constituent of tobacco smoke responsible for altering DNA structure and initiating the cancer process remains controversial, but the relationship between smoking and lung cancer has been confirmed by numerous epidemiological studies. Compared with non-smokers, passive smokers also have a 20–25% increased risk of lung cancer.

Psychological effects. The psychological effects of smoking are substantial, as indicated by the difficulties experienced by those 'giving up smoking'.

- Decreased appetite, with weight gain on stopping smoking.
- Emotional dependence on nicotine and the physical act of smoking is powerful. Physical withdrawal is less marked but includes restlessness, irritability, anxiety, depression, difficulty concentrating, decreased heart rate and increased appetite.

Cardiovascular effects. The risk of cardiovascular disease is increased and it occurs at a younger age. The overall risk of death from coronary artery disease is doubled in smokers compared with non-smokers, but the magnitude of the effect is related to the numbers of cigarettes smoked. The risk falls over the first 3–5 years after stopping smoking to a level close to that of non-smokers. Peripheral vascular disease and stroke are also increased. Even passive smokers have an excess risk of vascular disease of 25%. Contributory effects to the increased risk include increased plasma fatty acids and enhanced platelet aggregability.

Other effects. Nicotine and smoking have a number of other effects:

- peptic ulceration is twice as common in smokers
- smoking during pregnancy has several effects, the most important of which is an increased risk of a low-birthweight child
- smoking induces a number of the cytochrome P450 isoenzymes (Ch. 2) and increases the clearance of drugs such as theophylline (Ch. 12) and imipramine (Ch. 22)
- nicotine patches are sometimes used to reduce the symptoms of ulcerative colitis; they have no effect in Crohn's disease.

Withdrawal from nicotine

Withdrawal is often difficult to achieve unless motivation is high. Patients should be supported by counselling about health gains and advice on overcoming problems.

Nicotine replacement therapy. Smokers adjust their smoking habit to maintain plasma nicotine concentrations just above a threshold. The concentration falls within 1 h of the last cigarette and the craving for a cigarette can be reduced by nicotine replacement. This can be delivered from transdermal patches, by nicotine gum or via an inhaler or nasal spray. Established cardiovascular disease is a caution for, but not a contraindication to, nicotine replacement therapy. Behavioural therapy enhances the success rate achieved by nicotine replacement therapy. Use of nicotine replacement therapy doubles the chance of achieving abstinence.

Bupropion. This is an atypical antidepressant that is effective for enhancing tobacco withdrawal and is additive to the effect of nicotine patches, producing a modest increase in the chance of stopping. It is a weak inhibitor of neuronal reuptake of noradrenaline, 5HT and dopamine. It is used in a slow-release formulation and has a long half-life, with hepatic metabolism to active metabolites. Treatment is usually started 1 week before a 'quit date'. Unwanted effects include insomnia and dry mouth.

Alcohol (ethyl alcohol)

Mechanism of action and effects

It is unclear how alcohol (ethyl alcohol, ethanol) achieves its CNS effects. Non-specific actions such as increased

Possible mechanisms of action of alcohol

Inhibition of monoamine oxidase B in neurons
Inhibition of Na^+/K^+-ATPase in neuronal membranes
Increased neuronal adenylate cyclase activity
Decreased intracellular phosphatidylinositol system
    activity, leading to reduced Ca^{2+} availability
Enhanced opioid δ-receptor activation

Alcoholic content of alcoholic drinks

1 unit alcohol is about 10 g and is found in
½ pint of beer, lager, cider
1½ pints low-alcohol beer, lager, cider
⅓ pint strong beer, lager, cider
⅕ pint extra strong beer, lager, cider
1 glass of wine (8 units per 75 cl bottle)
1 small measure of sherry (13 units per bottle)
1 standard measure of spirits (30 units per bottle)
⅔ bottle of 'alcopop'

fluidity of neuronal cell membranes (cf. general anaesthetics) may reduce Ca^{2+} flux across the cell membrane but several other actions have been described (Box 54.1). Overall, alcohol facilitates central inhibitory neurotransmission, particularly via enhancing the effects of gamma-aminobutyric acid (GABA). Alcohol is a general CNS depressant. There is initial depression of inhibitory neurons, which produces a sense of relaxation, followed by progressive depression of all CNS functions. Mental processes that are modified by education, training and previous experience are affected first, while relatively 'mechanical' tasks are less impaired. Despite subjective impressions, there is no increase in mental or physical capabilities unless anxiety had previously reduced performance. All effects are closely related to blood alcohol concentration (Table 54.1).

Tolerance to many of the psychological effects of alcohol is seen in chronic alcoholics. Alcohol intake is usually measured in units (Box 54.2).

Pharmacokinetics

Although some ethanol is absorbed from the stomach, the majority is absorbed from the small intestine. High concentrations of alcohol (above 20%) and large volumes inhibit gastric emptying and delay absorption, as do foods high in fat or carbohydrate. Peak blood alcohol concentrations, therefore, depend on the dose and strength of the alcohol and on whether or not it was taken with food. Once absorbed, distribution of alcohol is fairly uniform and the ready passage across the blood–brain barrier and high cerebral blood flow ensure rapid access to the CNS. The effects on the brain are more marked when the concentration is rising, indicating a degree of acute tolerance.

Metabolism occurs mainly in the liver (Fig. 54.1), more than 90% being oxidised by alcohol dehydrogenase at a fixed rate that averages 10 ml h^{-1}. Acetaldehyde is produced and then further metabolised by aldehyde dehydrogenase (Fig. 54.1). Intracellular accumulation of acetaldehyde is responsible for many of the unpleasant effects of a hangover. Small amounts of alcohol are metabolised via the microsomal ethanol oxidising system (CYP2E1), the activity of which is increased by enzyme inducers such as alcohol itself (which does not affect the activity of alcohol dehydrogenase) (Ch. 36). Only 2–5% of alcohol is excreted unchanged, some in exhaled air, which is the basis of the breathalyser test.

Some drugs inhibit aldehyde dehydrogenase, leading to acetaldehyde accumulation if alcohol is taken with them. Typical 'hangover' effects of flushing, sweating, headache and nausea then occur after small amounts of alcohol. These drugs include metronidazole (Ch. 51) and chlorpropamide (Ch. 40). Genetic deficiencies in alcohol and aldehyde dehydrogenases occur particularly among Asians, leading to low levels of alcohol or aldehyde metabolism.

Table 54.1
The effects of alcohol at various plasma concentrations

Plasma concentration (mg 100 ml⁻¹)	Effects
30	Mild euphoria owing to suppression of inhibitory pathways in the cortex; the individual is more talkative, emotionally labile with loss of self-control; the risk of accidental injury is increased
80	The legal limit for driving in the UK; the risk of serious injury in a road accident is more than doubled
100–200	Speech becomes slurred and motor coordination is impaired
> 300	Often produces loss of consciousness
> 400	Frequently fatal as a result of respiratory and vasomotor centre depression

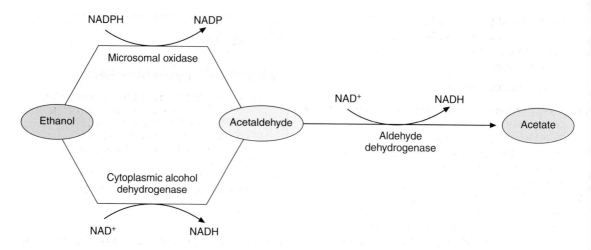

Fig. 54.1
The metabolism of alcohol. Alcohol dehydrogenase is responsible for 80–90% of the metabolism of ethanol.

Other effects of alcohol

Alcohol has a range of effects:

Cardiovascular effects

- A modest alcohol intake may have protective effects on the circulation, by inhibiting platelet aggregation and increasing high density lipoprotein cholesterol. The form in which the alcohol is taken is probably not important. The extent of this beneficial effect may have been overestimated; it is probably greatest at 1 unit per day and is lost when intake exceeds 3–4 units per day.
- Higher intake of alcohol has pressor effects that raise blood pressure, possibly through increased vascular sensitivity to catecholamines. This increases the risk of coronary artery disease and stroke.
- Cardiac arrhythmias can be provoked by high alcohol intake, particularly atrial fibrillation. This can occur after an alcoholic binge ('holiday heart') or following more chronic abuse.
- Alcoholic cardiomyopathy is a dilated cardiomyopathy that is only partially reversible with abstinence, and can lead to heart failure. An average intake of 10 units alcohol daily for 8–10 years can produce this condition.

Liver

- Hypoglycaemia occurs as a consequence of the metabolism of alcohol in the liver. The metabolic process generates excess protons, which encourages the conversion of glucose via pyruvate to lactate and predisposes to lactic acidosis. Alcoholics often have a low-carbohydrate diet, which compounds the hypoglycaemia. Hypoglycaemia tends to occur several hours after heavy alcohol intake and can contribute to convulsions on alcohol withdrawal.
- The lactic acidosis created by alcohol metabolism in the liver impairs the renal excretion of uric acid, which predisposes to gout.
- Lactic acidosis also facilitates synthesis of saturated fatty acids, which accumulate in the liver, leading to a fatty liver, possibly with altered liver function. Plasma triglycerides are also increased.
- Alcoholic hepatitis is usually a consequence of short-term heavy alcohol abuse. It can be fatal.
- Cirrhosis occurs with prolonged alcohol abuse, but individual susceptibility varies widely. On average, consumption of more than 8 units per day for at least 10 years is required for cirrhosis to occur in men. About two-thirds of this amount creates the same risk for women. Established cirrhosis reduces the first-pass metabolism and clearance of drugs eliminated by the liver.
- Chronic intake of alcohol induces several hepatic drug-metabolising enzymes from the cytochrome P450 family, which decreases the effectiveness of some therapeutic drugs, for examples warfarin, phenytoin and carbamazepine.

Other gastrointestinal consequences

- Erosive gastritis can occur as a result of stimulation of gastric secretions.
- Pancreatitis is probably caused by raised triglycerides or by pancreatic duct obstruction by proteinaceous secretions induced by alcohol.

Sexual function

- Sexual desire is often increased by alcohol, but the ability to sustain penile erection is reduced, possibly because of the vasodilator actions of alcohol.
- Direct damage to the Leydig cells of the testis reduces the circulating testosterone, leading to reduced libido, infertility and a loss of the male

distribution of body hair. Altered steroid metabolism in the liver leads to an increase in circulating oestrone in males, which causes gynaecomastia.

Neuropsychiatric effects

- A combination of alcohol toxicity with vitamin B_6 and thiamine deficiency in the diet of alcoholics predisposes to peripheral neuropathy and dementia. Specific mid-brain damage can result and produces the syndromes of Wernicke's encephalopathy and Korsakoff's psychosis.
- Alcohol has anticonvulsant properties and withdrawal predisposes to convulsions, even in individuals without a history of epilepsy.
- Alcohol can disturb sleep patterns, with decreased REM (rapid eye movement) sleep and increased stage 4 sleep during intoxication. Withdrawal increases REM sleep with associated nightmares (Ch. 20).
- Dose-related memory impairment can be caused by suppressed hippocampal function.
- Subdural haematoma is more common after head injury in heavy drinkers, perhaps as a consequence of cerebral atrophy.
- Depression or anxiety states are more common in heavy drinkers.

Carcinogenesis and teratogenesis

- Cancer of the mouth, oesophagus and liver are more common with heavy alcohol use. Colon and breast cancer may also be increased.
- The fetal alcohol syndrome is believed to be caused by the effects of alcohol on neuronal adhesion molecules that regulate neuronal migration. Heavy maternal drinking during pregnancy leads to impaired learning and memory in the child. Genetic factors may be involved in the susceptibility of the fetus to these problems.

Alcohol abuse and dependence

There are no reliable estimates of the number of people in the UK with alcohol-related problems although estimates suggest that they are 1–2% of the population. The distribution curve for alcohol consumption is continuous but skewed at the upper end; the risk of alcohol-related problems rises with the average alcohol intake. Up to 30% of hospital admissions are for alcohol-related problems, although the contribution of heavy drinking is often unrecognised. Screening for alcohol abuse can be carried out by obtaining a complete history of alcohol intake and, if necessary, using the CAGE questions (Box 54.3). Abnormal measurements of both the mean corpuscular volume (MCV) of red cells (which is raised with increasing alcohol intake because of an effect of alcohol on the cell membrane) and the liver enzyme

---

Box 54.3

The CAGE questionnaire for alcoholism

Have you ever felt you could Cut down on your drinking?
Have people Annoyed you by criticising your drinking?
Have you every felt bad or Guilty about your drinking?
Have you ever had a drink first thing in the morning to steady your nerves or get rid of a hangover (Eye-opener)?
A score of yes to one question or more should lead to further evaluation of the patient for alcoholism.

γ-glutamyl transpeptidase (γGT) will identify about 75% of people with an alcohol problem.

Psychological dependence on alcohol is common but physical dependence also occurs. Withdrawal symptoms occur 6–24 h after the last drink in dependent persons. If mild, these are related to autonomic hyperactivity and include anxiety, agitation, tremor, sweating, anorexia, nausea and retching. Convulsions can occur through neuronal excitation. Insomnia, tachycardia and hypertension are common with more severe withdrawal reactions. The most severe form of withdrawal is *delirium tremens*, with confusion, paranoia, visual and tactile hallucinations. Delirium tremens can cause death from respiratory and cardiovascular collapse.

If an individual is drinking excessively, controlled drinking may be an option. However, if there is alcohol dependence or alcohol-related problems, then abstinence is usually preferable.

Controlled detoxification is usually undertaken with a sedative agent, such as a benzodiazepine (Ch. 20) to attenuate withdrawal symptoms. Chlordiazepoxide is usually used, decreasing the dose over 7–10 days. Clomethiazole (Ch. 20) is sometimes used as an alternative but carries a greater risk of dependence. Multivitamin preparations containing an adequate amount of thiamine should be given for 1 month to prevent Wernicke's encephalopathy. Relapse is common after withdrawal from alcohol.

Two drugs are licensed in the UK to assist in the management of chronic alcoholism. Disulfiram, which inhibits acetaldehyde dehydrogenase, causes unpleasant hangover symptoms after small amounts of alcohol. Either alone or with psychosocial rehabilitation it can help to maintain abstinence. Acamprosate inhibits excitatory amino acids such as glutamate and has a number of other effects on neurotransmission by reducing transneuronal Ca^{2+} fluxes, increasing GABA uptake, increasing 5HT levels and antagonising noradrenergic neurotransmission. It is not toxic, is nonaddictive and can be used to reduce craving for alcohol.

FURTHER READING

Ashworth M, Gerada C (1997) Addiction and dependence – II: alcohol. *Br Med J* 315, 358–360

Balfour D, Benowitz N, Fagerström K et al. (2000) Diagnosis and treatment of nicotine dependence with emphasis on nicotine replacement therapy. *Eur Heart J* 21, 438–445

Barlecchi CE, MacKenzie TD, Schrier RW (1994) The human cost of tobacco. *N Engl J Med* 330, 907–912, 975–980

Davis RM (1997) Passive smoking: history repeats itself. *Br Med J* 315, 961–962

Garbutt JC, West SL, Carey TS et al. (1999) Pharmacological treatment of alcohol dependence. *JAMA* 281, 1318–1325

Gerada C, Ashworth M (1997) Addiction and dependence. I: Illicit drugs. *Br Med J* 315, 297–299

Hall W, Solowij N (1998) Adverse effects of cannabis. *Lancet* 352, 1611–1616

Hall W, Zador D (1997) The alcohol withdrawal syndrome. *Lancet* 349, 1897–1900

Leshner AI (1996) Molecular mechanism of cocaine addiction. *N Engl J Med* 335, 128–129

Mendelson JH, Mello NK (1996) Management of cocaine abuse and dependence. *N Engl J Med* 334, 965–972

O'Connor PG, Schottenfeld RS (1996) Patients with alcohol problems. *N Engl J Med* 338, 592–602

Raw M, McNeill A, West R (1999) Smoking cessation: evidence based recommendations for the health care system. *Br Med J* 318, 182–185

Schaffer A, Naranjo CA (1998) Recommended drug treatment strategies for the alcoholic patient. *Drugs* 56, 571–585

Swift RM (1999) Drug therapy for alcohol dependence. *N Engl J Med* 340, 1482–1490

Self-assessment

In the following questions, the first statement, in italics, is true. Are the following statements also true?

1. *Cocaine potently inhibits the uptake of noradrenaline into nerve terminals and this is the explanation for its mydriatic effect.*

   a. 'Crack' cocaine is the free base form of cocaine.
   b. Cocaine can be given topically into the eye to test for Horner's syndrome.
   c. Prolonged use has little damaging effect on the cardiovascular system.
   d. Tolerance to the euphoric and anorexic effects of cocaine rapidly develops.

2. *MDMA (Ecstasy) causes release of 5HT (5-hydroxytryptamine) from nerve endings while inhibiting 5HT uptake.*

   a. A toxic effect of taking Ecstasy in some individuals is hyperthermia and dehydration.
   b. Ecstasy suppresses appetite.
   c. Amphetamines are not banned in sporting events.

3. *Cannabis may impair driving ability and complex mental tasks and psychotic reactions can occur in predisposed individuals.*

   a. The euphoria caused by cannabis lasts for 24 h.
   b. Tetrahydrocannabinol (THC), the active ingredient of cannabis, causes nausea and vomiting.
   c. Cannabis acts on specific receptors in the brain.

4. *Nicotine induces very strong dependence.*

   a. Tolerance to the effects of nicotine develops very slowly.
   b. Nicotine causes tachycardia and reduced gut motility.
   c. Cotinine, a metabolite of nicotine, has a long half-life and can be measured in serum to determine smoking habits.
   d. Nicotine patches given alone are the optimum method for someone giving up smoking.
   e. A physical withdrawal symptom does not occur when giving up smoking.

5. *Ethanol is metabolised to a toxic substance, acetaldehyde, in the liver and then to acetic acid.*

   a. Chronic intake of alcohol induces hepatic drug-metabolising enzymes.
   b. A modest intake of alcohol increases the incidence of cardiovascular disease.
   c. Some individuals have a genetically determined low ability to metabolise ethanol.

6. *One part of a therapy to reduce alcohol intake is to inhibit acetaldehyde metabolism with disulfiram, causing sickness, headache and hangover symptoms following a small amount of alcohol intake.*

   a. Acamprosate, which is used to encourage abstinence, acts to reduce alcohol metabolism in a similar way to disulfiram.
   b. The severity of symptoms of withdrawal from ethanol consumption (detoxification) cannot be controlled by pharmacological means.

7. *Up to one-third of hospital admissions are for alcohol-related problems.*

   a. Ethanol can cause a macrocytosis.
   b. Ethanol enhances antidiuretic hormone secretion.
   c. The liver enzyme γ-glutamyl transpeptidase is depressed with heavy ethanol intake.

The answers are provided on pages 632.

Drug compendium

Drugs of abuse

Drug	Half-life (h)	Elimination	Comments
Amphetamine	8–10	Renal + metabolism	*Dextro*-isomer (dexamfetamine) is the active form and is sometimes used for treatment of hyperactivity in children (especially in the USA); rapidly absorbed (within 3 h); half-life is dependent on the urine pH (basic drug)
Cocaine	1–1.5	Metabolism + renal	Oxidised and hydrolysed in the liver; about 10% excreted unchanged in urine
Ecstasy (3,4-methyl-enedioxymetham-phetamine; MDMA)	6 (*R*), 4 (*S*)	Metabolism + renal	Peak plasma concentrations occur about 2 h after dosage; half-lives differ slightly between the enantiomers; oxidised by CYP2D6 (polymorphism of which may explain in part the idiosyncratic cases of intoxication); saturation of metabolism may contribute to the risk of overdose; the amphetamine analogue (MDA) and ethylamphetamine analogue (MDE or 'Eve') show similar properties
Alcohol (ethyl alcohol, ethanol)	Zero order	Metabolism + renal	Oxidation is saturated at normal intakes
Lysergic acid diethylamide (LSD)	5	Metabolism + renal	Few data are available; LSD is detectable in urine after oral dosage; 2-oxo-3- hydroxy-LSD is a major urinary metabolite
Metamphetamine (methamphetamine)	10–12	Renal + metabolism	Rapidly absorbed after ingestion; about 40% excreted in urine unchanged; oxidised by CYP2D6; few data available; renal excretion is pH dependent (metamphetamine is a metabolite of selegiline)
Nicotine	0.5–2	Metabolism + renal	Very rapidly absorbed after inhalation; the kinetics are absorption rate-limited when given as a patch, with peak plasma concentrations at 5–9 h; the main metabolite, cotinine, has a half-life of 10–40 h (and can be used to assess exposure)
Psilocybin	? (minutes)	Metabolism	Oxidised very rapidly by dephosphorylation to psilocin and also in the intestine to 4-hydroxyindole-3-acetic acid; few data available
Opioids			See Chapter 19
Benzodiazepines			See Chapter 20

Prescribing, compliance and information for patients

About 80% of medicines are prescribed in general practice (primary medical care). On average, men visit their general practitioners 3.5 times each year and women visit five times. A little over two-thirds of consultations end with the issuing of a prescription. Prescribing is particularly frequent for elderly people, who are likely to continue treatment for long periods of time. For these reasons, regular review of prescribed treatment should take place to determine whether it is still appropriate or necessary, and to ensure that important drug interactions and unwanted effects are not overlooked. Some drugs also require regular monitoring of efficacy (e.g. warfarin, antihypertensive treatment), blood concentrations (e.g. lithium) or for unwanted effects (e.g. amiodarone, thiazide diuretics).

Duties of the prescriber

There are certain legal requirements that must be met when a medicine is prescribed. The minimum are:

- the patient's name (surname and initial) and address; in the case of children up to 12 years, the patient's age must be specified.
- drug name
- dose
- route of administration
- frequency of administration
- duration of therapy
- doctor's name address and signature
- date.

Generic prescribing

In most situations, the generic name (the officially accepted chemical name) of the drug is preferred to the proprietary trade name (a 'Brand' name approved for use by a specific pharmaceutical company). One advantage of the generic name is that it is likely to indicate the nature of the drug. For example, all β-blocker drugs end with either -olol or -alol: atenolol, labetalol, metoprolol and sotalol. Similarly, tricyclic antidepressants end with -tyline or -pramine, for example amitriptyline, nortriptyline, clomipramine, imipramine, lofepramine. By contrast, the trade names for these drugs give little idea of the active ingredient: Tenormin, Trandate, Lopressor and Sotacor; Tryptizol, Allegron, Anafranil, Tofranil and Gamanil. Another problem with trade names is that they rarely give any indication when there is more than one active ingredient. For example, Parstelin contains both tranylcypromine and trifluoperazine. The generic names for many compound preparations have this indicated by the term 'co-', for example co-amilofruse indicates the presence of both amiloride and furosemide (frusemide) while co-proxamol contains both dextropropoxyphene and paracetamol.

Another advantage of generic prescribing is that pharmacists can dispense any product that meets the necessary specifications rather than having to buy in a specific brand. This helps to simplify stock holding and avoids unnecessary delays when dispensing for patients. Generic prescribing is sometimes cheaper than prescribing by trade name although the difference depends very much on pack size and other commercial factors and is sometimes marginal (Table 55.1). In recent years, there has been an increasing tendency for doctors to prescribe by generic name. It is likely that economic arguments have been the chief factor leading to this change. Despite these advantages, generic prescribing can create problems. It is possible that the patient may be confused or concerned if a different brand of the same medicine is issued when a prescription is renewed (tablet sizes may differ, as can their colour and whether or not they are scored). For drugs with a narrow therapeutic index, for example anticonvulsants, oral anticoagulants, oral hypoglycaemic agents and theophylline preparations (especially modified-release ones) a change to one that has a greater bioavailability could lead to toxicity, whereas one with a lesser bioavailability can lead to loss of therapeutic control. Recent stringent control both by the Medicines Control Agency and by pharmaceutical companies has almost eliminated this problem, except for some modified-release formulations such as those for lithium or theophylline. In these situations, brand prescribing is recommended.

Dosage

The total treatment is related to the individual dose size, its frequency and the duration of therapy. The route of administration is also important.

Dose. This is an essential item on all prescriptions and should be written in grams (g), milligrams (mg) or micrograms (which should not be abbreviated).

The route of administration. The route should be identified: oral, rectal or by various forms of injections, for example intravenous, intramuscular or subcutaneous. Considerable confusion can arise with intravenous administration of drugs since there are numerous systems for delivery. Drugs can be given by direct injection into a vein or can be infused, for example through the side-arm of a continuously running intravenous drip, via a motor-driven pump or added to intravenous infusion fluid. It is particularly important when prescribing drugs for intravenous administration to make clear the precise intentions.

Frequency and times of administration. Sometimes drugs are administered once only while others must be given on a regular basis, in which case the frequency or times of administration should be specified, for example twice daily or 9 a.m. and 9 p.m.

Duration of therapy. Duration can be specified in a number of ways, one being to complete the box near the top of the prescription sheet. Alternatively, it can be written on the prescription or the total number of tablets/capsules can be specified. Medicines are now dispensed in original (patient) packs with tablets individually packed by the pharmaceutical company. The duration of therapy is essential in the case of controlled drugs, such as opioids, for which the total amount to be dispensed must be written in both figures and in words.

Other items on a prescription

Other essential items on prescriptions include the doctor's signature and the address of his or her place of work. The latter is effectively waived for hospital prescriptions since it is assumed that the medical practitioner is based at the hospital in question. The prescription must be dated. Increasing use is now made of computer-issued prescriptions. The specific requirements for these are essentially similar to those outlined above and these avoid handwriting problems, assist in record keeping and data accumulation.

Table 55.1
Examples of comparative (net ingredient) costs of prescribing by generic or trade names

Generic name	Proprietary (trade) name	Cost per tablet/capsule (p)[a]	
		Generic	Proprietory
Ranitidine (150 mg tablets)	Zantac (Glaxo Wellcome)	28.7	32.5
Ampicillin (250 mg capsules)	Penbritin (Smithkline Beecham)	7.25	8.07
Naproxen (500 mg tablets)	Naprosyn (Roche)	14.50	17.45

[a] The proprietary product was the same tablet size but pack sizes may also vary.
Source: British National Formulary (2000) number 40.

Abbreviations

Directions for prescribing should preferably be in English (rather than Latin) without abbreviation. However, there are a number of abbreviations that are widely accepted. They include the following for route of administration: o or p.o., oral; i.v., intravenous; i.m., intramuscular; s.c., subcutaneous; and p.r., per rectum. Others such as intrathecal must not be abbreviated because of the potential seriousness of inappropriate administration: intrathecal vincristine, for example, has led to the death of several patients. Besides the abbreviations already listed for quantities, ml or mL are acceptable. Quantities of less than 1 g should be written in milligrams, that is 400 mg rather than 0.4 g, whereas quantities of less than 1 mg should be written in micrograms, that is 500 micrograms, rather than 0.5 mg. If decimals are unavoidable, a zero should precede the decimal point when there is no figure, for example 0.5 ml not .5 ml.

Concerning timing of doses, od (omni die) is acceptable but there is nothing wrong with saying once daily! Om (omni mane) stands for in the morning, and on (omni nocte) for at night. Ac is short for ante cibum (before food) and pc for post cibum (after food). Twice daily can be abbreviated to bd (bis die), thrice daily to tds (ter die sumendus) and four times daily to qds (quater die sumendus).

Compliance

The term 'compliance' is used to describe the extent to which a patient takes his or her medicine. Other terms such as adherence and concordance are now preferred since they emphasise the partnership between the patient and health professions in the process of taking medicines, rather than simply following instructions. It is frequently assumed that once a prescription has been given, the patient will automatically comply with the doctor's instructions. There is, however, abundant evidence that this is often not the case. Indeed, many prescriptions are not even taken to the pharmacist for dispensing and the very substantial proportion that are collected are not taken in the manner intended. Prescriptions are sometimes not presented to a pharmacist because of cost or because the doctor failed to discuss the 'hidden agenda' for which the presenting complaint was a front.

The degree of patient compliance is affected by many factors, which include the duration of treatment. Less than 50% of patients comply fully with long-term therapy such as that for high blood pressure or psychotic illness.

The frequency of dosing is a major influence. Few patients like taking their medicines with them to work. Therefore, compliance with twice daily regimens tends to be better than that for more frequent administration. There is a further improvement in the extent of compliance with once rather than twice daily dosing.

Unwanted effects can reduce the likelihood of a patient complying with therapy but at times can be turned to advantage. For example, giving all of the dose of tricyclic antidepressant at night means that the sedation can be used to aid sleep. Giving the patient advanced warning of likely unwanted effects such as dry mouth with this compound may earn their trust and encourage him or her to continue therapy.

A proportion of non-compliance is caused by patients forgetting whether or not they have taken their medicine on a particular day. Use of calendar packs can be helpful in this situation.

The patient's health beliefs are also particularly important. Compliance can be improved by involving the patient in monitoring his or her disease and its control by therapy, for example home monitoring of blood pressure, blood sugar in diabetes mellitus, or peak flow measurements in asthmatics. Supplying patients with accurate information about their medicines can improve their level of satisfaction, and satisfied patients are more likely to take their medicines.

Informing patients about their medicines

It is almost incredible to think that at one time doctors were reluctant to allow the name of a medicine to be shown on the container in which it was dispensed. However, paternalistic attitudes amongst the medical profession have been slow to disappear. Several surveys carried out in the early 1980s showed that patients felt that neither doctors nor pharmacists gave sufficient explanations about the medicines they receive. This situation was summarised by Leighton Cluff in the USA in his comment 'Better instructions are provided when purchasing a new camera or automobile than when a patient receives a life-saving antibiotic or cardiac drug'. More than 60% of patients prescribed a medicine in the previous month remember being told only very little or nothing about it. Patients are particularly keen to know when and how to take their medicine; about unwanted effects and what to do about these; precautions to take, such as possible effects on driving; problems with alcohol or other drugs; the name of the medicine; the purposes of treatment; how long to take it and what to do if a dose is missed.

Manufacturers of pharmaceuticals now produce printed leaflets about medicines which are included in

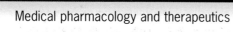

Medical pharmacology and therapeutics

original (patient) packs. Patients who receive leaflets about their medicines are better informed and more satisfied than others who have not been given this information. However, leaflets are complementary to, and not a substitute for, discussion with the medical practitioner, pharmacist, practice nurse, etc. Several books on medicines have been written for those with little specialist knowledge. A good example is the BMA *Guide to Medicines and Drugs*. The Internet provides an increasingly rich source for patients about their medicines and the variety of treatments available for their conditions.

Drug therapy in special situations

Prescribing in pregnancy

Guidelines for prescribing during pregnancy are set out in the *British National Formulary* and only general points are made below. Pregnancy can be associated with medical problems that require treatment, but exposure of the fetus to any unnecessary drugs is undesirable, particularly in the first trimester. The placenta provides a potential barrier to entry of drugs from the maternal circulation, but lipid-soluble drugs do cross, particularly if they are of low molecular weight. Limited metabolism of drugs can occur in the placenta and this will further restrict fetal exposure. The fetal liver has only a modest ability to metabolise drugs. The problem is illustrated by the statistics that approximately 90% of women take medication during pregnancy and an unrecorded number will take over-the-counter medication without guidance from a medical practitioner or a pharmacist.

Unequivocal teratogenic activity of drugs in man is limited to a relatively small number of compounds but their actions can be catastrophic. The list includes ethanol, thalidomide, some anticonvulsants, some chemotherapeutic drugs (e.g. alkylating agents and antimetabolites), warfarin, androgens, danazol, diethylstilbestrol, lithium and retinoids. Retinoids can result in teratogenesis even if the course of treatment in the mother is stopped before pregnancy occurs. Although teratogenesis is commonly thought of in terms of structural abnormalities or dysfunctional growth in utero, by definition it also refers to long-term functional defects. For example, maternal consumption of alcohol during pregnancy can cause behavioural and cognitive abnormalities in childhood, despite the birth of a seemingly unaffected infant. Some drugs exhibit a long latency period yet initially appear harmless. Diethylstilbestrol, which was given during pregnancy between the 1940s and early 1970s, resulted in abnormalities in the children when they reached adulthood.

Notwithstanding the limited list of drugs that are known to cause teratogenesis, there is a much larger number that should be avoided or used with caution in pregnancy because of their pharmacologic potential to produce biochemical dysfunction leading to detrimental effects in the fetus. The reader is referred to the *British National Formulary* for a detailed list of drug effects on the fetus. Examples of drugs that cause potentially serious pharmacological effects in the fetus following placental transfer of drug include:

- warfarin-induced anticoagulation (Ch. 11) that may predispose to cerebral haemorrhage in the fetus during delivery; by contrast heparin is effective in the mother and does not cross the placenta
- non-steroidal anti-inflammatory drugs (Ch. 29), which prevent closure of the ductus arteriosus after delivery; this is a prostaglandin-mediated action and is impaired by inhibition of cyclooxygenase
- amiodarone (Ch. 8), which impairs iodine incorporation into thyroxine, and maternal use of which can cause neonatal goitre.

Drugs can be given during pregnancy to affect uterine contraction. However, the prostaglandin analogue misoprostol (Ch. 33) can produce uterine contractions and lead to abortion. Conversely calcium antagonists (Ch. 6) can inhibit or delay labour by reducing uterine contraction.

Drugs and breast feeding

The *British National Formulary* states 'For many drugs insufficient evidence is available to provide guidance and it is advisable to administer only essential drugs to a mother during breast feeding'. However, most drugs penetrate into breast milk in quantities too small to be of concern. Several factors influence transfer including the characteristics of the milk (which changes in the first few days of lactation), the physicochemical properties of the drug, and the amount of drug in the maternal circulation. In general, drugs licensed for use in children can be safely given to the nursing mother. Drugs known to have serious toxic effects in adults should be avoided. If drugs have to be used, compounds with short half-lives are preferred since they are less likely to accumulate in neonates (who have lower drug clearance, see below). The feed should also ideally be timed to coincide with the trough blood concentration in the mother, which is just before taking a dose, in order to minimise neonatal exposure.

The reader should refer to the up-to-date lists in the *British National Formulary*. The American Academy of Pediatrics has published guidelines and categorised drugs into: (A) breast feeding compatible; (B) breast feeding compatible but with concern; (C) breast feeding – no data available; (D) breast feeding discouraged; (TX) breast feeding temporarily discouraged after the drug; (X) breast feeding contraindicated (taken from Larimore and Petrie 2000).

Prescribing for children

Both the pharmacokinetics and responses to drugs may differ between neonates, infants and children compared to adults. There are considerable differences between neonates (<1 month), infants (1 month to 12 months) and children, because many metabolic and physiological processes are immature at birth and develop rapidly in the first months of life.

Absorption. Slow rates of gastric emptying and intestinal transit may reduce the rate of drug absorption in neonates, but total absorption may eventually be more complete because of longer contact with the intestinal mucosa.

Distribution. Neonates and young children have a lower body fat content and higher total body water compared to adults; this influences the distribution of both lipid- and water-soluble drugs. The newborn have a lower plasma albumin concentration which also has a lower affinity for drug binding. In addition, the higher plasma concentrations of free fatty acids and bilirubin compete with drugs for plasma protein binding sites and vice versa (Ch. 2). The overall effect is reduced plasma protein binding, which increases the apparent volume of distribution of the drug, but also increases the proportion of drug available for metabolism. Drugs that are strongly bound to albumin should not be used during neonatal jaundice because the drugs may displace bilirubin (which is mostly in the unconjugated form) from protein binding sites, and increase the risk of kernicterus.

Metabolism. The liver drug-metabolising enzyme systems are immature in the neonate, and first-pass metabolism and hepatic drug clearance are low, especially for substrates of CYP1A2 and glucuronidation. When the enzyme systems mature, these processes become more extensive in young children than in adults because the relative liver mass and hepatic blood flow are higher.

Elimination. Renal function in the neonate and infant is much less developed than in children or adults. The glomerular filtration rate in the newborn is about 40% of the adult level and tubular secretory processes are poorly developed. Elimination of drugs such as digoxin, gentamicin and penicillin will therefore be delayed.

In neonates, inefficient metabolism and renal clearance mean that lower doses of all drugs are needed after allowing for body weight. Overall, in children, the larger volume of distribution and faster hepatic elimination mean that weight-related doses of metabolised drugs need to be higher in children than in adults. Prescribed doses are most accurately judged by considering both age and body surface area. Body surface area is a better guide to appropriate drug dosage than body weight (see Self-assessment section of Ch. 52).

Prescribing for the elderly

The elderly (usually taken to mean those over 70 years old) comprise a heterogeneous group who show considerable variation in 'biological' age. Changes occur in both the pharmacokinetics and pharmacodynamics of drugs with increasing age.

Pharmacokinetics

Drug absorption is unchanged by ageing, although bioavailability may be increased due to reduced first-pass metabolism.

Older people have a lower lean body mass and a relative increase in body fat compared to young adults. The apparent volume of distribution of water-soluble drugs is therefore lower in the elderly and a smaller loading dose of a drug such as digoxin may be needed. Conversely, lipid-soluble drugs may be eliminated more slowly due to their increased volume of distribution because of the relative increase in body fat.

The size of the liver and its blood flow decrease with age. Although enzyme activity per hepatocyte probably shows little change, the overall capacity for drug metabolism, particularly phase 1 reactions, is reduced. This is particularly important for lipid-soluble drugs such as nifedipine or propranolol that undergo extensive first-pass metabolism.

Increasing age is also associated with a progressive reduction in glomerular filtration rate. Elimination of polar drugs and metabolites is therefore slower; this can produce toxicity when drugs have a low therapeutic index, for example lithium, digoxin or gentamicin. Creatinine clearance is an estimate of glomerular filtration rate which usually correlates well with the clearance of drugs that are eliminated in the urine unchanged (as the parent drug). The elderly have a lower muscle mass than younger people, and so the plasma creatinine concentration (which is dependent on lean body mass) is a poor guide to the level of renal glomerular function. Plasma creatinine in the elderly frequently remains within the 'normal' laboratory reference range even when renal function is substantially reduced. The Cockcroft and Gault equation, which relates plasma creatinine to creatinine clearance, contains elements reflecting sex- and age-dependent differences in muscle mass.

Creatinine clearance (ml min^{-1}) equals:

$$\frac{1.23 \times (140 - \text{age in years}) \times (\text{weight in kg})}{\text{plasma creatinine } (\mu\text{mol l}^{-1})}$$

for males and

$$\frac{1.04 \times (140 - \text{age in years}) \times (\text{weight in kg})}{\text{plasma creatinine } (\mu\text{mol l}^{-1})}$$

for females.

Pharmacodynamics

The response to drugs can also be influenced by age.

The density or numbers of receptors may be reduced with age; for example β-adrenoceptors are decreased in number, reducing the response to agonist drugs. The elderly are often more susceptible to sedatives and hypnotics, possibly because of changes in receptor numbers and/or changes in the efficiency of the blood–brain barrier.

Altered structure and function of target organs can also influence the effects of drugs. For example, baroreceptor function is impaired in the elderly and vasodilator drugs are more likely to provoke postural hypotension. The high peripheral resistance and less distensible arterial tree found with increasing age also respond less well to arterial vasodilators.

These changes in patients reflect the ageing process itself; however, they are often complicated by the presence of chronic disease (frequently involving multiple pathological processes) and variation due to both genetic and environmental influences. As a consequence of these changes, and the frequent simultaneous use of several drugs, the risks of unwanted effects are higher in the elderly. For all these reasons it is usual to start drug treatment in the elderly with the smallest effective dose. Rational prescribing should also seek to minimise the numbers of drugs used.

Prescribing in renal failure

Pharmacokinetics

A reduction in drug dosage in renal failure is usually necessary only if a high proportion of the drug is eliminated by the kidney and also the compound has a low therapeutic index. Maintenance dosage may be lowered by either reducing the dose or increasing the dose interval; loading doses do not usually require any modification. Drugs that do not have dose-related unwanted effects rarely need large dose modifications. A further important consideration is the avoidance of drugs that have toxic effects on the kidney. Use of these in renal impairment can sometimes produce an irreversible decline in renal function.

The kidneys provide the major route of elimination for water-soluble drugs and water-soluble metabolites (see Ch. 2). Renal elimination of drugs can be affected indirectly by abnormal renal perfusion, such as might occur in shock, or directly by changes in the kidney, for example renal tubular necrosis. Reduced renal function may increase the risk of toxicity from the parent drug and/or its metabolites due to their accumulation in the body, although in some cases sensitivity may be increased in renal failure in the absence of obviously impaired elimination of the drug per se. Impaired renal function does not affect the majority of drugs, because most drugs are eliminated by hepatic metabolism.

Elimination of drugs by the kidney is significantly impaired only when the glomerular filtration rate is reduced below 50 ml min^{-1}. For some drugs, clinically important accumulation does not occur until much lower filtration rates. Changes in renal tubular secretion of drugs in renal disease are less well established.

For practical prescribing and dosage adjustment, renal impairment can be divided into three grades:

1. mild, with a glomerular filtration rate of 20–50 ml min^{-1}
2. moderate, with a glomerular filtration rate of 10–20 ml min^{-1}
3. severe, with a glomerular filtration rate of <10 ml min^{-1}.

The corresponding serum creatinine levels are 150–300, 300–700 and >700 µmol l^{-1} respectively, although serum creatinine is not always a reliable indicator of renal function (see 'Prescribing for the Elderly', above). For some drugs, only severe renal impairment needs to be considered (for example, a reduction in dosage is recommended for ampicillin), while for other drugs even mild impairment may be important (for example, dosage reduction and haematological monitoring are recommended for carboplatin whereas cisplatin should be avoided).

There are several other ways in which renal impairment may influence the handling of drugs.

- Metabolism in the liver can be altered in uraemic patients; although most oxidative metabolism is unchanged, other processes such as reduction, acetylation and ester hydrolysis are impaired.
- Metabolism in the kidney is important for the 1-α hydroxylation of vitamin D and also for the degradation of insulin, both of which can be impaired in renal failure.
- The distribution of drugs can be affected by changes in fluid balances in renal failure, and more importantly by altered protein binding. Circulating concentrations of albumin are decreased in severe renal failure with proteinuria. In addition, retained endogenous metabolites, such as the tryptophan metabolite indican, may compete for drug-binding sites on plasma proteins.
- The greater concentration of free drug in the circulation can lead to increased elimination (by filtration and/or metabolism) so that the active unbound drug concentration may be unchanged (see 'Drug Interactions', below).
- Tissue binding of digoxin is reduced in renal failure so that a lower loading dose should be given to compensate for the reduced volume of distribution.

Pharmacodynamics

Altered responses to drugs are found in uraemic patients. Drugs acting on the CNS in particular produce enhanced responses, possibly because of increased permeability of the blood–brain barrier.

Prescribing in liver disease

Changes in both pharmacokinetics and drug responses can occur in liver disease. The severity of the liver disease is important, as is whether the disease is decompensated, for example jaundice, hypoproteinaemia or encephalopathy.

Pharmacokinetics

The rate of absorption of drugs from the gut is not greatly affected, but other aspects of drug handling may be altered. The liver has characteristics that facilitate the rapid and extensive uptake and metabolism of lipid-soluble drugs (Fig. 56.1). These include:

- fenestrations in the endothelium allowing ready access to extracellular fluid
- rapid diffusion across the space of Disse (which is a matrix consisting primarily of type 4 collagen)
- a brush border on hepatocytes allowing rapid uptake
- high intracellular enzyme activity for both phase 1 and phase 2 metabolism.

During chronic liver disease a number of changes may occur which reduce the capacity of the liver to metabolise drugs (Fig. 56.2):

- Fenestrations in the endothelium are lost.
- Diffusion across the space of Disse may be reduced in fibrosis/cirrhosis as type 4 collagen is replaced by type 1 and type 3 collagen (which can form dense fibrils).
- The brush border on hepatocytes is lost.
- Intracellular enzyme activity is reduced.
- Intrahepatic vascular shunts may reduce the perfusion of hepatocytes.

Reduced hepatic uptake and metabolism or biliary excretion of drugs may result in a greater proportion of the drug and/or metabolites being eliminated via other routes, such as the urine.

First-pass metabolism may be considerably reduced in conditions such as liver cirrhosis. This primarily affects drugs that undergo extensive hepatic first-pass metabolism in patients with normal liver function. Bioavailability may increase considerably and approach 100% so that the bioavailability could change 5-fold or more (e.g. from <0.2 to 1.0).

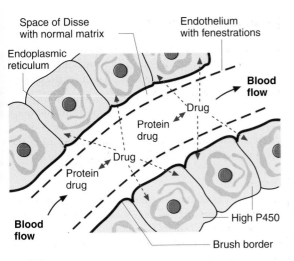

Fig. 56.1
Schematic for the uptake of a drug from the sinusoid of a normal healthy liver.

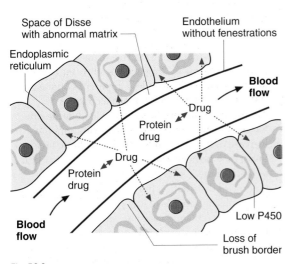

Fig. 56.2
Schematic for the uptake of a drug from the sinusoid of a liver showing the features characteristic of cirrhosis.

Biliary excretion is impaired in conditions giving reduced formation or elimination of bile. A correlation between drug clearance and bilirubin would be expected for drugs eliminated unchanged in bile, such as rifampicin and fusidic acid. Reduced elimination of drug metabolites in bile could affect enterohepatic circulation (Ch. 2).

Systemic clearance may be reduced for drugs eliminated by hepatic metabolism. This affects both high-clearance drugs, where the elimination rate is dependent on effective liver blood flow, and low-clearance drugs, where it is dependent on hepatic extraction and enzyme activity.

Distribution may be affected if protein synthesis is reduced, because the plasma albumin concentrations are decreased, resulting in a higher percentage of free drug in plasma and a greater apparent volume of distribution. An elevated plasma bilirubin may displace some drugs from their plasma protein binding sites, and this would also increase the apparent volume of distribution; examples of drugs that can be affected are lidocaine and propranolol.

Pharmacodynamics

The reduced ability to synthesise vitamin K-dependent clotting factors makes patients with chronic liver disease prone to clotting problems: they would be very sensitive to anticoagulant drugs, which are clearly contraindicated.

CNS depressant drugs, such as morphine and chlorpromazine, have an enhanced effect in patients with liver failure. This is caused by increased sensitivity of neuronal tissue (although the mechanism is not known) and can provoke encephalopathy in susceptible patients. Decreased plasma protein binding may contribute to the greater sensitivity by increasing the percentage of free drug so that more drug can cross the blood–brain barrier. Benzodiazepines may be used during investigational procedures, and the effects can be reversed by giving the benzodiazepine antagonist flumazenil.

Encephalopathy may also be triggered by drugs that cause constipation (which increases the formation of potentially toxic metabolites, such as ammonia, by the intestinal bacteria). Diuretics that produce hypokalaemia can precipitate hepatic encephalopathy in chronic liver disease, and therefore potassium-sparing diuretics such as spironolactone are usually used (spironolactone also blocks the effects of circulating aldosterone, which may be increased in liver disease).

Patients with pre-existing liver disease are likely to be more susceptible to potentially hepatotoxic drugs. This raises a problem for pain relief, since paracetamol is hepatotoxic at high doses, whereas NSAIDs can increase the risk of gastrointestinal bleeding and cause fluid retention, and opioids can precipitate encephalopathy. In practice, lower doses of paracetamol are usually given, taking care that the amounts do not exceed the reduced threshold for hepatotoxicity shown by such patients.

Prescribing in liver disease should therefore be carried out with care; drugs that are extensively metabolised by the liver should be given in smaller doses. The need for dose reduction arises primarily from an increase in bioavailability and a decrease in systemic clearance, both of which increase the average steady-state plasma concentration and the area under the plasma concentration–time curve for a single dose.

Drug interactions

Many patients receive more than one drug during a course of treatment because:

- Combination therapy is preferable or necessary for producing a single effect or response, such as the chemotherapy of malignant disease, or treatment of hypertension.
- A single condition or pathology may give rise to a variety of symptoms that are controlled by different drugs.
- The patient may suffer from more than one condition or pathology requiring treatment with drugs that are unrelated pharmacologically.

The term 'interaction' implies that the response to the combination of drugs is different to that which could be predicted from a simple summation of the effects produced by each drug if given singly. Interactions may result in either a decrease or increase in response compared with that predicted; this may be either beneficial or potentially harmful because of a lack of clinical response or the risk of toxicity.

Beneficial interactions are usually well recognised and are part of prescribing recommendations. In consequence the focus of this section, and of Appendix 1 of the *British National Formulary*, is those interactions that may give rise to adverse effects, especially when the interaction would not be readily predicted based on a knowledge of the sites and mechanisms of action.

Interactions are of greatest importance for drugs that have a narrow therapeutic index and for patient groups at increased risk such as the elderly (who are more likely or suffer multiple pathologies and may have decreased hepatic and renal function).

Drug interactions may arise from interference at the site or mechanism of action (pharmacodynamics) or from altered delivery of the drug to its site of action (pharmacokinetics).

Pharmacodynamic interactions

Pharmacodynamic interactions are usually predictable, based on the known actions of the drug. Interactions may relate to the principal site of action of the drug, or to secondary sites of action that are responsible for unwanted effects of the drug. In principle, drugs that are highly selective for a single site of action are less likely to produce pharmacodynamic interactions than drugs that show low selectivity.

Pharmacokinetic interactions

Absorption
Co-administration of two drugs could give an interaction if one drug affected the rate or extent of absorp-

tion of the other drug. Changes in the rate of absorption, for example by increasing or decreasing gastric emptying or intestinal motility, will affect the peak concentration but not usually the extent of absorption. Such interactions are less important than those that alter the extent of absorption, for example by retention of the drug in the gut lumen (e.g. tetracycline antibiotics plus divalent or trivalent metals, such as Ca^{2+}, Fe^{3+}) or by inhibition or induction of first-pass metabolism in the gut lumen, gut wall or liver.

Distribution
The main interaction affecting drug distribution arises from competition for the non-specific binding sites on plasma proteins, such as albumin (see Table 2.2). Interactions affecting plasma protein binding are of greatest importance when:

- the displaced drug is highly protein bound; if competition for protein binding sites reduces binding from 98% to 96% this will double the free drug concentration in plasma (from 2% to 4%); a 2% change in the binding of a drug which is 50% bound and 50% free would not be clinically or biologically significant
- the displaced drug has a narrow therapeutic index, so that a 2–3-fold change in free drug concentration gives an increase in drug actions
- the displaced drug has a low apparent volume of distribution, such that the plasma contains a significant proportion of the body load; if the drug has a high apparent volume of distribution, the increase in free drug in the plasma volume (about 3 litres) may be negligible after it has been distributed to (and 'diluted' in) a much higher apparent volume of distribution (for example 300 litres)
- the displacing drug is of low potency, such that large doses (on a mg basis) are given and protein binding sites become limiting.

In reality such interactions are of limited clinical relevance even when the above criteria are fulfilled. For example, the potentially important interaction between warfarin and aspirin is due to their combined pharmacodynamic effects rather than the displacement of warfarin (which is 99% bound and has an apparent volume of distribution of 0.1 l kg^{-1}) from its protein binding sites. One reason for this is that the additional free drug that has been displaced from protein binding sites may undergo rapid elimination by metabolism or glomerular filtration. When this occurs a new 'steady state' will be established when the combination is given, with similar amounts of free drug but reduced amounts of bound drug. Therefore, the total (free and bound) plasma concentration of the drug (which is measured in most drug assays) will be lower, and measured concentrations may be misleadingly low and indicate an inappropriate increase in drug dose. Examples of drugs displaying this problem are theophylline and phenytoin.

Metabolism

Interactions affecting metabolism could theoretically arise from simple competition for the same enzyme, but this would only be important if the combination resulted in saturation of the enzyme system. The doses of most drugs are such that the concentrations do not approach the K_m of the enzymes involved in their metabolism so that first-order kinetics (Ch. 2) apply. Under these circumstances the presence of two substrates is no different to the presence of increased amounts of single substrates; in consequence the clearance and half-lives are the same in combination as when given alone. A clinically useful exception is the administration of ethanol to prevent the metabolism of methanol (in overdose) to formate in order to reduce the risk of blindness.

Important interactions can occur when one drug in a combination induces or inhibits the enzymes involved in the metabolism of the other drug. This has been well recognised for drugs affecting the cytochrome P450 enzyme system (Table 2.9), largely because of the importance of this enzyme system for most drugs and the potential for induction of different isoenzymes. Enzyme inhibition occurs as soon as the drug concentration is sufficiently high, and inhibition can occur after a single dose (e.g. cimetidine). In contrast, enzyme induction requires the synthesis of additional enzyme and it takes a few days (or longer) for the elevated enzyme activity to reach a new equilibrium between synthesis and degradation. Induction or inhibition of hepatic enzymes can affect both systemic clearance and bioavailability after oral dosage.

Co-administration of two drugs, one of which is an enzyme inducer, will reduce the concentrations of the other drug. This may decrease the response to the second drug (if the parent compound is active), but could also increase the response to a prodrug, if the induced enzyme was responsible for this bioactivation. A problem can also arise when drug dosage has been optimised for the combination and treatment with the inducer is then stopped. Under such circumstances the enzyme activity decreases (usually over a period of 2–3 weeks) and plasma levels of the parent drug increase, possibly giving a risk of toxicity.

Excretion

Each of the three processes that are important in the renal elimination of drugs, i.e. glomerular filtration, pH-dependent reabsorption and renal tubular secretion, could be a site for a drug interaction.

Glomerular filtration depends on renal perfusion and removes free or non-protein bound drug only. In consequence, drugs affecting renal perfusion or plasma protein binding (see above) could give rise to interactions.

pH-dependent reabsorption could be altered by drugs that affect urine pH, either directly or via metabolic effects; the pH changes associated with aspirin overdose could affect the excretion of drugs taken concurrently.

Renal tubular secretion can give rise to interactions when there is competition for the transporter. Probenecid was developed specifically for co-administration with penicillins in order to inhibit their renal tubular secretion. Aspirin can interfere with the transport of both endogenous compounds (e.g. uric acid) and drugs (e.g. methotrexate).

The biliary excretion of drugs is not an important site for drug interactions, but the enterohepatic recycling of drugs can be affected by the co-administration of poorly absorbed broad-spectrum antimicrobials, which affect the hydrolysis of drug conjugates in the lower bowel (Fig. 2.13).

FURTHER READING

Briggs GG, Freeman RK, Yaffe SJ (1998) *Drugs in pregnancy and lactation. A reference guide to fetal and neonatal risk*, 5th edn. Baltimore, Williams and Wilkins

Ito S (2000) Drug therapy for breast-feeding women. *N Engl J Med* **343**, 118–126

Koren G, Pastuszak A, Ito S (2000) Drugs in pregnancy. *N Engl J Med* **338**, 1128–1137

Larimore WL, Petrie KA (2000) Drug use during pregnancy and lactation. *Primary Care* **27**, 35–53

Self-assessment answers

Chapter 2

1. Multiple choice answers

   1a. **False**. An increase in dose results in an increase in the concentrations of the drug in plasma and body tissues. A twofold increase in drug concentrations gives twofold higher concentrations available to elimination processes; consequently, the rate of elimination increases proportionately. Since clearance is given by the rate of elimination/plasma concentration, this ratio is not altered. A decrease in clearance with increase in dose occurs when the elimination process is saturated and an increase in concentration cannot give an increase in the rate of elimination. Few drugs show saturation kinetics (zero order) at therapeutic doses.

   b. **True**. This statement is true for all 'pre-systemic' sites of metabolism of the oral dose, e.g. gut lumen, gut wall and liver. Low bioavailability may also arise from poor absorption.

   c. **True**. If the liver is able to 'mop up' a high proportion of the drug as it is absorbed from the gastrointestinal tract, it will also clear a high proportion of drug from the blood after it has entered the general circulation. For example, if 80% of an oral dose undergoes first-pass liver metabolism during absorption (Fig. 2.2), then 80% of all drug delivered to the liver via the systemic blood flow will also be cleared; systemic clearance will equal 80% of liver blood flow.

   d. **True**. A longer half-life can arise from a higher apparent volume of distribution or a lower clearance; babies (under 6–12 months) show lower systemic clearance because of both reduced hepatic metabolism and lower renal excretion.

   e. **False**. A decrease in renal function could affect systemic clearance, providing that renal clearance of the drug was a significant part of total plasma clearance. However, bioavailability is simply the fraction of the oral dose that reaches the general circulation, and the kidneys are not part of the route between gut lumen and general circulation. (Although the AUC of an oral dose may be increased in renal disease, the AUC of an intravenous dose will show a similar increase and bioavailability is not altered.)

   f. **False**. Benzathine benzylpenicillin is a depot injection of penicillin in which the prolonged half-life results from prolonged and sustained release from the site of injection. Once absorbed into the blood, the circulating penicillin is handled by the kidneys as normal.

   g. **False**. Nifedipine is metabolised by CYP3A4; no interaction would occur because smoking induces CYP1A2. Our increased understanding of the cytochrome P450 isoenzymes has allowed more rational predictions of 'drug–drug' and 'drug–environmental chemical' interactions.

   h. **False**. Phenobarbital is a potent inducer of cytochrome P450 enzymes, which can increase the ability of the liver to extract the drug from the blood. This can increase the systemic clearance but decreases the oral bioavailability of co-administered drugs.

   i. **True**. A loading dose is designed to produce the body load that will be present during chronic treatment (at steady state) without the time delay while the drug accumulates during chronic treatment. Drugs with short elimination half-lives do not accumulate significantly and therefore the body load after the first normal (non-loading) dose will be the same as during chronic treatment (see also the answer to the data interpretation question 3d below).

   j. **False**. The influence of body composition on the apparent volume of distribution depends on the nature of the drug. Lipid-soluble drugs would show an increased apparent volume of distribution (V) in an obese patient (when expressed per kilogram body weight) but the converse would apply to water-soluble drugs. However, the V and clearance (CL) of drugs are independent variables; there is no reason why the different distribution in the body should affect the ability of the liver to extract the drug from the blood. Students sometimes can get confused about V and CL and think that if more drug enters the fat this will lower the

597

blood concentration and hence must lower CL. It is important to appreciate that V and CL are independent variables. If more drug enters adipose tissue (because there is more of it), then plasma concentration (C_p) will tend to be lower and therefore V (V = the amount in the body/C_p), will be higher. Because the plasma concentration at any time is lower and CL is a constant for that drug, then the rate of elimination at any point in time will be lower (CL = rate of elimination/C_p). The elimination half-life is related to both V and CL (half-life is 0.693 V/CL) and an increase in V without a change in CL would result in an increase in half-life. Because the steady-state plasma concentration (C_{ss}) depends on CL but not V ($C_{ss} = D \times F/CL \times t$, where D is administered dose, F is bioavailability and t is the interval between doses) there would not be any need to modify a chronic dosage regimen because of an increase in V. However, the steady-state body load ($C_{pss} \times V$) would be higher and, therefore, it could take longer to reach steady-state conditions (as indicated by the increase in half-life). [If you have understood this answer then you have 'cracked' pharmacokinetics!]

k. **False**. This statement is true for some drugs but not for all drugs: it depends on the drug. Administration of drugs with food will generally decrease the rate of absorption (because of effects on gastric emptying and/or absorption rate) and this will often reduce the peak plasma concentration. This may in some cases reduce unwanted effects. Another advantage of taking medicines with meals is that it can increase compliance with a three times daily (tds) dosage schedule. Potential disadvantages are the delay in absorption and in some cases interference with absorption, giving a decrease in bioavailability; for example, the absorption of tetracycline antimicrobials is almost completely abolished if they are taken with milk.

2. Drug bioavailability

a. The *rate* of absorption is determined by the rate of increase after oral dosing (providing that the elimination rates or oral and intravenous doses are parallel). Drug A is absorbed very rapidly while drug B takes about 6 h to reach a peak concentration.

b. The *extent* of absorption (bioavailability or F) is determined by the AUC$_{oral}$/AUC$_{iv}$. For drug A the AUC$_{oral}$ is much smaller than AUC$_{iv}$ and therefore F is much less than 1. In contrast, for drug B the AUC$_{oral}$ approximately equals AUC$_{iv}$ and so F is approximately 1.

c. The *rate* of distribution is given by the rate of decrease between the administration of the intravenous bolus dose (at time 0) and the establishment of the terminal elimination phase. The terminal phase for drug A starts at about 1 h whereas that for drug B starts at about 4 h. Therefore, A distributes more rapidly. The *extent* of distribution is given by the apparent volume of distribution, V which is indicated by the intravenous dose divided by the intercept (C_{p0}) obtained on back-extrapolation of the terminal phase of the plasma concentration–time curve (intravenous dose/C_{p0}). Both A and B give a similar intercept and, therefore, have similar apparent volumes of distribution.

d. The elimination half-life is given by 0.693/terminal slope (0.693/k or 0.693/β) and it is obvious that drug B has a longer half-life than drug A. The reason for the longer half-life of B is the lower clearance (CL) of B (since the volume of distribution is similar for A and B). This is also apparent by visual inspection of the graphs; CL = Dose$_{iv}$/AUC$_{iv}$ and the AUC$_{iv}$ for B is much greater than that for A (the doses were the same).

e. The potential for accumulation depends on the difference between half-life and dose interval. It is clear that nearly all of drug A has been removed from the plasma (and therefore the body) by 24 h, whereas considerable amounts of B remain at 24 h. Therefore, B would show significant accumulation on daily dosage.

3. Parameter calculations

a. The extent of absorption (note units cancel to give a fraction)

$$F = \frac{AUC_{oral}}{AUC_{iv}} \times \frac{Dose_{iv}}{Dose_{oral}}$$

A $F = \dfrac{2}{16} \times \dfrac{20\,000}{20\,000} = 0.125$

B $F = \dfrac{995}{1000} \times \dfrac{20\,000}{20\,000} = 0.995$

C $F = \dfrac{26}{40} \times \dfrac{20\,000}{20\,000} = 0.65$

b. The extent of distribution is given by V, which equals clearance, CL (calculated from intravenous data) divided by k, the terminal elimination rate constant, i.e.

$$CL = \frac{Dose_{iv}}{AUC_{iv}} \quad then \quad V = \frac{Dose_{iv}}{AUC_{iv} \times k}$$

The units are

$$\frac{\mu g}{\mu g\ ml^{-1}\ min \times min^{-1}} = ml$$

A $V = \dfrac{20\,000}{16 \times 0.0063} = 198\,413\ ml = 198\,l$

B $V = \dfrac{20\,000}{1000 \times 0.000\,22} = 90\,909\ ml = 91\,l$

C $V = \dfrac{20\,000}{40 \times 0.014} = 35\,714\ ml = 36\,l$

c. The rate of elimination is reflected in $t_{1/2}$:

$$t_{1/2} = \frac{0.693}{k}$$

A $t_{1/2} = \dfrac{0.693}{0.0063\ min^{-1}} = 110\ min = 2\ h$

B $t_{1/2} = \dfrac{0.693}{0.00022\ min^{-1}} = 3150\ min = 53\ h$

C $t_{1/2} = \dfrac{0.693}{0.014\ min^{-1}} = 49.5\ min = 1\ h$

These values were calculated using the intravenous data. The terminal half-lives of A and B are the same after both oral and intravenous dosage; the half-life for C is $(0.693/0.003) = 231\ min$ (4 h) after oral administration, suggesting an absorption rate-limited terminal phase (i.e. absorption is slower than elimination).

The clearance (CL) is the volume of blood cleared per minute

$$CL = \frac{Dose_{iv}}{AUC_{iv}} = \left(\frac{\mu g}{\mu g\ ml^{-1}\ min} = ml\ min^{-1} \right)$$

A $CL = \dfrac{20\,000}{16} = 1250\ ml/min$

B $CL = \dfrac{20\,000}{1000} = 20\ ml/min$

C $CL = \dfrac{20\,000}{40} = 500\ ml/min$

The route of administration is indicated by the percentage dose in urine as the parent drug, after the intravenous dose. Drug A is cleared by non-renal routes and is all metabolised. Drug B is cleared mostly (95%) by metabolism and drug C is cleared almost totally by renal elimination.

$$Renal\ clearance\ (CL_r) = \frac{amount\ excreted\ in\ urine_{(0-t)}}{AUC_{(0-t)}}$$

A $CL_r = \dfrac{20\,000 \times 0.00}{16} = 0\ ml\ min^{-1}$

B $CL_r = \dfrac{20\,000 \times 0.05}{1000} = 1\ ml\ min^{-1}$

C $CL_r = \dfrac{20\,000 \times 0.98}{40} = 490\ ml\ min^{-1}$

d. The potential for accumulation during chronic dosage is determined by comparison of the amount in the body during chronic dosage with that following a single dose.

$$Accumulation = \frac{\substack{Steady\ state \\ body\ load}}{\substack{Single\ dose \\ body\ load}} = \frac{C_{ss} \times V}{Dose \times F} = \frac{Dose \times F \times V}{Dose \times F \times CL \times t}$$

where t is dose interval during chronic intake and C_{ss} is $Dose \times F/CL \times t$. Since V/CL is $1/k$ or $t_{1/2}/0.693$ ($t_{1/2} \times 1.44$), this equation is simply

$$Accumulation = \frac{t_{1/2} \times 1.44}{t}$$

Therefore, the potential for accumulation with any proposed dose interval is directly proportional to the half-life, and the accumulation potential is B >> A > C. (In reality A and C would not show any significant accumulation on chronic dosage.)

e. To discuss factors that may influence the drugs, we need to be able to interpret what the numerical values mean in physiological terms. **Drug A** is eliminated by metabolism with no renal excretion of the parent drug. It is therefore very lipid soluble (hence the very high value for V). The short half-life results from the very high clearance, which approximates to liver blood flow. The low oral bioavailability is also consistent with high hepatic first-pass metabolism.

Absorption rate. This is probably very rapid because of the drug's high lipid solubility; a modified-release formulation may be required because of this rapid absorption and short half-life.

Bioavailability. If liver is the main site of first-pass metabolism, then bioavailability could be greatly increased by liver disease. Enzyme inducers would decrease bioavailability still further; inhibitors would increase it.

Distribution. This would mainly be influenced by the proportion of body fat.

Elimination. Hepatic clearance will depend largely on effective liver blood flow; therefore, perfusion abnormalities (e.g. hepatic cirrhosis) would have a major influence. Age may affect liver function. Enzyme induction would have little effect (since clearance is largely determined by liver blood flow); inhibitors could decrease hepatic metabolism of the drug and hence clearance. Pharmacogenetic differences in metabolising enzymes could be important if poor metabolisers showed low clearance (this would depend on the importance of the genetically determined enzyme in the overall clearance).

Drug B is eliminated mostly by metabolism but clearance is low and some is excreted in the urine as the parent drug.

Absorption rate. This is probably rapid (terminal phase is the same after oral and intravenous dose but elimination is very slow for both routes). Modified-release formulation would not be needed because of the long half-life.

Bioavailability. This would be high because of the drug's slow metabolism/low clearance; it is unlikely to be influenced by induction or inhibition of hepatic enzymes (even if first-pass metabolism doubled, the bioavailability would only decrease to 0.99).

Distribution. The slightly greater water solubility, compared with drug A, gives a lower volume of distribution.

Elimination. Renal function will not greatly influence total clearance. Renal clearance is only 1 ml min⁻¹, which is negligible compared with glomerular filtration rate; therefore nearly all filtered drug is reabsorbed from the tubule. Urine pH could affect this reabsorption, but renal clearance (1 ml min⁻¹) is only 5% of total clearance (20 ml min⁻¹). The main factor influencing the clearance of this drug will be the activity of the metabolising enzymes. Liver blood flow will not be important since the metabolic clearance (19 ml min⁻¹) is only a very small fraction of liver blood flow. Factors influencing the enzyme activity could include inducers/inhibitors, age and pharmacogenetics.

Drug C is eliminated almost exclusively by renal excretion without metabolism. The pharmacokinetics of this drug are dominated by its high water solubility.

Absorption rate. The drug shows 'flip-flop' kinetics and the elimination rate after oral dosage is determined by the absorption rate of this polar drug. The half-life after oral dosage (4 h) means that a modified-release oral formulation is not really needed despite the rapid elimination half-life (seen after intravenous administration).

Bioavailability. The low bioavailability is a reflection of the high water solubility and the slow rate of absorption from the gut. The non-

bioavailable fraction of the oral dose is probably simply lost in the faeces. (Note, it is not likely to undergo first-pass metabolism because the drug is not metabolised.)

Elimination. The renal clearance (490 ml min⁻¹) is greatly in excess of the glomerular filtration rate and approaches renal blood flow. The drug must, therefore, undergo renal tubular secretion. Factors influencing this drug will be renal blood flow (e.g. age and renal disease) and inhibitors of renal tubular secretion. Urine pH is unlikely to be a major influence (there is incomplete absorption from the gut despite the range of pH values in the gut lumen, which suggests that the water solubility of the drug is not influenced by pH).

Chapter 4

1. **False**. Noradrenaline is the transmitter substance at the postganglionic nerve endings. Adrenaline is released only from the adrenal medulla and acetylcholine is the transmitter in sweat glands and hair follicles.

2. **False**. Although acetylcholine is the transmitter at all ganglia and the neuromuscular junction, at sensible doses ganglion-blocking drugs block the nicotinic N_1 receptors in autonomic ganglia but not N_2 receptors at the neuromuscular junction.

3. **True**. Plasma or pseudocholinesterase can also metabolise acetylcholine but does so more slowly. Plasma cholinesterase, however, has a broader spectrum of activity and can metabolise drugs such as suxamethonium (succinylcholine).

4. **True**. Dopamine is predominantly an important transmitter in the CNS but is also a transmitter in selected situations in the periphery, e.g. the renal vascular smooth muscle.

5. **True**. This is important as selective inhibitors of MAO-A used in the treatment of depression leave MAO-B unaffected and it can metabolise tyramine in food; therefore, avoiding the 'cheese reaction'.

6. **False**. Stimulation of α_1-adrenoceptors on resistance vessels causes constriction; therefore, their blockade lowers blood pressure. However, α_2-adrenoceptor (presynaptic) stimulation reduces noradrenaline release and blockade of these receptors would raise blood pressure.

7. **False**. Botulinum toxin inhibits acetylcholine release and can be used locally where there is skeletal muscle spasm or excessive sweating.

8. **False**. The β_3-adrenoceptor has been found in adipocytes, the heart, colon and some other tissues but is less widespread than the β_2-adrenoceptor.

The β_3-adrenoceptor on adipocytes is being investigated to see if its stimulation will be effective to treat obesity.

9. **True**. Propranolol is a non-selective blocker of β-adrenoceptors and the role of the presynaptic β_2-adrenoceptor is to increase noradrenaline release.

10. **True**. Selective reversible inhibitors of the uptake of noradrenaline or 5HT (fluoxetine) are available and are used in the treatment of depression.

11. **False**. Sympathetic nervous stimulation releases noradrenaline and inhibits motility but increases the tone of the sphincters.

12. **False**. When the sympathetic supply to the radial muscle of the iris is stimulated, the muscle contracts and the pupil size increases. This effect can be used to facilitate retinal examination.

Chapter 5

1 a. **False**. Nitric oxide increases cGMP synthesis to bring about vasodilation.

  b. **True**. Glyceryl trinitrate undergoes extensive first-pass metabolism after oral dosing since initial entry into the systemic circulation is via the portal circulation and the liver. Transdermal patches or sublingual administration avoid the portal circulation and the drug gains direct access to the systemic circulation.

  c. **False**. Glyceryl trinitrate does not increase total coronary blood flow. It can, however, treat angina by increasing flow to the ischaemic areas by dilating collateral blood vessels or reducing coronary vasospasm.

  d. **False**. A major component of the benefit of glyceryl trinitrate is its peripheral vasodilator action, reducing preload and to a lesser extent arteriolar dilation, peripheral vascular resistance, and afterload. These reduce workload on the heart. The reflex tachycardia that occurs through a fall in peripheral resistance can be reduced by concomitant treatment with a β-blocker.

  e. **False**. t-PA cleaves plasminogen to increase the formation of plasmin, which results in the degradation of the fibrin that forms the framework of the thrombus.

2. Case history answers

  a. For acute attacks, sublingual glyceryl trinitrate is used to give rapid relief.

  b. For prophylaxis, a β-blocker or calcium antagonist will often be the treatment of first choice and in this situation will also be useful because they lower blood pressure. A combination of both or addition of a long-acting nitrate could be used if symptoms are not well controlled with a single agent. For example, atenolol and nifedipine together significantly decrease the number of angina attacks compared with either used alone. Anti-anginal drugs have not been shown to reduce the risk of subsequent myocardial infarction.

  c. Additional therapy to improve prognosis includes low-dose aspirin (75–150 mg), which has been shown to reduce the risk of subsequent myocardial infarction. Lowering plasma cholesterol concentration by diet or drugs such as simvastatin can also reduce the risk of subsequent myocardial infarction.

  d. Smoking, lack of exercise and obesity are all risk factors for coronary heart disease. TK is exposed to these increased risks and should address these by life-style changes.

  e. In an 80-year-old patient, there is likely to be reduced hepatic metabolism of calcium blockers. Because they are significantly metabolised by first-pass metabolism, it is likely that they will produce a greater reduction in blood pressure at smaller doses.

  f. The most consistent evidence is for combined use of heparin and aspirin in unstable angina. Addition of a β-blocker produces a small additional benefit.

  g. Coronary artery occlusion at the site of an atheroma causing necrosis.

  h. The benefit of thrombolytic therapy is strongly dependent upon the delay between symptoms and administration. The benefit is particularly great if thrombolytic therapy can be administered within 6 h from the onset of pain but there is good evidence for benefit at least until 12 h.

  i. Allergic reactions to streptokinase are extremely rare. TK had not had a previous myocardial infarction and had not previously been administered streptokinase so would be unlikely to have high titres of streptokinase neutralising antibodies. It would, therefore, be safe to give TK streptokinase unless he had severe symptomatic hypotension.

  j. Aspirin and thrombolytic therapy have been shown to have additive benefit for treating acute myocardial infarction, reducing subsequent reinfarction or death.

  k. Low doses of aspirin reduce the production of the platelet aggregating agent thromboxane A_2 by platelets, while having less effect on the production of the platelet disaggregating agent prostaglandin I_2 from endothelial cells. Large doses of aspirin do not produce any additional benefit, and the risk of gastric irritation or ulceration is increased.

l.   This is incorrect. Streptokinase has a longer duration of action than rt-PA and it is generally unnecessary to administer heparin when streptokinase has been given. However, it is necessary after rt-PA when it improves the long-term patency of the artery.

m.   Low-dose aspirin, β-blockers and ACE inhibitors all reduce mortality and the risk of reinfarction. The β-blocker will need to be given under close observation, since it carries a risk of worsening heart failure. In patients who have signs of heart failure, verapamil and diltiazem may be detrimental. Warfarin reduces mortality and reinfarction to a similar extent as low-dose aspirin so is not required unless patients are unable to tolerate aspirin.

Chapter 6

1 a.   **False**. Thiazide diuretics cause growth retardation of the fetus and are not recommended. Methyldopa, nifedipine and labetalol are most often used.

b.   **True**. Calcium channel antagonists act by opening L-type voltage-gated Ca^{2+} channels and nifedipine is relatively selective for smooth muscle. Verapamil and diltiazem, which have intermediate selectivity, also have cardiodepressant properties that may contribute to their blood pressure-lowering actions.

c.   **False**. Selective stimulation of imidazoline receptor type I_1, in the ventrolateral medulla is the principle mechanism of action of moxonidine, which lowers blood pressure in hypertension by decreasing sympathetic outflow and increasing vagal outflow

d.   **True** for (i) and (ii); **False** for (iii). Only β-blockers, having partial agonist activity, e.g. pindolol, produce peripheral vasodilatation by stimulating β_2-adrenoceptors in skeletal muscle blood vessels.

e.   **True**. Spironolactone blocks the aldosterone receptor, which stimulates the Na^+/K^+-ATPase pump, facilitating uptake of Na^+ into the interstitium from the tubule and, therefore, conserving K^+ and losing Na^+. Amiloride, however, directly blocks the Na^+ channel on the luminal side of the tubule.

f.   **False**. Baroreceptor impulses to the vasomotor centre are inhibitory. Increased impulses, therefore, reduce sympathetic outflow, enhance vagal outflow and lower blood pressure.

g.   **False**. Prazosin is a selective α_1-adrenoceptor blocker and, therefore, dilates blood vessels. It does not block the presynaptic receptor, which is α_2-type and, therefore, stimulation of this receptor to limit further noradrenaline release can still take place.

h.   **True**. Longer-term vasodilation and blood pressure lowering may be because of inhibition of Ca^{2+} entry into vessel cells and synthesis of vasodilator prostaglandins.

i.   **True**. ACE breaks down bradykinin, which is found in endothelial cells and is a potent vasodilator.

j.   **False**. Minoxidil causes extrusion of K^+ from the cell which results in the stabilisation of the membrane potential and vasodilatation.

k.   **False**. Nitroprusside is converted to cyanide and then to thiocyanate. The toxicity of these limits its use to 3 days.

2.   Case history answer

a.   Thiazide diuretics can cause hyperglycaemia and are less suitable for diet-controlled diabetes. Both thiazides and propranolol increase plasma lipids.

b.   Furosemide is a less effective hypotensive agent than the thiazides in uncomplicated hypertension but could be useful if there was evidence of renal impairment.

c.   The potassium-sparing diuretics are less effective than thiazides in essential hypertension. They should not be used in combination with an ACE inhibitor.

d.   A calcium antagonist plus atenolol is the most suitable of the choices described. Calcium antagonists do not affect lipid levels.

e.   ACE inhibitors reduce angiotensin II formation and increase the formation of the vasodilator bradykinin and improve survival after a myocardial infarction, especially if there is left ventricular impairment. They could be given together with a β-blocker, which shows additional benefit if there is left ventricular impairment. Calcium antagonists are not of benefit given after a myocardial infarction. ACE inhibitors appear to protect the kidney in diabetic nephropathy and could be considered in this situation.

Chapter 7

1 a.   **True**. In the healthy heart, to maintain cardiac output, contractility rises when there is an increase in afterload, which is, in turn,

determined largely by peripheral resistance. In the failing heart contractility cannot increase so stroke volume falls.

b. **False**. The plasma osmotic pressure works to move fluid from the interstitium into the vessel and the hydrostatic pressure in the other direction. Therefore, oedema occurs when the hydrostatic pressure is greater than the plasma osmotic pressure.

c. **False**. In cardiac failure the baroreceptor reflex sensory input to the vasomotor centre is reduced, resulting in increased sympathetic outflow.

d. **False**. Although digoxin may be of benefit, the mainstay of treatment is diuretics such as furosemide (frusemide). If diuretics are given concurrently with digoxin, K^+-sparing diuretics may also be required as hypokalaemia resulting from urinary K^+ loss can increase the risk of digoxin-induced rhythm disturbances.

e. **False**. Potassium ions and digoxin compete for the pump; therefore, high extracellular K^+ inhibits the effect of digoxin and low K^+ can increase the arrhythmic potential of digoxin.

f. **False**. The effect of low therapeutic doses of digoxin is to stimulate the vagus, sensitise baroreceptor outflow and thereby increase vagal outflow from the vasomotor centre; overall this increases the refractory period of the atrioventricular node. This is the reason that digoxin is useful in some arrhythmias, such as atrial fibrillation.

g. **True**. Dobutamine acts through stimulation of β_1-adrenoceptors, which results in an increase in cAMP and thereby increased cardiac contractility. Desensitisation occurs because of downregulation of the receptors in response to prolonged stimulation by the drug. Desensitisation to milrinone does not occur because it 'bypasses' the receptor and increases cAMP by preventing its breakdown (phosphodiesterase inhibitors are, however, of limited use).

h. **False**. Dobutamine is a selective β-adrenoceptor agonist and does not produce vasodilation.

i. **True**. Digoxin is eliminated unchanged by the kidney. Its half-life can be increased markedly in renal failure.

j. **True**. ACE inhibitors decrease angiotensin II and decrease aldosterone output. This results in less reabsorption of Na^+ in the collecting ducts in exchange for K^+ efflux into the tubules, resulting in increased K^+ retention. Spironolactone can produce additional clinical benefit but care must be taken to avoid dangerous hyperkalaemia, with regular monitoring of plasma K^+ concentration.

2. Case history answers

a. The main direct consequences of reduced cardiac output are increased fatigue and reduced muscle perfusion. The body's compensatory mechanisms of activation of the sympathetic nervous system and the renin–angiotensin system try to overcome the low cardiac output.

b. The place of digoxin is well established in heart failure associated with atrial fibrillation and a rapid ventricular rate but its benefit in heart failure in sinus rhythm remained controversial until recently. However, evidence is now available for the use of small doses of digoxin combined with diuretics and ACE inhibitors when there is severe left ventricular systolic dysfunction and sinus rhythm. Beta-blockers used injudiciously may worsen heart failure by reducing cardiac output. Very careful administration of low doses of β-blockers can be useful, but only when the heart failure has been stabilised with diuretics and an ACE inhibitor. A β-adrenoceptor agonist such as dobutamine may be of use in symptomatic treatment in acute heart failure but is not usually used in chronic heart failure. The treatment of first choice for chronic heart failure fluid retention is a diuretic.

c. For mild symptoms, a thiazide diuretic may be adequate but in most patients a loop diuretic such as furosemide (frusemide) is used. The loss of renal function in the elderly and renal underperfusion in heart failure means that thiazide diuretics are less effective in older patients with this condition.

d. The addition of K^+-sparing diuretics to furosemide (frusemide) or thiazide diuretics is the best way to prevent or treat the hypokalaemia. The adverse metabolic effects of thiazides are of less concern in patients with a serious disorder such as heart failure.

e. ACE inhibitors slow the progression of heart failure and improve survival. There is a small risk of severe hypotension following the first dose and omission of the diuretic immediately prior to this may be helpful.

f. The cough is thought to be caused by increased concentrations of bradykinin, as ACE inhibitors prevent the breakdown of bradykinin by kininase II, which is the same enzyme that converts angiotensin I to angiotensin II. An alternative strategy is to use an angiotensin II receptor antagonist such as losartan. These drugs are well tolerated and can improve symptoms, but their effect on mortality is less well established.

Chapter 8

1 a. **True**. Gradual pacemaker depolarisation in pacemaker cells results from an influx of Na^+ and Ca^{2+}, possibly against a background of slowing K^+ efflux.

b. **False**. Calcium influx also occurs from outside the cell in the plateau phase. The plateau is further stabilised even at rather small levels of Ca^{2+} influx because the muscle cell membrane extrudes smaller amounts of K^+ from the cells.

c. **False**. Reducing phase 4 slope certainly diminishes pacemaker rate of firing, as it takes longer to reach the threshold potential. However, although β-adrenoceptor antagonists and vagal stimulation reduce phase 4 slope, adrenergic stimulation and hypokalaemia in particular increase the slope. This can also occur in cells that do not normally have pacemaker activity. This is part of the explanation for the arrhythmic effects of adrenergic stimulation and hypokalaemia.

d. **False**. Normally this is true, but if the intracellular Ca^{2+} concentration rises (e.g. under the influence of cardiac glycosides, noradrenaline (norepinephrine)) this can exchange with Na^+ passing inwards, causing membrane depolarisations. These are called after-depolarisations or 'triggered activity'.

e. **False**. Class Ib Na^+ channel blockers (e.g. lidocaine) bind and dissociate rapidly to channels in their activated and refractory state, that is in phases 0 and 2, but dissociate from the channel in its resting state. They are, therefore, useful in those ventricular arrhythmias that have a long refractory period and would be particularly beneficial in arrhythmias where the myocardium is influenced by high-frequency excitation. The class Ic Na^+ channel-blocking drug flecainide interacts slowly with Na^+ channels and does not show preference for channels in any particular state. It, therefore, causes a general reduction in excitation, blocking both Na^+ and K^+ channels. The class Ia blocking drugs seem to have intermediate actions between these two.

f. **True**. Beta-blockers reduce pacemaker depolarisation rate by indirectly (through β-adrenoceptors) blocking Ca^{2+} channels in sinus and atrioventricular nodal tissue.

g. **True**. Although the type of Ca^{2+} channels utilised in the plateau phase 2 is different from those utilised in the pacemaker depolarisation during phase 4 of the action potential cycle, verapamil will act both to slow the rate of rise of the pacemaker depolarisation and to reduce the plateau phase, thus shortening the action potential. With these effects, verapamil is useful in supraventricular tachycardias but not in ventricular arrhythmias.

h. **False**. Adenosine has no beneficial effect on ventricular arrhythmias. Its main effect involves enhancing K^+ conductance and inhibition of Ca^{2+} influx. The result is reduced atrioventricular nodal conduction and increase in atrioventricular nodal refractory period. Adenosine is useful because it has a high efficacy and a short duration of action.

2. Case history answers

a. The aim at this stage is to restore and maintain sinus rhythm in this patient, who appears to have no structural heart disease. Since the arrhythmia is of short duration, pharmacological cardioversion may be successful. This could be achieved by flecainide, propafenone, sotalol or amiodarone. Amiodarone is usually reserved for patients with significant cardiac dysfunction or those refractory to other agents. Flecainide and propafenone should be avoided in those with significant cardiac dysfunction or concomitant ischaemic heart disease. However, they are probably suitable for this patient. Digoxin, calcium antagonists and β-blockers are ineffective for terminating atrial fibrillation. Synchronised DC cardioversion is successful in up to 90% of patients who have no structural heart disease or heart failure, who are aged less than 50 years and whose duration of atrial fibrillation is less than 1 year. It could be considered if drugs are unsuccessful. About 50% of patients with recent-onset atrial fibrillation (less than 48 h) do spontaneously convert to sinus rhythm. In this patient, the atrial fibrillation could have been brought on by excess alcohol (so-called 'holiday heart'). If this patient moderates his alcohol intake, then prophylaxis would not be necessary after a single attack.

b. Anticoagulation with warfarin is essential for at least 3–4 weeks before and 4 weeks after a DC cardioversion to minimise the risk of a systemic embolus. For prophylaxis against recurrence, antifibrillatory drugs are usually given for 3–6 months following DC cardioversion since this is the period of highest risk of recurrence. Digoxin, verapamil and β-adrenoceptor antagonists are not effective for prophylaxis. After 5 years of recurrence of atrial fibrillation, sinus rhythm could not be restored. Therefore, the aim in this patient is to control ventricular rate. Digoxin suppresses atrioventricular nodal conduction and can reduce the ventricular response rate. This is mediated through potentiation of vagal effects on the heart and is less effective during exercise; therefore, the addition of a β-blocker or calcium antagonist (such as verapamil or diltiazem) may be necessary. However, β-blockers (in high doses), verapamil and diltiazem are negatively inotropic and if there is significant cardiac dysfunction or heart failure they are contraindicated. The positive inotropic action of digoxin might be helpful if there is coexisting left ventricular impairment. The major long-term consequence of atrial fibrillation is the risk of thromboembolism and this is greatest in those over 75 years of age. For Mr GH, aspirin is sufficient as he is at a relatively low risk of stroke because of his age and lack of any coexisting hypertension, diabetes or significant left ventricular impairment.

Chapter 9

1   a.   **False**. Aspirin has been shown to reduce the risk of a first embolic stroke in atrial fibrillation.
    b.   **True**. The immediate risk of intracranial haemorrhage with t-PA is high and could be compounded by simultaneous administration of antiplatelet or anticoagulant agents. These should be considered later when the effect of the thrombolytic has waned.
    c.   **True**. The excitatory amino acid glutamate can cause a substantial rise in intracellular Ca^{2+} causing Ca^{2+} overload. This causes cell death by generation of free radicals. However, trials of drugs that interfere with glutamate synthesis or effect have been disappointing.
    d.   **False**. Aspirin alone or possibly together with dipyridamole reduces the risk of stroke but warfarin increases mortality and morbidity in patients with recurrent transient ischaemic attacks or strokes.

2. Case history answer
    a.   There is no standard treatment for acute stroke. Although thrombolysis has been shown in some trials to be useful in the treatment of stroke, safe and effective use is determined by a rigid set of criteria as there is a significant risk of intracranial haemorrhage. Thrombolysis is inappropriate in this situation. His blood

pressure is high and it is a considerable time since the onset of symptoms. Thrombolysis has been approved for use within 3 h of the onset of symptoms. The rapid resolution of signs indicates a TIA, for which thrombolysis is not given.
His blood pressure must be brought under control. He should be started on a low dose of aspirin.
Antiplatelet therapy should be continued. The antiplatelet drug dipyridamole may show some added benefit when given with aspirin and can be used if patients continue to have TIAs despite treatment with aspirin.

Chapter 10

1   a.   **False**. There is a two- to fourfold increase in risk of developing coronary disease, stroke or heart failure compared with age-matched subjects who do not have intermittent claudication.
    b.   **True**. By reducing cholesterol synthesis, simvastatin increases hepatic LDL receptors, which results in reduced LDL-cholesterol in blood and a small accompanying increase in high density lipoprotein (HDL)-cholesterol. The main potential benefit of lowered LDL cholesterol in these patients is a reduction in coronary artery disease events.
    c.   **False**. Verapamil is ineffective in the treatment of Raynaud's phenomenon and the agent of choice is nifedipine.

2. Case history answer
    a.   The potential benefit of propranolol in lowering blood pressure is outweighed by blockade of $β_2$-adrenoceptors in the limb blood vessels impairing vasodilation.
    b.   Cardioselective β-blockers such as atenolol do not cause deterioration in walking distance when used alone.
    c.   Vasodilators will lower blood pressure but do not improve walking distance. In some patients they may redirect blood from the maximally dilated ischaemic tissues to healthy tissues (vascular steal). This can be particularly troublesome in critical limb ischaemia, or when the cardiac output is also reduced by concurrent use of a β-blocker.
    d.   Lowering LDL cholesterol can stabilise atherosclerotic plaques perhaps reducing the consequences of coexistent heart disease; it is not known if walking distance or limb survival is improved.

e. Low-dose aspirin inhibits platelet aggregation and reduces future cardiac events, which are common in this group of patients.

f. Intensive management of blood pressure control, control of diabetes and antiplatelet therapy will reduce the risk of cardiac events. An exercise programme can improve walking distance. Smoking is a major contributory factor to impaired walking distance and cardiac events.

g. Excessive warming of limbs may dilate normal arteries, 'stealing' blood from diseased tissues.

Chapter 11

1 a. **False**. Streptokinase is usually infused for 1 h and rt-PA for 3 h. rt-PA has a short duration of action but streptokinase has a longer half-life, permitting a shorter infusion time.

b. **True**. Warfarin can cause fetal abnormalities and should not be given in early pregnancy.

c. **False**. Clopidogrel prevents platelet aggregation induced by the release of ADP after platelet activation. Clopidogrel also inhibits thrombin-induced platelet aggregation.

d. **True**. The increased expression of GPIIb/IIIa receptors on platelets is essential for aggregation as fibrinogen links adjacent platelets by binding to GPIIb/IIIa receptors, thereby initiating aggregation.

e. **True**. Thromboxane A_2 (TXA_2) required for platelet aggregation is synthesised by the cyclo-oxygenase type 1 (COX 1) enzyme whereas prostaglandins synthesised during inflammation are synthesised by cyclo-oxygenase type 2 (COX 2) enzymes. Aspirin is 160 times more active at inhibiting COX 1 than COX 2. Therefore, at the low doses required to inhibit TXA_2 synthesis, it has no anti-inflammatory effect.

f. **False**. Vitamin K is produced by gut bacteria. Alteration of gut flora by broad-spectrum antimicrobials will reduce vitamin K formation and hence clotting factors. This will enhance the activity of warfarin.

g. **False**. Tranexamic acid inhibits plasminogen activation, reducing fibrin degradation and the risk of bleeding.

h. **False**. The action of unfractionated heparin but not LMWH can be reversed by the strongly basic protein protamine, which rapidly binds to it forming an inactive compound.

2. Case history answer

a. Postoperative venous thromboembolism occurs in 40–50% of patients undergoing hip replacement and fatal pulmonary embolism in 1–5% if prophylactic anticoagulant therapy is not given. This lady is also at increased risk because of obesity.

b. This is controversial. Initiating prophylaxis postoperatively allows more effective surgical haemostasis and does not reduce the effectiveness of treatment.

c. Heparin is not active orally. The onset of action of heparin is rapid whereas warfarin takes several days for full effectiveness but can be given orally. Heparin would, therefore, be chosen if started pre- or postoperatively.

d. The patient was obese, a risk factor for postoperative thrombosis. Daily self-administered subcutaneous prophylaxis with low-molecular-weight heparin (LMWH) could be used. LMWH has a better bioavailability, a longer half-life and lower risk of producing thrombocytopenia. Unlike unfractionated heparin, its effect is predictable.

Chapter 12

1 a. **True**. This is particularly important and the T helper type 2 cells are involved in the generation of cytokines that promote activation of eosinophils and expression of IgE receptors on mast cells and eosinophils. The T helper type 2 cells also express endothelial adhesion molecules that attract eosinophils.

b. **False**. Leukotriene C_4 is a bronchoconstrictor, increasing mucus secretion and oedema.

2 a. **True**. Salbutamol is effective taken before exercise but the longer acting β_2-adrenoceptor agonists are slower in onset. Cromoglycate taken prophylactically may also be effective.

3 a. **False**. Hyper-reactivity of airways is seen but epithelial cells show variable damage.

4 a. **True**. There is evidence of tolerance to β_2-adrenoceptor agonists that can be reduced by administration of corticosteroids.

5 a. **True**. Erythromycin and ciprofloxin inhibit liver cytochrome P450 enzymes, which metabolise theophylline.

b. **False**. The methylxanthines (present in coffee) increase alertness and can cause irritability and headache.

c. **True**. All methylxanthines have positive inotropic and chronotropic activity and a narrow therapeutic index.

6 a. **False**. Ipratropium is less effective against allergen challenge but can be useful as an adjunct and in the management of chronic obstructive pulmonary disease.

b. **False**. Ipratropium can cause a modest tachycardia owing to blockade of muscarinic receptors in the heart.

c. **True**. Ipratropium has a quaternary structure and is, therefore, poorly absorbed.

7 a. **False**. Montelukast inhibits receptors for the cysteinyl leukotrienes (C_4, D_4, E_4).

b. **True**. The leukotriene antagonists need to be administered orally on a regular prophylactic basis to reduce asthmatic attacks. They are much less effective once an attack has started.

8 a. **True**. Glucocorticoids affect several steps in the inflammatory pathways involved in the genesis of asthma.

Chapter 13

1 a. **True**. Diphenhydramine and chlorpheniramine are common constituents of compound cough mixtures.

b. **True**. Dextromethorphan has the same cough suppressant potency as codeine but is not analgesic.

2 a. **False**. Surfactant acts like a detergent and lowers the surface tension, enabling the alveoli to expand and retain an expanded shape.

b. **False**. Doxapram is used in hospitals for postoperative respiratory failure. It stimulates the respiratory centre and the carotid chemoreceptors but its precise mode of action is unknown.

c. **False**. Mecysteine breaks the disulfide cross bridges that maintain the polymeric gel-like structure of mucus.

Chapter 14

1. **False**. Much of the K^+ filtered at the glomerulus is reabsorbed in the proximal tubule and in the loop

of Henle. Secretory loss into the urine is mainly in exchange for Na^+ occurring through specialised K^+ channels in the collecting ducts.

2. **True**. Impermeability to water and an active $Na^+/Cl^-/K^+$ cotransporter in the thick ascending limb are pertinent to the generation of the hyperosmotic interstitium and the counter current mechanisms for concentrating urine.

3. **True**. These regions are permeable to water where an osmotic effect can be exerted.

4. **True**. As a result of extracting water from intracellular compartments and expanding extracellular and intravascular fluid volume they can precipitate pulmonary oedema.

5. **True**. Acetazolamide results in a mild metabolic acidosis and a reduced plasma bicarbonate concentration which limits the H^+/Na^+ exchange at the luminal membrane.

6. **False**. By inhibiting the $Na^+/K^+/Cl^-$ cotransporter the medullary interstitial hypertonicity falls. Because this hypertonicity provides the osmotic force for the absorption of water in the collecting ducts (in the presence of antidiuretic hormone, vasopressin), the reduced osmotic pressure results in less water reabsorption. Loop diuretics are highly protein bound and little is filtered at the glomerulus. The drugs reach the luminal membrane cotransporter by secretion into the proximal tubule via the organic acid transport mechanism.

7 a. **True**. Loop diuretics are widely used in the control of oedema in heart failure for the elimination of the excessive salt and water load. The direct venodilator activity of furosemide reduces central blood volume.

b. **False**. A thiazide diuretic or metolazone can be added to a loop diuretic to act sequentially at different sites in the nephron, thus producing a marked diuresis and natriuresis.

c. **False**. Delivery of greater concentrations of Na^+ to the collecting ducts increases the exchange for K^+ at that site, thus increasing K^+ loss.

d. **False**. Once the cotransporter mechanism is maximally inhibited, no further water or salt excretion can occur

e. **True**. When high doses are used, especially in the presence of renal damage, or when taken with an aminoglycoside antibiotic, ototoxicity can occur.

8 a. **False**. Like the loop diuretics, the thiazides have to act from the renal tubular lumen on the

cotransporter that is on the luminal membrane. The thiazides are secreted by the proximal tubule transport mechanism into the lumen.

b. **False**. The thiazide diuretics do not increase Ca^{2+} excretion, unlike the loop diuretics, which do cause urinary loss of Ca^{2+}.

c. **True**. Metolazone is more potent than other thiazide diuretics and when given together with furosemide produces an intense diuresis. Its greater effect is possibly a result of additional actions in the proximal tubule. Unlike other thiazide diuretics it also works in advanced renal failure.

d. **True**. Thiazide diuretics could exacerbate diabetes mellitus. The mechanism may be through inhibition of insulin synthesis.

9 a. **False**. Although both drugs ultimately reduce activity of the Na^+ reuptake channel, amiloride blocks the channel directly, whereas spironolactone prevents the actions of aldosterone-induced proteins which enhance the Na^+ channel numbers and activity.

b. **True**. ACE inhibitors by inhibiting aldosterone secretion will increase K^+ concentration in the interstitium and blood by reducing K^+ excretion.

10 a. **False**. Because the diuretics act at different sites an additional natriuresis is produced.

b. **False**. Canrenone is an active diuretic, responsible for most of the effects of spironolactone.

11. **True**. Some diuretics may act partly by the generation of prostaglandins. In addition, prostaglandins help to maintain renal blood flow. Therefore, NSAIDs can reduce diuretic activity.

Chapter 15

1 a. **False**. Atropine blocks muscarinic receptors inhibiting the parasympathetic effects on the detrusor muscle resulting in urinary retention.

b. **True**. The tricyclics act to reduce detrusor instability, in part by their antimuscarinic actions.

c. **False**. Distigmine contracts detrusor muscle, which is undesirable in the presence of urinary outflow obstruction.

2. Case history answer

a. Drugs may be used in mild disease and while awaiting a trans-urethral resection of the

prostate. Selective α_1-adrenoceptor blockers increase urine flow to a limited extent but also decrease urgency, frequency and hesitancy. Blockers selective for α_{1A}-adrenoceptors such as tamsulosin are claimed to have fewer unwanted effects. Finasteride, which inhibits conversion of testosterone to dihydrotestosterone, reduces prostate size slowly.

b. Alpha$_1$-adrenoceptor blockers can cause postural hypotension, especially with first dose. They cause dizziness and can interact with other drugs to lower blood pressure. Finasteride can reduce libido and cause impotence.

c. The outcome is variable; symptoms may not worsen appreciably for many years but moderate symptoms can lead to a poor quality of life. Complications include urinary retention, incontinence and renal insufficiency owing to hydronephrosis.

Chapter 16

1. **True**. Nitrates result in increased nitric oxide production and elevate cGMP. Sildenafil has a similar effect by preventing cGMP breakdown. This can lead to additive unwanted effects.

2. **False**. These two drugs can act together to cause hypotension.

3. **False**. Phosphodiesterase type V is found in other blood vessels and tissues which can result in unwanted effects when sildenafil is given.

4. **False**. Parasympathetic stimulation enhances erection. Drugs known to inhibit the parasympathetic outflow, e.g. tricyclic antidepressants, can cause erectile failure.

5. **True**. Painful priapism with erections lasting many hours can occur.

6. **False**. Testosterone can be useful if the impotence is due to hypogonadism.

7. **True**. Probably through vascular dysfunction.

Chapter 17

1 a. **False**. Because of the diversity of substances that produce anaesthesia, it is probable that

there are not distinctive receptors at which these drugs act, but rather they produce more general effects on constituents of the cell membrane such as lipids or proteins.

b. **False**. The inhalational anaesthetics are volatile liquids.

c. **False**. The main inhalational anaesthetics are halogenated compounds.

2 a. **False**. It causes cardiac arrhythmias, hepatotoxicity with repeated use and hypotension. It also sensitises the heart to catecholamine. It is, however, a potent anaesthetic.

b. **True**. This is particularly true with highly lipid-soluble agents, which will accumulate in body fat stores and be slowly released after the operation.

c. **False**. Even at higher concentrations than 50%, nitrous oxide is not potent enough to produce effective surgical anaesthesia on its own.

d. **True**. Nitrous oxide and oxygen are used concurrently with fluorinated anaesthetics. The other attribute of nitrous oxide is that unlike fluorinated compounds it has analgesic activity.

3. **False**. Halothane undergoes substantial metabolism, but the other halogenated anaesthetics do not.

4 a. **False**. The half-life of the rapid distribution phase of thiopental is only about 3 min, hence its short duration of action. However, the elimination of thiopental from the body is much slower and the half-life is approximately 12 h. This partially accounts for the hangover seen with this drug.

b. **True**. Propofol is useful for short operations where it has rapid elimination and little hangover effect. The hepatic clearance of propofol has a half-life of 1–2 h.

c. **True**. Either extravascular injections of thiopental or intra-arterial injections can have damaging consequences because its pH is approximately 9–10.

d. **False**. Ketamine does have analgesic action unlike other available intravenous anaesthetics. It can be useful when pain is difficult to control.

5 a. **False**. Fentanyl is increasingly given for intra-operative analgesia. It is short acting and with rapid recovery; consequently, it has a low incidence of hangover effects.

6 a. **True**. This was true when slow-acting anaesthetics were given, but it is less problematic with rapidly acting inhalational anaesthetics.

b. **True**. Most are negatively inotropic and they depress myocardial function by interfering with Ca^{2+} fluxes. Halothane also sensitises the heart to catecholamines and can lead to arrhythmias.

c. **True**. Inhalational anaesthetics reduce the ventilatory response to carbon dioxide and hypoxia and increase the arterial partial pressure of carbon dioxide.

d. **True**. Sevoflurane is rapid in onset and also is more rapidly eliminated than halothane or isoflurane.

7. Case history answer

a. Atropine or hyoscine block muscarinic receptors, blocking bronchial and salivary secretions. Modern anaesthetics have less irritant effect thus reducing this problem. Muscarinic antagonists can reduce the bradycardia caused by some inhalation anaesthetics and suxamethonium.

b. Atropine can cause central nervous system excitation whereas hyoscine causes sedation and has anti-emetic properties.

c. Relatively minor but frequent complications occur with suxamethonium including bradycardia, postoperative myalgia, transient elevation of the plasma K^+ concentrations and raised intraocular, intracranial and intragastric pressures. A rare, but potentially fatal, complication is malignant hyperthermia, which is genetically determined. The short-acting non-depolarising blocking drug rocuronium has a similar duration of action and does not cause these problems.

d. Pancuronium is probably not the ideal muscle relaxant to use. It does not cause histamine release, but it can cause tachycardia and hypertension and is long-acting (Ch. 27). An alternative would be vecuronium, which has an intermediate duration of action, does not release histamine and lacks cardiovascular effects. The short-acting rocuronium is more expensive but has rapid onset and short duration of action and a low risk of cardiovascular effects.

e. Opioid-induced apnoea. The use of pethidine followed by fentanyl is generous for a short operation, resulting in respiratory depression. The patient could be treated by the administration of naloxone. The dose of neostigmine given may have been insufficient to reverse the competitive blocking effect of the long-acting pancuronium. The patient could have a genetically determined deficiency of pseudocholinesterase (plasma cholinesterase), which metabolises suxamethonium. This is present in about 1 in 2000 individuals. If respiratory depression is caused by suxamethonium, administration of neostigmine would make it worse. Fresh frozen plasma containing pseudocholinesterase could be administered.

f. Although mivacurium is a short-acting muscle relaxant, it is metabolised by pseudocholinesterase and its effect would be prolonged if there is a reduced level of this metabolising enzyme.

g. Neostigmine inhibits acetylcholinesterase. It reverses the actions of competitive neuromuscular-blocking drugs acting at nicotinic type 2 receptors at skeletal muscle but also enhances the activity of acetylcholine at muscarinic receptors causing bradycardia and respiratory depression. Glycopyrrolate selectivity blocks muscarinic receptors, thus reducing excess muscarinic stimulation.

Chapter 18

1 a. **False**. If absorbed, systemic high doses of local anaesthetics can produce cardiovascular collapse and central nervous system depression.

   b. **False**. Initial decline in local activity is due to removal into the systemic circulation. The anaesthetic is then metabolised.

   c. **True**.

   d. **False**. Prazosin is a vasodilator and would increase the removal of the local anaesthetic from its injection site: adrenaline or other local vasoconstrictors are necessary.

2 a. **True**. It is a long-acting local anaesthetic similar to bupivacaine but may be less arrhythmogenic.

   b. **False**. Levobupivacaine is marketed and shows lower cardiotoxicity.

Chapter 19

1 a. **True**. In patients with pain, analgesia is often associated with wellbeing (μ-receptors) whereas in pain-free patients dysphoria can occur (κ-receptors).

   b. **False**. Tolerance to miosis and the constipatory effects of opioids develops much less than to the other biological effects including analgesia and respiratory depression. Cross-tolerance to opioids is common.

c. **False**. Because of its long half-life and less potential to cause euphoria, it is used in controlled withdrawal in patients with opioid dependence. It is orally well absorbed and has a slow onset of action. Patients exhibit slower and less intense withdrawal symptoms with methadone.

2 a. **True**. Because the opioid μ-opioid receptors subserve analgesia and the κ-receptors are involved in respiratory depression, it is claimed that meptazinol has less respiratory depressant action.

   b. **False**. Naloxone is short-acting opioid antagonist acting at μ-, κ- and δ-receptors. It is used in opioid overdosage. Severe withdrawal symptoms can occur in addicts following naloxone administration.

3 a. **True**. Tricyclic antidepressants can be effective for the treatment of pain of neuropathic origin. They may act by enhancing amine levels in the descending inhibitory pathways that control the pain gate mechanism (see Fig. 19.3, p. 226).

   b. **False**. Phenytoin, carbamazepine and sodium valproate are useful analgesics in neuropathic pain, probably by stabilising neuronal membranes and inhibiting neurotransmitter release.

4. **True**. Because it is a partial agonist it can actually reduce the effects of morphine.

5. Case history answer

   a. Morphine acts at specific opioid receptors at spinal and supraspinal sites to produce analgesia and unwanted effects. Morphine is a strong agonist at all μ-receptors that subserve analgesia, euphoria, respiratory depression and dependence.

   b. Morphine oral solution is used to control short-term breakthrough exacerbations of pain on a patient initiated basis. Repeated use of this form of morphine should signal a reassessment of the dose of the long-acting morphine. When the patient is unable to take oral medication because of weakness or vomiting, rectal or continuous subcutaneous infusion may be required (see d). Normally, 80% of patients require less than 200 mg per day to control severe pain. With terminally ill patients having persistent severe pain, the dose is gradually increased over a period of 1 to 2 weeks until an appropriate level of control is achieved. The maximum level may be as high as 2–3 g per day. Unwanted effects can occur; therefore, close monitoring is needed when treatment is first initiated or dosage altered.

c. For reasons that are not easily explained from a theoretical viewpoint, addiction seldom occurs in patients with a high degree of pain. Possible reasons may be a high natural opioid level or high catecholamine levels.

d. Diamorphine can be used instead of morphine. It is more potent, but is no more efficacious. Its major advantage in practice is its high solubility, which reduces the volume of intramuscular injections or continuous subcutaneous infusion if these are required. Infrequently an unusual response to morphine may require its replacement by other opioids. Fentanyl is a suitable replacement delivered via a transdermal patch and having fewer unwanted effects.

e. Diclofenac is an aspirin-like non-steroidal anti-inflammatory drug (NSAID) often used in the treatment of arthritic conditions. Unlike opioids it has both analgesic and anti-inflammatory actions. NSAIDs appear to have only a small central component to their actions.

f. The pain from metastases is compounded by local inflammation: in this case the bone metastases cause 'inflammatory pain' which may be reduced by diclofenac thereby reducing the requirement for morphine.

g. Dexamethasone is a potent glucocorticoid. Inflammation increases local pressure (and hence pain) within the bone; dexamethasone is a potent corticosteroid, reducing inflammation and swelling.

h. Nausea is an unwanted effect caused by morphine, occurring particularly during the first week of administration but may also be a consequence of the cancer itself or related complications such as hypercalcaemia. Tolerance to the nausea induced by morphine occurs.

i. Metoclopramide is a dopamine antagonist that acts on the chemoreceptor trigger zone (CTZ) to reduce chemical and radiation-induced nausea.

j. A centrally acting anti-emetic such as prochlorperazine can be used. They have the same mechanism of action as metoclopramide.

k. Gastric and/or duodenal inflammation (which may cause considerable discomfort) or even ulceration may occur with prolonged use of diclofenac and a corticosteroid. Cimetidine in this patient relieved the gastric discomfort associated with oral administration of diclofenac.

l. Cimetidine is a histamine H_2 receptor antagonist. Note cimetidine inhibits the enzymes that convert codeine into morphine and may reduce its analgesic effect. (Diclofenac is available in a combined formulation with the prostaglandin analogue misoprostil, which has gastroprotective activity.)

m. Constipation is a feature of morphine therapy. Tolerance does not develop to opioid-induced constipation. Peristalsis is reduced while the tone of the intestinal muscle is increased.

n. Docusate sodium is primarily a stimulant of intestinal smooth muscle, which restores peristalsis. It also has some faecal-softening properties.

o. In practice, terminally ill patients are often given danthron, in combination with either docusate sodium (co-danthrusate) or poloxamer (co-danthramer). Danthron is a stimulant drug and stool softener and is particularly useful when 'bowel movements must be by strain'. The irritant properties of danthron and its carcinogenic potential restrict its general use. The alternatives in use include senna preparations (stimulants) and magnesium sulfate (a bulk purgative). Other agents do exist but cost is a prime factor when cheap agents are as effective as their more expensive counterparts.

p. Temazepam is a short-acting benzodiazepine used to aid sleeping.

Note. Pain control must also take note of the psychological, social and spiritual condition of the patient. At all times if pain control is inadequate adjuvant treatments such as radiotherapy or transcutaneous electrical nerve stimulation should be considered. Where neuropathic pain is evident, tricyclic antidepressants or anticonvulsants should also be considered.

Chapter 20

1 a. **False**. Dependence, tolerance and withdrawal symptoms occur on long-term continuous usage.

b. **True**. Additional CNS depression can occur.

2 a. **True**. Benzodiazepines are metabolised largely by the liver and rate of metabolism is reduced in the elderly; the elderly are also more sensitive to the effects of the drugs.

b. **False**. Buspirone is not a benzodiazepine and has less sedative action than temazepam.

3. **False**. Benzodiazepines affect the structure of sleep with loss of REM sleep. Zolpidem has less effect than some other benzodiazepines.

4. Case history answer

a. Mrs FL's insomnia and anxiety are essentially a normal response to bereavement and should present fewer long-term problems than chronic 'endogenous' anxiety. Benzodiazepines are much safer as hypnotics than their predecessors (barbiturates and phenothiazines). The central concept in benzodiazepine therapy is nevertheless to use the minimal effective dose for the shortest possible period. A short-acting benzodiazepine (e.g. temazepam) taken at night should help to restore her sleep pattern and help Mrs FL cope with pressures at work. The relatively short half-life of temazepam (5–10 h) should minimise risk of sedation during the working day.

b. Benzodiazepines are $GABA_A$ agonists that enhance $GABA_A$-mediated inhibition of neuronal activity in the 'reticular activating system' in the brain and spinal cord. Benzodiazepines bind to $GABA_A$ receptors (at a site distinct from barbiturates) and increase frequency of channel opening, causing Cl^- entry into the cell and neuronal hyperpolarisation. Benzodiazepines are relatively free of serious unwanted effects (e.g. compared with respiratory depression with barbiturates) and are safe in overdose, but sedation and psychomotor impairment may interfere markedly with driving and operating machinery (worsened by interaction with alcohol, barbiturates, and older sedative antihistamines). Rebound wakefulness may occur in the morning. Other unwanted effects include headache, dry mouth, hypotension, anterograde amnesia, skin rashes, and blood dyscrasias. Psychotic reactions (hallucinations) have been reported with triazolam.

c. Rebound wakefulness may indicate a need for a longer-acting benzodiazepine such as nitrazepam or diazepam, which may also help to reduce Mrs FL's daytime anxiety and panic attacks. Conversely, daytime sedation may interfere with driving and work, exacerbated by long-acting metabolites of these drugs. An alternative may be to prescribe buspirone; however, this requires 1 to 2 weeks for a response.

d. Long-term use of a benzodiazepine is associated with dependence, manifested mainly as a withdrawal reaction, which may include rebound anxiety, tremor, nausea, irritability, anorexia, and dysphoria. Together with rapid development of tolerance (especially to hypnotic action), these contraindicate benzodiazepine treatment for more than 3 weeks. In the longer term, antidepressants may be indicated. Mrs FL's recovery from bereavement may be aided by psychological counselling and support from family and employer.

Chapter 21

1 a. **False**.
   b. **True**. Regular blood monitoring is required.
   c. **False**. Injections are at 1 to 3 month intervals.

2 a. **True**. Negative symptoms are more difficult to treat, 'atypical' antipsychotics may have greater activity against negative symptoms.
   b. **False**. The plasma levels of chlorpromazine are highly variable and do not correlate with clinical effect.

3 **True**. Their antimuscarinic activity may contribute to this.

4. Case history answers
   a. Schizophrenia is associated with overactivity of dopaminergic pathways in the mesolimbic area and median temporal lobe, e.g. hippocampus and amygdala, although evidence of biochemical or organic abnormalities is sparse. Pharmacologically, florid schizophrenia symptoms may be mimicked by dopamine agonists (e.g. amphetamines) and are improved by dopamine antagonists. Antipsychotic activity correlates most closely with antagonism of dopamine D_2 (and possibly D_3) receptors.
   b. Distinct from their antipsychotic activity, drugs also block dopamine D_2 receptors in nigrostriatal pathways. This upsets the 'balance' between dopaminergic and cholinergic activity, leading to extrapyramidal movement disorders (e.g. tremor, akasthisia, tardive dyskinesia). The movement disorders thus mimic those seen in Parkinson's disease, where they are caused by a *neurological* deficit in dopaminergic activity. As with Parkinsonian patients, anticholinergic drugs are sometimes used in schizophrenia to ameliorate extrapyramidal side-effects. Mr PS's movement disorders (problems with writing/typing) appear relatively mild, possibly because chlorpromazine (an early phenothiazine) also has antimuscarinic activity. Paradoxically, newer phenothiazines (e.g. fluphenazine) often produce worse movement disorders than chlorpromazine.

   Mr PS's weight gain may be cushingoid caused by chlorpromazine antagonising the dopamine-dependent suppression of adrenocorticotrophic hormone (ACTH) release from the hypothalamus.
   c. As well as the above caused by dopamine antagonism, many antipsychotic drugs (especially early ones) produce unwanted

effects due to blockade of histamine receptors (sedation, tiredness), muscarinic receptors (dry mouth, blurred vision, impotence) and α_1-adrenoceptors (vasodilation-postural hypotension). Chlorpromazine may also produce 'yellowing' or darkening of vision because of idiosyncratic deposition in cornea.

d. Possible use of long-acting depot preparations (decanoates, etc.), and importance of support from GP and patient's family in maintaining compliance. A principal cause of poor compliance is unwanted effects of antipsychotic therapy. Since adverse effects vary widely from drug to drug, the choice of drug may have major impact on compliance, e.g. a drug causing severe movement disorders may be least appropriate in elderly patient at risk from falls, a drug with strong antimuscarinic effect (e.g. sexual dysfunction) may be more resented in younger patients.

e. Mr PS may benefit from a different antipsychotic drug like fluphenazine or flupentixol, which produce less antagonism of histamine receptors (less sedation) and muscarinic receptors (less dry mouth, blurred vision etc.), even though movement disorders may be worse than with chlorpromazine. Negative symptoms (apathy, withdrawal) are relatively poorly controlled with most antipsychotics compared with 'positive' symptoms (delusions, hallucinations), and both types of symptoms may be particularly resistant in a proportion of patients. An 'atypical' antipsychotic drug (clozapine, sulpiride) may help with the apathy and withdrawal reported by Mr PS, with relatively little sedation and movement disorders. Clozapine can cause blood disorders (agranulocytosis and aplastic anaemia) and blood monitoring is mandatory.

Chapter 22

1 a. **True**. Downregulation of $5HT_2$ receptors parallels the time course of improvement of clinical condition, whereas the time course of the increase in amine transmitters does not.

b. **False**. Different TCAs vary widely in their abilities to independently affect noradrenaline and serotonin reuptake.

c. **True**. TCAs have a greater potential to produce serious unwanted effects, e.g. causing cardiac arrhythmias in acute overdose. Interestingly, patient acceptability is similar with both drug classes.

2 a. **False**. Lofepramine is among the least cardiotoxic of the tricyclic and related antidepressants.

b. **True**. MAOI and SSRI should not be combined. The combination can cause CNS excitation, tremor and hyperthermia. An MAOI should not be started until 1 to 5 weeks after stopping SSRI, depending upon which SSRI has been taken.

3 a. **True**. Trazodone is atypical since it blocks $5HT_2$ receptors

b. **False**. Although like tricyclic antidepressants venlafaxine inhibits both noradrenaline and 5HT reuptake, it lacks the sedative and antimuscarinic effects of tricyclic antidepressants.

c. **False**. Venlafaxine is claimed to produce improvement in about 1 week whereas other antidepressants can take many weeks for their effects to be seen.

4 a. **True**. Alcohol should not be consumed by patients taking tricyclic antidepressants.

b. **False**. The half-life of lithium is long (about 24 h).

c. **False**. Although it is most commonly used in bipolar affective disorder, it is also used in patients with severe recurrent depressive episodes that do not respond to other treatment.

5. Case history answer

a. The causes of depression are unknown. Although it can occur in reaction to a stressful situation, most cases do not have an obvious precipitant. It is a syndrome (a cluster of symptoms) several features of which DW was exhibiting. The symptoms had been developing for a long period of time.

b. Risk factors include gender (more frequent in women), age (peak age 20–40 years), family history of depression, marital status (higher rates in separated and divorced), stress. Can we be certain that any of these were contributory? Exercise obsession, weight loss? Potential anorexia?

c. There is a biological association of depression with reduced central nervous system (CNS) monoaminergic neurotransmission, notably noradrenaline and 5-hydroxytryptamine (5HT) but it is still unclear whether this is cause or effect. Drugs that deplete monoamines can induce depression and when monoamines are repleted symptoms decrease.

Probably because of the depletion of monoamines, there is an upregulation of postsynaptic monoamine receptors. These include $5HT_2$ and α_1-adrenoceptors;

β_1-adrenoceptors may also be upregulated. Drugs used to treat depression increase CNS 5HT and/or noradrenaline in the synaptic cleft, which eventually results in receptor downregulation and a return to normal in the postsynaptic receptor numbers.

d. TCAs may not be the most appropriate choice if DW was showing suicidal tendencies. Their therapeutic index is low and a better choice would be a selective serotonin reuptake inhibitor (SSRI).

e. Unwanted effects include muscarinic receptor blockade (dry mouth, blurred vision, constipation), cardiotoxicity, sedation (variable) and postural hypotension.

f. The onset of action is delayed for at least 2–4 weeks. Two-thirds of depressed people improve, one-third do not. One-third of depressed patients would have got better without drug therapy. Whether TCAs prevent recurrence is unknown. Alternative treatments include SSRIs such as fluoxetine (Prozac). This has fewer unwanted effects such as cardiotoxicity and antimuscarinic actions but causes nausea, insomnia and agitation in some patients. Its antidepressant action is no better than that of tricyclic antidepressants. Other possibilities are monoamine oxidase inhibitors (MAOIs), which have considerable unwanted effects and require dietary restriction of tyramine (cheese) intake; they are less used now. RIMAs (reversible inhibitor of monoamine oxidase A, e.g. moclobemide) are selective for inhibition of this isoenzyme, leaving type B unaltered, and this is able to metabolise tyramine. Drugs previously called atypical antidepressants act partially by blocking monoamine receptors. Trazodone blocks postsynaptic $5HT_2$ receptors and has only a small effect on the inhibition of 5HT reuptake.

Chapter 23

1. **False**. Absences, manifested by unawareness of surroundings without motor disturbance, occur in children.

2. **False**. In 'Jacksonian epilepsy' jerking localised to a particular group of muscles may occur which can then gradually involve many other muscles.

3. a. **False**. There are currently no glutamate antagonists that are useful in treatment of epilepsy.

b. **False**. GABA causes hyperpolarisation by increasing Cl⁻ influx into cells and cannot be given orally. However, several anti-epileptic drugs act by enhancing the effect of GABA.

4. **False**. Phenytoin exhibits 'use-dependent' blockade of Na^+ channels, i.e. the block increases with duration of contact with the receptors.

5. a. **False**. Salicylates and valproate displace phenytoin from plasma proteins to which 80–90% of the drug is bound. This increases the free plasma concentration and the effect of phenytoin.

b. **False**. Phenytoin exhibits first-order kinetics up to the lower parts of the therapeutic dose range but at higher doses the relationship switches to zero-order kinetics after the liver metabolising enzymes have become saturated.

6. **False**. Although vigabatrin is effective in all types of epilepsy, acting by specifically reducing the breakdown of GABA, it is reserved for patients resistant to other drugs.

7. a. Absence seizures usually respond well to sodium valproate or ethosuximide. Ethosuximide is effective only in absence seizures. Phenytoin and phenobarbital are ineffective in absences.

b. Sodium valproate causes nausea, reversible transient hair loss and weight gain. Uncommonly liver damage can occur. Ethosuximide causes nausea, anorexia and headache.

c. Monotherapy with ethosuximide or sodium valproate should be tried before combining therapies. Compliance should also be checked before combining therapies. Sodium valproate reduces the clearance of ethosuximide and may cause toxicity.

8 a. A variety of drugs could be used in this patient. First line drugs usually include carbamazepine, phenytoin or sodium valproate.

b. Non-hormonal contraceptives such as barrier or intrauterine device are effective and do not carry the risk of drug interactions. However, many women will want to use a hormonal method.

c. Carbamazepine, phenytoin, phenobarbital and topiramate all induce liver enzymes that increase the metabolism of sex steroids and reduce efficacy of oral contraceptives.

d. Injected medroxyprogesterone acetate is affected less than sex steroids administered orally. The interval between injection of medroxyprogesterone acetate should, however, be reduced to 10 weeks. Medroxyprogesterone acetate may also reduce the incidence of epileptic attacks.

e. It is recommended that at a minimum pills containing a high concentration of estrogen (50 μg) should be given. Up to 3 pills per day containing 35 μg estrogen may be required to prevent breakthrough bleeding. The pill-free period can also be reduced. If any change in medication for her epilepsy is made, additional barrier methods of contraception should be used until medication is stabilised.

f. No. The progestogen-only pill would be ineffective as its metabolism is increased.

Chapter 24

1 a. **False**. Symptoms develop when approximately 80% of neurons have been lost.

b. **True**. There is overactivity of glutaminergic neurons in parkinsonism and this exacerbates the excessive outflow of GABA nerves to the motor cortex.

c. **False**. Levodopa has a short half-life and this may contribute to end-of-dose movement disorders.

2 a. **True**. In clinical trials of up to 6 months' duration in early Parkinson's disease, ropinirole has been shown to be as effective as levodopa.

b. **False**. Benzhexol can cause minor unwanted effects but also can cause severe confusion particularly in the elderly.

3 a. **True**. Bromocriptine stimulates dopamine receptors and its half life of 6–8 h is longer than levodopa.

b. **True**. Particularly tremor and rigidity may be partially because of other transmitter substances.

c. **True**.

d. **False**. Selegiline only inhibits monoamine oxidase type B (MAO-B), leaving MAO-A intact to metabolise tyramine in cheese and some other foods.

e. **False**. Entacopone inhibits the enzyme catechol-*O*-methyl transferase, which breaks down about 10% of levodopa. It, therefore, helps to maintain concentrations of levodopa, which has a short half-life.

4 a. **False**. Baclofen is used in the treatment of spasticity by inhibiting excitatory synapses and stimulating responses of the inhibitory transmitter GABA.

b. **True**. Botulinum toxin is used in spasticity injected locally and inhibits acetylcholine release for up to 3 months.

5 a. The cause of Parkinson's disease is a selective degeneration of dopaminergic neurons in the corpus striatum and the substantia nigra. The cause is unknown but hypotheses include actions of reactive oxygen metabolites, neurotoxins or immune disturbances. The basal ganglia of patients with Parkinson's disease generally have less than 10% of the normal amount of dopamine. This results in complex neurochemical disturbances: an upregulation of dopamine D_2 receptors but a downregulation of D_1 receptors in the striatum. An excessive inhibitory GABA-ergic outflow from the striatum to the thalamus and motor cortex and to the substantia nigra produces the symptoms. Cholinergic overactivity results from the removal of the inhibition effect of dopamine on cholinergic neurons. There is also overactivity of glutamate neurons and control of this may be a target for useful future drugs for the treatment of parkinsonism.

b. Patients have akinesia, rigidity and tremor possibly from inhibition of the motor cortical system whereas the descending inhibition of the brainstem locomotor areas may contribute to abnormalities of gait and posture. Patients have difficulty getting going and problems with fine movement, particularly in writing.

c. Levodopa is the immediate precursor of dopamine and is transported into the CNS by an active transport mechanism. Dopamine does not gain access. Levodopa causes nausea and vomiting because of its effect on the chemoreceptor trigger zone (the blood–brain barrier is deficient in the area postrema). Co-beneldopa is a combination of levodopa and benserazide. Benserazide or another compound, carbidopa, are used because they inhibit peripheral dopa decarboxylase activity and, therefore, prevent the breakdown of levodopa to dopamine. They do not cross the blood–brain barrier so levodopa is still converted to dopamine in the brain. Protection against peripheral unwanted effects can also be achieved with the peripheral-acting dopamine antagonist domperidone. Unwanted effects of levodopa are nausea and vomiting, postural hypotension, hallucinations and confusion and unpredictable motor disturbances.

d. Levodopa remains the most effective treatment for Parkinson's disease. There has however been extensive debate about when to start therapy with levodopa. There is no convincing evidence that levodopa accelerates neurodegeneration and survival is reduced if treatment is delayed until greater disability is present. In time, and despite long-term treatment with levodopa, there is an increasing incidence of dyskinesias and on–off fluctuations of effect, although most patients continue to derive benefit throughout the duration of their illness. At the end of 5 years of treatment, approximately 50% of patients will be experiencing reduced effectiveness with levodopa. In patients with young-onset disease at about the age of 40, almost all have developed dyskinesias and on–off problems after 5 years. These motor fluctuations can be as a result of unpredictable pharmacokinetic changes such as unpredictable absorption across the blood–brain barrier or delayed gastric emptying, or because of progression of the disease process following further loss of dopaminergic neurons. Resolving these problems is highly individual with dosage adjustments (either up or down) and shortening the interval between doses sometimes being helpful. The dyskinesia and on–off effects may be helped by smaller more frequent doses of levodopa or perhaps by modified-release formulations. An antimuscarinic drug can be given with levodopa and is particularly useful in the treatment of tremor. However, they have the propensity to cause confusion and hallucinations particularly in the elderly so they are often reserved for patients suffering from severe tremor. Other drugs which inhibit dopamine metabolism can also be introduced. Selegiline is an inhibitor of monoamine oxidase type B. Its use has been questioned after a study which showed an increase in mortality; however a second large study has not confirmed this. The catechol-*O*-methyl transferase inhibitors such as entacapone have also been developed as another way of reducing the breakdown of levodopa and dopamine. These agents seem to be able to prolong the benefits of levodopa therapy. A direct dopamine agonist could also be added to levodopa treatment for Mrs FT. The ergot derivatives such as lysuride and pergolide are used. A new non-ergot drug, ropinirole, has recently been licensed for the treatment of early Parkinson's disease. Its ability to stimulate D_3 receptors may contribute to its action. Apomorphine given subcutaneously can also be used to counteract the off periods in advanced disease.

e. Vitamin B_6 reduces the central effectiveness of levodopa as it is a cofactor for conversion to dopamine and therefore dopamine formation in the periphery would be enhanced.

f. Beta-blockers have been found to be helpful to reduce tremor in some patients with Parkinsonism.

g. No currently available drug has been proven to reduce disease progression. Studies suggesting that selegiline may be protective have not been confirmed. It does not delay the onset of dyskinesias during levodopa treatment.

6. There is extensive debate about when to commence levodopa therapy. The goal should be to improve quality of life and limit long-term unwanted effects. If the degree of disability is not severe and the patient, carers and clinicians are in agreement, there may be no immediate need for therapy; however, this is controversial as survival is reduced if treatment with levodopa is delayed until disability develops. If treatment is required, dopamine agonists could be started. These are less likely to produce dyskinesias and could delay the need for levodopa until progressive disabilities start to occur. The possibility of brain damage caused by boxing injury should also be considered. This responds poorly to standard treatments for Parkinson's disease.

Chapter 25

1. **False**. Interferon-β is used in multiple sclerosis and may diminish the production of inflammatory interferon-γ.

2. **False**. Multiple sclerosis is usually characterised by relapses and remissions over a number of years, although after about 10 years a steady decline sets in.

3. **True**. Glutamate is an excitatory amino acid neurotransmitter but can cause cell damage and death by a number of mechanisms including an uncontrolled increase in intracellular calcium.

4. **False**. Riluzole reduces glutamate release and action thereby reducing its toxicity.

5. **True**. Possibly because of its immunosuppressive and anti-inflammatory actions.

Chapter 26

1 a. **False**. Because of habituation problems and unwanted effects, ergotamine should not be used more than twice a month for acute attacks.

b.   **False**. Sumatriptan is more rapidly absorbed when given by subcutaneous or nasal routes of administration. It gives slower relief when given orally.

2.   **True**. Plasma levels of 5HT fall but urinary levels of the 5HT metabolite increase dramatically.

3   a.   **True**. By inhibiting $5HT_2$ receptors, there is reduced perivascular inflammation, vasodilation and pain.

b.   **False**. Ergotamine causes vasoconstriction and should be avoided in patients with vascular disease.

c.   **False**. Although sumatriptan causes chest discomfort and is contraindicated in patients with ischaemic heart disease or angina, the chest discomfort and tightness in those without ischaemic heart disease is probably caused by oesophageal spasm not myocardial ischaemia.

d.   **False**. The prophylaxis of migraine is effective in only about 40% of individuals.

4.   **True**. Metoclopramide is an antiemetic, increases gastric emptying and improves paracetamol absorption.

5.   **False**. In some people stress, chocolate, cheese, alcohol, etc. can provoke migraine attacks.

Chapter 27

1   a.   **False**. The depolarising block is enhanced when body temperature is artificially lowered.

b.   **False**. Mivacurium and atracurium are the muscle relaxants with the greatest propensity to cause histamine release and haemodynamic effects.

2   a.   **True**. Dantrolene relaxes skeletal muscle by preventing Ca^{2+} release from the sarcoplasmic reticulum.

b.   **True**. Contraction is an all or none response of the fibre in response to nerve stimulation.

c.   **False**. The N_2 receptor at skeletal muscle is selectively blocked by non-depolarising and depolarising muscle relaxants. The N_1 receptor at ganglia is selectively blocked by ganglion-blocking drugs. Selectivity is lost if inappropriately large doses of these agents are administered.

3   a.   **False**. Short-acting non-depolarising neuromuscular blocking drugs such as rocuronium can be used for intubation.

b.   **False**. Because of the quaternary nature of their structure, they are not absorbed orally. They do not cross the blood–brain barrier or placenta.

4   a.   **False**. Botulinum toxin contains two subunits that promote presynaptic binding and long-lasting block of acetylcholine release.

b.   **True**. Botulinum toxin is extremely toxic on systemic absorption.

c.   **True**. Botulinum toxin only inhibits acetylcholine release. Although sweat glands are sympathetically innervated, the postganglionic neurons are cholinergic and release acetylcholine.

Chapter 28

1   a.   **False**. Respiratory depression is caused by blockade of nicotinic receptors by high doses of an anticholinesterase (AChE inhibitor) and is not treatable by atropine. Artificial ventilation may be required.

b.   **False**. Breakdown of anticholinesterase is not affected. Lack of responsiveness results from the inadequate numbers of responsive nicotinic N_2 receptors.

2   a.   **True**. The neuromuscular blockade with suxamethonium may be prolonged and prolonged apnoea may result.

b.   **False**. The cholinergic crisis results from the excessive effects of an acetylcholinesterase inhibitor and would be exacerbated by the long-acting pyridostigmine. Assisted ventilation and withdrawal of the treatment should be performed or, if any acetylcholinesterase inhibitor were to be used, edrophonium should be given.

3.   Case history answers

a.   Electromyography (Jolly test), single muscle fibre electromyography, anti-acetylcholine receptor antibody (AChR) titres, injection of a short-acting inhibitor of acetylcholinesterase (the Tensilon test, the proprietary name for edrophonium).

b.   AChR antibody blocks nicotinic N_2 receptors, receptors are destroyed and receptors are cross-linked, which causes them to be destroyed more rapidly. The decrease in functional receptors reduces motor endplate potentials and reduces the likelihood of the muscle contracting.

c.   It is short acting giving an effect in 30–60 s and effects subside in 4–5 min.

d. Symptomatic treatment with an acetylcholinesterase inhibitor. Immunosuppression with a corticosteroid, using azathioprine or ciclosporin in addition if necessary.

by COX-1 enzymes. Celecoxib is a selective COX-2 inhibitor.

b. **True**. Pyrexia is caused by elevation of prostaglandin E_2 levels under the influence of COX-2 enzymes.

Chapter 29

1 a. **True**. COX-2 can be induced by cytokines, endotoxins and other inflammatory mediators. Although COX-1 cannot generally be induced, there are some situations where this has been reported.

b. **True**. PGE_2 generated by COX-2 sensitises the sensory pain neurons to bradykinin and other mediators but does not itself stimulate sensory pain fibres.

c. **False**. There is a wide range in the ratios with which NSAIDs inhibit COX-1/COX-2. This relates approximately, but somewhat loosely, to the extent of their anti-inflammatory and gastrointestinal unwanted effects.

d. **False**. Paracetamol is analgesic and antipyretic but has only a weak anti-inflammatory effect. The reasons for this are unclear but it may have a selective effect on COX enzymes in the hypothalamus.

2 a. **True**. Reduced blood flow contributes to the gastric damage caused by NSAIDs. They also inhibit bicarbonate and mucus secretion.

b. **False**. An increase in the risk of haemorrhage can occur.

3 a. **False**. Long-term use of high doses of aspirin or paracetamol can result in renal ischaemia, sodium and water retention, papillary necrosis and chronic renal failure.

b. **True**. Particularly in those over 75 years of age and in whom there is a history of peptic ulcer.

c. **False**. Ibuprofen is good in mild-to-moderate arthritis but other NSAIDs such as indometacin or diclofenac have greater anti-inflammatory potential, although a greater propensity to cause unwanted effects.

d. **False**. In a subgroup of asthmatics, aspirin induces an asthmatic response through formation of the bronchoconstrictor leukotriene C_4. It is not clear if COX-1- or COX-2-dependent prostaglandins are involved, but COX-2 selective inhibitors may have less potential to cause asthmatic attacks.

4 a. **False**. Inhibition of platelet aggregation is partly through generation of thromboxane A_2

Chapter 30

1 a. **False**. NSAIDs do not slow disease progress, indeed some evidence suggests they may hasten the disease progress.

b. **True**. The second-line drugs take a long time to act (4–6 months) but they should be discontinued if there is no sign of improvement by that time.

2 a. **True**. Sodium aurothiomalate can be given intramuscularly and auranofin by mouth.

b. **True**. Proteinuria occurs associated with immune-complex nephritis. Only 15% of patients continue with treatment after 5–6 years because of unwanted effects.

3 a. **False**. Methotrexate prevents reduction of folic acid to dihydrofolate and tetrahydrofolate (essential for DNA production). Folic acid can be given daily to prevent gastrointestinal and haematological complications.

b. **True**. Although 5-aminosalicylic acid is the active moiety in the treatment of inflammatory bowel disease, it is less effective than sulfasalazine in treating rheumatoid arthritis.

c. **True**. More than 50% of patients continue with methotrexate for 5 years or more whereas with most other disease-modifying drugs 50% have to be stopped within 2 years.

4. **False**. The combination of methotrexate with ciclosporin, sulfasalazine or hydroxychloroquine has shown significant benefit; it is reserved for patients with severe disease.

5 a. **False.** Although corticosteroids can give dramatic relief of symptoms in rheumatoid arthritis, there is no evidence that they slow progression of the disease.

b. **True**. The atrophy can last for many months following treatment.

6. **False**. Chloroquine and hydroxychloroquine can cause remission of rheumatoid arthritis but do not slow the progression of joint damage.

Chapter 31

1 a. The treatment of choice for an acute attack is a non-steroidal anti-inflammatory drug (NSAID) *but not aspirin*. Indometacin is often used and is effective within 2 days. If patients cannot take an NSAID, colchicine or glucocorticoids can be used but both have significant unwanted effects. Salicylates should be avoided as at low doses they reduce uric acid excretion, although at high doses they are uricosuric.

   b. Plasma uric acid will be raised. An arthrocentesis sample will show uric acid crystals. Infection should be excluded in an acutely inflamed joint.

   c. Uric acid crystals in the joint space. People who develop gout have had hyperuricaemia for years. Uric acid is a metabolic product of purines. Sardines, liver and kidney are rich in purines and a diet rich in purines can contribute to gout in some people. In most people, hyperuricaemia is caused by impaired renal clearance of uric acid. Overproduction of uric acid as a result of excessive alcohol consumption can also contribute. Joint trauma, lead toxicity and cool temperatures can decrease uric acid solubility.

   d. NSAIDs are drugs of choice in acute attacks (see a).

   e. Hyperuricaemia is treated after resolution of the acute attack. Allopurinol reduces plasma uric acid by inhibiting xanthine oxidase. This increases concentrations of hypoxanthine and xanthine, which are more water soluble. Patients who overproduce uric acid are best treated with allopurinol. Those that have low renal excretion of uric acid may be treated with a uricosuric drug (probenecid, sulfinpyrazone). Both inhibit the reabsorption of uric acid in the proximal convoluted tubule.

   f. Untreated gout can lead to formation of kidney stones. A significant number of people with gout will have hypertension.

Chapter 32

1 a. **False.** The chemoreceptor trigger zone is outside the blood–brain barrier. Moreover, toxins can also cause vomiting by stimulating vagal afferents in the stomach.

   b. **True.** Common antihistamines like promethazine have antimuscarinic activity and inhibit activity in the vomiting centre and in the vestibular nuclei. It is not certain whether the antihistamine component plays a role.

2. **False.** Metoclopramide increases stomach and intestinal motility which can add to its anti-emetic effects.

3. Case note answers

   a. Yes. Cyclophosphamide induces nausea and vomiting in almost all patients, but vincristine is much less emetogenic.

   b. A serotonin receptor antagonist such as ondansetron, alone or together with a corticosteroid, would be beneficial.

   c. Ondansetron inhibits 5-hydroxytryptamine (5HT) receptors in the chemoreceptor trigger zone and *also* 5HT receptors in the stomach. In the stomach some cancer chemotherapeutic agents can cause damage and release of 5HT which stimulates vagal afferents to the vomiting centre. It is uncertain how corticosteroids work but they have an antiemetic effect with ondansetron.

   d. Anticipatory nausea and vomiting is poorly treated with anti-emetic drugs. Treatment with benzodiazepines prior to the course of treatment can be helpful.

Chapter 33

1 a. **True.** Although the organism only appears to live on gastric mucosa, it is known that gastric metaplasia develops in the duodenum in response to low pH and by this means duodenal colonisation can occur.

   b. **False.** Approximately 80% of duodenal ulcers recur if *H. pylori* is not eliminated.

   c. **True.** Although the relationship between *H. pylori* and gastric cancer is somewhat difficult to prove, it has been estimated from epidemiological studies that this infection may increase the risk of developing gastric adenocarcinoma by five to six-fold. It is possible that acquisition of the infection at a young age may be of relevance.

   d. **True.** The relevance of this to *H. pylori* is that when infection is associated with pangastritis glandular atrophy and reduced gastric acid secretion occurs. This can then result in bacterial overgrowth and the formation of *N*-nitroso compounds that are mutagenic.

   e. **False.** In some countries the resistance to metronidazole is as high as 90% and in some locations in France resistance to erythromycin is as high as 17%.

f.   **True.** Omeprazole has to be converted to its active sulfonide form by protonation in acid. This is why it is active on the proton pump in the parietal cell but not other proton pumps in the body that operate at higher pH. This contributes to its selectivity.

g.   **False.** Histamine acts on H_2 receptors on parietal cells to stimulate acid secretion. This is the basis for the selective action of histamine H_2 receptor antagonists such as ranitidine and cimetidine.

h.   **True.** Acetylcholine stimulates muscarinic receptors which by increasing Ca^{2+} causes increased acid secretion. Selective vagotomy is used to treat ulcer disease.

2. **False.** Antacids do heal peptic ulcers but their effects are slower than with proton pump inhibitors or histamine H_2 receptor antagonists.

3 a.   **False.** Cimetidine causes gynaecomastia. This is because of an antiandrogenic effect.

b.   **False.** Histamine H_2 antagonists reduce acid secretion by about 60%. The action of other agents that promote acid secretion, for example gastrin and acetylcholine, are unaffected by histamine H_2 receptor antagonists.

c.   **False.** The active metabolite irreversibly inhibits the proton pump and fresh protein must be synthesised to replace the inhibited pump. This is the explanation for the very long duration of action of omeprazole.

4. **True.** Omeprazole can inhibit the metabolism of drugs such as warfarin or phenytoin. Lansoprazole, by contrast, is only a weak enzyme inhibitor.

5 a.   **False.** Part of the way that prostaglandins protects the mucosa is by increasing gastric mucosal blood flow, removing back-secreted H^+ and providing HCO_3^-. Prostaglandins additionally increase mucus secretion, decrease acid secretion and increase HCO_3^- secretion.

b.   **False.** Prostaglandin E_2 in large doses can increase gastrointestinal motility and increase gastrointestinal secretions.

c.   **False.** Healing can be brought about by both of these anti-ulcer drugs. Omeprazole may produce more rapid healing since the rate of healing is probably related to the degree of acid suppression.

6. **True.** This is the mechanism for its usefulness in the treatment of oesophageal reflux disease. Metoclopramide and similar drugs are most effectively used as adjuncts to proton pump inhibitors and H_2 receptor antagonists.

7. Case history answer

a.   This man could be experiencing non-ulcer dyspepsia or have peptic ulceration. Whichever he has, if his symptoms are associated with *H. pylori* infection they will return, as *H. pylori* has not been eradicated. Ranitidine for only 2 weeks of treatment is available without prescription. If ranitidine had been continued the symptoms would probably have been suppressed for longer. Failure to eradicate *H. pylori* results in a recurrence of peptic ulcer disease in 80% of patients within a year. At this stage, of course, it is not known if peptic ulcer disease is present. However, even if he has non-ulcer dyspepsia and is *H. pylori* positive it is likely that he will develop peptic ulcer disease in the future.

b.   No. If *H. pylori* is present, the symptoms will still recur in a high percentage of individuals.

c.   It is recommended that any patient over 45 years of age should be endoscopically examined and he should be referred for this procedure. The GP could assess for *H. pylori* infection serologically using a skin prick test; alternatively this could be done in hospital with urea breath test or bacteriological culture on a gastric antral biopsy. Intake of any non-steroidal anti-inflammatory drugs, smoking or alcohol intake should be assessed as these are strongly contributory to ulcer disease. (An endoscopic examination revealed a duodenal ulcer.)

d.   The answer to this is complex and imperfectly understood. Patients with only antral inflammation and *H. pylori* produce more gastrin and excess acid resulting in duodenal ulcers. If a pangastritis exists it is associated with lower levels of acid secretion and gastric ulcers.

e.   Numerous treatment regimens are being evaluated. Seven days therapy with a proton pump inhibitor or ranitidine plus either metronidazole or tinidazole plus amoxicillin or clarithromycin results in 70–90% eradication rate. The use of a proton pump inhibitor or histamine H_2 antagonist increases the effectiveness of the antimicrobials.

f.   It is possible that the strain of *H. pylori* was resistant to metronidazole and erythromycin. In some places, metronidazole resistance is 90% and clarithromycin 17%. The patient should be tested to see if *H. pylori* are still present.

g.   Culture sensitivities of the *H. pylori* in a biopsy specimen could be sought. Resistance to tinidazole is currently less than that to metronidazole. Quadruple therapy which has 93–98% success could be used, for example a proton pump inhibitor or ranitidine plus tinidazole plus amoxicillin plus bismuth. Ranitidine bismuth substrate could replace a separate proton pump inhibitor or ranitidine plus bismuth providing the benefits of quadruple therapy but in triple formulation.

Chapter 34

1 a. **True.** Sulfasalazine consists of sulfapyridine and 5-ASA linked by an azo bond. The azo bond is cleaved by bacteria to release the active 5-ASA. Sulfapyridine probably produces many of the unwanted effects of sulfasalazine.

   b. **True.** Modified-release formulations are available for rectal administration to deliver the drug to distal colonic mucosa. About 20% of the mesalazine administered in this way is absorbed into the circulation.

2 a. **True.** There is increased risk of Crohn's disease in smokers but a slightly decreased risk of ulcerative colitis.

   b. **False.** Although mesalazine may be of some benefit in colonic Crohn's disease, it is less effective than for patients with ulcerative colitis. Mesalazine is not very effective for small bowel Crohn's disease.

   c. **False.** Although they are effective for inducing remission, there is little evidence that corticosteroids prevent relapse.

   d. **False.** Patients with chronic Crohn's disease can become corticosteroid dependent and immunosuppressives such as azathioprine can be useful in reducing the corticosteroid dependence. Many months of treatment are required before they are fully effective.

3. Case history answer

   a. The cause of Crohn's disease is unknown. Several hypotheses have implicated a number of risk factors including infection, altered immune state, combined measles, mumps and rubella (MMR) vaccine and local ischaemia. None of these has been confirmed.

   b. Initial treatment is with corticosteroids. In this man, the Crohn's disease is confined to the distal colon. Topical treatment with corticosteroids such as budesonide could be used to limit systemic unwanted effects. If, however, there was involvement of the proximal large bowel or small bowel it would be necessary to give an oral corticosteroid such as prednisolone.

   c. Corticosteroids have a variety of actions. They can alter the release of inflammatory mediators such as arachidonic acid metabolites, kinins and cytokines. They can alter cell mediated cytotoxicity, antibody production, adhesion molecule expression, phagocytic function, leucocyte chemotaxis and leucocyte adherence.

   d. Corticosteroids should be given until remission occurs. If possible, the corticosteroid should be administered locally to keep the plasma concentration low, but for patients who experience systemic symptoms (such as fatigue, anorexia or weight loss) oral therapy is indicated.

   e. Systemic corticosteroids suppress the hypothalamic pituitary adrenal axis and can reduce the circulating levels of endogenous adrenal glucocorticoids. Gradual reduction of the dose of therapeutically administered glucocorticoid allows recovery of the production of endogenous corticosteroids.

   f. If the colitis is restricted to the distal colon, topical administration of mesalazine or an oral formulation that delivers 5-ASA to the colon could be used. 5-ASA is, however, less effective in Crohn's disease, particularly if it involves the small bowel.

   g. Continuous corticosteroid therapy for periods of 6 months or longer is eventually required in 40–50% of cases of Crohn's disease. If this occurs, surgery and immunosuppression are the two major therapeutic approaches. Immunosuppressive therapy is with azathioprine or 6-mercaptopurine: prolonged treatment with these drugs is usually required (up to 6 months) before a clinical response occurs.

Chapter 35

1 a. **False.** Defecation once every 3 days or three times a day is not abnormal.

   b. **True.** Increased fibre intake and exercise will help in the majority of cases of 'simple' constipation.

   c. **False.** Chronic use results in deterioration of colonic function with damage to the myenteric plexus (cathartic colon).

2 a. **True.** Aluminium salts cause constipation as do many other drugs including some antidepressants, opioid analgesics and calcium antagonists.

b. **False**. Some laxatives (magnesium^{2+} salts) can act within 6 h whereas lactulose and docusate take considerably longer to exert their activity.

3 a. **False**. Viral gastroenteritis is a major cause of infant diarrhoea and rotavirus predominates.

b. **True**. Overgrowth of the anaerobe *Clostridium difficile* following usage of broad-spectrum antimicrobials can occur and is increasingly resistant to metronidazole treatment.

c. **True**. However, the clinical importance of this is debated.

4 a. **False**. There are now frequent epidemics of cholera that are resistant to tetracycline.

b. **False**. A hypertonic solution will have an osmotic action drawing water into the bowel; the formulated solution should be isotonic or slightly hypotonic.

Chapter 36

1. Case history answer

a. Spironolactone is a reasonable choice as any changes in serum K$^+$ should be avoided because such patients are easily tipped into encephalopathy/coma by electrolyte imbalances, therefore avoid furosemide (frusemide)/thiazides. There is an increase in circulating aldosterone probably because of decreased metabolism and renin stimulation secondary to low plasma volume. This probably contributes to fluid retention; therefore, spironolactone is usually chosen.

b. Diminished hepatic reserve is indicated by four factors: (i) increased plasma bilirubin, which will be a combination of unconjugated bilirubin (because of impaired glucuronidation) plus conjugated bilirubin (because of impaired biliary excretion); (ii) decreased plasma albumin, caused by decreased synthesis, will lower the osmotic pressure of blood and, therefore, draw less water back out of tissues, leading to oedema/ascites; (iii) decreased clotting factors caused by decreased synthesis, which may contribute to oesophageal bleeding (note: many patients take a proton pump inhibitor such as omeprazole to reduce risk of gastrointestinal bleed); (iv) increased oestrogenic activity, as evidenced by gynaecomastia and testicular atrophy, probably caused by decreased inactivation of oestrogenic steroids in the liver.

c. Patients with cirrhosis are more susceptible to all CNS depressant drugs and diazepam is likely to give an increased response. The general mechanism is not known (may be change in blood–brain barrier). The metabolism of diazepam by cytochrome P450 will be reduced and, therefore, there will be an increased plasma concentration. (Note: there will be decreased formation of the active desmethyl metabolite.) A short-acting benzodiazepine without active metabolites would be better, e.g. midazolam.

d. A much lower dose of diazepam than usually used should be given and slower recovery would be expected.

e. These will be decreased albumin and α_1-acid glycoprotein in the patient's blood; therefore less protein binding can occur and there will be more free drug in blood leading to an increased response. Decreased first-pass metabolism means that bioavailability will increase from about 30% up to 70–80%. This is because of decreased cytochrome P450 activity and increased portocaval shunting of blood. The elimination half-life is independent of bioavailability but it will be longer because of reduced cytochrome P450.

f. Colestyramine is a non-absorbed anion exchange resin that adsorbs bile acids in gastrointestinal lumen. In liver cirrhosis, the fibrosis reduces outflow from bile cannaliculi and there is decreased bile flow. This leads to a build up of bile salts in blood and deposition in the skin, which causes itching. Adsorption of bile salts in the gut by colestyramine lowers blood bile salts by reducing enterohepatic circulation. Lactulose is used to modify the gut flora. A possible cause of encephalopathy is the failure of the liver to detoxify bacterial products formed in the large bowel. (Encephalopathy is more common during constipation.) Possible metabolites of importance are ammonia and tyramine. Lactulose is not absorbed in upper gastroinestinal tract but is fermented in lower bowel; this lowers lumen pH and may act by altering the microbial metabolism, with decreased formation of ammonia and tyramine. It also prevents constipation.

g. Analgesia in cirrhosis is a problem and there is no ideal answer. Opioids should usually be avoided because of risk of encephalopathy but you could give reduced dose. Non-steroidal anti-inflammatory drugs are best avoided to reduce the risk of haemorrhage from oesophageal varices. Paracetamol is a possible risk because it is hepatotoxic: however, it is well tolerated in cirrhosis probably because the decreases in effective perfusion of hepatocytes and reduced activity of cytochrome P450 outweigh the decrease in conjugation with glucuronic acid, sulfate and glutathione.

Chapter 37

1. **True.**
2. **True.**
3. **False.** Phentermine increases the release of noradrenaline in the hypothalamus, thus suppressing appetite.
4. **False.** The hypothalamus controls appetite and an appetite stimulant neuropeptide Y has been identified in this area.
5. **False.** Leptin is produced in adipose tissue and reduces neuropeptide Y production.

Chapter 38

1.
   a. **False.** The parent drug terfenadine is associated with ventricular arrhythmias in high doses. Fexofenadine retains the parent drug's antihistamine activity without having unwanted effects on the heart.
   b. **False.** The histamine receptors on the parietal cell are H_2 subtype and are not affected by these antihistamines which act on H_1 receptors.
   c. **False.** Fexofenadine acts only on the H_1 receptors.

2.
   a. **False.** Nasal corticosteroids are very effective.
   b. **False.** Prostaglandins and leukotrienes can also be released from mast cells and contribute to symptoms.

3. Case history answer
   a. Allergic rhinitis after exposure to allergens probably from cat dander. The correlation with exposure to the cat and his fitness and lack of drug intake suggest that it is not non-allergic rhinitis, which may occur because of infections, drugs etc.
   b. *Avoidance of exposure to allergen.* If this is not possible and the cat has to remain and pharmacological therapy is considered necessary, a non-sedating antihistamine should reduce rhinorrhoea, sneezing and itching but will have little effect on nasal congestion. A short course (3–4 days) of a nasal decongestant such as oxymetazoline would help reduce the nasal symptoms. Nasal inhaled corticosteroids

can also be very effective in controlling allergic rhinitis symptoms.

Chapter 39

1.
   a. **True.**
   b. **True.** Ciclosporin is nephrotoxic.

2. **True.** This enhances the formation of anti-inflammatory proteins and a corticosteroid-sparing effect is possible.

3. **True.** Azathioprine has a toxic action on cells and proliferation of antibody producing cells is inhibited. Proliferation of cells involved in cell mediated immunity is also inhibited.

4. Case history answer
   a. Basiliximab given before and 4 days after surgery has been shown to reduce acute rejection by 35%. Reduction of acute rejection is also achieved with combination therapy and corticosteroids; a calcineurin inhibitor such as ciclosporin and an antiproliferative immunosuppressive such as azathioprine can be used. When used in combination, lower doses of the drugs can be administered than when giving the drugs alone. Intensive monitoring of liver and renal functions are important.
   b. Oversuppression of the immune response brings with it problems of opportunistic infections associated with reduced immunity. Additional 'steroid effects' as described for iatrogenic Cushings-like syndrome may be apparent.

Chapter 40

1.
   a. **False.** Glibenclamide stimulates insulin secretion from the beta cells of the islets and would be ineffective in the absence of any insulin-secreting ability.
   b. **True.** Sulfonylureas cause weight gain partly by stimulating appetite.
   c. **True.** Glibenclamide has a long duration of action and active metabolites can increase when renal function declines. Hypoglycaemia is a greater problem in the elderly.

2.
   a. **True.** These drugs act in part by different mechanisms. Additionally, metformin does not

stimulate appetite, indeed it may suppress appetite.

3 a. **True**. Neonates born to diabetic mothers who were given oral hypoglycaemics in pregnancy have problems associated with hypoglycaemia.

   b. **True**. Sulfonylureas have some structural similarities to the sulfonamides and trimethoprim and can produce severe hypoglycaemia when given together.

4 a. **False**. Isophane insulin is complexed with protamine and has a duration of action of 20 hours, whereas insulin lispro is modified structurally and has a faster onset of action and shorter duration.

5. Case history answers
   a. Type 1.
   b. An upper respiratory infection can be all that is necessary to tip someone into ketoacidosis. Aggravating factors: candidiasis in the throat, overbreathing causing dryness.
   c. There is a familial tendency, although neither type 1 nor type 2 diabetes mellitus is a single gene disorder, so there is no classic pattern of inheritance.
   d. Once tubular maximum for glucose reabsorption in the kidneys is exceeded, the glucose in the distal tubules causes an osmotic diuresis, leading to polyuria, and then to thirst.
   e. Insulin, antimicrobials, fluids and salts to correct dehydration, glucose levels, ketoacidosis and electrolyte imbalances. Ketoacidosis can lead to coma.
   f. A dietary regimen should be worked up by the patient and dietician to create a stable pattern of eating habits commensurate with the patient's life style. Diets low in animal fat and high in fibre are recommended, ideally with carbohydrate intake distributed throughout the day.
   g. With a stable pattern of eating habit and activity, twice daily subcutaneous injections before breakfast and evening meal. The insulins would contain a mixture of short and long-acting insulins, the ratios of which vary depending upon the patient's glucose levels. Insulins frequently used are soluble insulin and isophane insulin.
   h. The time to onset of activity of neutral soluble insulin is 30 minutes with peak activity at 1–3 hours.
   i. The percentage of glycosylated haemoglobin can be measured. High concentrations are indicative of increased risk for microvascular and neuropathic complications.
   j. Newer, rapid-acting monomeric insulin lispro may be helpful. This has a time to onset of only 15 minutes and a time to peak plasma levels of 0.5–0.75 hours. It should, therefore, be given immediately before a meal. A possible altered regimen may involve insulin lispro during the day with insulin isophane given in the evening. However, overall education about eating and life-style would probably provide better patient benefit than a change of insulin regimen.

Chapter 41

1 a. **False**. T_3 and T_4 are largely bound to thyroxin-binding globulin (TBG).
   b. **True**. Thyroxine is cleared in about 6 days.
   c. **True**. The T_3–receptor complex activates transcription and protein synthesis.
   d. **False**. Iodine is converted to iodide and inhibits T_3 and T_4 release.

2 a. **True**.
   b. **True**. Levothyroxine is the standard treatment.
   c. **True**. Thyroxine has a very long half-life.

3. Case history answers
   a. An autoimmune disease in which antibodies to TSH are generated and bind to and activate TSH receptors.
   b. TSH (thyrotrophin) levels will be low due to the negative feedback effect of elevated T_3 and T_4.
   c. Bound T_3 and T_4 levels may be high due to increased binding capacity of binding proteins or increased levels of binding proteins rather than actual elevated levels of T_3 and T_4.
   d. Drugs of choice for controlling symptoms are β-blockers, although they do not improve fatigue and muscle weakness. Digoxin should be given for the atrial fibrillation (Ch. 8) and anticoagulation with warfarin to prevent thromboembolism.
   e. Carbimazole is the drug of choice given in a high dose then reducing over 4–6 weeks.
   f. The clinical state should be stabilised with carbimazole and a β-blocker. Carbimazole is stopped 3–4 days before radioiodine is given.
   g. It can take several months for maximum benefit of ^{131}I to occur.

Chapter 42

1. a. **False**. Vitamin D deficiency leads to hyperparathyroidism which may assist in

reducing the worst excesses of vitamin D deficiency. PTH increases calcitriol formation and calcitriol has a negative feedback effect on PTH.

b. **True**. Calcitonin reduces Ca^{2+} resorption and inhibits bone turnover.

c. **False**. Bisphosphonates inhibit bone dissolution, and effects occur slowly; plasma concentrations fall slowly with a maximum effect after about a week.

2 a. **False**. Oestrogens inhibit the cytokines that recruit the bone-resorbing osteoclasts. Oestrogens also inhibit the actions of PTH.

b. **False**. Raloxifene has been licensed to reduce bone density loss in postmenopausal women. It is an oestrogen receptor stimulant selective for its actions on oestrogen receptors in bone and without stimulant effects on oestrogen receptors in breast and uterus.

3. Case history answers

a. Osteomalacia can be caused by lack of vitamin D, calcium or phosphates. Treatment is with vitamin D supplements. Ergocalciferol (vitamin D_2 is given).

b. With a deficiency of vitamin D there is poor gut absorption of Ca^{2+}. Ca^{2+} absorption is improved.

c. Too much vitamin D may lead to hypercalcaemia.

Chapter 43

1 a. **False**. Somatostatin is an inhibitor of growth hormone release.

b. **False**. Somatostatin is also produced from intestinal and pancreatic cells.

c. **True**. Because dopamine is a stimulant of growth hormone release in healthy individuals and bromocriptine is a dopamine receptor agonist.

d. **True**. Octreotide is a long-acting analogue of somatostatin.

2 a. **True**. It can be used to improve fertility in women with high levels of prolactin.

b. **False**. On continued administration gonadotrophin receptors are downregulated and steroid synthesis declines.

c. **False**. Gonadorelin will inhibit testosterone synthesis in prostate cancer and reduce the size of the prostate.

d. **True**. Gonadorelin, a gonadotrophin analogue, reduces oestrogen synthesis which inhibits endometriosis.

e. **True**.

3 a. **True**. Vasopressin is a nonapeptide released from the hypothalamus.

b. **False**. In nephrogenic diabetes insipidus the kidney is unresponsive to vasopressin.

c. **False**. Paradoxically, in diabetes insipidus, the response to thiazide diuretics is a reduction in polyuria.

4. Case history answers

a. No. Epiphyseal closure occurs much later, so treatment at this age can dramatically increase height.

b. Biosynthetic GH (somatropin) has a half-life of only 25 min but high protein binding means that three injections a week are sufficient to maintain IGF-1 at required levels.

c. Insulin-like effects can produce hypoglycaemia and there is pain at the site of injection.

Chapter 44

1 a. **False**. Fludrocortisone is a synthetic mineralocorticoid with a salt-retaining:anti-inflammatory ratio of about 12.5–25.1. The glucocorticoid prednisolone should be used orally.

b. **True**. Beclomethasone has a short half-life systemically and is used by inhalation for its local effects on the airways in the treatment of asthma.

2 a. **False**. Corticosteroids lead to reduced tissue uptake of glucose and increased gluconeogenesis leading to 'steroid diabetes'.

b. **True**. After prolonged administration it is possible that the hypothalamic–pituitary–adrenal axis (both secretion of CRF and ACTH) will be suppressed (Fig. 44.3), i.e. endogenous cortisol levels are low. Slow withdrawal allows the adrenals to recover their normal cortisol secretion and avoids corticosteroid deficiency.

3 a. **False**. Reduced plasma sodium results in stimulation of renin secretion which is converted to angiotensin II. This then stimulates aldosterone release from the adrenal cortex which acts to increase Na^+ reabsorption in the distal part of the distal tubule.

b. **True**. ACTH stimulates both cortisol and aldosterone secretion by the adrenal cortex.

4 a. **False**. Dexamethasone can inhibit vomiting and will add to the anti-emetic actions of agents such as ondansetron in vomiting caused by cancer chemotherapy (Ch. 32).

b. **True**. Because of their catabolic effect on proteins they delay the healing of wounds.

c. **True**. Immunosuppressive effects of glucocorticoids can exacerbate an underlying infection.

5. Case history answers

a. (i) A tumour of the adrenal cortex secreting cortisol.

(ii) Excess secretion of ACTH by a pituitary tumour.

(iii) Excess secretion of ACTH by a non-pituitary tumour (commonly small cell carcinoma of the lung, medullary or thyroid carcinoma).

(iv) Iatrogenic, from therapeutic administration of glucocorticoids or ACTH.

b. The cause could not be a primary cortisol-secreting adrenocortical tumour or glucocorticoid administration as the ACTH levels would be low due to negative feedback of glucocorticoid on the anterior pituitary and hypothalamus. The possibility is an ACTH-secreting pituitary adenoma or ACTH-secreting non-pituitary tumour.

c. The dexamethasone suppression test is not definitive; it can suppress ACTH of pituitary origin but not from ectopic ACTH-producing tumours or adrenocortical tumours.

d. Control by inhibitors of adrenal corticosteroid synthesis, e.g. trilostane or metyrapone. (Note: the patient would probably also be showing signs of excess mineralocorticoid activity which should also be treated in parallel with spironolactone.)

Chapter 45

1 a. **False**. Until the late part of the follicular phase, oestrogens do have a negative feedback effect but at a level of approximately 200 pg ml^{-1} oestradiol there is a switch to positive feedback and the mid-cycle LH and FSH surge results.

b. **True**. Although the LH levels fall precipitously after the mid-cycle surge, they are high enough to support the secretion of progesterone.

2 a. **False**. The inhibition of ovulation is seen in between 25% and 40% of women. In women administered medroxyprogesterone acetate by injection, however, the percentage in whom inhibition of ovulation occurs is almost 100%.

b. **False**. Progesterone inhibits the motility of the fallopian tube, whereas oestrogens have the opposite action. An imbalance of either may alter the chances of fertilisation and implantation.

c. **True**. Removal of the corpus luteum before 6–8 weeks of pregnancy results in abortion, whereas after that time the placental production of steroids under the influence of hCG is sufficient to maintain the pregnancy.

3 a. **False**. Although the progestogens in the second-generation pills have variable androgenic activity, the progestogens gestodene and desogestrel have weak or no androgenic activity.

b. **False**. Although there are some small variations, overall the biphasic and triphasic patterns of application mimic more closely the steroidal changes in the menstrual cycle. However, they do not reduce the steroid load overall.

c. **False**. The fact that ethinylestradiol undergoes first-pass metabolism serves to maintain plasma concentrations.

d. **False**. With the progesterone-only contraceptive, if there is a delay of only 3 h or more after the normal time of taking the pill, then contraceptive protection may be lowered.

4 a. **True**. By inducing liver microsomal enzymes, the effective concentrations may be reduced as metabolism is enhanced.

5 a. **True**. The excess risk of thromboembolic disease in women taking the combined contraceptive pill is significantly greater in those who smoke over the age of 35 years.

b. **True**. However, there is little evidence for a lesser effect of the third-generation progestogens on carbohydrate metabolism when compared with second-generation progestogens such as levonorgestrel.

6 a. **False**. Particularly in the first 6 months of treatment, breakthrough bleeding frequently occurs.

b. **True**. Both steroids undergo first-pass metabolism and this can be avoided by absorption through the skin.

c. **True**. Raloxifene stimulates oestrogen receptors in bone and liver but not breast and reproductive tissue.

d. **True**. Tibolone has weak oestrogenic and progestogenic activity and has been shown to reduce bone loss.

7 a. **False**. Oxytocin is less effective in earlier pregnancy compared with term. In this patient

it is probable that an intravaginal pessary of prostaglandin would be used as this causes uterine contractility and also softens the cervix. This may be followed by oxytocin.

b. **False**. Oestrogens increase the gap junctions in the uterus thus facilitating the transmission of the uterine contractility from the fundal region through the body of the uterus. Progesterone prevents the action of oestrogens.

c. **False**. The source of the prostaglandins during labour is the uterine amnion membranes and the decidua.

8 a. **False**. In some women hypertonus occurs with the administration of prostaglandins.

b. **False**. Ergometrine is given alone or together with oxytocin at the time of delivery to reduce postpartum haemorrhage. It should not be given for labour induction.

9 a. **False**. The reason is not known but the combined oral contraceptive does relieve dysmenorrhoea in some women.

10 a. **True**. Magnesium sulfate inhibits Ca^{2+} availability and uterine contractility and can delay preterm delivery for a short period of time.

Chapter 46

1 a. **True**. Testosterone is well absorbed orally but degraded by first-pass metabolism to inactive metabolites.

b. **True**. Other treatments are required including the administration of hCG and other gonadotrophins.

c. **True**. Nandrolone has fewer androgenic effects than testosterone but has many other unwanted effects.

2 a. **True**.

Chapter 47

1 a. **False**. Vitamin B_{12} is absorbed with the aid of intrinsic factor in the distal ileum.

b. **True**. It is given by intramuscular injection every 2–3 months for life.

c. **True**. Macrocytes (large red cells) are seen.

2 a. **True**.

b. **True**. Methotrexate, trimethoprim and phenytoin inhibit the enzymes that convert folic acid to dihydrofolate in the DNA synthesis pathway.

c. **False**. Folic acid is given daily for up to 4 months to replenish stores.

3 a. **True**. The main cause of erythropoietin deficiency is renal failure.

4 a. **False**. CSFs are used to enhance blood cell development, for example where damage to cell-producing systems has occurred due to cytotoxic drugs.

5. Case history answers
   a. The haemoglobin is low; it is less than 115 g l^{-1} and in a woman this indicates anaemia. The mean cell volume is 61 fl (normal 76–96). The common cause for low MCV is iron deficiency anaemia. Iron deficiency anaemia is common in menstruating women. The other common cause is gastrointestinal bleeding, including haemorrhoids.
   b. Serum ferritin should be low and iron binding capacity elevated.
   c. Oral ferrous salts (e.g. sulfate, the form most easily absorbed).
   d. Gastrointestinal distension and loose bowel movements are common.
   e. From the duodenum and upper jejunum.
   f. It is optimally absorbed as haem.
   g. No. The rise in haemoglobin should be about 10 g l^{-1} each week.
   h. Lack of compliance; continued bleeding, malabsorption.
   i. Intramuscular iron sorbitol injection. Ten to twenty injections required over 2–3 weeks.

Chapter 48

1 a. **False**. The relationship is between high LDL cholesterol and coronary risk of atherosclerosis. High LDL cholesterol is associated with lipid peroxidation, take-up into macrophages and formation of fatty streaks.

b. **True**. One in 500 of the population has a single recessive gene disorder causing reduced synthesis of LDL receptors.

c. **False**. The resins sequester bile acids that contain cholesterol. This decreases absorption of ingested cholesterol and also increases bile acid-cholesterol synthesis in liver leading to further elimination of cholesterol.

2 a. **False**. Reducing cholesterol synthesis results in increased LDL receptors in the liver and hence increased LDL clearance from plasma.

   b. **False**. Serum LDL cholesterol falls by 20–35%.

   c. **False**. The two classes of drugs act by different mechanisms and act synergistically. The combination of two drugs can be used where the response to the statins is inadequate.

3. Case history answers

   a. General advice would include avoidance of smoking. Determine if there are problems of obesity, diabetes, hypertension. Consider the use of aspirin where appropriate.

   b. A statin would be recommended as first-choice drug in preventing cardiovascular effects in patients at increased risk. This patient is at increased risk. Statins are of proven benefit using data from extensive investigations; they are also well tolerated (see f).

   c. The reduction would depend upon dosage of statins, but a reduction in the region of 25% should be aimed for. This could take more than a month to achieve.

   d. Statins inhibit HMG-CoA reductase and increase LDL receptors (Fig. 48.1).

   e. The target total cholesterol recommended is 5 mmol l^{-1} and an LDL cholesterol concentration of less than 3 mmol l^{-1}.

   f. Gastrointestinal upsets. Use of statins is not recommended in patients with liver disease or in pregnancy. Liver function tests need to be performed.

   g. In addition to the statins use fibrates or anion exchange resins. Because the sites of action are different to those of the statins an additive effect should be expected.

   h. Fibrates decrease VLDL production, increase hepatic LDL uptake and stimulate lipoprotein lipase. Anion exchange resins sequester bile acids in the intestine and reduce cholesterol uptake.

Chapter 49

1. In atopic dermatitis:

   a. **False**. Topical corticosteroids (e.g. hydrocortisone cream) are the mainstay of treatment of atopic dermatitis, used for up to 4 weeks.

   b. **True**. One of the sedative antihistamines (e.g. promethazine) may be of value although direct effect on itching may be limited. Topical antihistamines and topical doxepin are also available.

2. In psoriasis:

   a. **False**. In severe psoriasis ciclosporin or methotrexate can be used.

   b. **True**. Oral retinoids such as vitamin A and derivatives reduce cell growth and can be used in psoriasis, but they can be teratogenic. Oral and topical retinoids are also useful in acne.

3. In acne:

   a. **True**.

   b. **False**. Resistance is increasing. There is cross-resistance between erythromycin and clindamycin and when possible non-antibiotic antimicrobials (benzoyl peroxide or azelaic acid) should be used.

4. Case history answer

   a. Atopic dermatitis is possible because of the appearance of the rash and the child's atopy and the previous history of her mother.

   b. The following are the initial management approaches:
   - good skin hygiene
   - emollients in bath water and topically applied to moisturise the skin
   - short courses of topically applied hydrocortisone as the mainstay of treatment
   - if necessary, topically applied antihistamine or oral sedative antihistamine if the itch is severe, although there is not a consensus that antihistamines are beneficial.

   c. Assessment of contributory factors such as food allergies and other allergens, psychological factors and removal of irritants and allergens. Severe acute exacerbations may require rigorous topical measures and antimicrobial treatment.

Chapter 50

1 a. **False**. Epinephrine may cause mydriasis, which serves to narrow even further the angle between the iris and the cornea.

   b. **True**.

   c. **True**. Tropicamide blocks the muscarinic receptors in the circular muscle of the iris causing mydriasis, which narrows the anterior angle and may reduce aqueous draining.

2 a. **False**. Cocaine causes mydriasis as well as having a local anaesthetic effect.

   b. **True**. Cyclopentolate acts for 12–24 h whereas tropicamide has a duration of action of about 3 h.

c. **True**. Pilocarpine is a muscarinic receptor stimulant; it contracts the ciliary muscle causing the lens to shorten and bulge and accommodate for near vision.

3 a. Reduced drainage of aqueous humour through the trabecular meshwork into the canal of Schlemm and the episcleral veins.

b. β-blockers are the drugs of first choice. α_2-adrenoceptor stimulants, prostaglandin analogues, inhibitors of carbonic anhydrase enzymes and muscarinic agonists could also be used.

c. Beta-blockers: avoid if asthma, bradycardia, heart block, heart failure. α_2-stimulants: avoid if severe cardiovascular disease. Muscarinic agonists: avoid if conjuctival or corneal damage, cardiac disease, asthma. Carbonic anhydrase inhibitors: can cause hypokalaemia and electrolyte imbalance. They should be avoided in pregnancy.

Prostaglandin $F_{2\alpha}$ analogue: avoid in pregnancy and asthma.

Chapter 51

1 a. **True**. Benzylpenicillin is actively secreted into the proximal tubule. This can be inhibited by probenecid or by other drugs that use the same secretory mechanism such as aspirin.

b. **False**. Broad-spectrum penicillins in particular can cause diarrhoea.

c. **False**. Azlocillin is broken down by β-lactamase.

d. **False**. Penicillins bind to penicillin-binding proteins and disrupt cell membrane peptidoglycans.

2 a. **True**. Cefotaxime is a third-generation cephalosporin antibacterial that penetrates the CNS and is resistant to β-lactamases.

b. **False**. But cephalosporins should be given carefully. Between 8 and 16% of patients who are allergic to penicillins will exhibit allergy to cephalosporins.

3 a. **True**. Imipenem is rapidly metabolised by dihydropeptidases in the kidney and is given in combination with cilastin, which inhibits the metabolising enzyme.

b. **False**. Like all β-lactams given in correct doses, imipenem is bactericidal.

4 a. **True**. The quinolones have good activity against *Pseudomonas* species.

b. **False**. Ciprofloxacin inhibits the hepatic metabolism of theophylline and can increase its toxicity.

5 a. **True**. Erythromycin often causes nausea and diarrhoea. Azithromycin is better tolerated.

b. **False**. Gentamicin is nephrotoxic and ototoxic and its plasma levels should be monitored.

c. **True**. Gentamicin is poorly absorbed from the gastrointestinal tract and is given parenterally.

6 a. **True**. Most sore throats are caused by viruses; those with bacterial causes usually resolve without antibacterials. The selection of increasingly resistant organisms relates to unnecessary use of antibiotics.

b. **True**. Tetracyclines can chelate with Ca^{2+} and form permanent yellow-brown deposits on developing teeth.

c. **True**. It is reserved for multiple antibiotic-resistant *Staphylococcus aureus* (MRSA) and metronidazole-resistant *Clostridium difficile*, which causes pseudomembranous colitis.

7 a. **True**. Rifampicin is a broad-spectrum antibiotic and can be utilised in some serious diseases caused by Gram-negative organisms such as Legionella and mycobacteria and also in methicillin-resistant *Staphylococcus aureus* (MRSA).

b. **False**. Isoniazid has a highly selective action to inhibit the production of mycolic acids, which are unique to the cell wall of mycobacterium species.

c. **False**. There is a high degree of resistance to co-trimoxazole in the organisms causing hospital urinary tract infections and it is seldom used for this indication.

d. **True**. Trimethoprim inhibits the conversion of folate to products used in the construction of DNA. Deficiency can result in megaloblastic anaemia and this can be prevented by giving additional folinic acid.

8. Answer for case history 1

a. The most common cause of community-acquired infection is *Streptococcus pneumoniae* but other 'atypical' organisms could be involved. In JW, who was previously well, a recent stay in a hotel abroad might indicate the involvement of *Legionella*, which multiplies in warm water, for example in the tanks of air conditioning systems. (The incubation time is 5–10 days.) Co-amoxiclav (amoxicillin + clavulanic acid) plus erythromycin or another macrolide should be given before the diagnosis is confirmed. If his condition is severe, rifampicin should also be given. The treatment should be reviewed immediately the microbiology sensitivities are known.

b. Amoxicillin is bactericidal and acts by interfering with bacterial cell wall peptidoglycan synthesis. It also allows greater activity of enzymes that lyse bacterial cells. Clavulanic acid inhibits β-lactamase, thus extending the spectrum of activity of amoxicillin. Erythromycin inhibits bacterial protein synthesis by acting on the bacterial ribosome. Rifampicin, perhaps better known for its role in treating tuberculosis, inhibits DNA-dependent RNA polymerase in many Gram-positive and Gram-negative bacteria.

9. Answer for case history 2

a. *Staphylococcus aureus* is a likely cause of an acute of pneumonia following an attack of influenza. The organism commonly produces abscesses in the lungs. Pulmonary infection with *S. aureus* may also occur in patients with cystic fibrosis. A Gram stain of the sputum demonstrates Gram-positive cocci in clusters – typical of staphylococci. The production of coagulase and DNAase identifies the organism as *S. aureus*. Many different species of coagulase-negative staphylococci exist and are found as part of the normal skin flora. The coagulase-negative staphylococci are typical causes of prosthetic valve endocarditis, joint prostheses and infected venous catheters. Of concern is the large number of antibiotic-resistant staphylococci (MRSA), which pose a threat to frail or immunocompromised patients. The treatment must be guided by the sensitivity tests. Most *S. aureus* strains are sensitive to flucloxacillin and this is the most appropriate antibiotic. In the circumstances, it may be combined with fusidic acid or gentamicin.

b. A range of other second-choice antibiotics effective against β-lactamase-producing *S. aureus* might be useful. For example fusidic acid, gentamicin, a cephalosporin, a quinolone, or erythromycin may be effective. There are increasing concerns about MRSA. Vancomycin is a glycopeptide. It is bactericidal and acts by inhibiting cell wall synthesis. It is effective against some MRSA. A new group of drugs, the streptogramins, have recently become available and quinupristin with dalfopristin is effective against MRSA.

10. Answer for case history 3

a. Clinically the patient is likely to have *Pneumocystis carinii* pneumonia (PCP), which is the predominant respiratory illness in patients with acquired immune deficiency syndrome (AIDS). This organism, which is a protozoan, is believed to be acquired at a young age and reactivates with waning immunity. The organism is endemic in the community and multiplies within the lungs and causes symptoms. There is often a seasonal prevalence of pneumonia caused by PCP. Symptoms can be scant and if present consist of breathlessness and cough. Induced sputum or bronchoalveolar lavage specimens should be sent to laboratory for detection of PCP and routine culture.

b. PCP can be detected in sputum or lavage by staining with methenamine silver stain for typical casts. Can also be detected by use of the polymerase chain reaction, and on lung biopsy.

c. The treatment of choice is high-dose co-trimoxazole. Many patients with AIDS have hypersensitivity reactions to sulfonamides and are on multiple drug combinations. Alternative treatments for PCP are aerosolised or parenteral pentamidine, dapsone and trimethoprim, primaquine, etc.

d. Long-term treatment with corticosteroids or other immunosuppressives.

e. After an attack of PCP, a patient must be given a prophylactic regimen, for example nebulised pentamidine or oral trimethoprim 3 days per week.

11. Answer for case history 4

a. *Salmonella, Shigella, Proteus* and *Pseudomonas* species are non-lactose-fermenting and produce pale-coloured colonies on this medium. All were contenders. (The last three were excluded on biochemical screening. *S. enteritidis* phage type 4 was eventually identified.)

b. Antibiotics have *no* role to play in the management of the majority of cases of salmonella gastroenteritis. Exceptions are if the gastroenteritis occurs in an individual who is immunocompromised or if there is evidence of systemic invasion in any patient. Ciprofloxacin would be the antibiotic of choice; it can be given orally and is cheaper than intravenous preparations. Dehydration and electrolyte imbalance should be corrected by fluid replacement. Control of the diarrhoea by antidiarrhoeal drugs is contraindicated because of the risk of inducing paralytic ileus and causing septicaemia.

c. Food poisoning, as this case would seem to be from the history, is a notifiable condition and should be reported to the consultant in

Communicable Disease Control. Because the patient has attended a convention, it is very likely that this is part of an outbreak and all persons attending the convention should be contacted to find out if they have been symptomatic and to collect faecal specimens for culture. Specimens of food, if still available, should also be collected for culture. (*S. enteritidis* phage type 4 has been epidemiologically linked to the use of contaminated hens' eggs.)

Chapter 52

1. The criteria for combination therapy in cancer treatment are:

   - each drug should be active as a single agent (ethics of clinical trials means that new drugs are not usually tested for this criterion in clinical studies)
   - each drug should have a different target within the cell (increases cell kill and decreases drug resistance)
   - each drug should show different unwanted effects (ideally this will give additivity for effect (previous criteria) but not of toxicity and hence an increase in therapeutic index.)

   For each of the three drug regimens, the first criterion can be assumed to be met because all the agents are well used drugs. Table A1 summarises the sites of action and side-effects of the drugs in each regimen. As can be seen all three use drugs that have different actions although regimen (c) is targeted only at DNA function. Regimen (b) contains drugs that all have bone marrow toxicity. This will need careful monitoring during therapy.

2. Because many of the drugs used in cancer therapy have a therapeutic index of 1 (toxic dose is the therapeutic dose), it is important to tailor the dosage to the individual patient. Children have a higher cardiac output and greater hepatic and renal blood flows than adults on a body weight basis. (Such parameters are related to body weight to the power 0.65–0.75 ($W^{0.7}$).) Therefore, the clearance of drugs tends to be faster in children than in adults and a proportional *higher* dose is necessary to give the same blood levels. Surface area also correlates to $W^{0.7}$; therefore, it is usual to correct the doses to surface area (calculated by the formula given or by nomogram). For example, if an adult male ($W = 72.1$ kg) is given 100 mg of a drug, how much would you give a 1-year-old child ($W = 9.9$ kg)? Simple correction for W would suggest 13.7 mg ($100 \times 9.9/72.1$), but correction for surface area using a nomogram would give 23.2 mg ($100 \times 0.434/1.874$). If the relation to $W^{0.7}$ was used, the calculated dose would be $100 \times 9.9^{0.7}/72.1^{0.7} = 100 \times 4.98/19.98 = 24.9$ mg. Interestingly this goes against what you may have assumed, i.e. that children would be 'more sensitive' and be given lower doses. The organs of elimination are essentially mature by about 6–9 months of age.

Table A1
Effects of three treatment regimens

	Site of action	Principal toxicity
(a) Acute lymphoblastic leukaemia		
Vincristine	Binds to tubulin/metaphase arrest	BMS + peripheral neuropathy
Asparaginase	Depletes asparagine in blood	↓ Clotting factors/insulin/albumin
Prednisolone	DNA transcription of cytokines (etc.)	Steroid actions
(b) Hodgkin's lymphoma (MOPP regimen)		
Mustine	Alkylates DNA	BMS + nausea/vomiting
Vincristine	Binds to tubulin/metaphase arrest	BMS + peripheral neuropathy
Procarbazine	Inhibits synthesis of DNA, RNA and protein	BMS + nausea
Prednisolone	DNA transcription of cytokines (etc.)	Steroid actions; therefore monitor BMS toxicity
(c) Testicular teratoma		
Etoposide	↑ DNA cleavage by topoisomerase II	BMS, nausea, alopecia
Bleomycin	Oxidative damage to DNA	Pulmonary fibrosis, 'allergy'
Cisplatin	Cross-links DNA	Nausea, BMS, nephrotoxicity, ototoxicity

BMS, bone marrow suppression.

Chapter 53

1. Initial features would be those of opioid overdosage caused by the codeine with possible symptoms of respiratory depression, pinpoint pupils, coma and cardiovascular collapse. The opioid antagonist naloxone is a rapid reversible antagonist of opioids at μ-, κ- and δ-receptors. It has a short half-life and may have to be given repeatedly. Naltrexone is an alternative opioid antagonist with a longer half-life than naloxone. Later developing symptoms of nausea, abdominal pain and sweating, and, if untreated, jaundice are those owing to liver damage caused by the toxic metabolite of paracetamol. N-Acetylcysteine is given, which conjugates with the hepatotoxic metabolite of paracetamol, and is most effective when given early after overdosage; the risk of liver damage is related to the time of ingestion before treatment and the plasma paracetamol concentrations. Alcohol consumption would increase the toxic effects of codeine and paracetamol. It enhances the central depressant actions of the opioid. Alcohol also induces cytochrome P450 enzymes, increasing formation of the toxic metabolite of paracetamol and causing toxicity at lower levels of paracetamol ingestion. Co-dydramol contains a lower concentration of codeine phosphate. Paracetamol with methionine could be considered as an alternative.

Chapter 54

1. a. **True**. Unlike the salt form of cocaine, the free base can be illicitly smoked.
   b. **True**. In the absence of sympathetic supply to the iris in Horner's syndrome, cocaine will not cause mydriasis.
   c. **False**. Acute actions are cardiac arrhythmias and chronic use can lead to heart failure.
   d. **True**. In only a few days tolerance develops to euphoria and appetite suppression.

2. a. **True**. Malignant hyperthermia is observed in some individuals after ingesting Ecstasy. This resembles heat stroke and dehydration.

   b. **True**. Like other amphetamines, Ecstasy has a short-term effect to suppress appetite.
   c. **False**. They produce increases in performance and are banned substances.

3. a. **False**. The psychic effects last only 2–3 h.
   b. **False**. THC is used to inhibit nausea and vomiting in patients taking cytotoxic drugs.
   c. **True**. Cannabis acts on cannabinoid receptors in the brain and periphery. The natural ligand for these receptors is anandamide.

4. a. **False**. Tolerance develops rapidly.
   b. **True**. These effects are caused by stimulation of autonomic ganglia.
   c. **True**. Cotinine is stable and inactive and can be measured.
   d. **False**. Nicotine patches and counselling are required.
   e. **False**. Irritability, sleep disturbances, reduced psychomotor test performance occurs on giving up smoking.

5. a. **True**. The induction of enzymes can decrease the effectiveness of some drugs such as warfarin and phenytoin.
   b. **False**. Moderate ethanol intake can increase high density lipoprotein concentrations, which has cardiovascular protective effects.
   c. **True**. Some individuals have a genetically determined variant of alcohol dehydrogenase that has reduced ability to metabolise ethanol.

6. a. **False**. Acamprosate acts to reduce craving for alcohol and not by inhibiting its metabolism.
   b. **False**. Benzodiazepines or clomethiazole can attenuate withdrawal symptoms but a risk of dependence to these agents exist.

7. a. **True**. Ethanol intake is a common cause of macrocytosis (large red cell volume) in the absence of anaemia.
   b. **False**. The diuresis resulting from ethanol intake is partly caused by inhibition of release of antidiuretic hormone.
   c. **False**. Gamma-glutamyl transpeptidase is elevated.

Index

Index

Index

Index